CARDIOVASCULAR PHARMACOLOGY

Third Edition

Cardiovascular Pharmacology

Third Edition

Editor

Michael J. Antonaccio, Ph.D.

Vice President
Cardiovascular Research and Development
Bristol-Myers Squibb Company
Wallingford, Connecticut

Raven Press ⬧ New York

Raven Press, Ltd., 1185 Avenue of the Americas, New York, New York 10036

Made in the United States of America

Library of Congress Cataloging-in-Publication Data
Cardiovascular pharmacology / editor, Michael J. Antonaccio — 3rd ed.
    p. cm.
    Includes bibliographical references.
    Includes index.
    ISBN 0-88167-644-6
    1. Cardiovascular pharmacology. I. Antonaccio, Michael J.
    [DNLM: 1. Cardiovascular Agents—therapeutic use.
  2. Cardiovascular Diseases—drug therapy. 3. Cardiovascular System—
drug therapy.   QV 150 C275]
RM345.C376 1990
615'.71—dc20
DNLM/DLC
for Library of Congress   90-8549
                                              CIP

9 8 7 6 5 4 3 2 1

To my parents, Frances and Mario Antonaccio,
My wife, Patty, and son, Nick,
For their love and support through the years

Preface

The evolution of cardiovascular medicine has been dramatic and rapid during the time span of the three editions of *Cardiovascular Pharmacology*. The fundamentals of this science have remained secure and the first chapter by Thomas Baum remains untouched—a fitting memorial to a superb pharmacologist, an inspiring teacher, and a close friend taken too soon from all of us.

The third edition contains several new chapters on new subjects or updated chapters on still important areas of research. New chapters include those on antihypertensive agents interacting with the sympathetic nervous system, vascular smooth muscle and vasodilators, modulation of neuroeffector transmission, and the pathophysiology and therapy of hyperlipidemia. Expanded and updated chapters deal with calcium antagonists, the renin-angiotensin system, ischemic heart disease, congestive heart failure, antiarrhythmic drugs, and thrombosis and antithrombotic agents.

The spirit of this book remains the same. It is a convenient single source of the elements of cardiovascular pharmacology, the important new research in this area, and the drugs that are contained within it. Although each chapter is an entity unto itself, there is also an interrelationship among them that weaves throughout the text and binds the chapters into a whole. The extensive use of figures and tables provides a concise summary of the information presented and will be particularly useful to teachers and students.

This book will be a useful adjunct in teaching cardiovascular pharmacology as well as serve as a source of information to professionals in pharmacology and other related areas of medicine.

Michael J. Antonaccio

Preface to Second Edition

The first edition of *Cardiovascular Pharmacology* sought to fill a need for a single text containing the basic elements of cardiovascular pharmacology useful to both graduate students and experienced investigators. The success of the first edition clearly demonstrated the existence of such a need, and the second edition is intended to build and expand upon the original publication.

Most of the original chapters have been retained and brought up to date. Others have been divided where appropriate so that topics that have grown in importance could be adequately covered. For instance, there are now entire chapters devoted to the topics of hypertensive vascular pathophysiology, antihypertensives, calcium antagonists, and the control of renin release. Recent findings in presynaptic modulation of neurotransmitter release are considered important enough to be treated independently. In 1977, this area of research was in its infancy.

This volume, like the first edition, will be of interest to both new and established investigators in cardiovascular pharmacology who wish to broaden their general knowledge, as well as to practicing and teaching clinicians.

Michael J. Antonaccio

Acknowledgments

Special acknowledgment is given to the contributing authors who have made the book a success.

Contents

1   Fundamental Principles Governing Regulation of
Circulatory Function
Thomas Baum

37   Antihypertensive Drugs Interacting with the Sympathetic Nervous
System and Its Receptors
P. A. van Zwieten

75   Vascular Smooth Muscle and Vasodilators
George B. Weiss, Raymond J. Winquist, and Paul J. Silver

107   Calcium Antagonists
David J. Triggle

161   Central Neurotransmitters Involved in Cardiovascular Regulation
Robert B. McCall

201   Renin-Angiotensin System, Converting Enzyme, and
Renin Inhibitors
Michael J. Antonaccio and John J. Wright

229   Modulation of Neuroeffector Transmission
Michael J. Rand, Henryk Majewski, and David F. Story

293   Ischemic Heart Disease: Pathophysiology and
Pharmacologic Management
Judith K. Mickelson, Paul J. Simpson, and Benedict R. Lucchesi

341   Congestive Heart Failure: Pathophysiology and Therapy
Gary S. Francis and Jay N. Cohn

369   Antiarrhythmic Drugs
Benedict R. Lucchesi

485   Pathophysiology and Therapy of Hyperlipidemia
Henry N. Ginsberg, Yadon Arad, and Ira J. Goldberg

515   Platelets, Thrombosis, and Antithrombotic Therapies
Yves Cadroy and Laurence A. Harker

541   Subject Index

Contributors

Michael J. Antonaccio *Cardiovascular Research and Development, Bristol-Myers Squibb Company, 5 Research Parkway, Wallingford, Connecticut 06492*

Yadon Arad *Department of Medicine, Columbia University, College of Physicians and Surgeons, 630 West 168th Street, New York, New York 10032*

*Thomas Baum *Pharmaceutical Research Division, Schering Corporation, Bloomfield, New Jersey 07003*

Yves Cadroy *Division of Hematology and Oncology, Emory University School of Medicine, Atlanta, Georgia 30322*

Jay N. Cohn *Cardiovascular Division, Department of Medicine, University of Minnesota Medical School; and the Veterans Administration Medical Center, One Veterans Drive, Minneapolis, Minnesota 55417*

Gary S. Francis *Cardiovascular Division, Department of Medicine, University of Minnesota Medical School; and the Veterans Administration Medical Center, One Veterans Drive, Minneapolis, Minnesota 55417*

Henry N. Ginsberg *Department of Medicine, Columbia University, College of Physicians and Surgeons, 630 West 168th Street, New York, New York 10032*

Ira J. Goldberg *Department of Medicine, Columbia University College of Physicians and Surgeons, 630 West 168th Street, New York, New York 10032*

Laurence A. Harker *Division of Hematology and Oncology, Emory University School of Medicine, Atlanta, Georgia 30322*

Benedict R. Lucchesi *Department of Pharmacology, The University of Michigan Medical School, 6322 Medical Sciences Building I, Ann Arbor, Michigan 48109-0626*

Henryk Majewski *Department of Pharmacology, University of Melbourne, Parkville, Victoria 3052, Australia*

Robert B. McCall *Cardiovascular Diseases Research, The Upjohn Company, Kalamazoo, Michigan 49001*

Judith K. Mickelson *Department of Pharmacology, The University of Michigan Medical School, 6322 Medical Sciences Building I, Ann Arbor, Michigan 48109-0626*

Michael J. Rand *Department of Pharmacology, University of Melbourne, Parkville, Victoria 3052, Australia*

Paul J. Silver *Department of Pharmacology, Sterling Research Group, 81 Columbia Turnpike, Rensselaer, New York 12144*

---

*Deceased.

xv

Paul J. Simpson   *Department of Pharmacology, The University of Michigan Medical School, 6322 Medical Sciences Building I, Ann Arbor, Michigan 48109-0626*

David F. Story   *Department of Pharmacology, University of Melbourne, Parkville, Victoria 3052, Australia*

David J. Triggle   *School of Pharmacy, State University of New York, C126 Cooke-Hochstetter Complex, Buffalo, New York 14260*

P. A. van Zwieten   *Departments of Pharmacotherapy and Cardiology, Academic Medical Center, University of Amsterdam, Meibergdreef 15, 1105 AZ Amsterdam, The Netherlands*

George B. Weiss   *Research Department, Pharmaceuticals Division, CIBA-GEIGY Corporation, 556 Morris Avenue, Summit, New Jersey 07901*

Raymond J. Winquist   *Department of Pharmacology, Boehringer Ingelheim Pharmaceuticals, Inc., Ridgefield, Connecticut 06877*

John J. Wright   *Cardiovascular Research and Development, Bristol-Myers Squibb Company, 5 Research Parkway, Wallingford, Connecticut 06492*

Cardiovascular Pharmacology, Third Edition, edited by Michael Antonaccio.
Raven Press, Ltd., New York © 1990.

Fundamental Principles Governing Regulation of Circulatory Function

Thomas Baum

Pharmaceutical Research Division, Schering Corporation, Bloomfield, New Jersey 07003

Editor's note. This chapter has been intact from previous volumes. The primary reason for this is that the chapter still contains all the appropriate information necessary to provide the background required for a sound understanding of the more detailed chapters that follow. It is fitting that this chapter has remained as timely now as it was several years ago because it demonstrates sound thinking and vision on Dr. Baum's part. It gives me great sadness to inform you that Tom died suddenly and unexpectedly in 1983, but it is with tribute to and fond personal memories of him that his chapter remains as it was when he was living.

AUTONOMIC NERVOUS SYSTEM

The autonomic nervous system plays a central role in the regulation of cardiovascular function. Although the system is not essential to life, it does enable organs to respond rapidly and efficiently to changing requirements. In its absence, overall adaptation to stressful situations may be severely compromised, although function at rest may remain within normal limits.

The system consists of two major divisions: the parasympathetic and the sympathetic (1,2). Autonomic outflow originates from "centers" (i.e., nuclei or more diffusely arranged groups of cells) in the midbrain and hypothalamus. These regions are closely interrelated and are further subject to excitatory and inhibitory input from afferents and from higher brain structures and the cerebellum. Preganglionic fibers emerge from the brainstem or cord and synapse or relay in ganglia (Fig. 1). These structures contain cell bodies of postganglionic fibers that innervate target organs. Activation of autonomic fibers results in the release of chemical substances (transmitters, mediators) from their terminals. The transmitter binds to a sensitive region (receptor) on the membrane of the target cell and initiates a complex series of events resulting in a response. Many organs (e.g., the viscera) are innervated by both divisions of the autonomic nervous system, which may exert opposing actions either directly or by modifying mediator release from opposing fibers. Other structures, such as most blood vessels, are predominantly supplied by fibers from only the sympathetic system. Some cells receive both sympathetic and parasympathetic innervation (e.g., in the sinoatrial node). Other organs, such as the iris, are also innervated by both systems, but sympathetic fibers supply the radial muscle and parasympathetic fibers the circular muscle. During the resting state, individual autonomic nerves may be quiescent or may fire at a relatively low rate. Activity of an organ may be initiated or enhanced by increasing the "tone" (i.e., firing rate) of the excita-

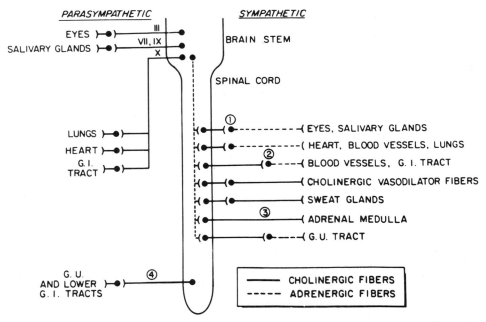

FIG. 1. Schematic representation of autonomic outflow. Various outflow patterns are illustrated in a highly schematic form. Roman numerals refer to cranial nerves. (1) Synapses in ganglia of the paravertebral sympathetic chain. (2) Synapses in more distal ganglia (e.g., celiac, superior and inferior mesenteric). (3) Preganglionic fibers in the splanchnic nerve. (4) Sacral parasympathetic outflow.

tory system and/or by reducing the activity of the inhibitory system. Cell bodies of afferent fibers lie in dorsal root ganglia or in the sensory ganglia of cranial nerves.

Parasympathetic Nervous System

Preganglionic fibers arise from the midbrain, medulla oblongata, and the sacral portion of the spinal cord (Fig. 1) (1). The third, seventh, ninth, and tenth cranial nerves contain fibers emanating from the brainstem. The sacral outflow forms the pelvic nerve and innervates the bladder, sexual organs, and terminal portions of the intestinal tract. Preganglionic parasympathetic fibers synapse in ganglia located in proximity to the target innervated. Consequently, postganglionic nerves are relatively short. On activation, both preganglionic and postganglionic fibers release acetylcholine (ACh) from their terminals.

Choline is transported into nerve terminals by an active process (2). Choline acetyltransferase catalyzes its synthesis into ACh, which is then stored in discrete vesicles within nerve endings. The enzyme is synthesized in the perikaryon and transported along the axon to the terminal by the microtubules. Small quantities of ACh are continuously released. Nerve activation results in dramatic changes in the permeability characteristics of the neuronal membrane, with consequent influx of ions (predominantly sodium and calcium) and depolarization (3). These events cause the migration of ACh-containing vesicles toward and fusion with the neurolemma, and extrusion of their contents (exocytosis). The released ACh combines with its receptors on target cells (*vide infra*). Acetylcholine esterase rapidly degrades free ACh. The enzyme is located on the postsynaptic membrane and, in some structures, also on the presynaptic side.

The cholinergic transmission process has a high degree of efficiency. Prolonged stimulation does not reduce tissue ACh content. The ACh release process is subject to modulation by numerous factors. It is highly dependent on calcium influx and can be inhibited by agents that depress nerve transmission (tetrodotoxin) or calcium entry. Several substances, including morphine, enkephalins, prostaglandins, botulism toxin, and adenosine triphosphate (ATP), diminish exocytotic release of ACh. Hemicholinium inhibits ACh synthesis by blocking its membrane transport system.

Sympathetic Nervous System

Anatomy

Descending tracts originating primarily from the medulla oblongata but also from the hypothalamus innervate, directly or via interneurons, cell bodies of preganglionic neurons located in the intermediolateral column of the thoracolumbar spinal cord (C-8 to L2–3). Preganglionic myelinated fibers emerge via the anterior roots and white rami and synapse in the paravertebral sympathetic chain or traverse the chain and relay in more peripheral ganglia (1,2). The former consists of 22 pairs of ganglia lying parallel to the vertebral column and extending from the superior cervical ganglion to the lumbar region. Individual segments carry descending and ascending efferent and afferent fibers. Gray rami convey postganglionic fibers from the chain to spinal nerves. Preganglionic fibers not synapsing in the paravertebral chain usually do so in more peripheral ganglia in the abdomen (i.e., celiac, superior and inferior mesenteric, and aorticorenal). Some fibers may synapse in even more distal ganglia lying in proximity to the organs innervated (e.g., genitourinary tract, rectum). Fibers to the adrenal medulla do not synapse on route. Most sympathetic postganglionic fibers release norepinephrine (NE, noradrenaline) at their endings and consequently are considered "adrenergic" or "noradrenergic" (4–7). These fibers form an extensive terminal plexus in the organ innervated. Varicosities appear periodically along the terminal network. Some sympathetic fibers liberate ACh (e.g., fibers to sweat glands and vasodilator fibers to skeletal muscle). Sympathetic cholinergic vasodilator pathways originate in the cortex and hypothalamus.

Adrenergic Synthesis, Storage, and Release Mechanisms

NE synthesis, storage, and release occur in the varicosities of the terminal fibers (2,5). These structures contain mitochondria as well as catecholamine-containing vesicles (Fig. 2). The vesicles are formed within the cell body and are transported peripherally.

Hydroxylation of tyrosine to form 3,4-dihydroxyphenylalanine (DOPA) initiates the enzymatic synthesis of NE and occurs in the axoplasm of the varicosity (2,5–9). The reaction is catalyzed by tyrosine hydroxylase utilizing a pteridine cofactor and constitutes the rate-limiting step. DOPA is decarboxylated to form dopamine, which is then transported into the vesicle, where β-hydroxylation to form NE occurs. Dopamine β-hydroxylase (DBH), a copper-containing enzyme, catalyzes the latter step. NE is stored within vesicles partially as a complex with ATP and the protein chromogranin, as well as in a more loosely bound form in both the vesicle and cytoplasm. Turnover studies have demonstrated that newly synthesized NE is incorporated into a more mobile pool and is preferentially released by nerve stimulation.

Uptake of catecholamines into vesicles is an active transport process requiring ATP and magnesium (10). NE can be highly concentrated within these structures and thereby protected from degradative enzymes. Several substances, including reser-

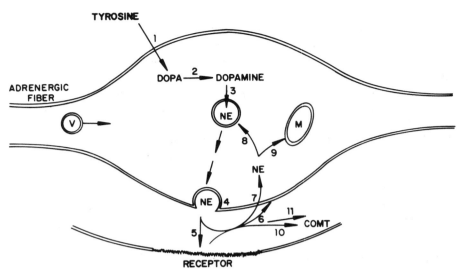

FIG. 2. Schematic representation of the adrenergic transmission process. The diagram illustrates a varicosity in a terminal sympathetic fiber and the effector cell. Tyrosine is transported across the axoplasmic membrane into the cytoplasm and hydroxylated to form DOPA by tyrosine hydroxylase (1). DOPA is then decarboxylated by DOPA decarboxylase to form dopamine (2). The latter is transported into the vesicles (V), where it is hydroxylated to form NE by dopamine β-hydroxylase (3). Vesicles are synthesized within the cell body and transported peripherally. NE is stored in vesicles partly in association with ATP and the protein chromogranin. An action potential results in the extrusion of the contents of the varicosity into the synaptic cleft (4). The released NE may then activate α- or β-adrenergic receptors on the effector cell (5). It also participates in a negative-feedback loop by activating α receptors on the presynaptic membrane, resulting in inhibition of the release process (6). NE is also returned to the fiber by the uptake-1 process (7). Free intracellular NE may then be transported into vesicles (8) or metabolized by mitochondria (M, 9). NE in the synaptic cleft is susceptible to metabolism by catecholamine-o-methyltransferase (COMT, 10), or it may diffuse away from the synaptic region (11).

pine, tetrabenazine, and prenylamine, inhibit the uptake mechanism into vesicles and consequently prevent storage of NE.

Conducted action potentials induce influx of sodium and calcium into adrenergic nerve endings. As in cholinergic terminals, calcium promotes the migration of vesicles toward the neurolemma, fusion of the vesicular membrane with the neurolemma, and extrusion of the vesicular contents (NE, ATP, DBH, and chromogranin) into the extracellular space (2,7). Autonomic fibers can release more than one type of transmitter (e.g., an amine and a peptide) (11).

Released NE can exert a negative feedback on its own liberation (7,12,13). Receptors (α_2) (*vide infra*) on the presynaptic membrane mediate this inhibition (Fig. 2). The process is probably physiologically relevant at low rates of sympathetic firing. However, contradictory views have been offered (14). A β-receptor-mediated facilitatory mechanism also exists on the presynaptic membrane (7,12). Its physiologic role remains uncertain, but it may be activated by circulating epinephrine. Angiotension II (AII) can also facilitate NE release (7,15). Several other substances, including ACh, dopamine, prostaglandins of the E series, 5-hydroxytryptamine (serotonin, 5HT), adenosine, and opiate peptides, attenuate NE release. Their contribution to the regulation of adrenergic transmission is even more speculative. In the heart, however, vagally released ACh can inhibit responses to sympathetic stimulation, probably by a presynaptic mechanism (6,7), as well as by physiologic postsynaptic antagonism.

In contrast to the situation with action-potential-induced NE liberation, tyramine and similar substances release NE most probably by displacement from the cytoplasmic pool rather than by exocytosis (2,5). These agents do not simultaneously liberate DBH, ATP, and chromogranin along with NE. Further, the process does not depend on availability of extracellular calcium.

The adrenergic transmission mechanism is remarkably efficient. Prolonged physiologic or electrical activation of sympathetic nerves does not reduce tissue NE levels (9). Enhanced turnover, in conjunction with a highly effective reuptake process of released transmitter and accelerated synthesis, maintains tissue concentrations. Tyrosine hydroxylase is subject to feedback inhibition by free NE in the cytoplasm (9). Nerve activation accelerates synthesis partially by attenuating this feedback. More prolonged periods of enhanced sympathetic activity result in the synthesis of additional quantities of enzymes (9,17,18).

A major factor contributing to the overall efficiency of sympathetic transmission is a mechanism for the reuptake of released mediator. An active process in the axoplasmic membrane termed "uptake-1" transports NE from the extracellular space back into the nerve terminal (10). The carrier requires energy, is linked to Na-K ATPase, and exhibits stereospecificity. However, other phenolic phenethylamines in addition to NE (e.g., metaraminol, α-methyl NE, α-methylepinephrine, tyramine, and octopamine) are also transported across the nerve membrane, although at slower rates. Several classes of compounds inhibit uptake-1. These include phenethylamines lacking a phenolic hydroxyl group (e.g., amphetamine), as well as structurally diverse substances such as ouabain, cocaine, imipramine, and guanethidine. Inhibitors of the axoplasmic transport system also attenuate the actions of agents capable of gaining access to the interior of the nerve ending and subsequently causing the release of NE (i.e., indirectly acting sympathomimetic amines such as tyramine). 6-Hydroxydopamine is also a substrate for the membrane pump. After uptake, it causes the destruction of the adrenergic fiber.

In contrast to the normal state, continuous sympathetic activation rapidly leads to depletion of tissue stores of NE after blockade of the membrane pump. On the other hand, pump inactivation can lead to potentiation and prolongation of effects of sympathetic nerve stimulation and injected NE.

NE can also be taken up into extraneuronal sites in smooth muscle, heart, glandular tissue, and other organs ("uptake-2") (10). The capacity of this mechanism to store NE exceeds that of uptake-1; however, its affinity for NE and epinephrine is more limited. Consequently, uptake-1 predominates at relatively lower concentrations. Amines taken up by the second process are rapidly metabolized. Uptake-2 can be blocked by drugs such as phenoxybenzamine and metanephrine.

Several drugs inhibit action-potential-evoked release of NE. Both guanethidine and bretylium rapidly attenuate NE release, but probably by different mechanisms (19). In addition, guanethidine produces a long-lasting depletion of tissue stores of NE, probably by blocking both the axoplasmic and vesicular uptake mechanisms. The initial short-latency inhibitory action of guanethidine can be rapidly reversed by administration of substances that have an affinity for uptake-1, such as amphetamine (20). Displacement of guanethidine from its inhibitory site probably accounts for restoration of the transmission process. The efficacy of these release inhibitors varies with the frequency of nerve activation.

Certain substances can affect the transmission process by acting as "false transmitters." For example, α-methyldopa is incorporated into storage vesicles after transformation into α-methylnorepineph-rine, which in turn is released by physio-logic impulses (19). Octopamine, formed by β-hydroxylation of tyramine, and, indeed, guanethidine, can be released in a similar fashion. The end-organ response to the false transmitter may be subnormal and may lead to reduced responsiveness, as in the case of octopamine.

Reduction or depletion of tissue stores of NE can alter organ responses to sympa-thetic nerve activation. Reserpine dimin-ishes the NE content of nerve endings by inhibiting the vesicular membrane pump (10). NE not sequestered into vesicles is exposed to the action of degradative enzymes. However, total tissue NE content must be greatly reduced in order to de-press transmission. For example, organ re-sponses to nerve stimulation recover much more rapidly after reserpine than do tissue stores of NE.

As discussed earlier, reuptake of released NE is the major process for terminating the response to sympathetic nerve activation. NE is metabolized by two major pathways (7). Extracellular NE is subject to *o*-methylation by catechol-*o*-methyltransfer-ase. Monoamine oxidase also deactivates NE rapidly; the enzyme resides primarily within mitochondria in nerve terminals and participates in the control of levels of free NE within nerve endings. NE may also dif-fuse from the synaptic site into the circula-tion.

Autonomic Ganglia

Activation of preganglionic fibers initi-ates a complex series of events in postgan-glionic neurons. An initial fast negative po-tential (excitatory postsynaptic potential, EPSP), a positive potential (inhibitory post-synaptic potential, IPSP), a late negative potential, and a late-late negative potential can be recorded from autonomic ganglia (21–23). ACh, the primary excitatory trans-mitter in ganglia, induces the initial fast EPSP and the late EPSP by activating ni-cotinic and muscarinic receptors, respec-tively (*vide infra*). The nature of the IPSP remains uncertain; it may be generated either monosynaptically by ACh or by ACh-induced release of dopamine or NE from interneurons (22,23). Exogenous do-pamine and NE can hyperpolarize postgan-glionic membranes under appropriate cir-cumstances. Preganglionic stimulation can elevate cyclic adenosine 3′,5′-monophos-phate (cAMP) levels in ganglia. The late-late EPSP may be mediated by a peptide (22).

Adrenal Medulla

Synthetic processes in the adrenal me-dulla follow the scheme outlined earlier for catecholamines. Final methylation of NE to epinephrine by phenylethanolamine-*N*-methyltransferase occurs in the cyto-plasm. Activation of preganglionic nerves results in the liberation of ACh, depolari-zation of the chromaffin cells, calcium in-flux, and release of the contents of the stor-age granules: catecholamines (primarily epinephrine), ATP, chromogranin, and en-kephalins (24). Although epinephrine can markedly influence many organ systems, the precise physiologic role of the adrenal medulla remains obscure.

Receptors

Biologically active substances (transmit-ters, hormones, some drugs) interact with specific proteins called "receptors," result-ing in various biophysical, biochemical, and ultimately physiologic consequences (25–27). Three general classes of receptors have been identified: (a) receptors located on the external surface of the plasma mem-brane in nerves, muscle, and glands acti-vated by amines and peptides; chemically, these are glycoproteins associated with lipids; (b) receptors for steroids that are located intracellularly in the soluble compartment; (c) receptors located within the cell nucleus (e.g., for thyroid hormone). In some instances, the agonist-receptor complex (e.g., peptides, insulin, growth hormone, prolactin, as well as low-density lipoproteins) can be internalized by endocytosis to form a vesicle within the cell (25–28).

Ligands interact with receptors by highly specific binding processes resulting in changes in the conformation or charge distribution of the receptor or neighboring region. These, in turn, result in changes in membrane permeability, alteration of the conformation of enzymes, or alteration of their associated regulatory subunits. Quantitatively, binding of agonists to membrane receptors depends on the number of receptors present and their affinity state. Binding of several classes of agonists (β-adrenergic, opiate) is markedly attenuated by guanosine triphosphate (GTP) and by sodium. GTP converts these receptors from high-affinity states to low-affinity states. In contrast, GTP does not alter binding of antagonists.

Physiologic responses vary with the number of receptors occupied. However, activation of a relatively small proportion of membrane receptors usually results in maximal physiologic responses.

The number and affinity of receptors are subject to negative feedback, leading to desensitization (down-regulation) or supersensitivity (up-regulation). Down-regulation may involve reduced synthesis of receptors. Not all agonist-receptor interactions are subject to down-regulation (e.g., aldosterone release by AII). Binding can alter the conformation of receptors in such a manner that the affinity of remaining receptors decreases (negative cooperativity). Large numbers of receptor systems utilizing amines, peptides, and steroids as agonists have been identified. These include receptors for NE, epinephrine, dopamine, ACh, 5HT, histamine, adenosine, AII, vasopressin, oxytocin, γ-aminobutyric acid, enkephalins, substance P, glycine, glutamate, etc. (25–30).

Antagonists can inhibit the actions of agonists by combining with agonist binding sites on the receptor or by binding to adjacent (allosteric) sites. Competitive blockade is surmountable, and the usual organ responses are obtained if the concentration of the agonist is increased; i.e., the dose–response curve is shifted to the right, but the maximum obtainable response remains unaltered. Noncompetitive blockade involves covalent binding to receptors. Maximum responses are depressed, and restoration of activity requires synthesis of new receptors.

Cholinergic Receptors

Acetylcholine is an agonist for two major types of receptors. These were originally classified as "muscarinic" or "nicotinic" on the basis of their similarities to responses to the alkaloid muscarine and nicotine. Cholinergic receptors in skeletal muscle and most of those on the cell bodies of postganglionic neurons and on nonmyelinated C fibers respond to nicotine and are considered "nicotinic." In contrast, receptors innervated by postganglionic cholinergic fibers, such as in smooth muscle and glands, are termed "muscarinic" (Table 1). Nicotinic receptors in ganglia and skeletal muscle are inhibited by competitive blockers such as hexamethonium and *d*-tubocurarine, respectively. Atropine exemplifies a blocker of muscarinic receptors (Table 2).

Activation of cholinergic receptors results in changes in cell membranes ultimately leading to various responses such as hyperpolarization of cells in the sinoatrial node or depolarization of ganglia (as indicated earlier) and intestinal smooth muscle. Biochemically, muscarinic receptors (e.g., in the heart) may be negatively coupled to

TABLE 1. *Organ responses to autonomic mediators*[a]

Organ	Adrenergic	Cholinergic
Heart		
Sinoatrial node	Rate + (β)	Rate −
Atrioventricular node	Automaticity + (β)	Automaticity −
	Conduction + (β)	Conduction −
His-Purkinje system	Automaticity + (β)	
Atria	Contractile force + (β)	Contractile force −
Ventricles	Contractile force + (β)	Contractile force −
Blood vessels		
Skeletal muscle	Constriction (α)	Dilatation
	Dilatation (β)	
Skin	Constriction (α)	Slight dilatation
Kidney, intestine	Constriction (α)	Dilatation
	Slight dilatation (β)	
Intestine	Motility and tone −	Motility and tone
Urinary bladder		
Detrussor	Relaxation (β)	Contraction
Trigone and sphincter	Contraction (α)	Relaxation
Uterus	Relaxation (β)	
	Contraction (α)	
Eye		
Radial muscle	Contraction (α)	
Sphincter		Contraction
Lacrimal glands		Secretion
Salivary glands	Viscous secretion (α)	Watery secretion
Sweat glands		Secretion
Metabolic	Glycogenolysis, lipolysis +	

[a]A plus sign indicates an increase or enhancement; a minus sign indicates a decrease or slowing; α and β refer to the type of adrenergic receptor that mediates the response. Constrictor responses in blood vessels are mediated by α receptors and dilator responses by β receptors. Epinephrine usually reduces vascular resistance of skeletal muscle, because the β-response predominates. Norepinephrine exerts relatively weak effects on vascular β receptors. As a result, sympathetic stimulation usually results in constriction. Responses of the uterus vary greatly and depend on the stage of the menstrual cycle, etc. Activation of both α and β receptors in the intestine results in inhibition of motility and tone. Species variation exists in the type of receptor involved in metabolic responses.

TABLE 2. *Receptor agonists and antagonists*

Receptor	Agonist	Antagonist
Adrenergic		
α_1	NE, phenylephrine, tramazoline	Prazosin, corynanthine
α_2	NE, guanabenz, clonidine	Rauwolscine
β_1	NE, isoproterenol	Metoprolol, atenolol
β_2	NE, isoproterenol, terbutaline	Propranolol (nonselective)
Dopamine$_1$	Dopamine, aminotetralins	Bulbocapnine, bromocriptine
Dopamine$_2$	Dopamine, apomorphine	Haloperidol, *S*-sulpiride
5HT$_1$	5HT	Methysergide
5HT$_2$	5HT	Ketanserin
Cholinergic-muscarinic	ACh	Atropine
Cholinergic-nicotinic	ACh	Tetraethylammonium, hexamethonium, curare
Histamine$_1$	Histamine, 2-methylhistamine	Mepyramine
Histamine$_2$	Histamine, 4-methylhistamine, dimaprit	Cimetidine
Angiotensin II	Angiotensin II	Saralasin

adenylate cyclase and indirectly linked to guanylate cyclase, resulting in elevated concentrations of cyclic guanosine monophosphate (cGMP).

Adrenergic Receptors

On the basis of qualitative and quantitative organ responses to various sympathomimetic amines, Ahlquist concluded that two distinct adrenergic receptors, α and β, exist (33). Subsets of these (α_1, α_2, β_1, β_2) have been identified by binding studies and the use of appropriate antagonists.

Both α_1- and α_2-adrenoceptors subserve arterial vasoconstriction. The finding that constrictor responses to sympathetic nerve stimulation are selectively attenuated by α_1 blockers, whereas parenterally administered NE is most susceptible to α_2 blockers, has led to the hypothesis that neuronally released NE gains access primarily to α_1 receptors at postjunctional sites but that circulating NE activates both (12,34). Activation of α_2 receptors on adrenergic, cholinergic, and tryptaminergic nerve terminals can inhibit the release of these transmitters (7,12). Adrenergic inhibition of intestinal motility is partially mediated by reduction of ACh release from cholinergic fibers.

NE and phenylephrine are potent agonists for α_1 receptors, which can in turn be blocked relatively selectively by prazosin and corynanthine (Table 2); α_2 receptors are activated by norepinephrine and guanabenz and blocked by rauwolscine.

Numerous biophysical and biochemical consequences of α-adrenoceptor activation have been observed, including inhibition of adenylate cyclase in some organs (e.g., platelets), elevation of cAMP in the brain, and indirect linkage to guanylate cyclase (12,31). α_1 receptor activation has been shown to augment the breakdown of phosphatidyl inositol (35). α_2 stimulation may specifically enhance calcium influx in vascular smooth muscle.

Activation of β_1-adrenoceptors causes augmentation of cardiac rate and contractility and relaxation of intestinal tone (37). Stimulation of β_2 receptors results in vasodilatation and bronchial and uterine relaxation (Table 1). Propranolol blocks both receptors, whereas metoprolol and atenolol block β_1 receptors relatively selectively (Table 2).

Adrenergic receptors are subject to feedback phenomena characteristic of receptors in general, such as up- and down-regulation and interaction with other systems (e.g., stimulation of α receptors can lower the affinity of β receptors) (25–28). Receptor density can vary widely among and within organs. Within the heart, the left atrium contains the highest concentration, followed by the right atrium and right and left ventricles (38).

Biochemical consequences of β receptor activation have been extensively studied (25–27). The β receptor, a guanine nucleotide regulatory protein, and the enzyme adenylate cyclase exist as a complex in the cell membrane. Binding by agonists to β receptors results in conformational changes that promote the exchange of guanosine diphosphate (GDP) bound to the regulatory protein for GTP. The regulatory-protein–GTP complex combines with the inactive catalytic subunit of the enzyme, forming an active complex capable of catalyzing the conversion of ATP to cAMP. The latter promotes the dissociation of regulatory subunits of protein kinases from their catalytic subunits, thereby activating them. Protein kinases, in turn, phosphorylate various proteins, leading to activation or inactivation of particular enzymes. The enzyme phosphodiesterase degrades cAMP and thereby participates in the regulation of its tissue levels.

GTP decreases the affinity of β receptors as well as other adenyl-cyclase-linked receptors for their agonist.

Dopamine

Ascending dopaminergic tracts originating in the brainstem have been identified (6). Peripherally injected dopamine stimulates the heart and constricts blood vessels by β- and α-adrenoceptor activation, respectively. In addition, it can activate distinct receptors in the renal and mesenteric beds, leading to vasodilation (39). Dopamine receptor activation can inhibit NE release and ganglionic transmission, as indicated earlier.

Dopamine receptors have been classified according to their linkage to adenyl cyclase. DA_1 receptors are linked, whereas DA_2 receptors are not. Agonists and antagonists are listed in Table 2 (39–42). Renal and mesenteric receptors resemble the DA_1 subgroup, but their linkage to adenyl cyclase remains uncertain.

Interactions of Other Endogenous Substances with the Cardiovascular and Autonomic Nervous Systems

AII, which will be discussed again later, can release epinephrine from the adrenal medulla, stimulate autonomic ganglia and intramural nerves in various organs, and enhance release of NE during sympathetic nervous stimulation (7,16,43,44).

Members of the prostaglandin family, particularly of the E series, inhibit NE release from sympathetic nerves by a presynaptic action in some organs (7,45–47). However, under certain circumstances they may potentiate the response of smooth muscle to various agonists, including NE, ACh, and 5HT, and at other times may diminish responses (34–36). Prostaglandins may play a physiologic regulatory role at sympathetic nerve endings, because inhibitors of their synthesis enhance organ responses to sympathetic nerve stimulation under appropriate conditions. Prostaglandins have also been reported to inhibit cardiac responses to vagal nerve stimulation (45).

5HT-containing neurons and tracts exist in the brain and spinal cord and in the intestinal tract. 5HT both constricts and dilates blood vessels by direct actions, and it can enhance the pressor effects of other agonists. Dilatation resulting from inhibition of sympathetic tone can also occur. 5HT receptors have also been subclassified: $5HT_1$ and $5HT_2$ (Table 2) (48,49). The former is adenylate-cyclase-linked.

Histamine stored in mast cells and platelets can be released by several agents, including compound 48/80, morphine, and curare. Histamine exerts numerous actions, including release of adrenal epinephrine, ganglionic stimulation, and contraction or relaxation of various smooth-muscle cells. Activation of H_2 receptors leads to gastric secretion and cardiac stimulation. Blood vessels contain H_1 as well as H_2 receptors. Both must be blocked in order to completely obtund the vasodilator action of histamine.

Purinergic Nerves

A nonadrenergic inhibitory system has been demonstrated in the intestine (50). Activation of the system results in hyperpolarization and relaxation of smooth-muscle cells. Cell bodies of these neurons originate in Auerbach's plexus and, in at least some portions of the intestine, are subject to control by preganglionic vagal nerves. Evidence suggests that ATP serves as the inhibitory mediator.

PERIPHERAL CIRCULATION

Tissue perfusion is the primary role of the circulation. The heart generates the force required to propel blood throughout peripheral vessels and must also provide an output adequate for the widely varying and rapidly changing demands of the organism.

Characteristics of Vascular Smooth Muscle

Vascular smooth-muscle cells possess characteristics generally typical of excitable cells. Their plasma membrane contains several specific ion channels and a number of active transport systems. These result in differences in ionic concentration and a potential difference across the membrane (50–70 mV, inside negative). Changes in the conformation or charge distribution within channels form "gating" mechanisms that regulate ion fluxes. The number of open channels and their kinetics are influenced by membrane voltage, mediators, hormones, cyclic nucleotides, and drugs (50–56).

The association of electrical membrane phenomena and mechanical activity has been demonstrated in several types of smooth muscle (51,52). Spontaneous rhythmic electrical activity and associated contractions occur in several isolated vessels, including mesenteric arteries and veins and portal veins. Slow fluctuations appear in the membrane potential, and spikes resembling action potentials arise from the peaks of the slow waves. Action potentials of long duration (up to 30 sec) have been observed in the turtle aorta and vena cava. Electrical activity arises in pacemaker areas in numerous isolated preparations, such as the rabbit portal vein, and then spreads over the entire tissue. Constrictor substances usually produce depolarization and initiate or increase the frequency of action potentials in spike-generating tissue.

Some tissues appear to respond to excitatory stimuli by graded depolarization rather than by spike generation. NE has been shown to produce depolarization and contraction in rat caudal, cat basilar, and rabbit pulmonary arteries (57–59). Papaverine and isoproterenol exert opposite effects (hyperpolarization and relaxation) (60). Inhibition of the sarcolemmal sodium pump by inhibition of Na-K ATPase results in depolarization.

Contractile mechanisms in vascular smooth muscle bear numerous similarities to those in skeletal and cardiac muscle (55,56,62–66). All contain the major proteins myosin and actin, but the arrangement of these two filaments is not as regular in smooth muscle, resulting in the absence of clear cross-striations. Myosin is composed of two "heavy" chains and two pairs of "light" chains. Extensions of the myosin molecule containing the light chains form cross-bridges toward the actin filament. The cross-bridges also possess a magnesium-dependent ATPase and an actin binding site.

Calcium binds to the protein calmodulin during initiation of the contractile process in vascular smooth muscle. The calcium-calmodulin complex then binds to the inactive catalytic subunit of myosin light-chain kinases, resulting in its activation. This enzyme phosphorylates the myosin light chain, permitting the activation of the magnesium-dependent ATPase on the myosin cross-bridges by actin. Hydrolysis of ATP ensues and results in tension development due to conformational changes in the cross-bridges and the relative movement of the myosin and actin filaments. Tension varies with the number of active cross-bridges and their cycling rate. Myosin light-chain phosphatase removes phosphate from the light chain and restores the two filaments to their "dormant" state. An alternative mode of activating myosin ATPase by the protein leiotonin has been proposed.

In cardiac and skeletal muscle the proteins tropomyosin and the troponins are associated with actin and exert an inhibitory role on its activity. Binding of calcium to troponin C removes this inhibition and permits activation of myosin ATPase.

Thus, calcium assumes a central role in the contractile process of all forms of muscle. During the resting state its concentration approximates 10^{-7} M or less. Concentration related activation occurs at 10^{-7} to 10^{-5} M. This calcium derives primarily from the sarcoplasmic reticulum (SR) in skeletal muscle. In cardiac muscle, influx of calcium occurs during the plateau of the action potential and is also released from the SR. In smooth muscle, calcium enters the cells through "voltage"-activated channels that become operative on membrane depolarization or through receptor-activated channels. Calcium can also be released from the SR and other intracellular binding sites. The contributions of these sources of calcium vary in different blood vessels and also depend on the mode of activation (53,55).

Biologically active substances such as NE, AII, and 5HT contract vascular smooth muscle by enhancing calcium influx through receptor-operated channels as well as release from intracellular stores. Agonist-induced depolarization provides another mechanism for calcium entry through the voltage-sensitive channels.

Relaxation occurs on sequestration of calcium into the SR or other stores or by efflux. Relaxant substances can act by influencing one or more of these processes. cAMP promotes the uptake of calcium by the SR and has also been shown to inhibit myosin light-chain kinase. Vasodilation produced by nitroglycerin and nitroprusside correlates with increases in cGMP (67,68).

Characteristics of Blood Vessels and Vascular Beds

Vascular smooth-muscle cells are arranged in series and in parallel with elastic components (69–71). Their contraction generates tension within the vessel wall. Tension generation and velocity of shortening vary with muscle length up to an optimal value (e.g., 150% of resting length in some vascular tissue) and then declines. Stretch affects the number of myosin cross-bridges capable of interacting with actin. Compared with skeletal and cardiac muscle, smooth muscle contracts very slowly but can generate great force at a relatively low energy cost.

Vascular smooth muscle is subject to influences by numerous local and extrinsic factors and at any one time may be in a relaxed state (i.e., possess little "tone"), whereas in other circumstances it may be contracted and possess a high degree of tone. Basal tone (i.e., the degree of intrinsic contraction in the absence of known external factors) varies considerably among different vessels.

Blood vessel caliber is determined by the interplay of two opposing forces: transmural distending pressure and tangential wall tension (71). Laplace described the relationship between the radius and wall tension in hollow circular structures as follows: tension = pressure × radius. Neither his formulation nor equations incorporating an additional factor relating to wall thickness are totally applicable to the circulation. However, they provide an extremely useful concept in describing vessel behavior as well as cardiac behavior.

Poiseuille studied the flow of liquids through rigid tubes and concluded that flow (F) varies directly with effective driving pressure (P) and the fourth power of the vessel radius (R) and inversely with the viscosity (V) of the fluid and the length (L) of the tube: $F = \pi PR^4/8\ VL$. Again, this formulation serves only as an approximation for the circulation, because blood vessels are distensible rather than rigid, flow is pulsatile, and blood consists of liquid as well as corpuscular components. Nevertheless, the equation highlights the critical factors influencing flow in a vascular bed, such that (other factors remaining constant) flow varies directly with driving pressure and inversely with resistance.

The content of contractile and elastic elements in arterial and venous vessels varies. Relative smooth-muscle content increases progressively from the aorta to precapillary sphincters. Veins contain a higher proportion of elastic elements than arteries and have a smaller wall/lumen ratio. Arterial and arteriolar segments control the resistance of vascular beds. However, under certain circumstances, postcapillary vessels can assume a relatively large proportion of the total resistance in some beds.

Compliance or distensibility represents a passive property of blood vessels that depends primarily on the elastic constituents of the vessel wall and accounts for the change in radius in response to altered distending pressure (74). Smooth-muscle tone, as well as disease processes, can influence overall elasticity and compliance. Venous capacitance greatly exceeds that of precapillary vessels. Thus, small changes in intravascular pressure can produce large changes in vein radius. Veins contain approximately 65% of total blood volume. Consequently, small changes in venous tone can translocate relatively large quantities of blood. Events on the arterial side are also capable of influencing venous mechanics. At constant systemic pressure, arterial constriction results in a fall in transmural pressure in postcapillary vessels. The latter, in turn, causes a reduction of venous volume as a result of passive recoil of the venous wall.

Small precapillary vessels and sphincters relax and contract spontaneously (74). This vasomotion persists after denervation but is under the influence of local metabolic factors. The opening and closing of sphincters results in intermittent flow in individual capillaries, and only a fraction are patent at any instant. During increased metabolic activity of an organ, the proportion of open capillaries increases markedly.

Bidirectional fluid movement occurs across capillaries and consists of filtration into the interstitial space and reabsorption into the capillary. Several factors influence these fluxes (74). The pressure gradient across the vessel walls tends to drive fluid out. whereas the colloid osmotic pressure difference favors reabsorption. At a given aortic pressure, the ratio of precapillary re-sistance to postcapillary resistance determines capillary pressure in individual beds. Thus, arteriolar dilation unaccompanied by venous relaxation tends to increase capillary pressure and enhance filtration. Venous constriction produces a similar change. Filtration predominates at the arterial end of a capillary, and reabsorption predominates at the venous end. However, because of periodic opening and closing of precapillary sphincters, filtration may occur across the entire length of an individual capillary at any one time, whereas reabsorption may predominate in others. The lymphatic system returns excess filtrate to the main circulation.

Arteriovenous anastomoses or shunts connecting small arteries to small veins and bypassing capillaries occur in some tissues, particularly in skin (74). Blood flowing through these channels serves no metabolic function. Closure of cutaneous shunts by sympathetic stimuli diverts flow into capillaries and facilitates heat loss during exercise.

Control of Flow in Vascular Beds

The peripheral circulation consists of numerous vascular beds connected in parallel. The relative resistance of each bed determines the proportion of cardiac output it will receive. As in a parallel electrical circuit, the reciprocal of total resistance ($1/R$) equals the sum of the reciprocals of individual resistances ($1/r_1 + \ldots + 1/r_n$). At rest, the kidneys and intestinal organs each receive approximately 20% of cardiac output, the brain and skeletal muscle 15%, and heart and skin 5%. During exercise, flow to muscle increases greatly. On the other hand, proportional (although not necessarily absolute) flow to some other organs (e.g., intestinal tract and kidneys) declines. Other activities that augment individual organ requirements for blood can also result in flow redistribution.

The state of vascular smooth-muscle contraction or tone is the major determinant of resistance. In vessels with minimal ability to constrict or relax, flow will tend to depend on the arterial–venous pressure gradient. The magnitude of intrinsic precapillary vessel tone varies considerably in different organs. Therefore, a given stimulus will not produce the same degree of dilatation or constriction in all beds.

Numerous local, neurogenic, and humoral factors influence vascular resistance. Trophic factors (e.g., NE) produce more long-term effects (75). Vascular smooth-muscle cells readily respond to alterations in tissue Po_2, Pco_2, and pH (73–75). Hypoxia, hypercarbia, and reduced pH result in vasodilatation, whereas changes in the opposite direction cause constriction. Overall, a correlation exists between metabolic activity and blood flow or vascular resistance under normal conditions. Venous blood emerging from normally perfused organs usually is vasodilator relative to arterial blood. However, the perfusion of various vascular beds with hypoxic blood results in dilatation only when Po_2 is greatly reduced; i.e., to approximately 40 mm Hg (73). Thus, tissue oxygen, carbon dioxide, or hydrogen ion concentrations cannot individually be responsible for resistance regulation. However, carbon dioxide tension is of critical importance in the cerebral circulation (77–79). Other factors contributing to local regulation include metabolites, nucleotides such as adenosine, potassium ion, and changes in osmolarity (73,75,80,81). Metabolic vasodilation in skeletal muscle also results in the opening of additional capillary channels. In contrast, postcapillary vessels appear to remain unaffected by local regulatory mechanisms. The pulmonary circulation displays a somewhat atypical response to hypoxia in that pulmonary arterial pressure increases. Augmented blood flow may contribute to the pressure elevation. Numerous other locally generated factors (prostaglandins, bradykinin, 5HT, histamine, etc.) also influence vascular tone.

The power of local regulatory mechanisms is illustrated by the phenomenon of autoregulation of blood flow. Changes in arterial transmural pressure or inflow result in changes in smooth-muscle tone and vessel resistance in the same direction, and these, in turn, tend to maintain blood flow constant (82). Autoregulation usually prevails in the pressure range of 60 to 140 mm Hg in most organs. Regulatory mechanisms become inadequate at the extremes, and flow will vary in proportion to driving pressure. The degree of autoregulation varies in different organs, being particularly powerful in the kidney and brain, somewhat less so in skeletal muscle, and almost negligible in skin. Passive mechanisms tend to counteract autoregulation to some extent, because changes in distending pressure modify vessel radius and, thereby, resistance.

At least three major mechanisms have been proposed to account for the process. The tissue-pressure hypothesis suggests that increasing perfusion pressure leads to increased capillary filtration and an elevation of extravascular pressure, and thus an increase in resistance. However, most evidence supports the metabolic and myogenic theories. The former is based on the supposition that a decrease in perfusion pressure will initially lower blood flow and reduce tissue Po_2 and cause an accumulation of metabolites. These factors, in turn, dilate smaller arterial vessels, reduce resistance, and tend to raise blood flow toward original levels. Myogenic theories of autoregulation extend the original observations of Bayliss and are based on the hypothesis that vascular smooth muscle responds to changes in distending pressure by contraction or relaxation. Isolated strips of small mesenteric and cerebral arteries have been shown to contract when quickly stretched. Distension also increases rhythmicity of isolated strips that normally display periodic contractions. Further, elevation of distending pressure increases vasomotion in small arterial vessels.

The relative roles of metabolic and myogenic factors in autoregulation remain controversial, and neither can account for the phenomenon alone. Their respective contributions probably vary from organ to organ as well as from time to time as circumstances change. Normal vascular tone is a prerequisite for autoregulation, because reactive hyperemia or the administration of vasodilators or metabolic inhibitors obtunds the process.

The cerebral circulation is principally under the control of intrinsic factors, with only minor contributions by extrinsic, including nervous, factors (77–79,83). A unique feature of the cerebral circulation is the highly selective permeability of the capillary endothelium, establishing a "blood-brain barrier." The barrier apparently depends on glial cells. Large arteries contribute significantly to the total resistance of this bed. Renal blood flow, unlike that to other organs, greatly exceeds metabolic requirements; yet the organ displays vigorous autoregulation.

Autonomic Control of the Peripheral Circulation

Adrenergic Influence

Most blood vessels are richly innervated by sympathetic nerves. Nerve terminals form a network of anastomosing filaments that run along the periphery of vessels. Adrenergic innervation is usually limited to the junction of the adventitia and the media. However, neurons have been demonstrated to penetrate for a short distance into the media in some vessels (e.g., the proximal saphenous artery of the rabbit) (4,84–86). In general, arteries are more densely innervated than veins. However, the density of innervation of individual arteries and veins varies considerably. Terminal axons have also been shown to innervate precapillary sphincters.

The preponderant limitation of adrenergic fibers to the adventitial-medial junction raises the question of the mode of activation of the more medial smooth-muscle cells. This could be accomplished by (a) diffusion of the mediator, (b) inward electrotonic spread of the excitatory potential from innervated cells, and (c) conduction by smooth-muscle cells along low-resistance pathways (84). The relative importance of these mechanisms remains unsettled. It has been demonstrated that impulse propagation can occur in isolated vascular tissue but that vessels differ greatly in their ability to conduct (86).

Stimulation of sympathetic nerves to most organs, or intraarterial administration of NE, results in vasoconstriction and an increase in vascular resistance, as indicated by a reduction in blood flow or by an increase in perfusion pressure when flow is maintained by a pump. Sympathetic stimulation also causes venous constriction, resulting in a reduction in venous capacitance and an increase in resistance (74). Maximal responses usually appear at frequencies of 10 to 20 Hz or less (74). Even lower frequencies result in peak effects in venous preparations. It has been estimated that stimulation at 0.5 to 2 Hz approximates the level of spontaneous tonic activity usually encountered in anesthetized animals.

Sympathetic stimulation may affect vessels in different organs or even vessels within an organ differentially. For example, blood is distributed away from the renal cortex during stimulation. Along similar lines, stimulation at equivalent frequencies produces larger increases in resistance in the kidney than in the forelimb (87).

The preponderant role of local factors in the regulation of the cerebral circulation was indicated earlier. In general, cerebrovascular responses to sympathetic nerve stimulation are weak (77,78,83). Coronary arteries are innervated by sympathetic fibers, stimulation of which can produce vasoconstriction. However, local metabolic factors predominate (88). Stimulation of sympathetic fibers to the intestine can result in intense vasoconstriction, which then "escapes" because of accumulation of locally produced dilator factors.

The ability to record pressures from small vessels has permitted more detailed studies of vascular responses to sympathetic nerve stimulation. These methods have revealed that the initial increment in total vascular resistance of the gastrocnemius muscle during sympathetic nerve activation results from constriction of the more distal arterial vessels. During continued stimulation, however, the distal vessels tend to relax while the larger proximal segment constricts progressively (89).

Responses to sympathetic stimulation in the perfused dog forelimb have also been studied in detail and have demonstrated even greater complexity (87,90). It was found that stimulation increased the overall vascular resistance, but changes in the constituent muscle and cutaneous beds differed considerably. Vascular resistance of the large arterial segments increased in muscle and particularly in skin. Small-vessel resistance, comprising effects in small arteries, arterioles, and smaller veins, did not change greatly in muscle but fell markedly in skin. Resistance of the venous segment composed of the larger veins increased very greatly in skin, but the increase was considerably smaller in muscle. These responses resulted in a net redistribution of blood flow from skin to muscle.

Sympathetic stimulation has also been shown to cause a net constriction of precapillary sphincters, resulting in reduced capillary surface area. During prolonged stimulation, accumulation of metabolites overcomes the decline in capillary filtration. In contrast, tonic sympathetic activity may not influence precapillary sphincters greatly or play a role in the regulation of capillary filtration surface area (91).

Arterial and venous constrictor responses to sympathetic stimulation and NE are mediated predominantly by α_1-adrenoceptor activation, as indicated earlier, but α_2 receptors may assume a greater role in large veins (92). Arterial smooth-muscle cells also possess β receptors (β_2). These probably are not innervated or do not respond greatly to neuronally released NE but may be activated by circulating epinephrine (93).

Intravenous infusion of NE elevates total peripheral resistance. On the other hand, total resistance usually falls during epinephrine infusion, mainly because of β-mediated dilation of vessels in skeletal muscle. NE has been reported to exert a trophic effect on vascular smooth muscle (76). Dopaminergic vasodilator receptors exist in the mesenteric and renal beds, as indicated earlier (39).

Sympathetic Vasodilator Fibers

Sympathetic nerves to skin and skeletal muscle also contain vasodilator fibers. The latter compose a system that originates in the cerebral cortex, relays in the hypothalamus and midbrain collicular region, but not in the medulla, and emerges from the thoracolumbar cord. Activation of the system by hypothalamic stimulation results in dilatation in muscle, but constriction in most other beds, as well as cardiac augmentation (94,95). Stimulation of these sites in conscious animals produces sham rage. Cholinergically mediated vasodilatation can be readily demonstrated in muscle on sympathetic nerve stimulation after pretreatment with adrenergic neuron blocking agents (96–98).

Parasympathetic Vasoactive Fibers

Cholinergic vasodilator fibers emerge from the sacral cord and innervate the genitals, bladder, and large intestine. Control of penile erection is one of the primary functions of this system. Activation of cholinergic fibers dilates resistance vessels in the penis, leading to greatly augmented blood flow and filling of the cavernous tissue under high pressure (99). Parasympathetic stimulation results in local vasodilatation in salivary glands through the mediation of bradykinin (*vide infra*).

Other Vasodilator Systems

Complex vasodilator systems exist in cutaneous beds such as the canine paw. After administration of adrenergic neuron blockers, sympathetic nerve stimulation results in a "sustained" noncholinergic vasodilator response that exceeds the duration of nerve activation (96–98). Transmural stimulation of isolated cerebral arterial causes relaxation that cannot be attributed to known mediators (100).

Histamine is widely distributed in the body in mast cells, leukocytes, and platelets and can be released from these depots by drugs and other stimuli. The substance dilates precapillary vessels and may also increase capillary filtration rate. It has been postulated that a histaminergic vasodilator system may participate in the reflex regulation of resistance of muscle beds (96,101).

Other Regulatory Systems

Renin-Angiotensin System

Renin is a proteolytic enzyme found principally in the kidney; it forms the decapeptide angiotensin I from a circulating α_2-globulin. Angiotensin converting enzyme (ACE), an exopeptidase, splits two amino acids from the decapeptide and forms the octapeptide AII. Juxtaglomerular cells located at the vascular pole on renal glomeruli form and release renin into the circulation (44,102). Renin is also present in numerous other organs, including blood vessels, the brain, uterus, etc. (103,104). Several mechanisms control renin release from juxtaglomerular cells. Release is inversely related to the distension of "baroreceptors" or stretch receptors in the afferent arteriole. Mechanisms in the macula densa sense the amount of sodium in the distal tubule and regulate renin release. Ac-

tivation of β-adrenoceptors on juxtaglomerular cells causes elaboration of renin. Prostaglandins also release renin and may constitute a critical link in several of the foregoing mechanisms. AII exerts negative feedback on release. Dopamine and vasopressin also inhibit.

AII is a powerful constrictor of vascular smooth muscle, probably mediated by influx and intracellular release of calcium. Infusion of subpressor quantities of AII can increase blood pressure in experimental animals after a latency of a few days (105). The peptide is one of the principal regulatory mechanisms for aldosterone release. In the kidney, AII affects the distribution of blood flow and the glomerular infiltration rate and enhances tubular sodium reabsorption (44,106,107). AII also facilitates release of NE at adrenergic neuroeffector junctions (7,15,44). The various components of the renin-angiotensin system are present in the brain. Central mechanisms will be discussed later.

In intact humans and animals, stress (e.g., sodium depletion, upright posture, hemorrhage, etc.) elevates plasma renin activity (PRA). The AII generated participates in cardiovascular adjustments to these interventions.

Several peptide competitive blockers of AII receptors have been synthesized, e.g., the 1-sarosine-8-alanine analogue (saralasin). Inhibitors of ACE have also been developed (108). The renin-angiotensin system is discussed in greater detail elsewhere in this volume.

Prostaglandins

Two families of highly active substances are derived from arachidonic acid: prostaglandins and leukotrienes (109–111). Prostaglandins (PGs) are a group of unsaturated acidic lipids containing a 20-carbon skeleton. Arachidonic acid is released from membrane phospholipids by phospholipases. In the PG pathway, cyclo-oxygenase forms the intermediate endoperoxides PGG$_2$ and PGH$_2$ from arachidonic acid. These, in turn, and depending on the tissue, are transformed into thromboxane A$_2$ (TxA$_2$) (e.g., in platelets), into prostacyclin (PGI$_2$) (in the walls of blood vessels), or into PGE$_2$ or PGF$_{2\alpha}$.

In the lipoxygenase pathways, arachidonic acid is converted into hydroxyperoxy eicosatetraenoic acid (HPETE) and then into several leukotrienes. Leukotrienes have been found in leukocytes, in mast cells, and in lung tissue. These substances compose the "slow-reacting substance of anaphylaxis" (SRS-A). Their cardiovascular role remains to be elucidated. However, they have been shown to constrict coronary arteries (112).

TxA$_2$ is the major metabolite of arachidonic acid in platelets and may also be formed in the lungs and spleen. It is an extremely potent aggregator of platelets, an effect probably mediated by reduction of cAMP levels (109,110,113). Prostacyclin, the principal metabolite of arachidonic acid in blood vessels, inhibits platelet aggregation and produces vasodilatation (109,110,114). Locally formed PGs may participate in regulation of blood flow. Their role in modulation of sympathetic transmission and renin release was discussed earlier.

Kinins

Kinins are potent vasodilator peptides formed from globulins (kininogens) by kininases (e.g., kallikrein). Salivary glands, pancreas, kidney, and plasma contain high concentrations of kallikrein (115,116). Glandular kallikrein forms kallidin (lysyl-bradykinin), which in turn is converted to the nonapeptide bradykinin by an aminopeptidase. Bradykinin is inactivated by kininase II, an enzyme identical with ACE. Kinins affect blood clotting mechanisms, fibrinolysis, and capillary permeability, in addition to participating in local control of blood

flow. In the kidney, kinins influence water and electrolyte excretion. AII and PGs can release bradykinin in organs such as the kidney. Bradykinin, in turn, is capable of releasing PGs.

Vasopressin

The nonapeptide vasopressin (antidiuretic hormone, ADH) is formed in the hypothalamus and stored and released from the posterior pituitary (117). Its primary physiologic role involves renal water reabsorption by controlling the permeability of collecting ducts to water. Although vasopressin exerts potent vasoconstrictor activity, its role in circulatory control remains unsettled, because much higher doses are required to raise blood pressure than to produce antidiuresis (118). However, this difference may be attributable to buffering by the baroreceptors. Nevertheless, vasopressin probably contributes to circulatory regulation in stressful states such as hemorrhage and may provide a backup mechanism to the renin-angiotensin system (118–120). Development of hypertension in models using sodium overload involves vasopressin (121).

5-Hydroxytryptamine

5HT is released from aggregating platelets. It is concentrated in the lungs, in the gastrointestinal tract, and in various brain pathways. 5HT has complex vascular actions (49,122). Vasoconstriction predominates, but dilatation can occur through direct means or secondary to inhibition of sympathetic-mediator release. 5HT can also enhance the constrictor actions of other agonists.

Other Vasoactive Substances

A substance released from the endothelium of isolated blood vessels has been shown to mediate the relaxant responses to ACh and bradykinin (123). Expansion of blood volume causes the release of a circulating natriuretic factor that increases renal sodium excretion subsequent to inhibition of Na-K ATPase. Inhibition of this enzyme also affects intracellular ion concentrations in cardiac and vascular smooth muscle. The hormone has been implicated in the development of hypertension (124,125). Evidence indicates that it may be released from the anterior hypothalamus. It may also be related to the postulated endogenous digitalislike substance "endoxin."

THE HEART

The primary function of cardiac muscle is generation of the force required to propel blood into peripheral organs. The actual volume of blood pumped by the heart results from the interplay of numerous complex factors.

Mechanical Properties of Cardiac Muscle Fibers

Depolarization of cardiac tissue results from rapid but brief influx of sodium. Calcium influx occurs during the plateau phase of the action potential, and repolarization is caused by potassium efflux (126). Contractile mechanisms in cardiac muscle resemble those outlined earlier for smooth muscle in regard to the general interaction of myosin and actin. However, activation results from the binding of calcium to troponin C and negation of its inhibitory influence on actin. The transverse tubular system and the SR are highly developed in cardiac muscle, and intracellular calcium stores play a greater role in the contractile process than in smooth muscle. Depolarization releases calcium from the SR (62,65,127).

Cardiac muscle consists of contractile and elastic elements arranged in series and in parallel. The contractile elements shorten on activation and stretch the series elastic elements. The external length of the muscle will diminish when the tension generated exceeds the imposed load.

Increasing the length of cardiac muscle up to its optimum maximizes the possibility for cross-bridge interaction and augments the extent and rate of force generation. This length–tension relationship forms the basis for the Frank-Starling "law of the heart," which states that the energy of contraction, however measured, is a function of the length of the muscle fiber prior to contraction (Fig. 3).

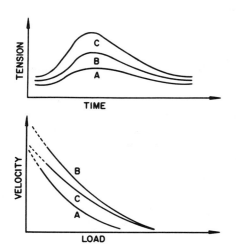

FIG. 3. Tension generation during isometric contraction and characteristics of the force–velocity relationship of isolated ventricular muscle. **Top panel:** Schematic representation of tension development during isometric contraction. Resting muscle length was increased progressively from *A* to *C*, causing rises in resting tension, rate of tension development, and peak tension during contraction. The time to peak tension did not change. **Bottom panel:** Schematic representation of the force–velocity relationship during shortening. Increasing the afterload reduces the peak velocity of shortening (curve *A*). Increasing the resting length shifts the curve upward (*C*) so that the velocity of shortening at a given afterload rises. However, extrapolation of the curve back to zero load provides the same value for V_{max}. A positive inotropic intervention shifts the curve upward, as from *A* to *B*. Under these circumstances, peak observed velocity, as well as V_{max}, increases. (Adapted from Sonnenblick et al., ref. 128, with permission.)

As just indicated, increasing the resting length (up to a point) augments the rate of tension development of isometric contraction and the velocity of shortening of isotonic contraction (128–131). On the other hand, an increase in the afterload (i.e., the load against which the muscle contracts) reduces the shortening velocity (Fig. 3). Isometric contraction results when the afterload is so great that the velocity of external shortening equals zero. Shortening velocity becomes maximal rapidly after initiation of contraction but then declines as the muscle decreases in length. The velocity of shortening at any time during contraction varies with muscle length at that instant and is no longer dependent on the initial length of the muscle. Theoretically, the maximal velocity of shortening (V_{max}) occurs when muscle contracts against no external load. V_{max} can be approximated by extrapolation of the velocity–load curve to zero. V_{max} varies with the contractile state of the muscle but, according to several investigators, is independent of preload and afterload (Fig. 3).

Force generation depends on its rate of development and the duration of the active state. The rate of tension development or the intensity of the active state depends critically on the concentration of calcium in the vicinity of the contractile proteins. Changes in resting length do not alter the basic "contractility" of cardiac muscle, which can be defined as the force developed at a given fiber length or, alternatively, as the rate of tension development or the velocity of contraction at a given length, or as V_{max}.

Increasing the number of contractions per unit time up to an optimum rate will augment contractility, as exemplified by the extent and velocity of shortening and the V_{max} of muscle. Relaxation also accelerates. The rate of tension development of an isometric contraction also rises, but the total tension generated may not increase, because the time to peak tension declines. Appropriately timed extrasystoles tend to potentiate the ensuing regular beats. The interpolation of a second stimulus soon after the termination of the refractory period of every regular beat (i.e., "paired pacing") usually results in only a small distinct increase in tension in its own right, but it greatly enhances the force generated by the subsequent primary beat (114,115).

Chemical substances that exert a positive inotropic effect increase the extent and velocity of shortening, V_{max}, and, in isometrically contracting muscle, the rate of force development. The total tension generated depends on both the rate of its development and the time to peak tension.

Mechanical Properties of the Intact Heart

The properties of myocardial fibers just outlined apply in principle to the whole heart. However, the geometry of the organ and the complex arrangement of muscle fibers introduce complicating factors. Nevertheless, the intact ventricle can be considered to function as a preloaded and afterloaded muscle. End-diastolic pressure (EDP), in conjunction with diastolic compliance, determines the resting length of muscle fibers (preload). Activation results in the development of force or tension within the myocardial wall and elevation of intracavity pressure. When intraventricular pressure exceeds aortic pressure (afterload), ejection ensues, and the ventricular volume declines. Prior to opening of the outflow valves, the ventricular volume remains unaltered, but the ventricle changes shape; i.e., the base-to-apex length shortens, and circumferential dimensions increase. Thus, some muscle fibers shorten even at this time. Wall tension follows the Laplace relationship during contraction: tension = pressure × radius. However, it must be emphasized that the Laplace formulation was developed for thin-wall vessels. During ejection, the ventricular radius shortens, and the myocardial tension re-

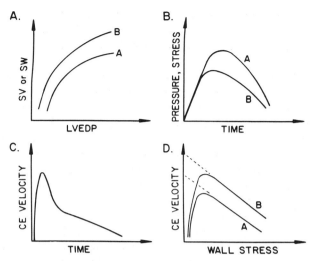

FIG. 4. Schematic representation of determinants of stroke volume, wall stress, intraventricular pressure, and contractile-element velocity in the intact heart. **A:** The Frank-Starling relationship between LVEDP or fiber length and stroke volume (SV) at constant outflow resistance or stroke work (SW). A positive inotropic intervention shifts the control curve (A) upward and to the left (B), so that greater SV or SW results from a given or even lower LVEDP. **B:** The time courses of left ventricular pressure development (A) and wall stress (B) during contraction. Wall stress declines as ventricular diameter shortens during ejection. **C:** The time course of the velocity of shortening of contractile elements (CE). Velocity rises rapidly after activation and reaches its peak early during the isovolumic phase. Velocity then declines as wall tension or stress rises. **D:** Relationships between CE velocity and wall stress or tension. After reaching an initial peak, an inverse relationship exists between CE velocity and wall stress. V_{max}, the theoretical maximal value for CE velocity, can be derived by extrapolating the descending portion of the curve back to the zero-stress axis. A positive inotropic intervention shifts the curve, as well as V_{max}, upward (B). (Adapted from Sonnenblick et al., ref. 128, with permission.)

quired to maintain internal pressure declines according to the Laplace relationship (Fig. 4) (110,132,134).

Length–Tension Relationship and Starling's Law of the Heart

The mechanical properties of the intact heart can be viewed in terms of the rate of tension development and the force–velocity relationship of contractile elements. However, because the function of the heart is to contract and propel blood into the periphery, the more obvious parameters of pressure, flow, work, and force of contraction can also be used to evaluate mechanical activity. Just as in isolated muscle, the resting or diastolic length of the ventricle determines the force generated during contraction. The latter can be expressed as stroke output at constant outflow pressure or as stroke work: stroke volume × (systolic pressure–EDP). Segment length is difficult to determine precisely in many circumstances; therefore, EDP has been used instead. EDP and segment length vary in the same direction, but discrepancies occur at higher pressures (e.g., above 12–15 mm Hg) or after changes in compliance.

A hyperbolic relationship exists between EDP or fiber length and stroke volume at constant afterload, as a consequence of the Frank-Starling relationship (Fig. 4) (132). Up to a point, the healthy heart will eject whatever quantity of blood flows into it by altering its EDP and fiber length. Increasing inflow elevates EDP, which, within limits, increases fiber length, resulting in a more forceful ventricular contraction and increases in stroke volume and ejection velocity. An elevation of outflow resistance results in incomplete emptying of the ventricle, leading to an increase in EDP, which in turn will tend to return stroke volume to its original level. In addition, it has been suggested that an increased afterload may produce a small augmentation of contractile force in its own right (homeometric autoregulation) (135,136). At very high EDP, particularly in diseased hearts, stroke volume or work may diminish. The heart may then function on the "descending limb" of the Starling curve (not illustrated in Fig. 4).

Many factors, such as heart rate, temperature, autonomic impulses, drugs, and disease states, influence the basic Frank-Starling mechanism and indeed may obscure it in conscious animals and humans. In the normal conscious reclining dog, left ventricular end-diastolic diameter is near maximum, so that further lengthening will not necessarily augment force. Loading with intravenous infusions in conscious dogs with low prevailing heart rate does not increase stroke volume (137).

Factors controlling ventricular filling also contribute to performance. These include atrial pressure, ventricular compliance, and duration of diastole. Changes in compliance occur in disease states (e.g., hypertension) (138,139).

Rates of Pressure Development and the Force–Velocity Relationship in the Intact Heart

As intraventricular pressure rises during isovolumic contraction, the rate of pressure development (dP/dt) mounts steadily. Maximum dP/dt occurs before or at valve opening, provided that aortic pressure is not excessive. A rise in aortic pressure will delay valve opening and lead to an increase in dP/dt (132,140–142). Maximum dP/dt depends on left ventricular EDP (LVEDP) as well as peak ventricular pressure.

The velocity of shortening of contractile elements (V_{ce}) can be calculated from the stresses and velocities of change in ventricular geometry during contraction (128,132,134). Wall stress can be derived from intraventricular pressures and contours using the Laplace relationship: tension = (pressure × radius)/(2 × wall thickness). Stress increases quickly during isovolumic contraction, but then starts to decline, whereas pressure may continue to rise (Fig. 4). Calculated V_{ce} increases very rapidly after the onset of activation, but after reaching an early peak it diminishes as wall tension rises. During this period, an inverse relationship exists between V_{ce} and tension or stress. Extrapolation of this force–velocity relationship to the velocity axis (zero force) provides a maximum value for V_{ce}: i.e., V_{max}. Increases in LVEDP or in aortic pressure elevate the force–velocity curve but alter its shape, so that extrapolated V_{max} remains constant.

Several indices of contractility employing aspects of the force–velocity relationship have been developed for use in humans and intact animals: the maximum of the continuously computed dP/dt/instantaneous P, comparison of dP/dt at a given pressure (e.g., at 40 mm Hg), or V_{ce}. These indices attempt to minimize the influences of changes in preload and afterload (128,132).

Inotropic Interventions

Numerous factors, including pH and other ions, tissue oxygen and metabolite concentrations, temperature, pacing rate and sequence, drugs, etc., influence the cardiac contractile state. Positive inotropic interventions alter the force–velocity relationship. They increase the rate of force development at equivalent muscle length or augment pressure development at a given LVEDP (or end-diastolic diameter) and speed the rate of relaxation. Indices of contractility, such as $V_{ce\ max}$, $dP/dt/P$, etc., are increased, and the Frank-Starling curve is shifted upward and to the left by positive inotropic interventions (128,132, 134,140,142). Total force may not change if the increase in force development is matched by an equivalent reduction in the duration of the active state. In general, inotropic stimuli produce more profound responses in anesthetized animals than in conscious animals and in depressed hearts than in normal or healthy hearts.

Function of the Atrium

Atrial muscle has properties similar to those of ventricular muscle. The atrium has been likened to a "booster pump" in that it augments the transfer of fluid from the feeder line or venous bed into the main pump, permitting adequate ventricular filling at relatively low venous pressure. An increase in atrial pressure enhances contractile force according to the Frank-Starling relationship and results in the transfer of greater amounts of blood into the ventricle (135,143,144). Atrial contraction produces a small elevation in ventricular EDP and usually a larger change in fiber length. At low ventricular rates, the atrial contribution to ventricular stroke volume may be relatively minor in normal hearts. At elevated rates and in diseased hearts, appropriately timed atrial systole assumes greater importance (144,145). In addition, atrial contraction promotes the closure of A-V valves.

Factors Regulating Cardiac Output

Cardiac minute volume represents the product of heart rate and stroke volume. Isolated changes in rate produce variable changes in cardiac output. In the midrange (i.e., 80–140 beats/minute), output usually remains independent of rate in humans as well as animals (142,146,147). Output diminishes at much slower or faster rates. However, an increase in rate contributes greatly to the elevation of output during exercise or, as shown in conscious dogs, during infusion of a volume load (137). Stroke volume declines progressively above optimal rates of about 60 to 90 beats per minute, all other factors remaining constant.

Numerous factors, including preload (EDP, end-diastolic volume, fiber length), afterload (outflow impedance), cardiac contractility, activation sequence, etc., influence stroke volume.

As stated earlier, the healthy heart can readily accommodate an increased inflow. Increased "venous return" resulting from an elevated pressure gradient from the venous capacity vessels to the right atrium tends to enhance stroke volume by the Starling mechanism. A fall in atrial pressure also augments the gradient for venous return. However, changes in preload (e.g., during blood infusion) do not always elevate cardiac output, because of countervailing reflex mechanisms.

Changes in outflow impedance can influence steady-state stroke volume. This effect is probably minimal in healthy hearts, but it assumes much greater importance in disease states such as congestive failure (132). On the other hand, outflow impedance influences end-systolic and end-diastolic dimensions and ejection fraction.

The force of contraction in a healthy heart usually accommodates adequately to changing preload and afterload and is not the limiting factor in determining stroke volume. Slight or even relatively moderate changes in contractility usually do not modify cardiac output. Thus, cardiac glycosides or paired ventricular pacing most often fail to augment output in healthy humans or animals (148).

The sequence of activation of cardiac muscle assures its optimum function as a pump. The importance of appropriately timed atrial contraction, particularly at rapid heart rates, was stressed earlier. Major disturbances in ventricular conduction, such as bundle branch block or ventricular extrasystoles, can reduce output.

Postural changes can influence cardiac output and dimensions partly as a result of reflex mechanisms. Output usually declines as the subject moves from the supine to the sitting and standing positions. Heart size diminishes during anesthesia and even more so after thoracotomy.

Numerous compensatory mechanisms exist that enable a weakened heart to meet metabolic demand (132). Initial or short-term adjustments include the Frank-Starling mechanism and reflexly induced changes in autonomic outflow. Cardiac output may be restored to acceptable levels, but indices of contractility remain depressed. Excessive volume loads or increases in outflow resistance can rapidly lead to ventricular dilatation and failure. Long-term compensatory adjustments result in hypertrophy due to the synthesis of additional myofibrils and contractile units. Hypertrophy reduces ventricular compliance and thus can modify the Frank-Starling mechanism. Dilatation augments myocardial oxygen consumption according to the Laplace relationship because the internal ventricular diameter increases. Hypertrophy also tends to encroach on oxygen supply. Autonomic adjustments to cardiac weakness or failure result in tachycardia and arterial and venous constriction, leading to redistribution of available cardiac output to the most vital organs.

Autonomic Influence

Atria and junctional tissues are richly innervated by parasympathetic and sympathetic fibers, whereas the latter predominate in ventricles (149,150). Vagal stimulation reduces sinus rate and depresses atrial contractility and conduction through the atrioventricular node (135,143). Cholinergic fibers also exert negative inotropic effects on the ventricles, but the magnitude of the response tends to be rather small. These fibers also have the capability of depressing ventricular automaticity.

Sympathetic activation augments contractility of atria and ventricles by β-adrenoceptor- and cAMP-mediated elevation of intracellular calcium concentration that is due, in part, to an increase in the number of calcium channels, as indicated earlier. Sympathetic stimuli increase the sinus rate, as well as that of other automatic tissues, and enhance transmission through the atrioventricular node and can constrict veins, leading to increased "venous return." Cholinergic and adrenergic stimuli react in a complex manner as outlined earlier. In addition, simultaneous excitation of both systems can produce cardiac dysrhythmias.

The relative contributions of parasympathetic and sympathetic systems to reflex changes in heart rate in conscious and anesthetized subjects vary considerably (149). Neurally mediated increases in rate may occur as a result of augmented sympathetic tone and/or reduced vagal tone, whereas opposite changes in firing of these fibers reduce the heart rate. Although considerable evidence exists for simultaneous and reciprocal changes in the two systems, increases in rate occur predominantly as a result of augmented sympathetic activity, whereas enhanced vagal firing is mainly responsible for reducing the rate. However, different levels of sympathetic tone and vagal tone exist under varying circumstances. Pentobarbital-anesthetized dogs have high sympathetic tone but relatively low vagal tone. Consequently, reduction of vagal activity plays a lesser role in raising heart rate in these animals than in conscious animals.

Elevated sympathetic tone contributes to the increases in heart rate and output during exercise. However, cardiac denervation does not seem to greatly diminish the running performances of dogs. Heart rate and output still increase in these animals, although changes may occur more slowly and may not reach the same peak levels as before denervation. However, propranolol has been shown to reduce the capacity for strenuous exertion in humans and to attenuate the accompanying increases in heart rate and output (151). Further, it was found that cardiac denervation combined with β blockade reduced the running performances of greyhounds considerably, whereas β blockade alone exerted only a slight effect (152). Thus, the autonomic nervous system plays an important but by no means indispensable role in the cardiovascular response to exercise.

Cardiac Energetics

Myocardial cells consume oxygen in their resting state to maintain their integrity, as do all other cells. Contraction necessitates far greater oxygen utilization. Major determinants of oxygen consumption in cardiac fibers are the rate and extent of shortening and, in the intact heart, systolic tension and its rate of development. The latter will vary with preload, afterload, end-diastolic dimensions, and inotropic state (132,153). Cardiac dimensions influence oxygen consumption, because more wall tension is required to generate a given intraventricular pressure in a large heart than in a small heart (Laplace relationship). Thus, inotropic drugs may reduce the oxygen consumption of dilated hearts because they diminish heart size. Heart rate is also one of the major determinants of oxygen consumption.

Overall, increases in stroke volume require relatively less oxygen than increases in pressure. Thus, "volume work" is more efficient than "pressure work."

Coronary Circulation

Coronary blood flow is subject to the same regulatory factors prevalent in other beds, i.e., driving pressure and vascular resistance. However, myocardial systole produces a high extravascular pressure gradient from the epicardium toward the endocardium (154). Consequently, flow occurs mainly during diastole in the deeper regions. Perfusion of subendocardial areas of the left ventricle may be particularly compromised during stress in patients with coronary atherosclerosis. Partial occlusion of a coronary vessel by mechanical measures or disease causes progressive dilatation of the resistance vessels in the subservient area. Under these conditions, flow becomes more and more dependent on the pressure gradient across the bed (arterial minus atrial or ventricular end-diastolic), as well as on the degree of extravascular compression. Dilatation of resistance vessels in normally perfused areas can divert blood away from the ischemic regions (coronary "steal").

Coronary vessels respond to autonomic stimuli directly, as do other beds, but cardiac oxygen consumption is the major determinant of coronary resistance. Adenosine may serve as a link in the metabolic regulation of resistance (81).

Spasm of coronary arteries, due to either local or exogenous factors, has been demonstrated angiographically and can precipitate episodes of angina pectoris (155).

BLOOD VOLUME

The volume and composition of blood greatly influence the circulation. Hematocrit, viscosity, and vascular resistance are intimately related, as outlined earlier. Plasma volume, in relation to the tone of resistance and capacitance vessels, determines the pressures within these compartments and thus, secondarily, modifies most aspects of circulatory function. For example, blood pressure of anephric patients is markedly sensitive to changes in plasma volume.

The balance between ingestion and excretion determines body water content. In turn, blood volume is determined by (a) fluid exchange between plasma and the interstitial space, (b) exchange between plasma and the external environment, and

(c) erythrocyte volume. Factors responsible for capillary fluid fluxes were outlined earlier.

Numerous regulatory mechanisms exist for the maintenance of optimal plasma volume. These operate primarily by modifying renal excretion of sodium and water. "Osmoreceptors" in the hypothalamus detect variations in plasma osmolality and respond by initiating appropriate changes in the rate of ADH (vasopressin) secretion (117). Increases in left atrial pressure activate stretch receptors in the atrial wall that result in a vagally mediated reduction in ADH secretion, leading to enhanced renal elimination of water and sodium (*vide infra*). Baroreceptor reflexes also affect ADH release. Aldosterone plays a major role in plasma volume control by regulating renal handling of sodium. Aldosterone secretion, in turn, is controlled by numerous factors, including plasma potassium concentration, angiotensin, ACTH, etc. The "natriuretic factor" discussed earlier also influences blood volume. Disease states can alter blood volume by many mechanisms, such as modifying secretion and degradation rates of aldosterone and ADH.

NEURAL CONTROL OF THE CIRCULATION

The nervous system has the ability to rapidly and profoundly modify cardiovascular function. Emotional stress tends to elevate blood pressure and heart rate, whereas the opposite changes occur during sleep. The central nervous system regulates the circulation primarily by varying sympathetic and parasympathetic outflow and by modifying the release of numerous hormones.

Central Pathways and Mechanisms

Neurons in the hypothalamus and medulla oblongata predominate in central cardiovascular regulation, but higher brain areas, the midbrain, pons, cerebellum, and spinal cord participate. Groups of nuclei subserving excitatory and inhibitory functions exist in the anterior and posterior hypothalamus. Nuclei and more diffusely grouped cells in the dorsal and ventrolateral regions of the medulla predominate in cardiovascular control. The dorsal vagal nuclei and the nuclei ambiguus contain cell bodies of cardiac vagal efferents (156–159).

Descending excitatory and inhibitory fibers form discrete tracts within the spinal cord (159,160). These impinge, either monosynaptically or polysynaptically, on preganglionic neurons located primarily in the intermediolateral column of the cord. Some descending hypothalamic tracts project directly to the cord without synapsing in the medulla.

It has been proposed that oscillatory circuits in the medulla generate firing with a periodicity of 2 to 6 Hz and that spinal neurons generate oscillatory activity with a periodicity of 10 Hz (161). It has been further suggested that input from other areas entrains these basic rhythms.

Baroreceptor afferents (*vide infra*) terminate in the nuclei of the solitary tracts (NTS), which in turn project to other cardiovascular "regions" in the medulla, as well as the hypothalamus, pons, and spinal cord (159–162). Baroreceptor reflexes are integrated at both supraspinal levels and spinal levels (159).

A large and diverse group of putative neurotransmitters modulate central cardiovascular mechanisms. Noradrenergic fibers originating in various cell groups in the brainstem innervate "cardiovascular" neurons in the hypothalamus, medulla, and spinal cord (158,159,163–165). Depletion of brain NE does not disrupt normal central regulatory mechanisms but does prevent the development of several forms of experimental hypertension (166).

Excitatory as well as inhibitory functions for noradrenergic fibers have been postulated (156,159,163,167). NE applied iontophoretically inhibits firing of spinal preganglionic neurons (168). Injection of NE into the NTS or anterior hypothalamus lowers blood pressure (156,163). Epinephrine-containing fibers originating in the brainstem also contribute to central control (164).

Ascending and descending serotonergic fibers originate in the raphe nuclei. Evidence indicates that spinal 5HT pathways are excitatory to preganglionic neurons, although contradictory views have been offered (156,165,168–170).

The various components of the renin-angiotensin system, including renin, its substrate, ACE, and AII receptors, exist in the central nervous system and are intimately involved with thirst mechanisms (133). Infusion of AII into the vertebral artery or its administration into the brain ventricular system elevates blood pressure by augmenting sympathetic outflow and by vasopressin release (44,171). Neural structures in the midbrain and medulla mediate the response in dogs and cats. Cells in the anterior hypothalamus (i.e., periventricular tissue in the anterior and ventral regions of the third ventricle, AV3V) participate in thirst mechanisms as well as centrally mediated responses to AII and several forms of experimental hypertension in rats (166). This region may directly or indirectly regulate elaboration of the natriuretic factor.

Other systems and mediators participate in central cardiovascular mechanisms: cholinergic, opiate peptide, γ-aminobutyric acid, substance P, glycine, glutamate, etc. (172–178). The great complexity of these is illustrated by evidence indicating that opiate peptides may mediate the hypotensive response to central α_2-adrenoceptor stimulation by clonidine (179).

Sensors exist within the circulation that detect changes in pressure, wall stretch, pH, P_{CO_2}, P_{O_2}, etc., and initiate compensatory reflex adjustments.

High-Pressure (Baroreceptor) Reflexes

The carotid sinuses and aortic arch contain specialized sensory fibers that are activated by distension of the vessel wall. Changes in luminal pressure alter the strain on these fibers and influence their firing rate in direct proportion to the distension. An increase in intraluminal pressure augments the firing rate of individual fibers and also recruits additional elements. The rate of change of pressure also determines the level of nerve firing. Thus, pulsatile pressure results in greater nerve activity than steady pressure at comparable mean levels. Changes in the ionic environment (sodium, potassium, calcium) of the nerve endings can alter their sensitivity (181). In dogs and cats the carotid sinus mechanism has a lower threshold and operates at a lower range of pressures than aortic receptors. Myelinated afferents have a lower threshold than nonmyelinated fibers (181,183).

Carotid sinus and aortic depressor afferents project to the NTS and result in inhibition of sympathetic outflow and frequently enhancement of vagal outflow. These lead to vasodilatation, reduction in blood pressure, and usually a decrease in heart rate. Thus, an increase in sinus and aortic arch pressure reflexly inhibits sympathetic outflow, whereas a fall in pressure produces opposite effects.

Baroreceptor reflexes modify cardiac contractility in anesthetized animals (132,135, 157,180). However, experiments in conscious animals and humans suggest that these reflexes do not have a great influence on the mechanical activity of the heart (184,185). Venous tone and venous capacity are subject to baroreceptor control (186). However, studies in conscious animals and in humans suggest only minimal participation of the venous system in baroreceptor reflexes (184).

Baroreceptors adapt relatively slowly (i.e., in a matter of hours or days) to sustained changes in pressure. Prolonged changes, however, result in a shift in the sensitive range. Upward resetting of baroreceptors in chronic hypertension probably results from reduced distensibility of the vascular wall (187). Reduction of pressure by long-term drug administration has been shown to return sensitivity to normal levels (188).

Sectioning of carotid sinus and aortic arch fibers results in an acute rise in blood pressure, which then tends to decline slowly. Blood pressure in conscious dogs after sinoaortic baroreceptor denervation is exquisitely sensitive to external stimuli, and continuously monitored pressure varies to a much greater extent over a 24-hr period in these animals than in controls. However, pressures are not greatly elevated in a quiet environment (189). These results have led to the conclusion that the primary function of the baroreceptors is not to set the long-term level of blood pressure but to minimize short-term fluctuations.

Pressure-sensitive areas along the common carotid and subclavian arteries and in the descending aorta have also been described, but their physiologic roles remain uncertain.

Cardiopulmonary Receptors

Reflexes originate from numerous cardiopulmonary regions (182,190). Receptors in tracheobronchial passages detect irritant substances and trigger the cough reflex. Pulmonary stretch receptors sensitive to inflation and deflation participate in the Hering-Breuer reflex. Deflation or "J" receptors can be activated by forced deflation or pulmonary congestion. Activation of these receptors can lower blood pressure and heart rate, but they are primarily concerned with respiration.

Three major groups of afferent fibers (two vagal, one sympathetic) emanate from the heart. Myelinated vagal fibers (A and B fibers) arising from the junctions of venae cavae and the right atrium and the pulmonary arteries and the left atrium compose one of these (182,190,191). The A fibers are activated by tension in the atrial wall, and they fire during atrial systole. The B fibers are more sensitive to changes in volume, and they discharge during rapid inflow.

Mechanical distension of these junctional areas, particularly on the left side, reflexly increases heart rate (Bainbridge reflex) (191). Volume loading raises the heart rate when it is low in conscious baboons, but it exerts the opposite effect when the prevailing rate is high (192). Left atrial distension also inhibits ADH release.

Nonmyelinated vagal afferents originate from throughout the atrial and ventricular walls. They are activated by distension and cause sympathoinhibition and vagal firing. Although they exhibit a low rate of spontaneous discharge, they contribute to cardiovascular regulation and assume considerable importance in adjustments to hemorrhage and venous pooling (190,193,194). Myelinated fibers also originate from the ventricular myocardium. Vagal fibers with similar function originate from the pulmonary artery.

Coronary artery occlusion can stimulate nonmyelinated fibers and initiate reflex bradycardia and hypotension. A similar reflex response can occur during myocardial infarction.

Afferent impulses from the heart are also carried over sympathetic nerves (181,190). Activation of these fibers by mechanical or chemical means enhances efferent sympathetic outflow to the heart.

Chemoreceptors and Chemoreflexes

Medullary hypoxia profoundly enhances sympathetic overflow to blood vessels and the heart, resulting in vasoconstriction and cardiac augmentation (157). Discrete chemosensitive organs exist in the carotid sinus and aortic arch regions (195,196). Afferent fibers run with the carotid sinus and aortic depressor nerves. Reduced pH and Po_2 and elevated Pco_2, as well as chemical substances such as cyanide, nicotine, and phenyldiguanide, activate the carotid and aortic bodies, resulting in stimulation of respiration and complex cardiovascular effects. The respiratory response is probably the most important.

Perfusion of the carotid and aortic bodies with hypoxic blood usually elevates peripheral resistance but reduces heart rate and atrial and ventricular contractility. Variable changes in systemic blood pressure occur. Injection of nicotine and cyanide into carotid arterial blood activates chemoreceptors and generally produces similar cardiovascular responses. These agents have also been shown to constrict muscular beds and dilate cutaneous and coronary beds (197).

Intravenous or intra-coronary-artery injection of veratrum alkaloids initiates the coronary chemoreflex or Bezold-Jarisch reflex, leading to decreases in blood pressure and heart rate. These substances have the ability to activate or sensitize numerous myelinated and nonmyelinated mechanoreceptor fibers. Other compounds, such as 5HT, bradykinin, lobeline, nicotine, phenyldiguanide, and aconitine, can also activate these fibers (198,199).

Spinal Reflexes

Somatic afferents can also modify cardiovascular function by facilitating or inhibiting preganglionic neurons at spinal levels (200). In addition, ascending projections from segmental levels influence bulbar control of sympathetic outflow and thus modulate input from other areas. Purely spinal cardiovascular reflexes can be demonstrated in experimental preparations and in paraplegic humans.

OVERALL REGULATION OF THE CIRCULATION

Guyton and associates have analyzed overall circulatory control critically and evaluated the roles of the baroreceptors, the chemoreceptors, the central and autonomic nervous systems, the renin-angiotensin-aldosterone system, capillary

fluid shifts, and renal excretory function (201). Nervous control mechanisms are ideally suited to short-term circulatory control because they respond very quickly and can profoundly affect function. They are directed predominantly toward maintenance of systemic blood pressure rather than cardiac output. For example, blood pressure will tend to remain relatively constant in the face of induced changes in cardiac output or during infusion of fluids as a consequence of reflexly mediated changes in vascular resistance. After baroreceptor denervation or destruction of the central nervous system, these interventions result in wide variations in pressure. Local regulatory factors then control vascular resistance, and the circulation is transformed from a pressure-regulated system to a flow-regulated system. Thus, the primary function of nervous mechanisms probably is to mediate the rapid circulatory adjustments to changing situations rather than long-term setting of blood pressure levels.

The renin-angiotensin-aldosterone system participates in short- as well as longer-term blood pressure control by influencing renal sodium reabsorption and by direct and possibly centrally mediated effects on blood vessels, as discussed earlier. According to Guyton and associates, the kidney is the primary regulator of blood pressure in the long term. A direct relationship exists between systemic blood pressure and sodium and urine outputs. Thus, any variation in pressure initiates a compensatory change in urinary volume and, in turn, plasma volume, which will tend to return pressure to normal levels. These adaptations, of course, imply adequate renal function. Disease states that compromise renal function may severely strain this homeostatic process.

There are numerous other examples of cardiac and vascular adaptation to changing internal environment and to disease. Cardiac dilatation and hypertrophy in response to chronically increased volume and pressure loads were mentioned earlier. Blood vessels also hypertrophy in the presence of persistently elevated pressure (202).

Numerous cardiovascular control mechanisms are outlined in the foregoing, and it is evident that considerable redundancy exists. The autonomic nervous system contributes to the rapid adjustment to exercise. Yet animals or humans subjected to cardiac denervation or pharmacologic blockade increase their output markedly during exercise, although the response may not be as great or occur as rapidly as in the normal situation. Although extensively studied, the importance of the adrenal medulla in normal circulatory control remains uncertain. However, its role may be crucial after inhibition of sympathetic vasoconstrictor responsiveness (203). The renin-angiotensin system assumes a critical regulatory role during sodium depletion and hemorrhage. Vasopressin probably provides an additional backup system.

Responses to Drugs

Many of the mechanisms outlined earlier can be modified by drugs. However, responses to equivalent doses may vary widely under differing physiologic conditions and in disease states. Effects of autonomic blocking agents will naturally depend greatly on prevailing levels of sympathetic and parasympathetic outflow. Sympathetic tone is very low in a quietly resting dog; therefore, sympatholytic drugs will exert negligible effects on blood pressure and cardiac function. On the other hand, animals anesthetized with barbiturates exhibit a high degree of sympathetic tone but low vagal tone. Under these conditions, sympatholytics affect function markedly. Drugs that depress cardiac contractility slightly probably do not influence cardiac output in healthy conscious animals or humans, because of considerable reserve capacity. However, in hearts depressed by disease or anesthesia, these substances can produce pronounced effects. It is clear that the state of the circulation at any instant will profoundly influence the qualitative and quantitative nature of drug responses. Regulatory mechanisms will attempt to nullify drug-induced changes.

REFERENCES

1. Kuntz A. *The autonomic nervous system.* Philadelphia: Lea & Febiger, 1953.
2. Mayer SE. Drugs acting at synaptic and neuroeffector junctional sites. Neurohumoral transmission and the autonomic nervous system. In: Gilman AG, Goodman LS, Gilman A, eds. *The pharmacological basis of therapeutics.* New York: Macmillan, 1980;56–90.
3. Ceccarelli B, Hurlbut WP. Vesicle hypothesis of the release of quanta of acetylcholine. *Physiol Rev* 1980;60:396–434.
4. Fuxe K, Sedvall G. The distribution of adrenergic nerve fibers to blood vessels in skeletal muscle. *Acta Physiol Scand* 1965;64:75–86.
5. Smith AD. Mechanisms involved in the release of noradrenaline from sympathetic nerves. *Br Med Bull* 1973;29:123–129.
6. Livett BG. Histochemical visualization of peripheral and central adrenergic neurons. *Br Med Bull* 1973;29:93–99.
7. Vanhoutte PM, Verbeuren TJ, Webb RC. Local modulation of adrenergic neuroeffector interaction in the blood vessel wall. *Physiol Rev* 1981;61:151–247.
8. Cotten M deV. ed. Regulation of catecholamine metabolism in the sympathetic nervous system. *Pharmacol Rev* 1972;24:161–434.
9. Weiner N, Cloutier G, Bjur R, Pfeffer RI. Modification of norepinephrine synthesis in intact tissue by drugs during short-term adrenergic nerve stimulation. *Pharmacol Rev* 1972;24: 203–221.
10. Iversen L. Catecholamine uptake processes. *Br Med Bull* 1973;29:130–135.
11. Pelletier G, Steinbusch HWM, Verhofstad AAJ. Immunoreactive substance P and serotonin present in the same dense-core vesicles. *Nature* 1981;293:71–72.
12. Langer SZ. Presynaptic regulation of the release of catecholamines. *Pharmacol Rev* 1981; 32:337–362.
13. Weiner N. Multiple factors regulating the release of norepinephrine consequent to nerve stimulation. *Fed Proc* 1979;38:2193–2202.
14. Kalsner S, Suleiman M, Dobson RE. Adrenergic presynaptic receptors: an overextended hypothesis? *J Pharm Pharmacol* 1980;32:2990–2992.
15. Zimmerman BG. Adrenergic facilitation by angiotensin: does it serve a physiological function? *Clin Sci* 1981;60:343–348.
16. Muscholl E. Peripheral muscarinic control of

norepinephrine release in the cardiovascular system. *Am J Physiol* 1980;239:H713–H720.
17. Pletscher A. Regulation of catecholamine turnover by variation of enzyme levels. *Pharmacol Rev* 1972;24:225–232.
18. Zigmond RE. The long-term regulation of ganglionic tyrosine hydroxylase by preganglionic nerve activity. *Fed Proc* 1980;39:3003–3008.
19. Laverty R. The mechanism of action of some antihypertensive drugs. *Br Med Bull* 1973;29:152–157.
20. Day MD, Rand MJ. Evidence for a competitive antagonism of guanethidine by dexamphetamine. *Br J Pharmacol* 1963;20:17–28.
21. Volle RL, Hancock JC. Transmission in sympathetic ganglia. *Fed Proc* 1970;29:1913–1918.
22. Dunn NJ. Ganglionic transmission: electrophysiology and pharmacology. *Fed Proc* 1980;39:2982–2989.
23. McAfee DA, Hennon BK, Whiting GJ, Horn JP, Jarowsky PJ, Turner DK. The action of cAMP and catecholamines in mammalian sympathetic ganglia. *Fed Proc* 1980;39:2997–3002.
24. Wilson SP, Klein RL, Chang K-J, Gasparis MS, Viveros OH, Yang WS. Are opioid peptides cotransmitters in noradrenergic vesicles of sympathetic nerves? *Nature* 1980;228:707–709.
25. Baxter JD, Funder JW. Hormone receptors. *N Engl J Med* 1979;304:1149–1161.
26. Lefkowitz RJ, Caron MG, Michel T, Stadel JM. Mechanisms of hormone receptor-effector coupling: the α-adrenergic receptor and adenylate cyclase. *Fed Proc* 1982;41:2664–2670.
27. Pollet RJ, Levey GS. Principles of membrane receptor physiology and their application to clinical medicine. *Ann Intern Med* 1980;92:663–680.
28. Snyder SH, Goodman RR. Multiple neurotransmitter receptors. *J Neurochem* 1980;35:5–15.
29. Demeyts P, Rousseau GG. Receptor concepts. A century of evolution. *Circ Res [Suppl I]* 1980;46:I-3–I-9.
30. Snyder SH, Bruns RF, Daly JW, Innis RB. Multiple neurotransmitter receptors in the brain: amines, adenosine and cholecystokinin. *Fed Proc* 1981;40:142–146.
31. Sabol SL, Nirenberg M. Regulation of adenylate cyclase of neuroblastoma × glioma hybrid cells by α-adrenergic receptors. *J Biol Chem* 1979;254:1913–1920.
32. Rosenberger LB, Yamamura HI, Roeske WR. The regulation of cardiac muscarinic cholinergic receptors by isoproterenol. *Eur J Pharmacol* 1980;65:129–130.
33. Ahlquist RP. A study of the adrenotropic receptors. *Am J Physiol* 1948;153:586–600.
34. Drew GM, Whiting SB. Evidence for two distinct types of postsynaptic α-adrenoceptor in vascular smooth muscle in vivo. *Br J Pharmacol* 1979;67:207–215.
35. Jacobs KH, Schultz G. Signal transformation involving adrenoceptors. *J Cardiovasc Pharmacol* 1982;4:S63–S67.
36. VanMeel JCA, DeJonge A, Kalkman HO, Wilffert B, Timmermans PBMWM, Van Zwieten PA. Vascular smooth muscle contraction initiated by postsynaptic α-adrenoceptor activation is induced by an influx of extracellular calcium. *Eur J Pharmacol* 1981;69:205–208.
37. Lands AM, Arnold A, McAuliff JP, Luduena FP, Brown TG, Jr. Differentiation of receptor systems activated by sympathomimetic amines. *Nature* 1967;214:597–598.
38. Baker SP, Boyd HM, Potter LT. Distribution and function of α-adrenoceptors in different chambers of the canine heart. *Br J Pharmacol* 1980;68:57–63.
39. Goldberg LI, Kohli JD, Kotake AN, Volkman PH. Characteristics of the vascular dopamine receptor: comparison with other receptors. *Fed Proc* 1978;37:2396–2402.
40. Creese I, Sibley DR, Leff S, Hamblin M. Dopamine receptors: subtypes, localization and regulation. *Fed Proc* 1981;40:147–152.
41. Brodde O-E. Vascular dopamine receptors: demonstration and characterization by in vitro studies. *Life Sci* 1982;31:289–306.
42. Cavero I, Massinghamn R, Lefèvre-Borg F. Peripheral dopamine receptors, potential targets for a new class of antihypertensive agents. *Life Sci* 1982;31:939–948.
43. Regoli D, Park WK, Rioux F. Pharmacology of angiotensin. *Pharmacol Rev* 1974;26:69–123.
44. Peach MJ. Renin-angiotensin system: biochemistry and mechanisms of action. *Physiol Rev* 1977;57:313–370.
45. Hedqvist P. Autonomic neurotransmission. In: Ramwell PW, ed. *The prostaglandins.* New York: Plenum Press, 1973;101–131.
46. Moncada S, Vane JR. Pharmacology and endogenous roles of prostaglandin endoperoxides, thromboxane A₂, and prostacyclin. *Pharmacol Rev* 1979;30:293–331.
47. Brody MJ, Kadowitz PJ. Prostaglandins as modulators of the autonomic nervous system. *Fed Proc* 1974;33:48–60.
48. Leysen JE, Awouters F, Kennis L, Laduron PM, Vandenberk J, Janssen PAJ. Receptor binding profile of R 41 468, a novel antagonist at 5-HT receptors. *Life Sci* 1981;28:1015–1022.
49. VanNeuten JM, Janssen PAJ, VanBeek J, Xhonneux R, Verbeusen TJ, Vanhoutte PM. Vascular effects of ketanserin (R41 468), a novel antagonist of 5-HT₂ serotonin receptors. *J Pharmacol Exp Ther* 1981;218:217–230.
50. Burnstock G. Purinergic nerves. *Pharmacol Rev* 1972;24:509–581.
51. Somlyo AP, Somlyo AV. Vascular smooth muscle. I. Normal structure, pathology, biochemistry, and biophysics. *Pharmacol Rev* 1968;20:197–272.
52. Holman ME. Electrophysiology of vascular smooth muscle. *Ergeb Physiol* 1969;61:137–177.
53. Casteels R. Electro- and pharmacomechanical coupling in vascular smooth muscle. *Chest [Suppl]* 1980;78:150–156.
54. Katz AM, Messineo FC, Herbette L. Ion

channels in membranes. *Circulation [Suppl I]* 1982;65:I-2–I-10.

55. VanBreemen C, Aaronson P, Loutzenhiser R, Meisheri K. Ca^{2+} movement in smooth muscle. *Chest [Suppl]* 1980;78:157–165.

56. Webb RC, Bohr DF. Regulation of vascular tone, molecular mechanisms. *Prog Cardiovasc Dis* 1981;24:213–242.

57. Hermsmeyer K, Abel PW, Trapani AJ. Membrane sensitivity and membrane potentials of caudal arterial muscle in DOCA-salt, Dahl, and SHR hypertension in the rat. *Hypertension [Suppl II]* 1982;4:II-49–II-51.

58. Harder DR, Abel PW, Hermsmeyer K. Membrane electrical mechanism of basilar artery constriction and pial artery dilatation by norepinephrine. *Circ Res* 1981;49:1237–1242.

59. Häusler G. α-Adrenoceptor mediated contractile and electrical responses of vascular smooth muscle. *J Cardiovasc Pharmacol* 1982; 4:S97–S100.

60. Itoh T, Kajiwara M, Kitamura K, Kurijama H. Effects of vasodilator agents on smooth muscle cells of the coronary artery of the pig. *Br J Pharmacol* 1981;74:455–468.

61. Brock TA, Smith JB, Overbeck HW. Relationship of vascular sodium-potassium pump activity to intracellular sodium in hypertensive rats. *Hypertension [Suppl II]* 1982;4:II-43–II-48.

62. Adams RJ, Schwartz A. Comparative mechanisms for contraction of cardiac and skeletal muscle. *Chest [Suppl]* 1980;78:123–139.

63. Hartshorne DJ. Biochemical basis for contraction of vascular smooth muscle. *Chest [Suppl]* 1980;78:140–149.

64. Stull JT, Sanford CF. Differences in skeletal, cardiac and smooth muscle contractile element regulation by calcium. In: Weiss GB, ed. *New perspectives on calcium antagonist.* Bethesda: American Physiological Society, 1981;35–46.

65. Bárány M, Bárány K. Protein phosphorylation in cardiac and vascular smooth muscle. *Am J Physiol* 1981;241:H117–H128.

66. Murphy RA. Myosin phosphorylation and cross-bridge regulation in arterial smooth muscle. *Hypertension [Suppl II]* 1982;4:II-3–II-7.

67. Axelsson KL, Wikberg JES, Andersson RGG. Relationship between nitroglycerin, cyclic GMP and relaxation of vascular smooth muscle. *Life Sci* 1979;24:1779–1786.

68. Keith RA, Burkman AM, Sokoloski TD, Fertel RH. Vascular tolerance to nitroglycerin and cyclic GMP generation in rabbit aortic smooth muscle. *J Pharmacol Exp Ther* 1982;221:525–531.

69. Rhodin HP. Architecture of the vessel wall. In: Bohr DF, Somlyo AP, Sparks HV, Jr, eds. *Handbook of physiology, section 2, the cardiovascular system, vol. 2, vascular smooth muscle.* Bethesda: American Physiological Society, 1980;1–31.

70. Somlyo AV. Ultrastructure of vascular smooth muscle. In: Bohr DF, Somlyo AP, Sparks HV, Jr, eds. *Handbook of physiology, section 2, the cardiovascular system, vol. 2, vascular smooth*

muscle. Bethesda: American Physiological Society, 1980;33–67.

71. Dobrin PB. Mechanical properties of arteries. *Physiol Rev* 1978;58:397–460.

72. Rüegg JA. Smooth muscle tone. *Physiol Rev* 1971;51:201–248.

73. Haddy FJ, Scott JB. Metabolically linked vasoactive chemicals in local regulation of blood flow. *Physiol Rev* 1968;48:688–707.

74. Mellander S, Johansson B. Control of resistance, exchange, and capacitance functions in the peripheral circulation. *Pharmacol Rev* 1968;20:117–196.

75. Sparks HR, Jr. Effect of local metabolic factors. In: Bohr DH, Somlyo AP, Sparks HV, Jr, eds. *Handbook of physiology, section 2, the cardiovascular system, vol. 2, vascular smooth muscle.* Bethesda: American Physiological Society, 1980;475–513.

76. Abel PW, Trapani A, Aprigliano O, Hermsmeyer K. Trophic effect of norepinephrine on the rat portal vein in organ culture. *Circ Res* 1980;47:770–775.

77. Kuschinsky W, Wahl M. Local chemical and neurogenic regulation of cerebral vascular resistance. *Physiol Rev* 1978;58:646–689.

78. Abboud FM. Special characteristics of the cerebral circulation. *Fed Proc* 1981;40:2296–2300.

79. Sokoloff L. Relationships among local functional activity, energy metabolism, and blood flow in the central nervous system. *Fed Proc* 1981;40:2311–2316.

80. Dobson JG, Jr, Rubio R, Berne RM. Role of adenine nucleotides, adenosine, and inorganic phosphate in the regulation of skeletal muscle blood flow. *Circ Res* 1971;29:375–384.

81. Berne R. The role of adenosine in the regulation of coronary blood flow. *Circ Res* 1980; 47:807–813.

82. Johnson PC. The myogenic response. In: Bohr DH, Somlyo AP, Sparks HV, eds. *Handbook of physiology, section 2, the cardiovascular system, vol. 2, vascular smooth muscle.* Bethesda: American Physiological Society, 1980; 409–442.

83. Heistad DD, Busija DW, Marcus ML. Neural effects on cerebral vessels: alteration of pressure-flow relationship. *Fed Proc* 1981;40: 2317–2321.

84. Burnstock G, Gannon B, Iwayama T. Sympathetic innervation of vascular smooth muscle in normal and hypertensive animals. *Circ Res [Suppl II]* 1970;27:5–23.

85. Bevan JA, Purdy RE. Variations in adrenergic innervation and contractile responses to the rabbit saphenous artery. *Circ Res* 1973;32:746–751.

86. Bevan JA, Ljung B. Longitudinal propagation of myogenic activity in rabbit arteries and in the rat portal vein. *Acta Physiol Scand* 1974;90:703–715.

87. Abboud FM. Control of the various components of the peripheral vasculature. *Fed Proc* 1972;31:1226–1239.

88. Mohrman DE, Feigl EO. Competition between

symptathetic vasoconstriction and metabolic vasodilatation in the canine coronary circulation. *Circ Res* 1978;42:79–86.

89. Folkow B, Sonnenschein RR, Wright DL. Loci of neurogenic and metabolic effects on precapillary vessels of skeletal muscle. *Acta Physiol Scand* 1971;81:4459–4471.

90. Abboud FM, Eckstein JW. Comparative changes in segmental vascular resistance in response to nerve stimulation and to norepinephrine. *Circ Res* 1966;18:263–277.

91. Honig CR, Frierson JL, Patterson JL. Comparison of neural controls of resistance and capillary density in resting muscle. *Am J Physiol* 1970;218:937–942.

92. Vanhoutte PM. Heterogeneity of postjunctional vascular α-adrenoceptors and handling of calcium. *J Cardiovasc Pharmacol* 1982;4: S91–S96.

93. Russell MP, Moran NC. Evidence for lack of innervation of β₂-adrenoceptors in the blood vessels of the gracilis muscle of the dog. *Circ Res* 1980;46:344–352.

94. Uvnas B. Cholinergic vasodilator nerves. *Fed Proc* 1966;25:1618–1622.

95. Folkow B, Lisander B, Tuttle RS, Wang SC. Changes in cardiac output upon stimulation of the hypothalamic defense area and the medullary depressor areas in the cat. *Acta Physiol Scand* 1968;72:220–233.

96. Beck L, Pollard AA, Kayaalp SO, Weiner LM. Sustained dilatation elicited by sympathetic nerve stimulation. *Fed Proc* 1966;25:1596–1606.

97. Ballard DR, Abboud FM, Mayer HE. Release of a humoral vasodilator substance during neurogenic vasodilatation. *Am J Physiol* 1970; 219:1451–1457.

98. Rolewicz TF, Zimmerman BG. Peripheral distribution of cutaneous sympathetic vasodilator system. *Am J Physiol* 1972;223:939–944.

99. Weiss HD. The physiology of human penile erection. *Ann Intern Med* 1972;76:763–799.

100. Lee TJ-F, Hume WR, Su C, Bevan JA. Neurogenic vasodilatation of cat cerebral arteries. *Circ Res* 1978;42:535–542.

101. Ryan MJ, Brody MJ. Neurogenic and vascular stores of histamine in the dog. *J Pharmacol Exp Ther* 1972;181:83–91.

102. Keeton TK, Campbell WB. The pharmacologic alteration of renin release. *Pharmacol Rev* 1980;31:81–227.

103. Ganten D, Schelling P, Ganten V. Tissue isorenins. In: Genest J, Koiw E, Kuchel O, eds. *Hypertension: pathology and treatment*. New York: McGraw-Hill, 1977;240–256.

104. Asaad MM, Antonaccio MJ. Vascular wall renin in spontaneous hypertensive rats. Potential relevance to hypertension maintenance and antihypertensive effect of captopril. *Hypertension* 1982;4:487–493.

105. McCubbin JW, Soares deMoura R, Page IH, Olmsted F. Arterial hypertension elicited by subpressor amounts of angiotensin. *Science* 1965;149:1395–1396.

106. Freeman RH, Davis JO. Physiological actions of angiotensin II on the kidney. *Fed Proc* 1979;38:2276–2279.

107. Ploth DW, Navar G. Intrarenal effects of the renin-angiotensin system. *Fed Proc* 1979;38: 2280–2285.

108. Antonaccio MJ, Cushman DW. Drugs inhibiting the renin-angiotensin system. *Fed Proc* 1981;40:2275–2284.

109. Moncada S, Vane JR. Pharmacology and endogenous roles of prostaglandin endoperoxides, thromboxane A₂, and prostacyclin. *Pharmacol Rev* 1979;30:293–331.

110. Moncada S. Biological importance of prostacyclin. *Br J Pharmacol* 1982;76:3–31.

111. Sirois P, Borgeat P. From slow reacting substance of anaphylaxis (SRS-A) to leukotriene D₄ (LTD₄). *Int J Immunopharmacol* 1980; 2:281–293.

112. Michelassi F, Landa L, Hill RD, Lowenstein E, Watkins WD, Petkau AJ, Zapol WM. Leukotriene D₄: a potent coronary artery vasoconstrictor associated with impaired ventricular contraction. *Science* 1982;217:841–843.

113. Gorman RR. Modulation of human platelet function by prostacyclin and thromboxane A₂. *Fed Proc* 1979;328:83–88.

114. Feigen LP. Actions of prostaglandins in peripheral vascular beds. *Fed Proc* 1981;40:1987–1990.

115. Regoli D, Barabé J. Pharmacology of bradykinin and related kinins. *Pharmacol Rev* 1980; 32:1–46.

116. Carretero OA, Scicli AG. Possible roles of kinins in circulatory homeostasis. *Hypertension* [*Suppl II*] 1981;3:I-4–I-12.

117. Bie P. Osmoreceptors, vasopressin, and control of renal water excretion. *Physiol Rev* 1980;60:962–1048.

118. Johnston CI, Newman M, Woods R. Role of vasopressin in cardiovascular homeostasis and hypertension. *Clin Sci* 1981;61:129s–139s.

119. Cowley AW, Switzer SJ, Guinn MM. Evidence and quantification of the vasopressin arterial pressure control system in the dog. *Circ Res* 1980;46:58–67.

120. Gavras H, Hatzinikolaou P, North WG, Bresnahan M, Gavras I. Interaction of the sympathetic nervous system and renin in the maintenance of blood pressure. *Hypertension* 1982;4: 400–405.

121. DiPette DJ, Gavras I, North WG, Brunner HR, Gavras H. Vasopressin in salt induced hypertension of experimental renal insufficiency. *Hypertension* [*Suppl II*] 1982;4:II-125–II-130.

122. VanNeuten JM, Janssen PAJ, deRidder W, Vanhoutte PM. Interactions between 5-hydroxytryptamine and other vasoconstrictor substances in the isolated femoral artery of the rabbit; effect of ketanserin (R41 468). *Eur J Pharmacol* 1982;77:281–287.

123. Chand N, Altura BM. Acetylcholine and bradykinin relax intrapulmonary arteries by acting on endothelial cells: role in lung vascular disease. *Science* 1981;213:1376–1379.

124. Panmani M, Huot S, Buggy J, Clough D, Haddy F. Demonstration of a humoral inhibitor of the Na^+-K^+ pump in some models of experimental hypertension. *Hypertension* [*Suppl II*] 1981;3:II-96–II-101.

125. Gruber KA, Rudel LL, Bullock BC. Increased circulating levels of an endogenous digoxin-like factor in hypertensive monkeys. *Hypertension* 1982;4:348–354.

126. Carmeliet E, Vereeck J. Electrogenesis of the action potential and automaticity. In: Berne RM, ed. *Handbook of physiology, section 2, the cardiovascular system, vol. 1, the heart.* Bethesda: American Physiological Society, 1979; 269–334.

127. Winegrad S. Electromechanical coupling in heart muscle. In: Berne RM, ed. *Handbook of physiology, section 2, the cardiovascular system, vol. 1, the heart.* Bethesda: American Physiological Society, 1979;393–428.

128. Sonnenblick EH, Parmley WW, Urschel CW. The contractile state of the heart as expressed by force-velocity relations. *Am J Cardiol* 1969;23:488–503.

129. Jewell BR. A reexamination of the importance of muscle length on myocardial performance. *Circ Res* 1977;40:221–230.

130. Brady AJ. Mechanical properties of cardiac fibers. In: Berne RM, ed. *Handbook of physiology, section 2, the cardiovascular system, vol. 1, the heart.* Bethesda: American Physiological Society, 1979;461–474.

131. Strobeck JE, Kreuger J, Sonnenblick EH. Load and time considerations in the force-length relation of cardiac muscle. *Fed Proc* 1980;39:175–182.

132. Braunwald E, Ross J, Jr. Control of cardiac performance. In: Berne RM, ed. *Handbook of physiology, section 2, the cardiovascular system, vol. 1, the heart.* Bethesda: American Physiological Society, 1979;533–580.

133. Weber KT, Hawthorne EW. Descriptors and determinants of cardiac shape: an overview. *Fed Proc* 1981;40:2005–2010.

134. Weber KT, Janicki JS. The dynamics of ventricular contraction: force, length, and shortening. *Fed Proc* 1980;39:188–195.

135. Sarnoff SJ, Mitchell JH. The regulation of the performance of the heart. *Am J Med* 1961; 30:747–771.

136. Vatner SF, Monroe RG, McRitchie RJ. Effects of anesthesia, tachycardia, and autonomic blockade on the Anrep effect in intact dogs. *Am J Physiol* 1974;226:1450–1456.

137. Vatner SF, Boettcher DH. Regulation of cardiac output by stroke volume and heart rate in conscious dogs. *Circ Res* 1978;42:557–561.

138. Janicki JS, Weber KT. Factors influencing the diastolic pressure-volume relation of the cardiac ventricles. *Fed Proc* 1980;39:133–140.

139. Rankin JS, Arentzen CE, Ring WS, Edwards CH, II, McHale PA, Anderson RW. The diastolic mechanical properties of the intact left ventricle. *Fed Proc* 1980;39:141–147.

140. Mason DT, Braunwald E, Covell JW, Sonnenblick E, Ross J, Jr. Assessment of cardiac contractility. The relation between the rate of pressure rise and ventricular pressure during isovolumic systole. *Circulation* 1971;44:47–58.

141. Peterson KL, Uther JB, Shabetai R, Braunwald E. Assessment of left ventricular performance in man. Instantaneous tension-velocity-length relations obtained with the aid of an electromagnetic velocity catheter in the ascending aorta. *Circulation* 1973;47:924–935.

142. Mason DT, Spann JF, Jr, Zelis R. Quantification of the contractile state of the intact human heart. Maximal velocity of contractile element shortening determined by the instantaneous relation between the rate of pressure rise and pressure in the left ventricle during isovolumic systole. *Am J Cardiol* 1970;26:248–257.

143. Mitchell JH, Gilmore JP, Sarnoff SJ. The transport function of the atrium. Factors influencing the relation between mean left atrial pressure and left ventricular end diastolic pressure. *Am J Cardiol* 1962;9:237–247.

144. Skinner NS, Jr, Mitchell JH, Wallace AG, Sarnoff SJ. Hemodynamic effects of altering the timing of atrial systole. *Am J Physiol* 1963;205:499–503.

145. Lister JW, Klotz DH, Jomain SL, Stuckey JH, Hoffman BF. Effect of pacemaker site on cardiac output and ventricular activation in dogs with complete heart block. *Am J Cardiol* 1964;14:494–503.

146. Ross J, Jr, Linhart JW, Braunwald E. Effects of changing heart rate in man by electrical stimulation of the right atrium. Studies at rest, during exercise, and with isoproterenol. *Circulation* 1965;32:549–558.

147. Bishop VS, Stone HL, Horwitz LD. Effects of tachycardia and ventricular filling pressure on stroke volume in the conscious dog. *Am J Physiol* 1971;220:436–439.

148. Vatner SF, Higgins CB, Patrick T, Franklin D, Braunwald E. Effects of cardiac depression and of anesthesia on the myocardial action of a cardiac glycoside. *J Clin Invest* 1971;50:2585–2595.

149. Higgins CB, Vatner SF, Braunwald E. Parasympathetic control of the heart. *Pharmacol Rev* 1973;25:119–155.

150. Levy MN, Martin PJ. Neural control of the heart. In: Berne RM, ed. *Handbook of physiology, section 2, the cardiovascular system, vol. 1, the heart.* Bethesda: American Physiological Society, 1979;581–620.

151. Epstein SE, Robinson BF, Kahler RL, Braunwald E. Effects of beta-adrenergic blockade on the cardiac response to maximal and submaximal exercise in man. *J Clin Invest* 1965; 44:1745–1753.

152. Donald DE, Ferguson DA, Milburn SE. Effect of beta-adrenergic receptor blockade on racing performance of greyhounds with normal and with denervated hearts. *Circ Res* 1968;22:127–134.

153. Gibbs CL. Cardiac energetics. *Physiol Rev* 1978;58:174–254.

154. Moir TW. Subendocardial distribution of coronary blood flow and the effect of antianginal drugs. *Circ Res* 1972;30:621–627.

155. Braunwald E. Coronary artery spasm as a cause of myocardial ischemia. *J Lab Clin Med* 1981;97:299–312.

156. Calaresu FR, Faiers AA, Mogenson GJ. Central neural regulation of heart and blood vessels in mammals. *Prog Neurobiol* 1975;5:1–35.

157. Korner PI. Central nervous control of autonomic cardiovascular function. In: Berne RM, ed. *Handbook of physiology, section 2, the cardiovascular system, vol. 1, the heart.* Bethesda: American Physiological Society, 1979; 691–739.

158. Smith OA, Astley CAS, DeVito JL, Stein JM, Walsh KE. Functional analysis of hypothalamic control of the cardiovascular responses accompanying emotional behavior. *Fed Proc* 1980;39:2487–2494.

159. Dampney RAL. Functional organization of central cardiovascular pathways. *Clin Exp Pharmacol Physiol* 1981;8:241–259.

160. Foreman RD, Wurster RD. Localization and functional characteristics of descending sympathetic spinal pathways. *Am J Physiol* 1973; 225:212–217.

161. Gebber GL. Central oscillators responsible for sympathetic nerve discharge. *Am J Physiol* 1980;239:H143–H155.

162. Ross CA, Ruggiero DA, Reis DJ. Afferent projections to cardiovascular portions of the nucleus of the tractus solitarius in the rat. *Brain Res* 1981;223:402–408.

163. Elliott JM. The central noradrenergic control of blood pressure and heart rate. *Clin Exp Physiol Pharmacol* 1979;6:569–579.

164. Chalmers JP, Blessing WW, West MJ, Howe PRC, Costa M, Furness JB. Importance of new catecholamine pathways in control of blood pressure. *Clin Exp Hypertens* 1981;3:396–416.

165. Loewy AD, Neil JJ. The role of descending monoaminergic systems in central control of blood pressure. *Fed Proc* 1981;40:2778–2785.

166. Brody MJ, Haywood JR, Touw KB. Neural mechanisms in hypertension. *Annu Rev Physiol* 1980;42:441–453.

167. Szabadi E. Adrenoceptors on central neurones: microelectrophoretic studies. *Neuropharmacology* 1979;18:831–843.

168. Coote JH, Macleod VH, Fleetwood-Walker S, Gilbey MP. The response of individual sympathetic preganglionic neurones to microelectrophoretically applied endogenous amines. *Brain Res* 1981;215:135–145.

169. Kuhn DM, Wolf WA, Lovenberg W. Review of the role of the central serotonergic neuronal system in blood pressure regulation. *Hypertension* 1980;2:243–255.

170. Franz DN, Madsen PW, Peterson RG, Sangdee C. Functional roles of monoaminergic pathways to sympathetic preganglionic neurons. *Clin Exp Hypertens* 1982;A4:543–562.

171. Phillips MI, Weyhenmeyer J, Felix D, Ganter D, Hoffman WE. Evidence for an endogenous brain renin-angiotensin system. *Fed Proc* 1979; 38:2260–2266.

172. Buccafusco JJ, Brezenoff HE. Pharmacological study of a cholinergic mechanism within the rat posterior hypothalamic nucleus which mediates a hypertensive response. *Brain Res* 1979;165:295–310.

173. Schaz K, Stock G, Simon W, Schlör K-H, Unger T, Rockhold R, Gant D. Enkephalin effects on blood pressure, heart rate, and baroreceptor reflex. *Hypertension* 1980;2:395–407.

174. Persson B. GABAergic mechanisms in blood pressure control. A pharmacologic analysis in the rat. *Acta Physiol Scand [Suppl]* 1980; 491:1–54.

175. Williford DJ, DiMicco JA, Gillis RA. Evidence for the presence of a tonically active forebrain GABA system influencing central sympathetic outflow in the cat. *Neuropharmacology* 1980; 19:245–250.

176. Häusler G, Osterwalder R. Evidence suggesting a transmitter or neuromodulatory role for substance P at the first synapse of the baroreceptor reflex. *Naunyn Schmiedebergs Arch Pharmacol* 1980;314:111–121.

177. Gillis RA, Helke CJ, Hamilton BL, Norman WP, Jacobowitz DM. Evidence that substance P is a transmitter of baro- and chemoreceptor afferents in the nucleus tractus solitarius. *Brain Res* 1980;181:476–481.

178. Reis DJ, Granata AR, Perrone MH, Talman WT. Evidence that glutamic acid is the neurotransmitter of baroreceptor afferents terminating in the nucleus of the tractus solitarius (NTS). *J Auton Nerv Syst* 1981;3:321–334.

179. Farsang C, Ramirez-Gonzales MD, Mucci L, Kunos G. Possible role of an endogenous opiate in the cardiovascular effects of central alpha adrenoceptor stimulation in spontaneously hypertensive rats. *J Pharmacol Exp Ther* 1980;214:203–208.

180. Downing SE. Baroreceptor regulation of the heart. In: Berne RM, ed. *Handbook of physiology, section 2, the cardiovascular system, vol. 1, the heart.* Bethesda: American Physiological Society, 1979;621–652.

181. Brown AM. Receptors under pressure. An update on baroreceptors. *Circ Res* 1980;46:1–10.

182. Paintal AS. Vagal sensory receptors and their reflex effects. *Physiol Rev* 1973;53:159–227.

183. Jones JV, Thorén PN. Characteristics of aortic baroreceptors with non-medulated afferents arising from the aortic arch of rabbits with chronic renovascular hypertension. *Acta Physiol Scand* 1977;101:286–293.

184. Epstein SE, Beiser GD, Goldstein RE, Stampfer M, Wechsler AS, Glick G, Braunwald E. Circulatory effects of electrical stimulation of the carotid sinus nerves in man. *Circulation* 1969;40:269–276.

185. Vatner SF, Higgins CB, Franklin D, Braunwald E. Extent of carotid sinus regulation of the myocardial contractile state in conscious dogs. *J Clin Invest* 1972;51:995–1008.

186. Shoukas AA, Sagawa K. Control of total sys-

temic vascular capacity by the carotid sinus baroreceptor reflex. *Circ Res* 1973;33:22–33.

187. Kezdi P. Resetting of the carotid sinus in experimental renal hypertension. In: Kezdi P, ed. *Baroreceptors and hypertension.* Oxford: Pergamon Press, 1967;301–308.

188. Sapru HN. Prevention and reversal of baroreceptor resetting in the spontaneously hypertensive rat. *Fed Proc* 1974;33:359.

189. Cowley AW, Jr, Liard JF, Guyton AC. Role of the baroreceptor reflex in daily control of arterial blood pressure and other variables in dogs. *Circ Res* 1973;32:564–576.

190. Brown AM. Cardiac reflexes. In: Berne RM, ed. *Handbook of physiology, section 2, the cardiovascular system, vol. 1, the heart.* Bethesda: American Physiological Society, 1979; 677–689.

191. Linden RJ. Function of cardiac receptors. *Circulation* 1973;48:463–480.

192. Vatner SF, Zimpfer M. Bainbridge reflex in conscious, unrestrained, and tranquilized baboons. *Am J Physiol* 1981;240:H164–H167.

193. Thorén PN. Characteristics of left ventricular receptors with nonmedullated vagal afferents in cats. *Circ Res* 1977;40:415–421.

194. Abboud FM, Eckberg DL, Johannsen UJ, Mark AL. Carotid and cardiopulmonary baroreceptor control of splanchnic and forearm vascular resistance during venous pooling in man. *J Physiol* 1979;286:173–184.

195. Biscoe TJ. Carotid body: structure and function. *Physiol Rev* 1971;51:437–495.

196. Coleridge JCG, Coleridge HM. Chemoreflex regulation of the heart. In: Berne RM, ed. *Handbook of physiology, section 2, the cardiovascular system, vol. 1, the heart.* Bethesda: American Physiological Society, 1979;621–652.

197. Hackett JG, Abboud FM, Mark AL, Schmid PG, Heistad DD. Coronary vascular responses to stimulation of chemoreceptors and baroreceptors. Evidence for reflex activation of vagal cholinergic innervation. *Circ Res* 1972;31:17–18.

198. Kaufman MP, Baker DG, Coleridge HM, Coleridge JCG. Stimulation by bradykinin of afferent vagal C-fibers with chemosensitive endings in the heart and aorta of the dog. *Circ Res* 1980;46:476–484.

199. Felder RB, Thames RD. Responses to activation of cardiac sympathetic afferents with epicardial bradykinin. *Am J Physiol* 1982;242: H148–H153.

200. Sato A, Schmidt RF. Somatosympathetic reflexes: afferent fibers, central pathways, discharge characteristics. *Physiol Rev* 1973;53: 916–947.

201. Guyton AC. *Arterial pressure and hypertension.* Philadelphia: W. B. Saunders, 1980.

202. Folkow B. Physiological aspects of primary hypertension. *Physiol Rev* 1982;62:347–504.

203. deChamplain J, Van Amerigen MR. Regulation of blood pressure by sympathetic nerve fibers and adrenal medulla in normotensive and hypertensive rats. *Circ Res* 1972;31:617–628.

Cardiovascular Pharmacology, Third Edition,
edited by Michael Antonaccio.
Raven Press, Ltd., New York © 1990.

Antihypertensive Drugs Interacting with the Sympathetic Nervous System and Its Receptors

P. A. van Zwieten

Departments of Pharmacotherapy and Cardiology, Academic Medical Center, University of Amsterdam, 1105 AZ Amsterdam, The Netherlands

Lowering blood pressure by reducing sympathetic activation of the circulatory system is the most classical approach in the drug treatment of hypertension. An impressive variety of drugs with different mechanisms allows the selective inhibition of sympathetic stimuli in virtually all the different structures of the sympathetic pathways, ranging from the central nervous system to the postsynaptic adrenoceptors at the target organs and all relevant neuronal components between these two extremes. Well-known antihypertensive drugs interacting with the sympathetic nervous system and its receptors are, for instance:

1. centrally acting antihypertensives (e.g., clonidine, guanfacine, and α-methyldopa), which are agonists with respect to central α_2-adrenoceptors predominantly in the brain stem;
2. ganglionic blocking agents (ganglioplegics), such as hexamethonium and trimetaphan;
3. peripheral adrenergic neuron-blocking agents, e.g., guanethidine and bretylium;
4. several *Rauwolfia* alkaloids (e.g., reserpine) (it should be noted that reserpine and related drugs display substantial central hypotensive activity as well);

these drugs cause depletion of norepinephrine stores;
5. antagonists of postsynaptic α- and β-adrenoceptors (α- and β-adrenoceptor antagonists or blockers).

The variety of different mechanisms involved emphasizes our current ability to deliberately influence the sympathetic pathway involved in circulatory control at almost every desired site, as illustrated in Fig. 1.

Apart from these various drugs, which directly interfere with sympathetic control of the circulatory system, several newer groups of drugs, like the calcium antagonists and possibly also the angiotensin-converting enzyme (ACE) inhibitors display a subtle interaction with peripheral α-adrenoceptors and with peripheral sympathetic neurotransmission, which probably contributes to their vasodilator and antihypertensive potency.

The aforementioned various categories of drugs will be dealt with in this chapter. Before discussing the drugs and their modes of action, the current views on the role of the sympathetic nervous system in circulatory regulation and in hypertensive disease are briefly summarized, with an emphasis on the classification and function

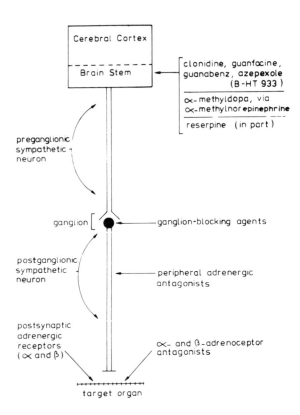

FIG. 1. Schematic representation of the influence of various antihypertensive drugs on the different structures in the central nervous system and the peripheral sympathetic system. Various drugs like clonidine and related agents as well as α-methyldopa and, to some degree, reserpine interfere with the central regulation of blood pressure at the level of the brain stem. The ganglion-blocking agents will interrupt sympathetic transmission at the ganglionic level. Various peripheral adrenergic antagonists, e.g., guanethidine and compounds with a similar pharmacological profile, interrupt sympathetic transmission at the postganglionic level. Various α- and β-adrenoceptor antagonists may lower arterial blood pressure because they diminish the activating influence of the sympathetic nervous system on the circulation.

of α- and β-adrenoceptors, which are particularly important targets of various antihypertensive drugs.

NEURONAL PATHWAYS IN THE SYMPATHETIC NERVOUS SYSTEM AS TARGETS OF ANTIHYPERTENSIVE DRUGS

Central Nervous Pathways

Peripheral sympathetic activity, which directly modulates the circulatory system and hence plays an important role in the regulation of blood pressure, is largely dominated by sympathetic pathways in the central nervous system. The most relevant centers involved in the central regulation of blood pressure are located in the pontomedullary region. As visualized schematically in Fig. 2, the main centers involved are the vasomotor center, the nucleus tractus solitarii, and the nucleus of the vagus nerve. These centers are interconnected and also connected with peripheral pathways and the pathways involved in the carotid sinus occlusion and baro/chemoreceptor reflexes. The connection with the periphery is predominantly subserved by the inhibitory bulbospinal neuron. It seems likely that the influence of higher functions and regions in the brain is mediated by the nucleus of the solitary tract. The brain stem region with the aforementioned centers and their neuronal interconnections contain a high density of adrenergic synapses and corresponding α-adrenoceptors of the α_2-subtype, which are presumed to be the targets of the centrally active antihypertensives, such as clonidine, guanfacine, and α-methyldopa (which acts via its metabolite α-methylnorepinephrine).

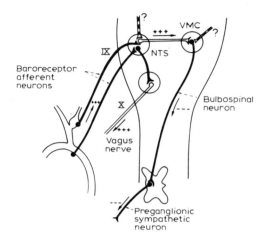

FIG. 2. Schematic representation of the neuronal connections between medullary centers, baroreceptors (aortic arch and carotid sinus), vagus nerve (X), nucleus, and the peripheral sympathetic system. NTS, nucleus tractus solitarii; VMC, vasomotor center; + + +, facilitating neuron; ---, inhibitory neuron; ▬▬▬, neuron where it is unknown whether it is a facilitating or inhibitory connection between the hypothalamic region and NTS/VMC.

Peripheral Sympathetic Ganglia

The sympathetic ganglia are the targets of the by now obsolete class of ganglionic blocking agents. The receptors involved are of the nicotinic cholinergic type. The ganglionic blockers are competitive antagonists of these cholinergic receptors. The same type of receptors is present in the parasympathetic ganglia of the autonomic nervous system. For this reason it is unavoidable that ganglionic blocking agents simultaneously block the cholinergic receptors in the parasympathetic system and hence disrupt ganglionic transmission in this system, with concomitant adverse reactions.

Postganglionic Sympathetic Neurons

Postganglionic neurons in the sympathetic nervous system are also the potential target of antihypertensive drugs, i.e., the adrenergic neuron blockers (guanethidine, bretylium, etc.). These drugs do not act via specific receptors but rather influence impulse propagation at the membrane in a rather unspecific manner (guanethidine) or cause depletion of the intracellular vesicles where norepinephrine, the neurotransmitter, is stored (reserpine, guanethidine) and

hence impair sympathetic neurotransmission.

CLASSIFICATION OF α- AND β-ADRENOCEPTORS: AGONISTS AND ANTAGONISTS

A schematic overview of the postganglionic sympathetic neuron and the corresponding synapse is shown in Fig. 3. Adrenoceptors, at both presynaptic (prejunctional) and postsynaptic (postjunctional) sites, are the main targets of drugs interacting with the sympathetic nervous system. These drugs comprise the α- and β-adrenoceptor antagonists. For these reasons, emphasis in this introduction will be on the postganglionic α- and β-adrenoceptors. In addition, some attention will be paid to central α_2-adrenoceptors, which are the targets of the classic centrally acting antihypertensives, like clonidine, α-methyldopa, and guanfacine. α-Adrenoceptors are located at the level of the membranes of the vesicles or varicosities, i.e., the storage sites of the endogenous neurotransmitter (see Fig. 3). The excitation of the presynaptic α-adrenoceptors by an agonist, either the endogenous neurotransmitter norepinephrine (or epinephrine) or a synthetic α-sympathomimetic drug, inhibits the release of endogenous norepinephrine from the vesicle (1–4).

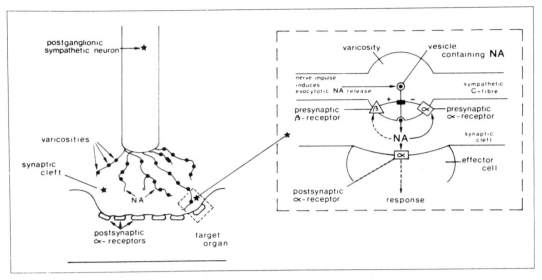

FIG. 3. Adrenergic synapse. Nerve activity releases the endogenous neurotransmitter norepinephrine (NA) and epinephrine from the varicosities. Norepinephrine and epinephrine reach the postsynaptic α- (or β-) adrenoceptors on the cell membrane of the target organ by diffusion. On receptor stimulation, a physiological or pharmacological effect is initiated. Presynaptic α_2-adrenoceptors on the membrane (insert), when activated by endogenous norepinephrine as well as by exogenous agonists, induce an inhibition and block a facilitation of the amount of transmitter norepinephrine released per nerve impulse. Conversely, the stimulation of presynaptic β_2-receptors enhances norepinephrine release from the varicosities. When norepinephrine has been released, it travels through the synaptic cleft and reaches both α- and β-adrenoceptors at postsynaptic sites, thus causing physiological effects such as vasoconstriction or tachycardia.

Accordingly, intrasynaptic norepinephrine inhibits its own release. This process might have a role as a physiological feedback phenomenon, but firm evidence for such a role for the presynaptic adrenoceptors is lacking so far. The concept of pre/postsynaptic receptors has been thoroughly investigated for α-receptors (1–4). In a later stage it has been recognized that β-adrenergic, cholinergic, dopaminergic, and angiotensin II receptors also occur at both pre- and postsynaptic sites. The concept of pre- and postsynaptic receptors was developed mainly by Langer and Starke and co-workers (for relevant reviews, see [1–4]).

More recently the existence of presynaptic β-receptors has been postulated, postsynaptic β-adrenoceptors having been accepted to exist (5) for many years. When stimulated by means of the appropriate agonist, presynaptic β_2-adrenoceptors will trigger an accelerated release of endogenous norepinephrine from presynaptic sites (5). The relevance of this mechanism in physiological regulation processes so far remains unclear.

α_1- and α_2-Adrenoceptors: Agonists and Antagonists

For many years, α-adrenoceptors have been subdivided into the subtypes α_1 and α_2, similar to the subdivision of the β-adrenoceptors. This subdivision is based on the different affinities of either receptor subtype for selective agonists and antagonists. Table 1 shows the most important agonists and antagonists of α_1- and α_2-adrenoceptors. Obviously the endogenous neuro-

TABLE 1. α-*Adrenoceptor agonists and antagonists: characterization with respect to their selectivity for* α_1- *and* α_2-*adrenoceptors*

Agents	Receptor stimulated or blocked
Agonists	
Norepinephrine (neurotransmitter)	$\alpha_1 + \alpha_2 + \beta_1$
Epinephrine (neurotransmitter)	$\alpha_1 + \alpha_2 + \beta_1 + \beta_2$
Methoxamine	α_1
Clonidine (Catapres, Catapresan)	$\alpha_2 > \alpha_1$
Guanfacine	$\alpha_2 > \alpha_1$
Azepexole (B-HT 933)	α_2
B-HT 920	α_2
UK 14,304	α_2
Antagonists	
Phentolamine (Regitine)	$\alpha_1 + \alpha_2$
Tolazoline	$\alpha_2 > \alpha_1$
Prazosin (Minipress)	α_1
Doxazosin	α_1
Terazosin	α_1
Trimazosin	α_1
Labetalol	$\alpha_1 + \beta_1 + \beta_2$
Corynanthine[a]	α_1
Rauwolscine[a]	α_2
Yohimbine	α_2
Idazoxan	α_2

[a]Diastereoisomers.

transmitters norepinephrine and epinephrine are nonselective agonists that stimulate both α_1- and α_2-adrenoceptors about equally well. Methoxamine, cirazoline, and to a lesser degree phenylephrine are prototypes of selective α_1-adrenoceptor stimulants. The experimental agents B-HT 920, B-HT 933 (azepexole), and UK 14,304 are the best examples of highly selective α_2-adrenoceptor agonists. With respect to the antagonistic drugs, the classic compound phentolamine is an example of a nonselective ($\alpha_1 + \alpha_2$)-blocker. The antihypertensive drug prazosin is a selective antagonist of α_1-adrenoceptors at postsynaptic sites as are its successors doxazosin, terazosin, and trimazosin. Rauwolscine and yohimbine, both Rauwolfia alkaloids, and the synthetic compound idazoxan, are examples of selective α_2-adrenoceptor antagonists (for reviews, see [6–10]).

β_1- and β_2-Adrenoceptors: Agonists and Antagonists

Approximately two decades after the subdivision of adrenoceptors into α- and β-subtypes by Ahlquist (11), Lands (12) proposed the subdivision of the β-adrenoceptors into β_1- and β_2-subpopulations. As for the α_1/α_2-adrenoceptors, we can divide these into the selective and mixed (nonselective $\beta_1 + \beta_2$) agonists and antagonists with respect to β_1/β_2-adrenoceptors (Table 2).

However, few selective β_1-adrenoceptor agonists are available. Dobutamine is usually characterized as a selective β_1-adrenoceptor agonist, which is more or less true as far as β-adrenoceptors are concerned. However, it should be realized that dobutamine is simultaneously an active α_1-adrenoceptor agonistic drug (13). Salbutamol and terbutaline are examples of selective β_2-adrenoceptor agonists. Norepinephrine is fairly selective as a β_1-adrenoceptor agonist, in addition to its $\alpha_1 + \alpha_2$-adrenoceptor agonistic activity. Epinephrine is nonselective with respect to both α- and β-adrenoceptors, because it simultaneously activates α_1 and α_2 as well as $\beta_1 + \beta_2$-adrenoceptors. Selective β-adrenoceptor blockers are available for both the β_1- and the β_2-subtypes (Table 2).

Distribution of α_1/α_2- and β_1/β_2-Adrenoceptors at Pre- and Postsynaptic Sites

It should be emphasized that the terms pre/postsynaptic, α_1/α_2, and β_1/β_2 are not necessarily associated. The question of which receptor subtypes are located at pre- and postsynaptic sites is discussed below. Presynaptic α-adrenoceptors are predominantly of the α_2-subtype. However, at postsynaptic sites both α_1- and α_2-adrenoceptors are found, in approximately equal proportions.

Presynaptic β-adrenoceptors are predominantly of the β_2-subtype. The functional

TABLE 2. β-*Adrenoceptor agonists and antagonists: characterization with respect to their selectivity for* β_1- *and* β_2-*adrenoceptors and to ISA*

Agents	Receptors stimulated or blocked	ISA
Agonists		
Norepinephrine (neurotransmitter)	$\beta_1 + \alpha_1 + \alpha_2$	
Epinephrine (neurotransmitter)	$\beta_1 + \beta_2 + \alpha_1 + \alpha_2$	
Dobutamine (racemate)	$\beta_1 > \beta_2 + \alpha_1$	
Prenalterol	β_1 (partial agonist)	
Xamoterol	β_1 (partial agonist)	
Isoproterenol	$\beta_1 + \beta_2$	
Orciprenaline	$\beta_1 + \beta_2$	
Fenoterol	$\beta_2 \gg \beta_1$	
Pirbuterol	$\beta_2 \gg \beta_1$	
Rimiterol	$\beta_2 \gg \beta_1$	
Ritodrine	$\beta_2 \gg \beta_1$	
Salbutamol	$\beta_2 \gg \beta_1$	
Terbutaline	$\beta_2 \gg \beta_1$	
Antagonists		
Propranolol[a]	$\beta_1 + \beta_2$	−
Alprenolol[a]	$\beta_1 + \beta_2$	±
Pindolol[a]	$\beta_1 + \beta_2$	+++
Oxprenolol[a]	$\beta_1 + \beta_2$	++
Timolol[a]	$\beta_1 + \beta_2$	−
Sotalol[a]	$\beta_1 + \beta_2$	−
Practolol	$\beta_1 \gg \beta_2$	+
Atenolol	$\beta_1 \gg \beta_2$	−
Metoprolol	$\beta_1 \gg \beta_2$	−
Acebutolol	$\beta_1 \gg \beta_2$	±
ICI 118,551	$\beta_2 \gg \beta_1$	−

[a]Nonselective.
−, none; ±, weak; +, demonstrable; +++, strong.

role of the various receptor subtypes involved may be summarized as follows:

1. *Presynaptic receptors.* Stimulation of presynaptic α_2-adrenoceptors causes an impaired release of norepinephrine from presynaptic sites; receptor blockade by α_2- or nonselective ($\alpha_1 + \alpha_2$) antagonists causes an enhanced release of the endogenous neurotransmitter. Conversely, the stimulation of presynaptic β_2-adrenoceptors causes an accelerated release of endogenous norepinephrine, whereas the blockade of presynaptic β_2-adrenoceptors by an appropriate antagonist inhibits norepinephrine release from the vesicles (5).

2. *Postsynaptic receptors.* Stimulation of vascular postsynaptic α_1-adrenoceptors causes vasoconstriction, increased peripheral resistance, and a rise in blood pressure. The same principle holds true for the stimulation of postsynaptic α_2-adrenoceptors (14,15). However, it should be realized that the contractile processes are probably rather different in the heart, with mainly α_1-adrenoceptors being present at postjunctional sites (16).

Recently obtained evidence (17,18) suggests that the vascular postsynaptic α_2-adrenoceptor is not under direct neuronal control because of its extrasynaptic position (Fig. 4). This situation is in contrast to that of the postsynaptic α_1-adrenoceptor, which is under direct neuronal control, owing to its position within the synapse. Accordingly, the postsynaptic α_2-adrenoceptor is considered to be noninnervated. As such it should be regarded as a hormone receptor that predominantly responds to circulating catecholamines, in particular epinephrine. The postsynaptic vascular β-receptor is virtually only of the β_2-subtype. Its stimulation by appropriate agonists, including circulating epinephrine, causes a modest degree of vasodilation. Its blockade, conversely, leads to modest vasoconstriction. As discussed for the postsynaptic α_2-adrenocep-

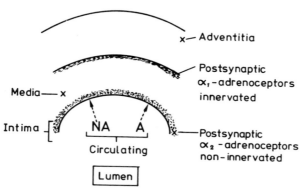

FIG. 4. Differential positions of postsynaptic (postjunctional) α_1- and α_2-adrenoceptors in vascular smooth muscle. The α_1-adrenoceptor is assumed to have an intrasynaptic position and is thus under direct neuronal control. The α_2-adrenoceptor is noninnervated, i.e., not under direct neuronal control, owing to its extrasynaptic position. It is closer to the vascular lumen and hence mainly influenced by circulating norepinephrine and epinephrine. As such, it should be considered a hormone receptor, similar to the noninnervated β_2-adrenoceptors.

tor, the postsynaptic β_2-adrenoceptor is not under direct neuronal control (noninnervated) and thus should be considered instead as a hormone receptor (19).

Distribution of α- and β-Adrenoceptors and Their Subtypes over Different Organs and Tissues

The distribution of α- and β-adrenoceptors and their subtypes (α_1/α_2, β_1/β_2) over

different organs and subtypes is summarized in Table 3. Only well-established data are shown, rather than attempting a complete survey.

Adrenoceptors in the Central Nervous System

Both α- and β-adrenoceptors of the current subtypes (α_1/α_2, β_1/β_2) can be shown to occur in various regions of the central ner-

TABLE 3. *Distribution of postsynaptic α_1/α_2- and β_1/β_2-adrenoceptors over various organs and tissues, and the effect of receptor stimulation and blockade*

Organ/tissue	Receptor	Stimulation causes	Blockade causes
Blood vessels (resistance vessels)	α_1	Constriction	Dilatation
	α_2	Constriction	Dilatation
	β_2	Dilatation	Constriction
Heart	α_1	Contractile force ↑	?
	$\beta_1 > \beta_2$	Heart rate ↑	Bradycardia
		AV conduction ↑	AV conduction ↓
		Contractile force ↑	Contractile force ↓
Spleen	α_1	Contraction	Relaxation
M. sphincter pupillae	α_2	Dilatation	Contraction
Thrombocytes	α_2	Aggregation	—
Adenylcyclase	$\beta_1 + \beta_2$	Hyperglycemia	Hypoglycemia
		Free fatty acid ↑	Free fatty acid ↓
Intestine	$\beta_1 + \beta_2$	Relaxation	—
Bronchi	$\beta_2 > \beta_1$	Relaxation	Constriction
Uterus	β_2	Relaxation	Contraction
Skeletal muscle	β_2	Tremor	Anti-tremor

AV, atrioventricular; ↑, increase; ↓, decrease.

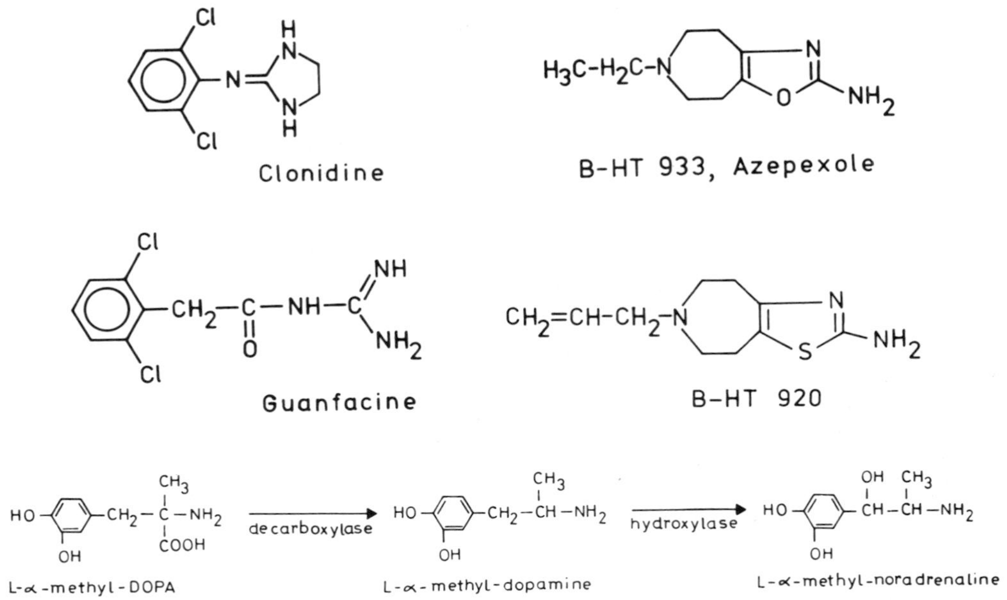

FIG. 5. Top: Chemical structures of various centrally acting hypotensive drugs interfering with central α_2-adrenoceptors. Note the structural dissimilarity between clonidine, an imidazolidine, and similar compounds on the one hand and the newer compounds, azepexole (B-HT 933) and B-HT 920 (which are oxazolo- and thiazolo-azepines, respectively), on the other hand. **Bottom:** L-α-Methyldopa (Aldomet) is converted into α-methyldopamine and then into α-methylnorepinephrine. The conversion takes place in the brain where the required enzymes are available in high concentrations. L-α-Methylnorepinephrine is the active drug that stimulates the central α_2-adrenoceptors.

vous system. The functional role of these receptors remains unknown in detail in many cases and cannot be discussed in the present context.

As discussed previously, the central α_2-adrenoceptors, located in the pontomedullary region, which contain a high density of (nor)adrenergic neurons and synapses. The central α_2-adrenoceptors are the targets of the centrally acting antihypertensives, which are α_2-adrenoceptor agonists. Stimulation of central α_2-adrenoceptors with appropriate agonists activates an inhibitory neuron and hence depresses peripheral sympathetic nervous activity and reduces blood pressure and heart rate (Fig. 5). Central α_1-adrenoceptors are probably functionally associated with the baroreceptor reflex system, as suggested by Huchet et al. (20,21). It seems unlikely that central α_1-adrenoceptors are directly involved in the

proposed but unproven central hypotensive activity of prazosin and related selective α_1-adrenoceptor antagonists (22,23).

CENTRALLY ACTING α_2-ADRENOCEPTOR AGONISTS AS ANTIHYPERTENSIVES

In view of the importance of the central regulation of blood pressure, heart rate, and other possible circulatory parameters, it can readily be imagined that certain drugs may influence the peripheral circulation via a primarily central mechanism. Centrally acting hypotensive drugs have indeed been developed in the course of the past three decades. Their hypotensive action is initiated at the central level, particularly in the pontomedullary region. Interference by centrally acting hypotensive drugs with certain receptors is known to lower blood pressure via the autonomic nervous system. Accordingly, a simultaneous reduction in sympathetic tone and enhanced parasympathetic activity will readily explain the decrease in blood pressure and heart rate induced by centrally acting drugs of this type (for reviews, see [24,25]).

Reserpine was the first drug for which central hypotensive activity was demonstrated convincingly in laboratory animals (26), although its peripheral effect on the adrenergic system in certainly more important as the basis of its antihypertensive potency (27).

Clonidine, guanfacine, and α-methyldopa (Fig. 5) have become and have remained the prototypes of centrally acting antihypertensives (for reviews, see [28–30]). They owe their central hypotensive activity to the stimulation of α_2-adrenoceptors in the pontomedullary region of the brain. These central α-receptors were postulated for the first time by Schmitt (31).

New approaches have been found in the development of experimental compounds that owe their hypotensive potency to their interaction with central cholinergic, dopaminergic, opiate, and possibly also γ-aminobutyric acid (GABA) receptors. So far, however, none of these compounds has ever reached the stage of clinical applicability. Only a few drugs, which owe part of their hypotensive activity to their interaction with central serotonergic receptors are clinically useful as antihypertensives. Examples of such drugs are urapidil (32,33) and ketanserin (34,35), which also have important peripheral pharmacodynamic activities.

Centrally Acting Drugs Interfering with α-Adrenoceptors in the Brain

The vast majority of compounds that lower blood pressure via a primarily central mechanism owe this activity to their interference with central α-adrenoceptors (Fig. 6). Vari-

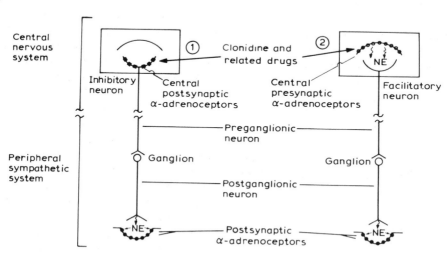

FIG. 6. Schematic representation of the interaction of clonidine (and related drugs) with post- and presynaptic α-adrenoceptors in the brain stem, as the basis of their central hypotensive effect. Two possibilities are shown: Clonidine stimulates central postsynaptic α-adrenoceptors; an inhibitor neuron is activated and the peripheral sympathetic activity is diminished, thus causing a hypotensive effect (1). Clonidine stimulates presynaptic α-adrenoceptors; central norepinephrine (NE) release is diminished, the facilitatory neuron is less activated, and peripheral sympathetic activity is diminished, thus causing a hypotensive effect (2). Mechanism (1) is more likely to be correct.

TABLE 4. *Drugs that lower blood pressure via interference with central α-adrenoceptors in the pontomedullary region*

Clonidine and congeners[a]
Lofexidine[a]
Compound 44549[a]
Guanfacine[a]
Guanabenz[a]
BAY c-6014[a]
Xylazine[a]
Azepexole (B-HT 933)[a]
B-HT 920
Reserpine
α-Methyldopa
Tricyclic antidepressants[b]
Cocaine[b]
Phenothiazine neuroleptics[b]
Monoamine oxidase inhibitors[b]
Amphetamine[b]
L-DOPA[b]
L-Dioxyphenylserine[b]

[a]For details, see Fig. 6 and text.
[b]For details, see ref. 24 and text.

ous drugs that can lower blood pressure due to interference with central α-adrenoceptors are listed in Table 4. Most of these are irrelevant as antihypertensive drugs but are mentioned for theoretical reasons.

From a historical point of view, reserpine was the first hypotensive compound for which a certain degree of acute central hypotensive activity was recognized (26), although its well-established antihypertensive potency is due mainly to peripheral mechanisms. Destruction of norepinephrine-containing vesicles will substantially increase the concentration of this neurotransmitter at the level of central α-adrenoceptors, hence inducing a fall in blood pressure via the mechanism discussed below.

Mode of Action of Centrally Acting α₂-Adrenoceptor Agonists

The concept of α-adrenoceptors as mediators of the hypotensive action of clonidine was proposed by Schmitt (31,36). This concept was based on the following facts:

1. Clonidine is known to activate peripheral α-adrenoceptors. In view of its struc-

tural similarity to naphazoline and related decongestant drugs, this influence of clonidine on peripheral α-adrenoceptors is not surprising.

2. The central hypotensive effect of clonidine is antagonized by yohimbine, piperoxan, and other α-adrenoceptor blocking drugs, which are sufficiently lipophilic to allow brain penetration. The antagonism is dose dependent and competitive in nature.

In this context, clonidine should be considered as the α-receptor agonist and the α-adrenoceptor blocking drug as the antagonist of these receptors (37).

The detailed explanation of the decrease in blood pressure as a result of central α-adrenoceptor excitation remains difficult. In his original concept, Schmitt (31,36) presumed that the excitation of central α-adrenoceptors would activate an inhibitory neuron (possibly the bulbospinal pathway), thus causing a depression of peripheral sympathetic activity and hence a fall in blood pressure and heart rate.

The reduced sympathetic tone has indeed been established in animal experiments (38). However, events at the level of the central α-adrenoceptors and the neuronal pathways between these receptors and the peripheral target organs remain obscure.

An alternative explanation on the basis of a presynaptic effect of clonidine on central α-adrenoceptors may also be considered. The question of whether post- or presynaptic mechanisms are involved in the central hypotensive action of clonidine and related drugs is discussed below. The concept of the central α-adrenoceptors is also the basis of the explanation of the hypotensive effect of α-methyldopa. It has already been argued that a variety of compounds interfering with catecholamine metabolism owe their central hypotensive activity to increases in the concentration of norepinephrine at the level of the central α-adrenoceptors. This type of indirect central hypotensive activity probably holds true for reserpine, monoamine oxidase inhibitors, cocaine, tricyclic antidepressants, tyramine, and possibly other drugs as well (37). The central hypotensive activity of clonidine and related imidazolidines, and also that of the indirectly acting agents discussed above, can be diminished or even abolished by yohimbine, piperoxan, idazoxane, and other α-adrenoceptor blocking agents that can penetrate the brain to a sufficient degree. In this context, clonidine, α-methylnorepinephrine (from α-methyldopa), and endogenous norepinephrine (mediated by the indirectly acting agents discussed above) are the receptor agonists, and the α-adrenoceptor blocking agents become the antagonists, as depicted in Fig. 7.

The central hypotensive activity of clonidine, α-methyldopa, and drugs with a similar action is also inhibited by tricyclic antidepressants and by phenothiazine neuroleptics because of the α-adrenoceptor

blocking potency of these psychotropic agents (39,40).

In spite of the similarity between the modes of action of the various α-adrenoceptor agonists discussed and which have led to the general scheme depicted in Fig. 7, certain subtle differences may still exist between the different types of drugs. It has been demonstrated, for instance, by De Jong (41) that the stereotactic injection of α-methylnorepinephrine (the active component in the effect of α-methyldopa) into the region of the brain stem where the central α-adrenoceptors are located causes a hypotensive effect. However, clonidine injected into the same brain region under identical circumstances has hardly any effect. This observation indicates that there may be a subtle difference between the modes of action of clonidine and α-methyldopa.

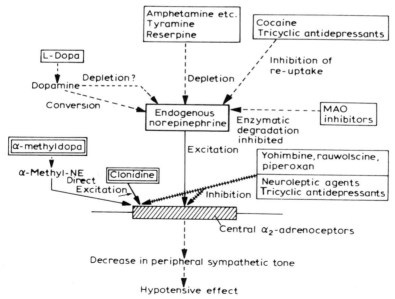

FIG. 7. Influence of various compounds that can excite or inhibit central α₂-adrenoceptors. Excitation is brought about by clonidine, α-methylnorepinephrine (α-methyl-NE) and endogenous norepinephrine. Various compounds can increase the level of norepinephrine by different mechanisms and hence induce α-receptor stimulation. α-Adrenolytic compounds such as yohimbine, phenothiazine, neuroleptic agents, and tricyclic antidepressants inhibit the central adrenoceptors. Consequently, the central hypotensive action of clonidine and related drugs is diminished via a competitive mechanism.

So far, interference between centrally acting hypotensive drugs and corresponding α-adrenoceptors has only been discussed with respect to the blood pressure-lowering effect. However, the hypotensive effect of most of the centrally acting drugs is accompanied by bradycardia. The bradycardia induced by clonidine is a rather complex phenomenon and is probably built up from several different components. At least part of the clonidine-induced bradycardia is mediated by the same central receptors and is due to the same type of mechanism as that involved in the hypotensive action (for reviews, see [28–30]). In addition, clonidine has been shown to enhance vagal reflex bradycardia (42). This effect is also initiated by the stimulation of central α-adrenoceptors by clonidine; it is diminished by pretreatment with a sufficiently lipophilic α-adrenoceptor blocking agent, such as yohimbine, or by phentolamine after intracisternal administration (in order to bypass the blood-brain barrier). Recently, De Jonge et al. (43) have provided evidence that a peripheral presynaptic mechanism also contributes to the bradycardia induced by clonidine in pentobarbitone-anesthetized rats. Accordingly, bradycardia induced by a series of clonidine congeners with considerable differences in lipophilicity, and thus differences in brain penetration, was investigated in bilaterally vagotomized, atropine-treated rats anesthetized with pentobarbitone. The inhibition of sympathetic tone in these animals by imidazolidines can be fully explained by the stimulation of cardiac prejunctional α_2-adrenoceptors as such. However, a centrally induced reinforcement of vagal reflex bradycardia also contributes to the decrease in cardiac frequency induced by clonidine and related drugs.

In spite of a considerable amount of neuropharmacological research, the precise location of the central α-adrenoceptors involved in the hypotensive activity of clonidine and related drugs has not yet been determined. However, it seems likely that these receptors are located in the pontomedullary region. This issue was discussed in the general introduction on α-adrenoceptors. Alternatively, Bousquet and Guertzenstein (44) have proposed the ventral part of the brain stem as the site of action of clonidine and related drugs. However, this conclusion was drawn by topical application of clonidine to that particular area and the fall in blood pressure thus obtained may well be explained by the local anesthetic activity of clonidine. Furthermore, the antihypertensive agent, guanfacine, which is similar to clonidine in every aspect of its central hypotensive action, does not cause a fall in blood pressure when applied topically to this region (45).

In conclusion, the pontomedullary region is the area that can be indicated with certainty as the main region of α-adrenoceptor localization.

Physiologically, this also makes sense in view of the presence of numerous adrenergic and noradrenergic synapses, the vasomotor center, the nucleus tractus solitarii, and the nucleus of the vagus nerve. These centers are interconnected and also connect with peripheral sympathetic pathways and the pathways involved in the carotid sinus occlusion and baroreceptor reflexes, as visualized in the scheme proposed by Chalmers (Fig. 2). It seems conceivable that the α-adrenoceptors required for the effect of centrally acting sympathoinhibitory drugs are integrated in the system of the various nuclei and neural connections. In this system, the nuclei involved should be regarded as an integrated circuit rather than as distinctly separated regions. This concept seems more acceptable than hypothalamic localization of the α-adrenoceptors. Their presence at the ventral surface of the brain stem also seems very unlikely.

At the cellular level the location of the central α-adrenoceptors involved is generally assumed to be at postsynaptic sites, as shown in Fig. 6, although the final evidence for this view is difficult to provide for methodological reasons.

A variety of experimental arguments supports the view that the central α-adrenoceptors that trigger the central hypotensive activity of clonidine, guanfacine, and α-methyldopa belong to the α₂-subtype. Experiments which strongly suggest the involvement of central α₂-adrenoceptors are the following.

Clonidine's central hypotensive activity can be demonstrated on injection into the left vertebral artery of the cat. This effect can be analyzed by means of the three diastereoisomers yohimbine, rauwolscine, and corynanthine, which display the same degree of brain penetration. In a very careful analysis (46) it was demonstrated that the central hypotensive effect of clonidine, obtained after injection of the drug into the cat left vertebral artery, is effectively antagonized by the α₂-adrenoceptor blocking agents yohimbine and rauwolscine injected via the same route prior to clonidine (see Fig. 8). However, corynanthine, the α₁-receptor blocking agent, had little influence on the central hypotensive effect of clonidine. Recent correlation studies are also in agreement with the involvement of α₂-adrenoceptors at the central level (47).

Application of the Hansch model in analysis of quantitative structure-activity relationships has made it possible to establish some of the structural demands of the α-adrenoceptor in the central nervous system, which is assumed to mediate the hypotensive action of clonidine and related imidazolidines. All studies on the quantitative structure-activity relationships in imidazolidines have revealed that lipophilicity is a major determinant of their hypotensive effect (48,49). Lipophilicity will determine the amount of drug penetrating the brain and hence the concentration that interacts with the central α-adrenoceptors. For this reason the lipophilicity of the various drugs studied was quantified and accounted for by multiple regression analysis, which is required for the exploration of quantitative structure-activity relationships by means of the Hansch model. Furthermore, steric and electronic factors were incorporated in the correlation studies. From these studies, a hypothetical working model visualizing the mode of interaction between clonidine-like imidazolidines and the central α-adrenoceptor has emerged (see Fig. 9). It demonstrates the necessity of a very definite substitution pattern at the phenyl ring and other steric requirements. The π-electrons of the phenyl nucleus will interact with the receptor structure's charge transfer. Hydrogen bonding at the bridge nitrogen atom is possible, as is electronic interaction between the imidazolidine nitrogen and the receptor.

Although no doubt remains with respect

Mean arterial pressure (%)

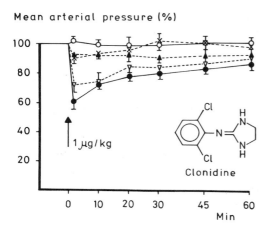

FIG. 8. Comparison of the hypotensive action of clonidine (1 μg/kg) infused intravenously (○) or via the left vertebral artery (●) of anesthetized cats. The central hypotensive effect of clonidine (1 μg/kg) is significantly inhibited by the α₂-adrenoceptor blocking agents, yohimbine (10 μg/kg) (X) or rauwolscine (10 μg/kg) (▲) injected into the left vertebral artery 15 min prior to clonidine (means ± S.E.M.; n=5–8). However, the selective α₁-adrenoceptor antagonist, corynanthine (10 μg/kg) (▽), given via the same route, is ineffective. (Data from ref. 46.)

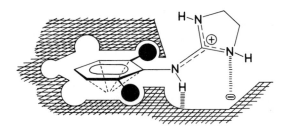

FIG. 9. Hypothetical working model showing the mode of interaction between clonidine-like imidazolidines and the central α-receptor. Note the steric requirements and position of the substituents at the phenyl nucleus (●), the hydrogen bonding between the bridge nitrogen and the receptor, the electrostatic interaction between the imidazolidine moiety and the receptor, and the charge transfer between phenyl ring and receptor. The receptor is represented by the hatched area. (From ref. 24.)

to the functional involvement of central α_2-adrenoceptors in the central hypotensive activity of clonidine and related drugs, a second receptor type has recently been proposed to play an additional role, as proposed by Reis and collaborators (50,51). The rostral portion of the ventrolateral medulla (RVL) has been proposed as a site of action of clonidine in the brain. This region is assumed to contain a novel type of imidazole receptor, which is different from α_2-adrenoceptors. These imidazole receptors appear to mediate the hypotensive effect of clonidine when injected by means of microtechniques into the RVL. Interestingly, an endogenous ligand for this receptor, called clonidine-displacing substance (CDS), has been identified. CDS, a biologically active substance extracted from brain mimics clonidine in the RVL by binding to both imidazole receptors and α_2-adrenoceptors (50,51). If CDS were indeed an endogenous ligand for the imidazole receptor, it might play a relevant role in the central regulation of blood pressure. As yet it cannot be judged whether there exist important links between α_2-adrenoceptors and imidazole receptors.

It seems preferable to consider the α_2-adrenoceptor as the main target of centrally acting drugs of the clonidine-type, whereas the imidazole receptor may be regarded as an auxiliary second target, which might somehow modulate the process triggered by α_2-adrenoceptor stimulation.

Centrally Acting Antihypertensives and Their Application

The clinically useful, centrally acting antihypertensives are limited, as mentioned previously, to the α_2-adrenoceptor agonists, which can achieve sufficiently high concentrations at the level of the central α_2-adrenoceptors. Accordingly, only those drugs will be discussed.

α-Methyldopa is one of the oldest of the centrally acting drugs, although its central mode of action was recognized several years after its introduction in the treatment of hypertension. Its central mechanism is brought about by its active metabolite α-methylnorepinephrine, which is formed *in vivo*. The peripheral false transmitter hypothesis as well as the inhibition of L-DOPA-decarboxylase were proposed in the 1960s as the explanation of the drug's antihypertensive effect, but at present the central mechanism is assumed to offer the most plausible explanation of the drug's antihypertensive effect.

α-Methyldopa causes a fall in blood pressure that is accompanied by a reduction of total peripheral resistance and modest bradycardia (52). Furthermore, an increased venous compliance has been proposed, causing reduced venous return and the maintenance of the cardiopulmonary volume. In spite of the fall in blood pressure caused by α-methyldopa, the glomerular filtration rate remains intact. Renal function is not influenced by treatment with this drug and may even be somewhat improved. α-Methyldopa is therefore understandably useful in the management of hypertension associated with renal impairment. α-Methyldopa is hardly used any more as a routine first-choice drug in the treatment of essential hypertension, although several older patients whose treatment was initiated with α-methyldopa are maintained on the drug, provided that they tolerate it satisfactorily.

α-Methyldopa has hardly any contraindications, and postural hypotension is usually mild or absent. For these reasons, it may still be useful in the elderly.

α-Methyldopa has been widely recommended for the antihypertensive treatment of pregnant women, although at present other drugs can be imagined as well. For reviews on α-methyldopa, see [52–54]).

Clonidine has become the prototype of centrally acting α_2-adrenoceptor agonists. It causes a decrease in mean arterial blood pressure, which is associated with a decrease in heart rate. The total peripheral resistance remains either unchanged or decreases with prolonged treatment. A decreased venous return is also presumed to occur during clonidine treatment. Plasma norepinephrine and plasma renin levels are significantly reduced by clonidine treatment (55,56). Clonidine is an effective and safe drug in the management of essential and less common forms of hypertension. The main drawback is the adverse reactions, which have limited its use in Western Europe. Also, many newer types of effective antihypertensives have been developed that are tolerated much better.

Apart from chronic therapy, acute administration of clonidine has proved effective in hypertensive emergencies. It should be realized, however, that clonidine, when administered intravenously as a bolus injection, causes a transient rise in blood pressure as a result of the stimulation of post-synaptic α-adrenoceptors (probably both α_2 and α_1) in peripheral blood vessels. This peripheral pressor effect does not occur during chronic treatment with clonidine, in which the central hypotensive effect is predominant.

Outside the field of hypertension there is some interest in clonidine in the treatment of hot flashes in menopausal women and as a useful drug in reducing narcotic withdrawal symptoms (heroin, morphine, methadone) in drug addicts (57).

Guanfacine has a mode of action that is identical with that of clonidine, and its hemodynamic pattern is also very similar (58). As a result of its pharmacokinetic profile, its duration of action, however, is longer than that of clonidine, thus allowing once daily administration of the drug in antihypertensive treatment. The slow development of the hypotensive effect and the absence of contraindications for guanfacine make it a potentially useful drug in the treatment of elderly hypertensives. The pattern of side effects is also similar to that of clonidine, but it appears that guanfacine causes less sedation (59). An advantage over clonidine is the virtual absence of a withdrawal syndrome on sudden cessation of treatment.

Guanabenz, lofexidine, tiamenidine, and azepexole (B-HT 933) are newer, centrally acting antihypertensives, which are also α_2-adrenoceptor agonists. No particular advantages over clonidine or guanfacine have been demonstrated for these drugs (60), despite the fact that some of these compounds (e.g., azepexole) are more selective for α_2-adrenoceptors than clonidine.

Rilmenidine (S 3341) is a new clonidine-like α_2-adrenoceptor stimulant with central hypotensive activity (61,62), which has been shown to cause little or no sedation, at least in animal experiments. This apparent dissociation between central hypotensive activity and sedation remains to be substantiated clinically.

Pharmacological Backgrounds of Adverse Reactions

Sedation, drowsiness, and a reduction in salivary flow with complaints of a dry mouth are the most frequently reported side effects for the centrally acting antihypertensives acting via central α_2-adrenoceptors, although there are differences in the intensity and incidence for these adverse reactions between the various drugs. Sexual impotence also occurs rather frequently, but this is only well documented for α-methyldopa and clonidine. Sedation caused by the centrally acting antihypertensives is mostly mediated by central α_2-adrenoceptors, probably located in the cortical region (46,63). The sedation can be antagonized by α_2-blockers like yohimbine and rauwolscine, but much less effectively by an α_1-blocker like corynanthine (46). Because both the central hypotensive activity and sedation are caused by the same type of receptors (α_2), although located in different brain regions, it is logically very difficult to develop α_2-adrenoceptor stimulants with central hypotensive activity that do not cause sedation. As mentioned previously, such a dissociation has been claimed for rilmenidine (S 3341), but as yet the clinical evidence for the absence of a sedative effect is weak. It has been speculated (62) that the absence of sedation in animal experiments may be caused by an unknown stimulatory process that counteracts α_2-receptor-mediated sedation. The reduction in salivary flow and dry mouth caused by clonidine and related drugs is probably mediated by the activation of presynaptic α_2-adrenoceptors at both peripheral and central levels. The stimulation of these presynaptic α_2-receptors by the centrally acting antihypertensives inhibits cholinergic transmission and hence impairs salivary flow (64). Sexual impotence is probably explained by the reduced sympathetic activity caused by the centrally acting antihypertensives.

Apart from these more generally observed adverse reactions to the centrally acting antihypertensives, a few adverse reactions that are more unique to the individual drugs should be mentioned here.

α-Methyldopa may incidentally cause an allergic reaction, reflected by a positive Coombs' antiglobulin test, in particular after at least 6 months of treatment, but hemolytic anemia is rare. Several types of skin rashes have been reported.

Clonidine may cause parotid pain and sometimes mental depression. Bradycardia caused by clonidine was already discussed from a mechanistic point of view. It should be considered as a phenomenon logically associated with its central sympathoinhibitory activity. For reviews on adverse reactions, see (65,66).

The Clonidine Withdrawal Syndrome

Several authors have described withdrawal symptoms after the abrupt cessation of prolonged treatment with clonidine (67–70). This withdrawal syndrome is mainly associated with symptoms suggestive of sympathetic overactivity such as agitation, sweating, headache, facial flushing, and tachycardia. It is mainly observed after interruption of prolonged treatment with rather high doses of clonidine. For ethical reasons, the withdrawal syndrome can hardly be studied in humans, but a suitable animal model is available at present (71,72). Continuous infusion of clonidine (or other drugs to be studied) via subcutaneously implanted ALZET-mini-osmopumps, followed by surgical extirpation of the pumps, allows mimicking of the withdrawal syndrome in conscious rats. After interruption of drug treatment, the withdrawal syndrome is characterized by severe tachycardia and spontaneously occurring, transient rises in blood pressure (upswings). The tachycardia appears to be triggered at the level of the presynaptic α_2-adrenoceptor in the heart, whereas the blood pressure upswings are initiated at the level of the presynaptic adenylate cyclase/α_2-adrenoceptor complex in the central nervous system (73).

Guanfacine, when interrupted after prolonged treatment, causes but a mild or almost no withdrawal syndrome because of its persistence in the organism, at the receptor level (72). Guanfacine, with a much longer half-life of elimination than clonidine, will be present at the receptors involved for a considerable time period, even after abrupt cessation of its administration. α-Methyldopa also causes a mild or no withdrawal syndrome after stopping its treatment. This is not a matter of pharmacokinetics, as mentioned for guanfacine, but rather the result of a protective effect by the β_2-adrenoceptor agonist activity of the active metabolite α-methylnorepinephrine (74), and is probably also partly explained by the depletion of endogenous norepinephrine caused by treatment with α-methyldopa.

Interactions Between Centrally Acting Antihypertensives and Other Drugs

As a general rule, the sedative effect of clonidine and other central α_2-adrenoceptor agonists will be enhanced by all kinds of central nervous depressant drugs (minor tranquilizers, antiepileptic agents, etc.). This phenomenon has been studied in detail in animal experiments but is not well-documented in humans. Tricyclic antidepressants of the imipramine type have been demonstrated to counteract the central hypotensive activity of clonidine and related drugs, both in hypertensive patients and in animal models (39). This relevant, competitive interaction is explained by the α-adrenoceptor antagonistic activity of the central α_2-adrenoceptor agonist, occurring at the level of α_2-adrenoceptors in the brain, which are the targets of the centrally acting antihypertensives. Clonidine as such can be safely combined with β-blockers, but it has been observed in patients and confirmed in animal studies that after abrupt cessation of treatment, the clonidine-withdrawal syndrome is exacerbated by the simultaneous blockade of β_2-adrenoceptors and the concomitant modulation of adenylate cyclase activity and desensitization of the α_2-adrenoceptor (73,75).

GANGLION-BLOCKING AGENTS (GANGLIOPLEGICS)

Ganglion-blocking agents inhibit the transmission across the synapses in both sympathetic and parasympathetic ganglia. Some well-known compounds are tetraethylammonium, hexamethonium, pentolinium, chlorisondamine, trimetaphan, and mecamylamine. Ganglionic blocking agents are competitive antagonists at the level of nicotinic cholinergic receptors in the autonomic ganglia. Because the same receptors and the same neurotransmitter (acetylcholine) are present in both the sympathetic and parasympathetic ganglia, ganglionic blockade in the parasympathetic system by ganglioplegics is unavoidable and the basis of severe adverse reactions. The sympathetic ganglionic blockade explains the fall in blood pressure, total peripheral resistance, and heart rate caused by these drugs. Blood pressure is only slightly decreased in the supine position but may fall severely and rapidly in the upright position. The orthostatic hypotension is the result of venous pooling of blood, in the absence of compensatory reflex vasoconstriction at the venous side of the circulation. The ganglionic blocking agents are effective antihypertensives in particular in the beginning of treatment, but usually tolerance develops when their application is prolonged. Tolerance is caused by a compensatory increase in intravascular volume, which can be counteracted by the simultaneous administration of diuretics.

Adverse reactions are severe. The blockade of sympathetic transmission is the background of the aforementioned severe postural hypotension. Simultaneously occurring parasympathetic ganglionic blockade explains other side effects like obstipation, paralytic ileus, urinary retention, impaired accommodation, and dry mouth. Disturbed sexual functions in men (impotence and/or inhibition of ejaculation) are also commonly observed. The severity and frequency of these side effects as well as the availability of effective antihypertensives that are tolerated much better have made the ganglionic blocking drugs obsolete as therapeutic agents in the management of hypertension. They are only of some interest in fundamental pharmacology and for historical reasons, because they were virtually the first drugs to be introduced for antihypertensive treatment. For reviews on ganglioplegics, see (76,77).

ADRENERGIC NEURON-BLOCKING AGENTS

Adrenergic neuron-blocking agents inhibit the function of sympathetic postganglionic neurons by impairing the release of norepinephrine from the varicosities in response to the conducted nerve impulse (Fig. 1). Accordingly, they suppress the excitability of the adrenergic nerve endings to the action potential. This effect is similar to that whereby these drugs cause local anesthesia. However, it is specific for the adrenergic nerves, because the adrenergic neuron-blocking drugs are taken up by the amine pump (uptake I) and hence accumulate in the neuron. Furthermore, some of them, e.g., guanethidine, also cause depletion of the norepinephrine stores, and this process will contribute to the reduction of sympathetic tone.

Guanethidine is the best-known example of an adrenergic neuron-blocking drug. Other compounds are, for instance, bretylium, debrisoquine, guanacline, and cyclazenine.

The hemodynamic profile of these drugs is similar to that of the ganglionic blockers. Accordingly, total peripheral resistance,

heart rate, and cardiac output are reduced, as a result of diminished sympathetic tone. The blood flow to the renal, splanchnic, cerebral, and other vascular beds is reduced significantly. As with the ganglionic blockers, venous return and compensatory sympathetic regulatory mechanisms are impaired, thus leading to postural hypotension. Tolerance develops, as for the ganglioplegic agents, because of the increase in plasma volume secondary to the retention of sodium and water. Simultaneous treatment with a diuretic may prevent this problem.

In many ways the adverse reactions to the adrenergic neuron-blocking drugs are similar to those of the ganglion blockers: postural hypotension and inhibition of ejaculation as well as an increase in body weight (volume expansion) and, as mentioned previously, tolerance.

In contrast to the ganglionic blocking agents, the adrenergic neuron blockers do not impair parasympathetic neurotransmission. Accordingly, several side effects may occur that are caused by unopposed parasympathetic activity, such as diarrhea and increased gastric secretion.

In summary, the adrenergic neuron blockers are drugs with several unpleasant side effects, and they have lost a great deal of their attraction in the management of hypertension, owing to the development of newer effective antihypertensives that are much better tolerated. For reviews on adrenergic blocking agents, see (78,79).

RESERPINE AND OTHER RAUWOLFIA ALKALOIDS

Several alkaloids from Rauwolfia serpentina were introduced in the drug treatment of hypertension in the 1950s. Reserpine was used most frequently as an antihypertensive. Other compounds are raubasine, rescinnamine, and syrosingopine. Reserpine and related compounds cause the depletion of norepinephrine stores by blocking the uptake system of the amine storage granules. For this effect, only a very small fraction of the administered reserpine is sufficient (80,81). This fraction of reserpine is bound irreversibly to the membranes of the granules. Reserpine causes considerable depletion of brain norepinephrine and somewhat less effectively depletes norepinephrine in the heart, whereas epinephrine from the adrenal stores is also depleted but a lesser extent (82,83), with the exception of the adrenals of the dog, which are very sensitive to reserpine (84). There is no simple relationship between the degree of depletion and the impairment of neuronal activity, but it has been shown that a loss of 75% or more of the norepinephrine stores for more than 4 hr will usually cause severe depression of sympathetic nervous activity. Parasympathetic activity is not impaired by reserpine. The pronounced depletion of brain catecholamine stores by reserpine would suggest that reserpine might also cause hypotension via a central effect. This presumption was confirmed by the experiments by van Zwieten et al. (26), in which very low doses of reserpine, injected into the brain (via the vertebral artery) reduced both blood pressure and central nervous system norepinephrine, without influencing norepinephrine levels in peripheral tissues. The impaired activity of the sympathetic system causes the following hemodynamic effects: reduced vascular resistance and a fall in blood pressure, as well as a modest fall in heart rate (85). Renal flow is moderately diminished. Reserpine has little effect on venous return, and postural hypotension does not appear to be a serious problem.

Reserpine causes several and sometimes most unpleasant side effects. Most of them can be explained on the basis of its mode of action. Unopposed parasympathetic activation causes nasal congestion, enhanced gastric secretion with ulcer formation, and diarrhea. Biochemical changes in the central nervous system mainly cause sedation and mental depression. At high doses, which are not required in antihypertensive treatment, extrapyramidal symptoms may occur, which are caused by the central nervous system depletion of dopamine.

Owing to the development of more specific, effective antihypertensives with fewer side effects, reserpine is used less and less frequently in the management of hypertension. It is still used regularly, usually combined with various other antihypertensives, in general practice in some continental European countries.

The other antihypertensive *Rauwolfia* alkaloids mentioned do not offer any advantage over reserpine. Because of the loss of interest in this type of therapeutics, the pharmacological differences between the various alkaloids are no longer relevant and will not be discussed here. For reviews on reserpine and other *Rauwolfia* alkaloids as antihypertensives, see (86,87).

α-ADRENOCEPTOR ANTAGONISTS (α-BLOCKERS)

Role of α-Adrenoceptors in Hypertensive Disease

To date, a clear and consistent picture regarding the characteristics and density of α-adrenoceptors in human hypertensive disease has not emerged. This limitation is explained so far by methodological shortcomings that do not allow radioligand-binding investigations on α-adrenoceptors in vascular smooth muscle, with virtually all studies being limited to α_2-adrenoceptors on *ex vivo* thrombocytes.

Conflicting results have been reported with respect to the α_2-receptor density in thrombocytes of hypertensives. Various groups reported an increase, others a decrease in α_2-receptor densities on platelets, and a few authors found no change at all (88–90).

In hypertensive subjects, the hyperreactivity that is known to exist in the systemic circulation was also found in the vascular bed of the human forearm. The hyperreactivity proved a general phenomenon for both α_1- and α_2-adrenoceptor-mediated vasoconstriction, as well as for both epinephrine and norepinephrine (91,92). These findings cast doubt on the specificity of the hyperreactivity phenomenon encountered in hypertensive subjects. Whether highly specific or not, the hyperreactivity to vasoconstrictor stimuli in hypertensives appears to be a logical basis for drug treatment with α-adrenoceptor antagonistic drugs.

Antihypertensive Activity of α-Adrenoceptor Blocking Agents: Mode of Action and Hemodynamic Profile

α-Adrenoceptor antagonists cause vasodilation and a fall in blood pressure because the endogenous agonists norepinephrine and epinephrine can no longer reach and stimulate the vascular α-receptor, which is occupied by the antagonist. Nonselective α_1- and α_2-adrenoceptor antagonists like phentolamine cause vasodilation, which is based on the blockade of both α_1- and α_2-adrenoceptors. The application of such drugs is accompanied by marked reflex

tachycardia, triggered by the baroreceptor reflex system and the autonomic nervous system. Owing to presynaptic α_2-receptor blockade, treatment with phentolamine is accompanied by enhanced release of catecholamines from the nerve endings. Probably as a result of reflex sympathetic activation, phentolamine treatment induces the stimulation of the renin-angiotensin-aldosterone system and plasma renin activity is increased, causing the retention of sodium and water. The reflex tachycardia is a serious drawback in the use of nonselective $(\alpha_1 + \alpha_2)$ adrenoceptor blocking agents as antihypertensives. The introduction of the selective α_1-adrenoceptor blocking agent prazosin as an antihypertensive offered much better possibilities for antihypertensive treatment, with reflex tachycardia being virtually absent.

Prazosin and related selective α_1-adrenoceptor antagonists (Fig. 10) owe their antihypertensive activity to the competitive blockade of postsynaptic α_1-adrenoceptors in resistance vessels. It has been suggested that the blockade of central α_1-adrenoceptors plays a role as well, as concluded from the hypotensive activity obtained on stereo-

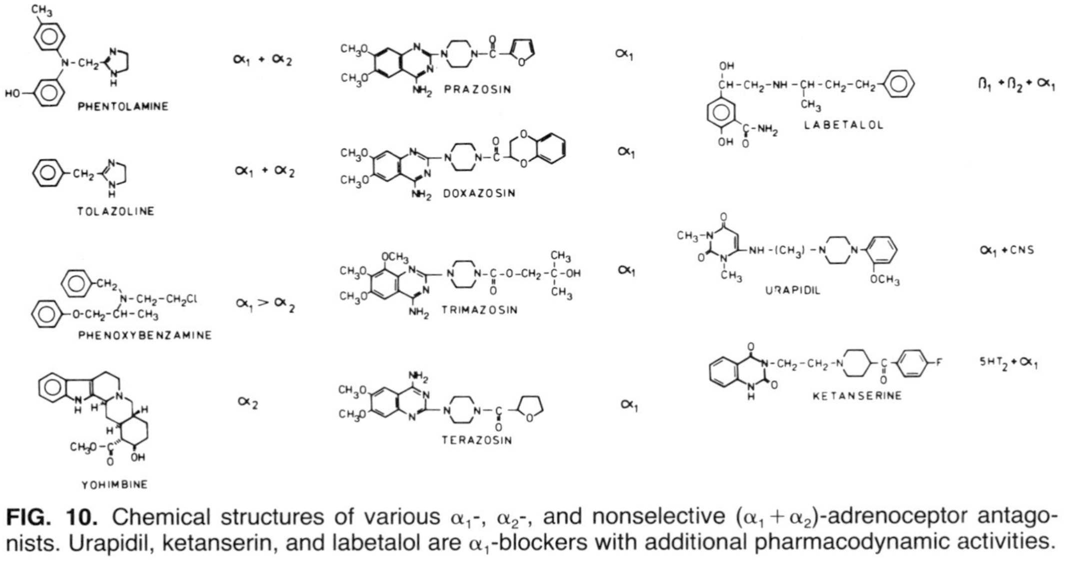

FIG. 10. Chemical structures of various α_1-, α_2-, and nonselective $(\alpha_1 + \alpha_2)$-adrenoceptor antagonists. Urapidil, ketanserin, and labetalol are α_1-blockers with additional pharmacodynamic activities.

tactic injection of prazosin into the nucleus tractus solitarii (93). However, several other groups of investigators using various experimental methods have provided solid evidence against a central hypotensive activity of prazosin (46,94), and it seems best to attribute prazosin's therapeutic efficacy to the blockade of peripheral postsynaptic α_1-adrenoceptors in resistance vessels. Various other mechanisms involved in the hypotensive effect of prazosin and related α_1-antagonists can be ruled out (95,96), for example, interference with peripheral sympathetic ganglia or neurons, inhibition of phosphodiesterase activity, and direct vasodilator activity. The absence of marked reflex stimulation of the heart despite the potent vasodilator activity of prazosin and related compounds may be explained by the two mechanisms: (a) The

first is the absence of norepinephrine release via a presynaptic (α_2) mechanism (cf. Fig. 3), because selective α_1-antagonists do not interfere with the modulating influence of presynaptic α_2-adrenoceptors; conversely, classical, nonselective α-adrenoceptor antagonists with an α_2-component are known to substantially enhance the release of norepinephrine from presynaptic sites. (b) Second, the blockade of central α_1-adrenoceptors by prazosin has been shown by Huchet et al. (20,21) to modulate baroreceptor reflex mechanisms, thus counteracting the reflex tachycardia evoked by peripheral vasodilation. For a schematic presentation of this mechanism, see Fig. 11.

Prazosin causes a relaxation of both resistance and capacitance vessels. The pronounced venous dilatation is understandable in view of the particular dependence of

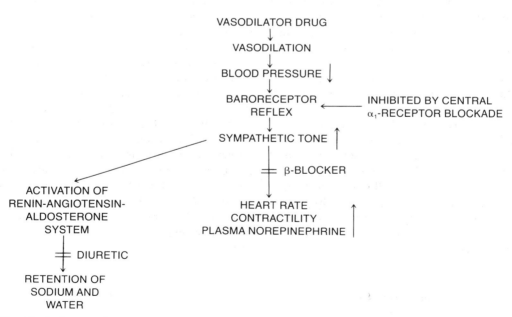

FIG. 11. Reflex mechanisms triggered by vasodilator drugs. Reflex activation of the sympathetic system is mediated by the baroreceptors. The increased sympathetic activity causes an elevation of plasma norepinephrine, a rise in heart rate, and contractility and activation of the renin-angiotensin-aldosterone system. This forms the basis for retention of sodium and water. The rise in cardiac activity is counteracted by a β-blocker. Diuretics (natriuretic agents) prevent the retention of sodium and water. The blockade of central α_1-adrenoceptors by selective α_1-adrenoceptor antagonists (provided that they penetrate the central nervous system) diminish baroreceptor reflex activation.

the veins on sympathetic stimulation (97). The venous dilatation is probably the cause of the "first-dose effect," i.e., the orthostatic hypotension observed after the first dose of prazosin. Prazosin causes a modest dilatation of the renal vascular bed in hypertensive patients that is not associated with an impairment of renal function. However, like most antihypertensives that are vasodilators, prazosin causes modest fluid retention that is counteracted by treatment with diuretic agents.

The successor drugs to prazosin, i.e., trimazosin, doxazosin, and terazosin (Fig. 10) appear to have globally the same mode of action and hemodynamic profile as prazosin. Clinically relevant differences between these drugs and prazosin mainly concern pharmacokinetic characteristics. The three aforementioned successor drugs to prazosin may be briefly characterized as follows.

Trimazosin is somewhat less selective for α_1-adrenoceptors than prazosin. In contrast to prazosin it shows weak direct vasodilator activity, which may contribute to the drug's antihypertensive activity, but to a moderate degree.

Doxazosin is a selective α_1-adrenoceptor antagonist, with a longer duration of action than prazosin.

Terazosin displays the same degree of selectivity for α_1-adrenoceptors as prazosin, but on a molar base its potency is threefold lower. Terazosin has a longer duration of action than prazosin, allowing once daily administration in the treatment of hypertension, and is more hydrophilic. For reviews on selective α_1-adrenoceptor antagonists, see (98–100).

to as the first-dose effect. Headache, dizziness, and occasionally palpitations, as well as fluid retention, are also the reflection of vasodilation caused by prazosin. After cessation of treatment, a withdrawal syndrome is usually not observed. Sexual dysfunction during prazosin treatment is rare and the association with the drug is not convincingly established. Respiratory function remains uninfluenced by prazosin and related drugs. Prazosin has been reported to favorably influence the profile of plasma lipids during long-term treatment of hypertension, with a tendency to improve the ratio HDL/LDL + VLDL, by increasing HDL and reducing the LDL + VLDL fractions (101,102). In some but not all studies prazosin was found to decrease plasma triglyceride levels. Most studies on the influence of prazosin on lipid levels have included only a small number of patients, and larger studies under carefully controlled conditions will be required to definitely establish the usefulness of prazosin as a hypolipidemic agent. Prazosin does not interfere with glucose metabolism and is considered to be safe in the treatment of hypertensives with concomitant diabetes (103).

The successor drugs trimazosin, doxazosin, and terazosin display a pattern of adverse reactions that is very similar to that of prazosin, although much less clinical experience is available than for prazosin. It appears that doxazosin and terazosin cause less postural hypotension than prazosin (104,105). This difference with prazosin may be explained by the slower onset of the hypotensive effects of doxazosin and terazosin.

Adverse Reactions

Adverse reactions to prazosin are directly related to its mode of action and hemodynamic profile. We already mentioned postural hypotension, explained by the venous vascular dilatation and referred

Therapeutic Use

The older α-blockers, such as phentolamine and phenoxybenzamine, are only used in the preoperative phase of pheochromocytoma and during surgery. They are usually combined with a β-blocker in order to normalize heart rate and to prevent the reflex tachycardia caused by these α-adrenoceptor antagonists.

Prazosin's efficacy in mild to severe hypertension has been demonstrated in numerous therapeutic trials, against placebo and in comparison with other drugs. Follow-up studies have shown continued efficacy after 2 to 5 years of treatment. Its efficacy as monotherapy has been shown, but prazosin is frequently combined with a diuretic, a β-blocker, or both. Comparative studies have shown prazosin to be as effective as α-methyldopa, clonidine, hydralazine, atenolol, indoramin, minoxidil, propranolol, and labetalol. Prazosin does not significantly change renal function or cause adverse effects on renal function in hypertensives with renal impairment. The virtual absence of reflex tachycardia was discussed previously. Orthostatic hypotension, probably caused by dilatation of the venous vascular bed, is the basis of the so-called first-dose effect. It can be largely avoided by starting the therapy with a very low dose of 0.5 mg, to be ingested at bed time and followed by a gradual build-up of the dosage schedule. For reviews on prazosin in the treatment of hypertension, see (98–100).

A certain efficacy of prazosin as an unloading drug in the treatment of congestive heart failure has been described, usually in trials with small numbers of patients.

Trimazosin resembles prazosin in many ways, but its onset of action is slower, probably because trimazosin is converted *in vivo* into pharmacologically active metabolites.

Terazosin and doxazosin are also very similar to prazosin, but their duration of action is longer. One daily dose of these drugs is usually sufficient to control blood pressure in hypertensive patients.

Drug interactions and combination with other drugs are usually not a problem in the application of selective α$_1$-adrenoceptor antagonists. Most other types of antihypertensives cause an additive antihypertensive effect when combined with α$_1$-blockers. A diuretic may be required to counteract fluid retention and/or a β-blocker to prevent reflex tachycardia, which is, however, usually modest or absent.

α$_1$-Adrenoceptor Antagonists with Additional Pharmacodynamic Properties

Urapidil, a derivative of uracil (Fig. 10), is a hybrid drug with at least two different modes of action, combined in the same molecule (which has no stereoisomers). It is a selective α$_1$-adrenoceptor antagonist that is less potent on a molar base and also somewhat less selective for α$_1$-receptors than prazosin. In addition, it displays substantial central hypotensive activity that, unlike clonidine and related drugs, is not mediated by central α$_2$-adrenoceptors. A few experimental arguments favor the view that this central mechanism is caused by stimulation of central serotonergic receptors of the 5HT$_{1A}$-subtype, but conclusive evidence for this mechanism is lacking. Urapidil is also a weak β$_1$-adrenoceptor blocker. Its efficacy in the treatment of essential hypertension is well documented and appears to be maintained during prolonged administration. Reflex tachycardia does not occur, and there is rather a tendency to bradycardia. Sedation is the main side effect, usually in the beginning of treatment and less pronounced or absent as the drug is continued. For reviews on urapidil, see (32,33).

Labetalol is a combined α$_1$- and β$_1$+β$_2$-blocker. Because it is more a β- than an α-blocker, its properties will be discussed later. Ketanserin (Fig. 10) is a selective antagonist of 5HT$_2$-serotonergic receptors with additional rather weak α$_1$-adrenoceptor affinity. Its antihypertensive activity is not well understood on a pharmacological basis. This activity cannot be explained by either 5HT$_2$- or α$_1$-adrenoceptor antagonistic activity alone. For reviews, see (34,35,106).

β-ADRENOCEPTOR ANTAGONISTS (β-BLOCKERS)

Role of β-Adrenoceptors in Hypertension

β-Adrenoceptors in the various tissues have been demonstrated to occur at both pre- and postsynaptic sites, and it therefore seemed logical to investigate not only their physiological role, but also their role and changes in hypertensive disease. The role of postjunctional β_1-adrenoceptors in triggering sympathetic activation of the heart is well-known, but it has also been recognized for a few years that β_2-adrenoceptors play a functional role in cardiac activity. This role of β_2-adrenoceptors becomes even more important in chronic congestive heart failure, when down-regulation of β_1- but not β_2-adrenoceptors changes the ratio β_1/β_2 considerably into the direction of the β_2-subtype (107,108). In the vascular system, postjunctional β_2-adrenoceptors are virtually the only two β-receptor subtypes present, but the functional role of these vascular β_2-receptors is rather weak, with their stimulation and blockade causing only weak vasodilator and vasoconstrictor effects, respectively. Most of the available experimental evidence suggests that presynaptic β-adrenoceptors belong to the β_2-subtype, although a few authors maintain that they are β_1 (5). When stimulated, the presynaptic β_2-adrenoceptors enhance the release of norepinephrine from the nerve endings. Because epinephrine, either circulating or released from the nerve endings after prior uptake, appears to be the naturally occurring agonist, it appears doubtful whether the presynaptic β_2-receptors may be considered a true feedback system.

In hypertension, both in animals and humans, a down-regulation of β_2-adrenoceptors has been established in a limited number of studies, mainly by means of ra-

dioligand-binding experiments with lymphocytes. Accordingly, the stimulation of vascular postsynaptic β_2-adrenoceptors appears to cause less vasodilation in hypertensive than in normotensive animals. Down-regulation of myocardial β-adrenoceptors has been demonstrated to occur in hypertensive rats. Such an effect would exacerbate rather than attenuate the elevated blood pressure. Accordingly, changes in vasodilator, postsynaptic β_2-receptors are more likely to be associated with development and maintenance of hypertension than to be the sequelae of the elevated pressure.

Stimulation of prejunctional β_2-adrenoceptors facilitates sympathetic transmission, and the "epinephrine hypothesis" in hypertension is based on this mechanism. The involvement of presynaptic β_2-adrenoceptors in the development of hypertension appears to be an attractive principle, which is, however, as yet not supported by sufficient experimental evidence. For a review on this subject, see (5).

In summary, the role of β-adrenoceptors in hypertensive disease is as such unclear and does not offer a logical basis for antihypertensive treatment.

Antihypertensive Activity of β-Adrenoceptor Blocking Agents

Mode of Action

β-Adrenoceptor blockers (for structures, see Fig. 12) were initially introduced as therapeutics in the management of some types of arrhythmia and angina pectoris. In both cases their beneficial activity is readily explained pharmacologically. The antihypertensive efficacy of β-blockers was demonstrated convincingly in patients by Prichard and Gillam in 1969 (109), and since then, these drugs have been used on a very large scale in the management of essential hypertension. Despite their very well-documented and widespread application as antihypertensive therapeutics, the

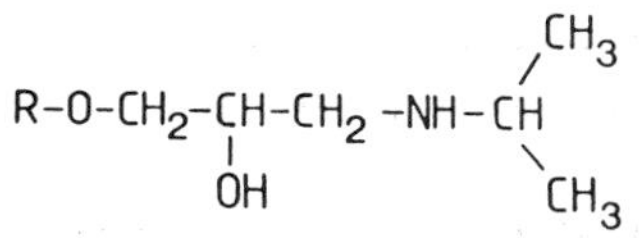

$$R-O-CH_2-CH-CH_2-NH-CH\begin{smallmatrix}CH_3\\\\CH_3\end{smallmatrix}$$

OH

β-adrenoceptor antagonist
(β-blocker)

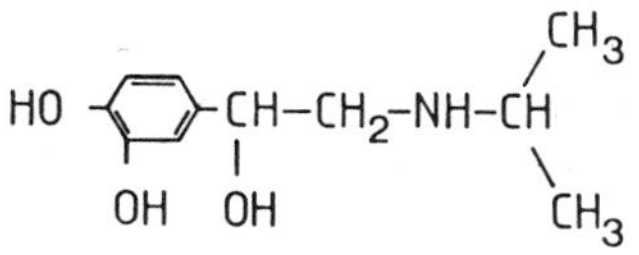

$$HO-\bigcirc-CH-CH_2-NH-CH\begin{smallmatrix}CH_3\\\\CH_3\end{smallmatrix}$$

OH OH

isoproterenol

FIG. 12. Basic chemical structure of β-adrenoceptor antagonists (β-blockers). Note the similarity to the $(\beta_1+\beta_2)$-adrenoceptor agonist isoproterenol. Virtually all β-blockers available at present contain an ether structure connecting the side chain, which is also characteristic of several β-adrenoceptor agonists (like isoproterenol) with the substituent R, which is an aromatic and/or heterocyclic nucleus. Only for the β-blocker sotalol is this situation different in this sense, in that the same side chain is directly connected with the substituent R, not involving an ether bond.

pharmacological explanation of their therapeutic potency remains unsatisfactory. The following hypotheses have been put forward to explain the antihypertensive activity of β-adrenoceptor antagonists.

1. A reduction in cardiac output. This explanation may hold for short-term treatment, but probably not for prolonged treatment, in which some β-blockers also cause a reduction in total peripheral resistance without greatly changing cardiac output. The cardiac output hypothesis certainly does not hold for the β-blockers with partial agonist activity (intrinsic sympathomimetic activity [ISA]).

2. Lowering of plasma renin. Most, but not all, β-blockers cause a reduction in plasma renin activity via β-receptor blockade, which has been proposed as an explanation for the hypotensive activity of these compounds (110). However, there are many experimental arguments that disagree with this hypothesis, for instance, the observation that β-blockers with ISA, such as pindolol, lower elevated blood pressure without influencing plasma renin activity at all (111).

3. Central hypotensive activity. Certain animal experiments in which β-blockers were injected into the brain by means of various techniques would favor a central hypotensive effect of these drugs, but many reports disagree with this presumption (for reviews, see [112,113]).

In human pharmacological experiments, β-blockers tend to increase plasma norepinephrine levels (as a measure of sympathetic activity) instead of lowering these levels, as would be expected for a centrally acting antihypertensive drug. A further argument against a central mechanism as an explanation for the antihypertensive activity is the observation that all β-blockers studied so far can cause a comparable degree of blood pressure lowering, irrespective of their ability to penetrate the brain. Accordingly, hydrophilic β-blockers like atenolol or sotalol, which hardly penetrate the brain, are as effective in the treatment of hypertension as lipophilic drugs such as propranolol.

4. A presynaptic mechanism has been proposed as an explanation for the antihypertensive activity of β-blockers. Since the weight of experimental evidence favors the β_2-character of the presynaptic β-receptor, this would imply that presynaptic β-receptor blockade, which may be expected to reduce presynaptic norepinephrine release, should cause a fall in plasma norepinephrine levels, which in reality does not occur (see above). A further problem with this hypothesis is the observation that selective β_1-blockers are effective antihypertensives, although they cannot be expected to antagonize presynaptic β_2-receptors. Furthermore, the selective β_2-adrenoceptor antagonist ICI 118,551 only attenuates the development of hypertension in young spon-

taneously hypertensive rats but does not appear to have a hypotensive effect in adult animals (5,114).

In summary, none of the various hypotheses proposed to explain the antihypertensive activity of β-blockers can be satisfactorily reconciled with the experimental findings. Although β-blockers have been used for many years and on a very large scale in the management of essential hypertension, their mode of action in this condition remains unknown. For reviews, see (5,112,113,115).

Hemodynamic Profile

The changes in hemodynamic profile caused by the various types of β-blockers are somewhat different, and some of these differences may be clinically relevant. Therefore, the hemodynamic properties of the β-blockers with and without ISA will be discussed separately. The background of the various categories of β-blocking drugs is largely determined by ancillary properties, like β₁-selectivity and ISA, which will be discussed.

Nonselective Blockers Without ISA

Propranolol is the typical example of this category of β-blockers. When injected intravenously, heart rate decreases as does the stroke volume, but to a lesser extent. Cardiac output is decreased and total peripheral resistance increases, but blood pressure remains almost unaltered. This hemodynamic profile after acute administration appears to be similar for all other nonselective β-blockers devoid of ISA investigated so far. The hemodynamic pattern established in steady state during long-term treatment of essential hypertension is rather different. As a result of the as yet unexplained readjustment mechanisms, total peripheral resistance and blood pressure

are lowered, whereas heart rate and cardiac output remain reduced, as in the acute experiments.

A similar hemodynamic profile as described for the nonselective blockers is generally observed for the selective β₁-blockers, but the readjustment of the total peripheral resistance seems to be more rapid with atenolol (β₁-selective) than with propranolol (β₁ + β₂).

Plasma volume and venous return are reduced by propranolol and probably also by other β-blockers. The reduction in plasma volume appears to be unrelated to the lowering of cardiac output. It may be important to prevent tolerance of the hypotensive activity in long-term treatment. The reduced venous return is explained by unopposed α₁-adrenoceptor stimulation, which will cause venoconstriction.

β-Blockers with ISA

The hemodynamic profile of the β-blockers with ISA differs from that of the β-blockers devoid of this property, in particular with respect to total peripheral resistance, which is adjusted more rapidly and to lower values, indicating a certain degree of vasodilator activity of these compounds. This vasodilator potency could be clearly demonstrated in plethysmographic experiments in the vascular bed of the human forearm (116). For reviews on the hemodynamic properties of the β-blockers, see (117,118).

Heart rate is much less depressed by β-blockers with ISA (pindolol, oxprenolol) than by those without this property, and in many patients treated with antihypertensive doses of pindolol, heart rate remains unchanged. Cardiac output remains reduced during treatment with ISA β-blockers, although usually somewhat less than during the administration of the non-ISA blockers.

Exercise does not greatly affect the hemodynamic properties of the various types of β-blockers. In general, the chronic depression of cardiac output is well tolerated, although in the kidneys, liver, and skeletal muscle, a reduction in blood flow is usually observed.

Ancillary Properties of Various Drugs

The competitive blockade of β_1-adrenoceptors appears to be the determinant and common mechanism of the antihypertensive activity of all β-blockers developed. Previously, the somewhat vague and uncertain role of presynaptic β_2-adrenoceptors was alluded to. Several β-blockers display ancillary pharmacodynamic properties in addition to their β_1-adrenoceptor antagonistic potency. The most important of these ancillary properties and their potential clinical consequences will now be discussed.

β_1-Receptor Selectivity

Several β-blockers are much more potent inhibitors of β_1- than β_2-receptor-mediated effects, although at sufficiently high doses this selectivity for β_1-receptors is lost and β_2-receptor blockade will then occur as well. A small difference in hemodynamic profile between selective (β_1) and nonselective ($\beta_1 + \beta_2$)-adrenoceptor blocking agents was discussed previously. The term β_1-*selective* is preferable to *cardioselective,* which would implicate any occurrence of noncardiac effects.

β_1-Selectivity is mainly relevant with respect to the incidence and severity of side effects, which are initiated by the blockade of β_2-receptors. Accordingly, bronchoconstriction, peripheral vasoconstriction causing cold extremities, and metabolic effects like hypoglycemia should be expected to occur less readily during treatment with selective β_1-blockers (119). Atenolol, metoprolol, and acebutolol are well-known examples of selective β_1-blockers. The newer compound bisoprolol (120) is assumed to be the most selective β_1-adrenoceptor antagonist developed so far.

Partial Agonism: ISA

β-Blockers with partial agonistic or ISA cause the same degree of β-receptor blockade as the compounds devoid of ISA, which implies that the accessibility of the β-receptors to endogenous catecholamines is reduced to the same degree by both categories of β-blockers. However, those with ISA cause a modest stimulation of the β-receptor as a result of their molecular structure, and as such they are partial agonists. The difference in hemodynamic profile between β-blockers with and without ISA was already discussed, with an emphasis on the modest vasodilator potency of ISA β-blockers. This vasodilator potency is the result of ISA toward β_2-adrenoceptors. The β_1-receptor ISA is reflected in the observation that heart rate at rest is reduced very little or not at all by β-blockers with ISA. When sympathetic drive is high, for instance, during exercise but also in conditions of heart failure, the β-blockers with ISA act as pure antagonists and hence cause the same reduction in heart rate and cardiac output as induced by the compounds devoid of ISA. β-Blockers with ISA may display, at least potentially, the following clinical advantages over the compounds devoid of this activity. There are fewer complaints of cold extremities, owing to the vasodilator component (β_2-ISA) and less bradycardia at rest (β_1-ISA). ISA insufficiently protects against β-blocker-induced bronchoconstriction. Furthermore, the modest increase in plasma lipids caused by β-blockers appears to be less pronounced or absent in compounds with ISA. For a review of β-blockers with ISA, see (121).

Membrane-stabilizing ("Quinidine-like") Activity

Several β-blockers (see Table 5) have been demonstrated to possess membrane-stabilizing activity. This appears to be a rather nonspecific effect causing reduced

TABLE 5. *Various β-adrenoceptor blocking agents and their differentiation with respect to β₁-selectivity, membrane stabilization, and ISA*

Drugs	β_1-Selectivity	Membrane stabilization	ISA
Acebutolol	$\beta_1 > \beta_2$	−	+
Alprenolol	$\beta_1 + \beta_2{}^a$	±	+
Atenolol	$\beta_1 \gg \beta_2{}^b$	−	−
Betaxolol	$\beta_1 \gg \beta_2$	±	−
Bopindolol	$\beta_1 + \beta_2$	−	+
Metoprolol	$\beta_1 \gg \beta_2$	−	−
Metipranolol	$\beta_1 + \beta_2$	−	−
Oxprenolol	$\beta_1 + \beta_2$	±	++
Penbutolol	$\beta_1 + \beta_2$	±	+
Pindolol	$\beta_1 + \beta_2$	−	+++
Practolol	$\beta_1 \gg \beta_2$	−	++
Propranolol	$\beta_1 + \beta_2$	+	−
Sotalol	$\beta_1 + \beta_2$	−	−
Timolol	$\beta_1 + \beta_2$	−	−

$^a\beta_1 + \beta_2$, a nonselective compound.
$^b\beta_1 \gg \beta_2$, β_1-selectivity.

membrane permeability for various ions (Na^+, K^+, Ca^{2+}), also called quinidine-like activity, which in fact is the same as that caused by various local anesthetics. However, this activity is only demonstrable in animal experiments and at dosages and concentrations that are considerably higher than those required to obtain an antihypertensive effect in human hypertensives. In addition, it has been found that the D-isomer of propranolol, which displays membrane-stabilizing activity but is devoid of β-receptor antagonistic potency, does not lower elevated blood pressure, in neither hypertensive subjects nor spontaneously hypertensive rats (122,123). Taken together, membrane-stabilizing activity is clinically irrelevant, with respect to both antihypertensive activity and adverse reactions.

Pharmacokinetic Differences

The various β-blockers have rather differential pharmacokinetic properties that have been studied in full detail (for review, see [124]). We shall only briefly mention here those differences that are clinically relevant. Globally, β-blockers can be differentiated from a pharmacokinetic point of view on the basis of their renal or hepatic clearance. The more water-soluble β-blockers, such as atenolol or sotalol, are predominantly eliminated via the kidney and have a rather long duration of action. Their elimination and duration of action are somewhat prolonged in patients with renal insufficiency. Conversely, lipid-soluble drugs like propranolol and alprenolol are subject to hepatic biotransformation and their duration of action is relatively short. Esmolol (125), an ester that is rapidly hydrolyzed in both the liver and circulating blood, has an extremely short action, which allows its acute application, for instance, when required in general anesthesia, but the drug is, of course, unsuitable as an antihypertensive. Once daily administration is an important, favorable feature of a β-blocker when applied as an antihypertensive drug, thus improving patient compliance. Table 5 gives a survey of several β-blockers and their different properties as discussed here.

Adverse Reactions

Most of the adverse reactions of the various β-blockers can be readily understood and even predicted on the basis of their β₁- or β₂-antagonistic activities. The blockade of β₁-adrenoceptors underlies the following adverse reactions: bradycardia, impaired atrioventricular (AV) conduction, and a reduction in cardiac output. At rest these effects, especially the bradycardia, are less pronounced for β-blockers with ISA, but during vigorous exercise, when sympathetic nervous activity and plasma norepinephrine levels are high, little or no difference remains between the β-blockers with and without ISA.

Vasoconstriction in the extremities (126) is a common and frequently reported adverse reaction to β-blockers, as reflected by patients complaining of cold hands and feet, particularly in the cold season. This adverse reaction is explained by the blockade of vascular β_2-adrenoceptors causing unopposed α_1-adrenoceptor stimulation and concomitant vasoconstriction. Accordingly, this adverse reaction is much more common for the non-selective $\beta_1 + \beta_2$-adrenoceptor blockers, as a result of their β_2-component, than for the selective β_1-adrenoceptor antagonists. The vasoconstriction in the vascular beds is also the reason that β-blockers, in particular the non-selective agents, should be avoided in patients with peripheral vascular disease, including both Raynaud's phenomenon and atherosclerotic disorders (claudication).

Pressor responses to β-adrenoceptor blocking drugs have been reported incidentally for various types of β-blockers, irrespective of ancillary properties like β_1-selectivity, ISA, or membrane stabilization (127). This rare phenomenon is difficult to explain, particularly because ancillary properties do not give any clue. Fluid retention might be a possible explanation, but the evidence for this view is inconclusive.

Muscular fatigue usually occurs at the beginning of treatment with a β-blocker, more so with the $\beta_1 + \beta_2$-nonselective than with the selective compounds. Various explanations have been offered for this harmless but unpleasant adverse reaction: a reduction in cardiac output during exercise, impaired release of lactic acid from muscular tissues, and the reduction of blood glucose during exercise (β_2 effect).

Respiratory side effects of β-blockers are predominantly the result of β_2-receptor blockade in the airways, although the role of β_1-adrenoceptors cannot be fully dismissed. There is certainly a quantitative difference between the β_1-selective and the nonselective drugs in this respect, but the β_1-selective blockers can also be harmful in asthmatic patients. This phenomenon is explained by the observation that the bronchi contain, besides the well-known majority of β_2-adrenoceptors, a significant number of functional β_1-receptors. The increase in airway resistance by β-blocker treatment is the reason that these drugs, including the β_1-selective compounds, are contraindicated in patients suffering from obstructive airways diseases.

Central nervous system side effects with β-blockers are common, in particular at the beginning of treatment. Sleep disturbances, increased dreaming and tiredness may occur. Hallucinations, vivid dreams, and depression have been reported incidentally. The pharmacological basis of these central nervous system side effects is unclear. It appears that the more hydrophilic compounds like atenolol and sotalol, which do not or hardly penetrate the brain, induce this type of adverse reaction less frequently than lipophilic drugs such as propranolol (128).

The lipid pattern has been reported to be unfavorably influenced by long-term β-blocker treatment, but the effect is moderate and probably reversible on prolonged administration of the drugs (129). A few reports suggest that β-blockers with ISA do not or hardly change plasma lipids (130).

Blood glucose is lowered as a result of β_2-receptor blockade, although this effect is usually modest (131). For this reason, the application of selective β_1-adrenoceptor blockers appears to be preferable in diabetic patients.

Various skin reactions, reflecting allergic phenomena, have been reported with β-blockers. The incidence of these reactions, however, is rare and not related to β-receptor blockade as such. Retroperitoneal fibrosis, sclerosing peritonitis, and severe skin reactions are reasons that practolol was taken from the market, but this severe syndrome, which is unrelated to β-receptor blockade, has fortunately been limited to the use of practolol and not any other β-blockers.

Withdrawal Syndrome

Sudden cessation of long-term β-blocker treatment is particularly relevant in patients with myocardial ischemia, in which the incidence of ischemic events may increase in the withdrawal phase (132). In antihypertensive treatment with β-blockers, such problems have not been described after abrupt withdrawal of the drugs, although gradual reduction of the dosage appears to be wise when β-blocker treatment is to end.

Interactions with Other Drugs

Impaired AV conduction by β-blockers is enhanced by verapamil and possibly also by diltiazem. The effect is additive because the lowered AV conduction is caused by different mechanisms.

The sympathetic hyperactivity caused by abrupt withdrawal of clonidine, following prolonged treatment, appears to be exacerbated by β-blockers (75). This interaction is probably explained by the blockade of vascular β2-adrenoceptors, thus causing enhanced vasoconstriction on stimulation of vascular α-adrenoceptors by circulating catecholamines.

On a pharmacokinetic basis, the following interaction may occur between β-blockers, which are metabolized substantially in the liver, and other drugs. The blood levels of these β-blockers are elevated significantly during concomitant treatment with, for example, cimetidine (which inhibits enzymatic degradation of the β-blockers).

Conversely, β-blocker treatment, which reduces cardiac output, will also reduce liver perfusion and hence impairs the metabolic degradation of lidocaine. For reviews on drug interactions with β-blockers, see (133,134).

Therapeutic Use in Hypertension

Since Prichard's demonstration in 1969 (109) that β-blockers are effective antihypertensives, these drugs have achieved and maintained an important position in the management of hypertension. The β-blockers are effective in various types of hypertension but most frequently used in essential hypertension, the most common form of hypertension.

The response to β-blockers cannot be predicted from cardiac output or plasma renin levels, as was originally believed, nor can it be maintained that the elderly hypertensives respond less to β-blocker treatment than younger adults. Whereas the response in elderly hypertensives is probably similar (122,124), it should be realized that β-blockers will cause more frequent and more serious adverse reactions in elderly patients, who therefore have more contraindications to these drugs than younger subjects.

β-Blockers, as discussed previously, may cause several adverse reactions. Most of these side effects can be predicted and, if necessary, avoided by careful selection of patients.

β-Blockers can be and are used as monotherapy and can be readily combined with diuretics and various types of vasodilators, including calcium antagonists and ACE inhibitors. No strict guidelines can be given with respect to the choice of β-blocker in individual patients. When given in appropriate doses, all β-blockers so far introduced cause a similar antihypertensive effect, and the same probably holds for the responder rate, although the latter issue has not been studied in detail yet.

Differences in adverse reactions, as discussed, are not impressive, although the ancillary properties cause some marginal variations. From a practical point of view, the choice of a β-blocker for an individual patient may be determined by the following principles:

1. A compound that has been used successfully and safely for a long time in many patients is preferable to a new compound (unless the latter offers obvious advantages).
2. Patient compliance is improved by using compounds that can be administered once daily.
3. Ancillary properties may offer certain advantages in particular cases. For instance, a diabetic patient should be treated preferably with a β_1-selective blocker; patients with a low heart rate should receive a β-blocker with ISA.

The cardioprotection that has been presumed to occur as a result of β-receptor blockade remains limited to the secondary prevention following a myocardial infarction (135,136). The various large-scale trials with β-blockers and other drugs in hypertension have not revealed any protective activity against coronary events; in other words, primary prevention is not achieved by β-blocker treatment (137,138).

β-Adrenoceptor Antagonists with Additional Antihypertensive Properties

During the past few years, several β-blockers have been developed that possess one or more additional pharmacodynamic properties that cause a lowering of blood pressure besides their β-adrenoceptor blocking potency. Except for labetalol, clinical experience with these drugs is very limited, and only mention of the pharmacodynamic backgrounds of these drugs, as summarized in Table 6, will be made here.

Most of the additional pharmacodynamic properties aim at lowering of total peripheral resistance, as a result of arteriolar vasodilation. This vasodilator effect can be achieved in various ways, such as

TABLE 6. *Examples of β-blockers with additional pharmacological properties*

Compound	Properties
Labetalol	$(\beta_1 + \beta_2)$-blocker + α_1-blocker
Celiprolol	β_1-blocker + vasodilator
Bevantolol	β_1-blocker + vasodilator
Dilevalol	β_1-blocker + β_2-agonist
BWA 575 C	β-blocker + ACE inhibitor

α-adrenoceptor blockade, β_2-adrenoceptor stimulation, direct vasodilator activity, or ACE inhibition. Because β-receptor blockade tends to increase total peripheral resistance (although it may be slightly reduced after long-term treatment), it seems useful to reduce this parameter, which is invariably elevated in patients with established hypertension. Conversely, β-receptor blockade will prevent any reflex tachycardia elicited by peripheral vasodilation.

Labetalol was the first example of this type of drug. It is a nonselective $(\beta_1 + \beta_2)$-blocker with additional, much weaker α_1-adrenoceptor activity. The α-adrenoceptor antagonism becomes manifest on acute intravenous administration and at the beginning of long-term treatment, as reflected by postural hypotension. The α-adrenoceptor effect appears to wear off in the course of prolonged treatment. In steady state, labetalol is probably very similar to other β-blockers that have no α-adrenoceptor blocking potency. Apart from the aforementioned postural hypotension at the beginning of treatment, the adverse reactions to labetalol are similar to those of the classic β-blockers, as discussed earlier. It should be realized that labetalol is a mixture of four stereoisomers. The β-blockade is contained in one stereoisomer, the α_1-adrenoceptor antagonism in a second stereoisomer, and the other two stereoisomers are pharmacodynamically inactive. Accordingly, labetalol is not a "true" hybrid drug and should instead be considered as a combination of different compounds. For a review on labetalol, see (139).

Because the various newer β-blockers with additional pharmacodynamic properties have hardly been studied clinically, they are only listed in Table 6.

CALCIUM ANTAGONISTS

Calcium antagonists are becoming more and more appreciated as effective antihypertensives, apart from their important application in angina pectoris and other cardiological disorders. They owe their antihypertensive activity to arteriolar vasodilation, induced by the selective blockade of specific calcium channels in the sarcolemma of arterial vascular smooth muscle. In addition, a second mechanism may contribute to the vasodilator potency of these drugs. Because this second mechanism involves the sympathetic nervous system, it is only briefly mentioned here. Accordingly, this mechanism may be summarized as follows. The stimulation of vascular α-adenoceptors by appropriate agonists, including endogenous catecholamines, triggers the transmembranous influx of extracellular calcium ions and hence contributes to the activation of contractile proteins. Calcium antagonists block this calcium influx and hence cause vascular relaxation and a fall in blood pressure. This interaction between calcium antagonists and α-adrenoceptors invariably occurs with α_2-adrenoceptors. Under certain conditions, this interaction also occurs with α_1-adrenoceptors. The subtle interaction with α-adrenoceptors was studied extensively in various animal models (for reviews, see [140–142]), and it could also

be demonstrated to occur in human hypertensives (143). For a schematic presentation, see Fig. 13.

ACE INHIBITORS

The vasoconstrictor effect of angiotensin II, although predominantly mediated by angiotensin-II receptors, also involves a complex interaction with the sympathetic nervous system. The following mechanisms may play a role: tyramine-like activity, i.e., the mobilization of endogenous norepinephrine from presynaptic sites; sensitization of vascular postsynaptic α-adrenoceptors; blockade of the neuronal reuptake of norepinephrine; prejunctional facilitation of sympathetic (adrenergic) neurotransmission in vascular smooth muscle by the enhancement of the amount of norepinephrine released per nerve impulse. The first three mechanisms are rather insensitive and not particularly specific. However, a prejunctional facilitation of sympathetic neurotransmission in vascular smooth muscle by angiotensin II has been demonstrated by Zimmerman et al. (144) and by Lokhandwala et al. (145). Recent experiments with captopril have confirmed that angiotensin II may facilitate sympathetic neurotransmission via a presynaptic mechanism, which may occur at very low levels of circulating angiotensin II. Accordingly, angiotensin II stimulates presynaptic angiotensin-II receptors and hence enhances the release of endogenous norepinephrine from the nerve endings, thereby facilitating sympathetic neurotransmission. Conversely, treatment

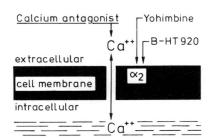

FIG. 13. Schematic presentation of the hypothesis by which calcium antagonists cause a reduction of α_2-adrenoceptor stimulation-induced vasoconstriction. The formation of the α_2-adrenoceptor-agonist complex is accompanied by an influx of extracellular calcium ions, which is inhibited by calcium antagonists.

with an ACE inhibitor such as captopril or enalapril will reduce the concentration of angiotensin II (by inhibiting the conversion of angiotensin I into angiotensin II) and hence depress the aforementioned angiotensin-II-induced facilitation of sympathetic neurotransmission. Accordingly, it may well be that part of the therapeutic efficacy of ACE inhibitors (as vasodilators in the treatment of hypertension and congestive heart failure) is owing to such a mechanism. For reviews on this subject, see (146,147).

REFERENCES

1. Langer SZ. Presynaptic regulation of the release of catecholamines. *Pharmacol Rev* 1981;32: 337–362.
2. Starke K. α-Adrenoceptor classification. *Rev Physiol Biochem Pharmacol* 1981;88:199–236.
3. Starke K. Presynaptic receptors. *Annu Rev Pharmacol Toxicol* 1981;21:7–30.
4. Timmermans PBMWM, van Zwieten PA. The postsynaptic α_2-adrenoceptor. *J Auton Pharmacol* 1981;1:171–183.
4a. Chalmers JP. Brain amines and models of experimental hypertension. *Circ Res* 1975; 36:469–472.
5. Borkowski KR. Pre- and postjunctional β-adrenoceptor and hypertension. *J Auton Pharmacol* 1988;8:153–171.
6. Berthelsen S, Pettinger WA. A functional base for classification of α-adrenergic receptors. *Life Sci* 1977;21:595–606.
7. van Zwieten PA, Timmermans PBMWM. Cardiovascular α_2-adrenoceptors. *J Mol Cell Cardiol* 1983;15:717–733.
8. van Zwieten PA. Receptors involved in the regulation of vascular tone. *Arzneimittelforschung* 1985;35:1904–1909.
9. Timmermans PBMWM, van Zwieten PA. α_2-Adrenoceptors: classification, location, mechanisms and targets for drugs. *Med Chem* 1982;25:1389–1401.
10. van Zwieten PA, Timmermans PBMWM, van Brummelen P. Role of alpha-adrenoceptors in hypertension and in antihypertensive treatment. *Am J Med* 1984;77:17–25.
11. Ahlquist RP. A study of the adrenotropic receptors. *Am J Physiol* 1948;153:586–600.
12. Lands AMK, Arnold A, McAuliff JP, Lunduena FP, Brown RG. Differentiation of receptor systems activated by sympathomimetic amines. *Nature* 1967;214:597–598.
13. Kenakin TP. An in vitro quantitative analysis of the α-adrenoceptor partial agonist activity of dobutamine and its relevance to inotropic selectivity. *J Pharmacol Exp Ther* 1981;216: 210–219.
14. van Zwieten PA, Timmermans PBMWM. Cardiovascular α_2-adrenoceptors. *J Mol Cell Cardiol* 1983;15:717–733.
15. van Zwieten PA, Timmermans PBMWM. Central and peripheral α-adrenoceptors. Pharmacological aspects and clinical potential. *Adv Drug Res* 1984;13:209–254.
16. Wilffert B. Adrenoceptors in the heart. *Prog Pharmacol* 1986;6:47–64.
17. Langer SZ, Massingham R, Shepperson N. Presence of postsynaptic α_2-adrenoceptors of predominantly extrasynaptic location in the vascular smooth muscle of the dog hind limb. *Clin Sci* 1980;59:225S–228S.
18. Wilffert B, Timmermans PBMWM, van Zwieten PA. Extrasynaptic location of α_2- and non-innervated β_2-adrenoceptors in the vascular system of the pithed normotensive rat. *J Pharmacol Exp Ther* 1982;221:762–768.
19. Hawthorn MH, Broadley K. Evidence from use of neuronal uptake inhibition that β_1-adrenoceptors, but not β_2-adrenoceptors, are innervated. *J Pharm Pharmacol* 1982;34:664–666.
20. Huchet AM, Doursout M, Ostermann G, Chelly J, Schmitt H. Possible role of α_1- and α_2-adrenoceptors in the modulation of the sympathetic component of the baroreflex. *Neuropharmacology* 1983;22:1243–1248.
21. Huchet AM, Velly J, Schmitt H. Role of α_1- and α_2-adrenoceptors in the modulation of the baroreflex vagal bradycardia. *Eur J Pharmacol* 1981;71:455–461.
22. Timmermans PBMWM, van Zwieten PA. The interaction between prazosin and clonidine at α-adrenoceptors in rats and cats. *Eur J Pharmacol* 979;55:57–61.
23. Laubie M, Schmitt H. Prazosin produces a sustained and reflex-mediated increase in renal sympathetic nerve activity in anesthetized dogs. *Eur J Pharmacol* 1988;151:75–82.
24. van Zwieten PA. Antihypertensive drugs with a central action. *Prog Pharmacol* 1975;1:1–63.
25. Kobinger W. Drugs as tools in research on adrenoceptors. *Naunyn Schmiedeberg's Arch Pharmacol* 1986;332:113–123.
26. van Zwieten PA, Bernheimer H, Hornykiewicz O. Zentrale Wirkungen des Reserpins auf die Kreislaufreflexe des Carotinussinus. *Naunyn Schmiedebergs Arch Exp Pathol Pharmak* 1966; 253:310–318.
27. Boura ALA, Green AF. Reserpine. In: van Zwieten PA, ed. *Handbook of hypertension, vol 3.* Elsevier, Amsterdam, 1984;220–227.
28. Kobinger W. Central alpha-adrenergic systems as targets for hypotensive drugs. *Rev Physiol Biochem Pharmacol* 1978;81:39–75.
29. van Zwieten PA, Thoolen MJMC, Timmermans PBMWM. The hypotensive activity and side-effects of methyldopa, clonidine and guanfacine. *Hypertension* 1984;6(suppl II):1128–1133.
30. Timmermans PBMWM. Centrally acting hypotensive drugs. In: Van Zwieten PA, ed. *Handbook of hypertension, vol 3.* Elsevier, Amsterdam, 1984;102–153.
31. Schmitt H. Actions des alpha-sympathomimé-

tiques sur les structures nerveuses. *Actual Pharmacologiques* 1971;24:93–131.

32. Amery A, ed. Treatment of hypertension with urapidil. Preclinical and clinical update. *R Soc Med Serv* 1986;101:1–186.

33. van Zwieten PA, de Jonge A, Wilffert B, Timmermans PBMWM, Thoolen MJMC. Cardiovascular effects and interaction with adrenergic receptors of urapidil. *Arch Int Pharmacodyn Ther* 1985;276:180–201.

34. Mylecharane EJ, Philips CA, Markus JK, Shaw J. Evidence for a central component to the hypotensive action of ketanserin in the dog. *J Cardiovasc Pharmacol* 1985;7(suppl 7):S114–S116.

35. van Zwieten PA, Mathy M-J, Boddeke HWGM, Doods HN. Central hypotensive activity of ketanserin in cats. *J Cardiovasc Pharmacol* 1987;10(suppl 3):S54–S58.

36. Schmitt H. The pharmacology of clonidine and related products. *Handbook Pharmacol* 1977;39:212–216.

37. van Zwieten PA, Thoolen MJMC, Timmermans PBMWM. The pharmacology of centrally acting antihypertensive drugs. *Br J Clin Pharmacol* 1983;15:455S–462S.

38. Schmitt H, Schmitt H, Fénard S. Action of α-adrenergic blocking drugs on the sympathetic centres and their interactions with the central sympathoinhibitory effect of clonidine. *Arzneimittelforschung* 1973;23:40–43.

39. van Zwieten PA. Reduction of the hypotensive effect of clonidine and α-methyldopa by various psychotropic drugs. *Clin Sci Mol Med* 1976;51:411–414.

40. van Zwieten PA. The interaction between clonidine and various neuroleptic agents and some benzodiazepine tranquillizers. *J Pharm Pharmacol* 1977;29:229–232.

41. de Jong W. A central noradrenergic inhibitory mechanism on blood pressure and heart rate in the nucleus tractus solitarii of the rat medulla. In: *Abstracts, 15th Dutch Federative Meeting.* Nijmegen, 219.

42. Kobinger W, Walland A. Modulating effect of central adrenergic neurones on a vagally mediated cardio-inhibitory reflex. *Eur J Pharmacol* 1973;22:344–350.

43. de Jonge A, Santing PN, Timmermans PBMWM, van Zwieten PA. Functional role of cardiac presynaptic α_2-adrenoceptors in the bradycardia of α-adrenoceptor agonists in pentobarbitone- and urethane-anesthetized rats. *J Auton Pharmacol* 1982;2:87–91.

44. Bousquet P, Guertzenstein PG. Localization of the central cardiovascular action of clonidine. *Br J Pharmacol* 1973;49:573–577.

45. Scholtysik G, Lauener H, Eichenbergen E. Pharmacological actions of the antihypertensive agent N-amidino-2-(2,6-dichlorophenyl-) acetamide-hydrochloride (BS 100-141). *Arzneimittelforschung* 1975;25:1483–1486.

46. Timmermans PBMWM, Schoop AMC, Kwa HY, van Zwieten PA. Characterization of α-adrenoceptors participating in the central hypotensive and sedative effects of clonidine, us-

ing yohimbine, rauwolscine and corynanthine. *Eur J Pharmacol* 1981;70:7–11.

47. Timmermans PBMWM, van Zwieten PA. Quantitative structure-activity relationships in centrally acting imidazolidines, structurally related to clonidine. *J Med Chem* 1977;20:1636–1639.

48. Hoefke W. Centrally acting antihypertensive agents. *Am Chem Soc Symp Series* 1976;27:28–35.

49. Timmermans PBMWM, Hoefke W, Staehle H, van Zwieten PA. Structure-activity relationship in clonidine-like imidazolidines and related compounds. *Prog Pharmacol* 1980;3(1):1–115.

50. Ernsberger P, Meeley MP, Reis DJ. An endogenous substance with clonidine-like properties: selective binding to imidazole sites in the ventral medulla. *Brain Res* 1988;441:309–318.

51. Atlas D, Diamant S, Fales HM, Pannell L. The brain's own clonidine: purification and characterization of endogenous clonidine displacing substance from brain. *J Cardiovasc Pharmacol* 1987;10(suppl 12):S122–S127.

52. Safar ME, London GM, Levenson JA. Effect of α-methyldopa on cardiac output in hypertension. *Clin Pharmacol Ther* 1979;25:266–270.

53. Reid JL, Elliott HL. Methyldopa. In: Doyle AE, ed. *Handbook of Hypertension, vol 5.* Elsevier, Amsterdam, 1984;92–112.

54. McMahon FG. Methyldopa. In: *Management of hypertension*, p. 252. Futura, Mount Kisco, NY, 252.

55. Wing LMH, Reid JL, Hamilton CA. Effects of clonidine on biochemical indices of sympathetic function and plasma renin activity in normotensive man. *Clin Sci Mol Med* 1977;53:45–48.

56. Pettinger WA, Keeton TK, Campbell WB, Harper DC. Evidence for a renal α-adrenergic receptor inhibiting renin release. *Circ Res* 1976;38:338–342.

57. Washton AM, Resnich RB. Clonidine for opiate detoxification: outpatient clinical trials. *Am J Psychiatry* 1980;137:1121–1124.

58. Mann S, Millar Craig MW, Melville DI. An ambulatory trial of guanfacine. *Br J Clin Pharmacol* 1980;10:103S–106S.

59. Jerie P. Clinical experience with guanfacine in long-term treatment of hypertension. *Br J Clin Pharmacol* 1980;10(suppl 1):375–379.

60. Reid JL, Zamboulis C, Hamilton CA. Guanfacine: effects of long-term treatment and withdrawal. *Br J Clin Pharmacol* 1980;10:183S–188S.

61. Dollery CT, Safar ME. A symposium: rilmenidine, a novel alpha$_2$-agonist antihypertensive agent. *Am J Cardiol* 1988;61(suppl D):1D–103D.

62. van Zwieten PA, Thoolen MJMC, Jonkman FAM, Wilffert B, de Jonge A, Timmermans PBMWM. Central and peripheral effects of S3341 [(N-dicyclopropylmethyl)-amino-oxazoline] in animal models. *Arch Int Pharmacodyn* 1986;279:130–149.

63. Delbarre B, Schmitt H. A further attempt to characterize sedative receptors activated by clonidine in chickens and mice. *Eur J Pharmacol* 1973;22:355–360.

64. Green GJ, Wilson H, Yates MS. The mechanism of the clonidine-induced reduction in peripheral parasympathetic submaxillary salivation. *Eur J Pharmacol* 1979;56:331–334.
65. Dollery CT, Davies DS, Draffan GH. Clinical pharmacology and pharmacokinetics of clonidine. *Clin Pharmacol Ther* 1976;19:11–15.
66. Jarrott B. Clonidine and related compounds. In: Doyle AE, ed. *Handbook of hypertension, vol 5*. Elsevier, Amsterdam, 1984;113–168.
67. Hökfelt B, Hedeland H, Dymling J. Studies on catecholamines, renin and aldosterone following Catapresan® (2-(2,6-dichlorphenylamine)-2-imidazolidine hydrochloride) in hypertensive patients. *Eur J Pharmacol* 1970;10:389–397.
68. Hansson L, Hunyor SH, Julius S, Hoobler SW. Blood pressure crisis following withdrawal of clonidine, with special reference to arterial and urinary catecholamine levels and suggestion for acute management. *Am Heart J* 1973;85:605–608.
69. Chrysant SG, Whitsett TL. Withdrawal of antihypertensive therapy. *JAMA* 1978;239:2241–2243.
70. Weber MA. Blood pressure rebound following withdrawal of antihypertensive therapy. *JAMA* 1978;239:833.
71. Thoolen MJMC, Timmermans PBMWM, van Zwieten PA. Discontinuation syndrome after continuous infusion of clonidine in spontaneously hypertensive rats. *Life Sci* 1981;28:232–235.
72. Thoolen MJMC, Timmermans PBMWM, van Zwieten PA. Cardiovascular effects of withdrawal of some centrally acting antihypertensive drugs in rats. *Br J Clin Pharmacol* 1983;15:491S–505S.
73. Jonkman FAM, Man PW, Thoolen MJMC, van Zwieten PA. Location of the mechanism of the clonidine withdrawal tachycardia in rats. *J Pharm Pharmacol* 1985;37:580–582.
74. Thoolen MJMC, Hendriks JCA, Timmermans PBMWM, van Zwieten PA. Continuous infusion and withdrawal of methyldopa in the spontaneously hypertensive rat. *J Cardiovasc Pharmacol* 1983;5:221–223.
75. Saarima S. Combination of clonidine and sotalol in hypertension. *Br Med J* 1976;I:810–812.
76. Green AF. Antihypertensive drugs. *Adv Pharmacol* 1962;I:161–192.
77. Boura ALA, Green AF. Depressants of peripheral sympathetic function. In: van Zwieten PA, ed. *Handbook of hypertension, vol 3*. Elsevier, Amsterdam, 1984;194–238.
78. Maxwell RA. Guanethidine after twenty years: a pharmacologist's perspective. *Br J Clin Pharmacol* 1982;13:35–39.
79. Maxwell RA, Wastila WB. Adrenergic neuron blocking drugs. In: Gross F, ed. *Handbook of experimental pharmacology, vol 39, antihypertensive agents*. Springer-Verlag, Berlin-Heidelberg-New York, 1977;161.
80. Carlsson A, Rosengren E, Bertler A, Nilsson J. Effect of reserpine on the metabolism of catecholamines. In: Garattini V, ed. *Psychotropic Drugs*. Elsevier, Amsterdam, 1957;363.
81. Muscholl E, Vogt M. The action of reserpine on the peripheral sympathetic system. *J Physiol (Lond)* 1958;141:132–138.
82. Shore PA, Giachetti A. Reserpine: basic and clinical pharmacology. In: Iversen LL, Ivensen SD, Snyder SH, eds. *Handbook of psychopharmacology*. Plenum Press, New York-London, 1977;197.
83. de Schaepdrijver AF. Hypertensive responses in reserpinized dogs. *Arch Int Pharmacodyn* 1960;124:45–52.
84. Shore PA. Release of serotonine and catecholamines by drugs. *Pharmacol Rev* 1962;14:531–549.
85. Kisin I, Yushakov S. Effects of reserpine, guanethidine and methyldopa on cardiac output and its distribution. *Eur J Pharmacol* 1976;35:253–258.
86. Carlsson A. Pharmacological depletion of catecholamine stores. *Pharmacol Rev* 1966;18:541–563.
87. von Euler S. Synthesis, uptake and storage of catecholamines in adrenergic nerves, the effect of drugs. In: Blaschko H, Muscholl E, eds. *Handbook of experimental pharmacology, vol. 33, catecholamines*. Springer-Verlag, Berlin-New York, 1972;186.
88. Brodde OE. Density and affinity of α-adrenoceptors in normal subjects and hypertensive patients. In: Hayduk K, Bock KD, eds. *Proceedings of clonidine workshop Essen 1982*. Steinkopff-Verlag, Darmstadt, 1983.
89. Brodde OE, Daul A, O'Hara N, Bock KD. Increased density and responsiveness of α_2- and β_2-adrenoceptors in circulating blood cells of essential hypertensive patients. *J Hypertens* 1984;2(suppl 3):111–114.
90. Motulsky HJ, O'Connor DT, Insch PA. Platelet α_2-adrenergic receptors in treated and untreated essential hypertension. *Clin Sci* 1983;64:265–272.
91. Amann FW, Bolli P, Kiowski W, Buhler FR. Enhanced α-adrenoceptor-mediated vasoconstriction in essential hypertension. *Hypertension* 1981;3(suppl 1):119–123.
92. van Zwieten PA, Jie K, van Brummelen P. Postsynaptic α_1- and α_2-adrenoceptor changes in hypertension. *J Cardiovasc Pharmacol* 1987;10(suppl 4):S68–S75.
93. Kubo T, Kihara M, Hata H, Misu Y. Cardiovascular effects in rats of alpha 1 and alpha 2 adrenergic agents injected into the nucleus tractus solitarii. *Naunyn Schmiedebergs Arch Pharmacol* 1987;335:274–279.
94. Gillis R, Dretchen K, Namath I, et al. Hypotensive effect of urapidil: CNS-site and relative contribution. *J Cardiovasc Pharmacol* 1987;9:103–108.
95. Cambridge D, Davey MJ, Greengrass PM. The pharmacology of antihypertensive drugs with special reference to vasodilators, α-adrenergic blocking agents and prazosin. *Prog Pharmacol* 1980;3:107.
96. Constantine JW, McShane WK, Scriabine A, Hess HJ. Analysis of the hypotensive action of prazosin. In: Onesti G, Kim KE, Moyer

JH, eds. *Hypertension: mechanisms and management.* Grune and Stratton, New York, 1973:429.

97. Robinson BF. Drugs acting directly on vascular smooth muscle: circulatory and secondary effects. *Br J Pharmacol* 1981;12:5S.

98. Brogden RN, Heel RC, Speight TM, Avery GS. Prazosin: a review of its pharmacological properties and therapeutic efficacy in hypertension. *Drugs* 1977;14:163–197.

99. Cavero I, Roach AG. The pharmacology of prazosin, a novel antihypertensive agent. *Life Sci* 1980;27:1525–1533.

100. Graham RM, Pettinger WA. Prazosin. *N Engl J Med* 1979;300:232–236.

101. Ferrier C, Beretta-Piccoli C, Weidmann P, Mordasini R. Alpha-1-adrenergic blockade and lipoprotein metabolism in essential hypertension. *Clin Pharmacol Ther* 1986;40:525–530.

102. Weidmann P, Uehlinger DE, Gerber A. Antihypertensive treatment and serum lipoproteins. *J Hypertens* 1985;3:297–306.

103. Konigstein RP. Treatment with prazosin in patients suffering from a maturity onset diabetes. *Wien Med Wochenschr* 1978;128:27–29.

104. Torvik D, Madsbu HP. An open one-year comparison of doxazosin and prazosin in mild to moderate essential hypertension. *Am J Cardiol* 1987;59:73G–77G.

105. Kyncl JJ. The pharmacology of terazosin. *Am J Med* 1986;80(suppl 5B):12–19.

106. Frohlich E, van Zwieten PA. Serotonin in cardiovascular regulation. *J Cardiovasc Pharmacol* 1987;10(suppl 3):S1–S137.

107. Bristow MR. Myocardial β-adrenergic receptor down-regulation in heart failure. *Int J Cardiol* 1984;5:648–652.

108. Bristow MR, Ginsberg R, Minobe W, et al. Decreased catecholamine sensitivity and β-adrenergic-receptor density in failing human hearts. *N Engl J Med* 1982;307:205–211.

109. Prichard BNC, Gillam PMS. Treatment of hypertension with propranolol. *Br Med J* 1969;I:7–9.

110. Buehler F, Laragh JL, Baer L, et al. Propranolol inhibition of renin secretion: a specific approach to diagnosis and treatment of renin dependent hypertensive diseases. *N Engl J Med* 1972;287:1209–1213.

111. Lancaster R, Goodwin TJ, Peart WS. The effect of pindolol on plasma renin and blood pressure in hypertensive patients. *Br J Clin Pharmacol* 1976;3:453–460.

112. Watson RDS, Eriksson BM, Hamilton CA. Effects of chronic beta-adrenoceptor antagonism on plasma catecholamines and blood pressure in hypertension. *J Cardiovasc Pharmacol* 1980;2:725–729.

113. Jones DH, Daniel J, Hamilton CA, Reid JL. Plasma noradrenaline concentration in essential hypertension during long-term β-adrenoceptor blockade with oxprenolol. *Br J Clin Pharmacol* 1980;9:27–31.

114. Borkowski KR, Quinn P. Adrenaline and the development of spontaneous hypertension in rats. *J Auton Pharmacol* 1985;5:89–100.

115. Frishman WH. β-Adrenoceptor antagonists: new drugs and new indications. *N Engl J Med* 1981;305:500–506.

116. Chang PC, Blauw GJ, van Brummelen P. Pindolol, a betablocker with vasodilating properties due to stimulation of vascular β₂-adrenoceptors. *J Hypertens* 1983;1(suppl 2):338–339.

117. Lund-Johansen P. Hemodynamic effects of antihypertensive agents. In: Freis ED, ed. *The treatment of hypertension.* MTP Press, Lancaster, 1978:61–90.

118. Lund-Johansen P. Hemodynamic effects of antihypertensive agents. In: Doyle AE, ed. *Handbook of hypertension, vol 5.* Elsevier, Amsterdam-New York-Oxford, 1984;39–66.

119. Deacon SP, Karunanayake A, Bamett D. Acebutolol, atenolol and propranolol and metabolic responses to acute hypoglycemia in diabetics. *Br Med J* 1977;2:1255–1258.

120. Buehler FR, Haeusler G. Optimization of β-blockers for cardiovascular care. *J Cardiovasc Pharmacol* 1986;8(suppl 11):1–23.

121. van Zwieten PA. Differential pharmacological properties of β-adrenoceptor blocking drugs. *J Cardiovasc Pharmacol* 1983;5:S1–S7.

122. Prichard BNC, Boakes AJ. The use of beta-adrenergic blocking drugs in hypertension: a review. *Curr Med Res Opin* 1977;4(suppl 5):51–59.

123. Prichard BNC. Aspects of the evaluation of antihypertensive drugs. In: Border P, ed. *Proceedings of the international symposium on clinical pharmacology.* Royal Academy of Medicine of Belgium, Brussels, 1970, 193–202.

124. Prichard BNC, Owens CWI. β-Adrenoceptor blocking drugs. In: Doyle AE, ed. *Handbook of hypertension, vol 5.* Elsevier, Amsterdam-New York-Oxford, 1984;169–224.

125. The Esmolol Multicenter Study Group. Efficacy and safety of esmolol vs. propranolol in the treatment of supraventricular tachyarrhythmias: a multicenter double blind clinical trial. *Am Heart J* 1985;110:913–918.

126. Zacharias FJ, Cowen KJ, Vickers J, Wall BG. Propranolol in hypertension: a study of long-term therapy 1964–1970. *Am Heart J* 1972;83:755–762.

127. Drayer JIM, Weber MA, Longworth DL, Laragh JL. The possible importance of aldosterone as well as renin in the long-term antihypertensive action of propranolol. *Am J Med* 1978;64:187–192.

128. Turner P. Beta-blockade and the human central nervous system. *Drugs* 1983;25(suppl 2):262–273.

129. Ames RP. The effects of antihypertensive drugs on serum lipids and lipoproteins. Part II: Non-diuretic drugs. *Drugs* 1986;32:335–357.

130. van Brummelen P, Buehler FR. Bopindolol-induced changes in plasma lipid fractions in hypertensive patients. In: van Zwieten PA, ed. *The position of bopindolol, a new β-blocker.* Royal Soc. Med. Serv., London-New York, 1986; 63–65.

131. Waal-Manning HJ. Can β-blockers be used in diabetic patients? *Drugs* 1979;17:157–160.

132. Prichard BNC, Walden J. The beta adrenergic

withdrawal phenomenon. *Br J Clin Pharmacol* 1982;13(suppl 2):337S–341S.

133. Kirch W, Kohler H, Spahn H, Mutschler E. Interaction of cimetidine with metoprolol, propranolol or atenolol. *Lancet* 1981;2:529–531.

134. Lilja M, Journela AJ, Justila H, Mattila MJ. Interaction of clonidine and β-blockers. *Acta Med Scand* 1980;207:173–179.

135. The Norwegian Multicenter Study Group. Six-year follow-up of the Norwegian multicenter on timolol after acute myocardial infarction. *N Engl J Med* 1985;313:1055–1060.

136. Furburg CD. Secondary prevention trials after myocardial infarction. *J Cardiovasc Pharmacol* 1988;12(suppl 1):S83–S87.

137. Medical Research Council Working Party. MRC trial of mild hypertension: principal results. *Br Med J* 1985;291:97–104.

138. Sever PS. 1985—The year of the hypertension trials: interpreting the results. *Trends Pharmacol Sci* 1986;8:134–139.

139. Louis WJ, McNeil JJ. Labetalol. In: Doyle AE, ed. *Handbook of hypertension, vol 5*. Elsevier, Amsterdam-New York-Oxford, 1984;225–245.

140. van Zwieten PA, van Meel JCA, Timmermans PBMWM. Pharmacological basis of the therapeutic effects of calcium entry blockers. Interaction with vascular α-adrenoceptors. *Hypertension* 1983;5(suppl II):II/8–II/17.

141. van Zwieten PA, Timmermans PBMWM. Pharmacological basis of the antihypertensive action of calcium entry blockers. *J Cardiovasc Pharmacol* 1985;7:S11–S17.

142. van Zwieten PA, Timmermans PBMWM. Receptor subtypes involved in the action of calcium entry blockers. *Ann NY Acad Sci* 1988;522:349–360.

143. Jie K, van Brummelen P, Timmermans PBMWM, van Zwieten PA. Influence of calcium entry blockade on α_1- and α_2-adrenoceptor mediated vasoconstriction in the forearm of hypertensive patients. *Eur J Clin Pharmacol* 1987;32:115–120.

144. Zimmerman BG, Syberts EJ, Wong PC. Interaction between sympathetic and renin-angiotensin system. *J Hypertens* 1984;2:581–586.

145. Lokhandwala MF, Amelang E, Buckley JP. Facilitation of cardiac sympathetic function by angiotensin II: role of presynaptic angiotensin receptors. *Eur J Pharmacol* 1978;52:405–410.

146. de Jonge A, Thoolen MJMC, Timmermans PBMWM, van Zwieten PA. Interaction of angiotensin converting enzyme inhibitors with the sympathetic nervous system. *Prog Pharmacol* 1984;5:25–34.

147. van Zwieten PA, de Jonge A. Interaction between the adrenergic and renin-angiotensin-aldosterone-systems. *Postgrad Med J* 1986;62(suppl 1):23–27.

Cardiovascular Pharmacology, Third Edition,
edited by Michael Antonaccio.
Raven Press, Ltd., New York © 1990.

Vascular Smooth Muscle and Vasodilators

*George B. Weiss, †Raymond J. Winquist, and ‡Paul J. Silver

*Research Department, Pharmaceuticals Division, CIBA-GEIGY Corporation,
Summit, New Jersey 07901; †Department of Pharmacology, Boehringer Ingelheim
Pharmaceuticals, Inc., Ridgefield, Connecticut 06877; ‡Department of Pharmacology, Sterling
Research Group, Rensselaer, New York 12144*

Increased contractile tone generated by hypertensive vascular smooth muscle cells has been generally considered the physiological end point in the sequence of events that occurs in hypertension. More specifically, hypertension, defined as an elevated blood pressure, can result when total peripheral vascular resistance is increased. Although a variety of mechanisms have been postulated for the causes and genesis of hypertension, there is clearly a convergence of pathways at the smooth muscle cells of the resistance vessels to elicit a directly related increase in contractility and blood pressure.

It is this end point in the hypertensive process that is affected by vasodilators. These agents do not act on the various putative regulatory systems that are believed to play important roles in control and/or modulation of vascular resistance. Instead, their action is directly on the vascular smooth muscle cell to interfere, in some manner, with the contractile response. The desired result is either a decrease in elevated contractile tone or prevention of an increased contractile response. Thus, vasodilators do not cure hypertension. The conditions that initiate events leading to vascular hypertension are not changed by vasodilators and, presumably, may persist or even progress. However, by either dilating or preventing constriction of resistance vessels, vasodilators will decrease elevated blood pressure or block the onset of increased vascular tone and, in doing so, prevent the variety of deleterious physiological consequences of overt maintained or intermittent hypertension.

The focus of this chapter is on the increasing level of information about how vasodilators act. During the past 6 years since the previous edition of this volume, a considerable amplification of our understanding of the mechanisms regulating vascular smooth muscle permeability and contractility has occurred. This rapid progress has been, in large part, related to significant improvements in experimental measurement of membrane ionic permeability parameters and of subcellular biochemical events. An increased specificity of mechanism of action can be attributed to different vasodilators, and, conversely, new approaches can be evaluated for potential for development of additional novel vasodilators.

THE VASCULAR SMOOTH MUSCLE CELL MEMBRANE

The vascular smooth muscle cell membrane contains a number of systems contributing to the regulation of Ca^{2+} mobilization into the intracellular compartment and subsequent induction and maintenance of contractile tone and tension. The resting smooth muscle cell membrane is polarized and ionic gradients regulate the degree of polarization (1,2). In particular, alterations in K^+ permeability and gradients have been extensively studied (3). Exposure of isolated smooth muscle preparations to elevated K^+ concentrations decreases the transmembrane K^+ gradient and, in this manner, induces depolarization, increased Ca^{2+} influx, and contraction (4). Conversely, agents that increase K^+ permeability without significantly affecting the transmembrane K^+ gradient hyperpolarize the cells and increase resistance to depolarization (5). Recently, based on improved smooth muscle electrophysiological techniques (whole cell voltage clamp, patch clamp), a new class of agents, the K^+ channel openers, has been identified (5). This

group of agents includes not only older drugs (diazoxide [6,7], minoxidil [7,8], pinacidil [9]) with previously unidentified "nonspecific" mechanisms of vasodilator action but also drugs currently in development (e.g., chromakalim [10]). A number of inhibitors of different K^+ channels (e.g., 4-aminopyridine, glyburide) have also been identified (5). Prevention of cell depolarization could impede not only Ca^{2+} uptake but also the release of Ca^{2+} from membrane sites, and this action, in turn, would decrease contractility and vasospasm.

A consistent model of Ca^{2+} release in smooth muscle has been developed from existing data (11) (Fig. 1). At least four different types of Ca^{2+} entry can be identified. The various entry mechanisms are differentiated on the basis of whether each leads directly to increased free intracellular Ca^{2+},

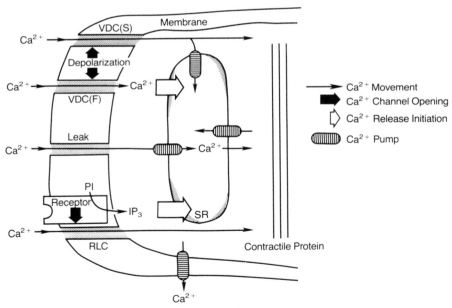

FIG. 1. Calcium movements in smooth muscle. Four different Ca^{2+} influx pathways are illustrated: the fast-inactivating, voltage-dependent Ca^{2+} channel (VDC(F)); the slow-inactivating, voltage-dependent Ca^{2+} channel (VDC(S)); the resting influx (leak) Ca^{2+} channel; the receptor-linked Ca^{2+} channel (RLC). Also indicated is storage site (SR) Ca^{2+} accumulation (Ca^{2+} pump) or release (Ca^{2+} release initiation). SR Ca^{2+} is released by a Ca^{2+}-induced Ca^{2+} release (after VDC(F) entry) or by a receptor-activated conversion of phosphatidylinositol (PI) to IP_3. Released SR Ca^{2+} or directly entering Ca^{2+} (RLC or some VDC(S) Ca^{2+}) activates contractile filaments and is then either extruded from the cell or reaccumulated in the SR. (From ref. 11.)

to increased Ca^{2+} accumulation in the sarcoplasmic reticulum (SR), or to release of Ca^{2+} from the SR. A complete discussion of the experimental basis of these interactions (11) is not appropriate within this context. However, the critical concept is that the Ca^{2+} important for increased intracellular Ca^{2+} levels originates from a variety of membrane and cellular sources that can be experimentally dissociated but, in many vascular tissues, are interrelated or even convergent (12).

The diagram in Fig. 1 can also be used to illustrate potential specific sites of action for vasodilators that act to prevent increases in intracellular free Ca^{2+} levels (or, by decreasing Ca^{2+} uptake or release, permit elevated intracellular Ca^{2+} levels to decrease). Agents could act by blocking any of the Ca^{2+} uptake mechanisms or by preventing release of Ca^{2+} from the SR. Alternatively, agents could stimulate membrane Ca^{2+} pumps that extrude cellular Ca^{2+}, inhibit release of Ca^{2+} from the SR, or inhibit SR Ca^{2+} pumps that accumulate Ca^{2+} (for subsequent release).

In fact, those agents known to be clinically effective vasodilators with Ca^{2+}-related mechanisms of action act on one of two different sites. The extensively studied Ca^{2+} channel blockers (verapamil, diltiazem, nifedipine, and their analogs) specifically block the slow-inactivating, voltage-dependent Ca^{2+} channel and prevent depolarization-induced increases in Ca^{2+} entry (13) and the accompanying maintained smooth muscle contraction. The therapeutic rationale that makes this mechanism an attractive one is that only the increased Ca^{2+} entry accompanying either transient (vasospastic) or maintained (vasoconstrictive) increases in vascular contractility is blocked. Resting Ca^{2+} levels and Ca^{2+} entry through other mechanisms are not affected and other Ca^{2+}-dependent cellular processes are not disrupted. Thus, these agents could be more strictly defined not as direct vasodilators but, rather, as direct blockers of vasoconstriction.

The other site of Ca^{2+} uptake inhibition by known vasodilators is the receptor-linked Ca^{2+} channel. The agents demonstrated to inhibit this Ca^{2+} uptake component include the organic nitrates (e.g., nitroprusside) (14,15), endothelium-derived relaxing factor (EDRF) (16), and atrial natriuretic factor (ANF) (17,18). The biochemical basis of the inhibitory action of this varied group of compounds (see section on second messenger systems) is an activation of cGMP (19). Inhibition of the receptor-linked channel appears to depend on this nucleotide (20). Thus, by preventing activation of the receptor-linked channel, this Ca^{2+} uptake component is blocked. The vasodilator actions of nitroprusside and EDRF are not linked to interactions at a specific receptor and appear, instead, to be direct effects on the receptor-linked channel (21).

If verapamil (or other agents of this class) and nitroprusside act as vasodilators by blocking different Ca^{2+} uptake mechanisms, their effects should be additive, and this has been demonstrated for rabbit aorta (14,15). In this extensively studied vascular preparation, the voltage-sensitive Ca^{2+} channel blockers inhibit the maintained contraction and accompanying ^{45}Ca uptake elicited with depolarizing concentrations of K^+ but do not block contractions induced by norepinephrine. Conversely, contractions obtained with nondepolarizing or only slightly depolarizing concentrations of norepinephrine are inhibited by nitroprusside but not by voltage-sensitive Ca^{2+} channel blockers. In a recent review (12) it was concluded that most vessels show some convergence of these two mechanisms. That is, a portion of the response to high K^+ is blocked by nitroprusside and a portion of the response to norepinephrine is blocked by voltage-sensitive Ca^{2+} channel blockers. The degree of overlap appears to vary among vessel types. Whether this convergence of vasodilator activity is due to either a decrease in Ca^{2+} channel specificity or some type of convergence of Ca^{2+} mobilization mechanisms, the result is that in many vessels (especially smaller resistance vessels) both types of vasodilator are active.

Agents that block the actions of stimulatory agents coupled to the receptor-linked channel by blocking relevant drug-receptor interactions (e.g., at some α-adrenergic receptors) inhibit vasoconstriction by this indirect action (22). Receptor-drug interactions are coupled to the receptor-linked channel as well as to Ca^{2+} release mechanisms in varied ways in different vessels (12) so that a physiological basis exists for differing vasodilator profiles for these agents as well as for those with direct vascular smooth muscle vasodilator activity.

CONTRACTILE PROTEINS AND REGULATION OF CONTRACTION OF VASCULAR SMOOTH MUSCLE

Contraction of vascular and other smooth muscles is regulated by the concentration of Ca^{2+} in the vicinity of the contractile proteins and thus is similar to regulation of contraction of striated muscle. However, the Ca^{2+} regulatory mechanism(s) at the contractile proteins is quite different when smooth muscle is compared with striated muscle. Whereas regulation is primarily thin-filament linked in striated muscle via the troponin system, Ca^{2+} regulation is primarily thick-filament linked in smooth muscle where the primary Ca^{2+} receptor protein is calmodulin.

The thin filament is composed mainly of the contractile protein, actin. G-actin monomers, which are single-chain globular proteins with a molecular weight of approximately 42,000 daltons, are arranged so that a two-stranded helical filament is formed (Fig. 2). Tropomyosin, a rod-like dimeric protein with a molecular weight of approximately 70,000 daltons, is another major protein constituent of the smooth muscle thin filament. A third major protein of the thin filament is caldesmon, which is a dimer with a molecular weight of 120,000 to 150,000 daltons. The stoichiometric distribution of actin : tropomyosin : caldesmon is 1 : 7 : 28 (23). Caldesmon is capable of binding Ca^{2+} and is phophorylatable.

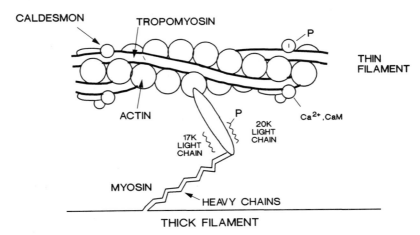

FIG. 2. Diagrammatic representation of the major contractile proteins of vascular smooth muscle. The thin filament is comprised of actin, tropomyosin, and caldesmon, whereas the thick filament is comprised of the MLCs and myosin heavy chains. Actin-myosin interactions are primarily regulated by Ca^{2+} via Ca^{2+}-calmodulin-stimulated phosphorylation (P) of the 20-dalton MLC. Caldesmon, which can also be phosphorylated and binds Ca^{2+}-calmodulin (CaM), may also play an important role in modulating force development and/or maintenance.

The thick filament of smooth muscle is comprised entirely of the contractile protein, myosin (Fig. 2). Myosin is a hexameric molecule consisting of two high molecular weight subunits (heavy chains) and four low molecular weight subunits (light chains). In native myosin, the overall configuration is that of an intertwined coiled tail region with two protruding "head" regions. These head regions project from the thick filament and contain the actin-binding regions. According to the sliding filament theory of muscle contraction, tension development and shortening occur as a result of actin-myosin interactions, causing thick and thin filaments to move past one another. Although smooth muscle lacks the well-ordered structure of the sarcomere that is present in striated muscle, careful ultrastructural and topographical analysis of the thin and thick filaments in smooth muscle reveals an organization that is consistent with a similar mechanism of contraction with dense bodies serving as the attachment sites for the thin and thick filaments (24,25). The light-chain subunits of myosin are associated with the head region of the molecule. In smooth muscle, two pairs of light chains, with molecular weights of approximately 17,000 and 20,000 daltons, are present. The 20,000-dalton light chain is of particular interest in that it can bind divalent cations and is capable of being phosphorylated in a calcium-dependent manner.

During excitation, intracellular levels of Ca^{2+} increase and Ca^{2+} binds to calmodulin. Ca^{2+} binding to calmodulin leads to Ca^{2+}-calmodulin-mediated activation of a specific protein kinase, myosin light-chain kinase (MLCK), which catalyzes the phosphorylation of serine −19 on the 20,000-dalton myosin light chain (MLC) (Table 1). When this MLC is phosphorylated, an increase in the rate of actin-myosin interactions occurs. Actin-myosin interactions can be quantitated by measuring changes in superprecipitation of actomyosin or by measuring the Mg-ATPase activity of myosin that is activated by actin. It is possible to

phosphorylate a second site (threonine) in smooth muscle by MLCK. Diphosphorylated MLC may be needed for further enhancement of actin-myosin interactions (26). Numerous MLC phosphatases have also been identified that dephosphorylate the MLC and thus reverse the effects of MLCK.

Substantial biochemical and physiological evidence supports the role of MLC phosphorylation in the regulatory process of vascular smooth muscle contraction (see [27–29] for reviews). However, it is also evident that MLC phosphorylation is not necessary for maintaining isometric force in intact vascular smooth muscle. These studies have shown that MLC phosphorylation increases during the initial development of force and then declines during the subsequent maintenance of isometric force. Initial force development by a variety of pharmacological interventions and neural stimulation is always accompanied by, and correlated with, varying extents of MLC phosphorylation. The rate and magnitude of the phosphorylation transient depend on the nature of the contractile stimulus and probably reflect declines in the concentration of intracellular free Ca^{2+} during maintained contractions (30,31). Murphy and co-workers (32,33) first observed that shortening velocity in intact arterial and tracheal smooth muscle is also transient and generally follows the same time course as MLC phosphorylation. A "latch-bridge" hypothesis has been proposed by these investigators, which suggests that isometric force may be maintained in smooth muscle with low cross-bridge cycling rates. Regulation of slow cross-bridge cycling rates is also Ca^{2+} dependent but may be independent of MLC phosphorylation.

These data have suggested that a second Ca^{2+} regulatory mechanism, in addition to MLC phosphorylation, is important in smooth muscle contractile regulation. In recent years, several hypotheses have been suggested. Nonomura and Ebashi (34) suggested that two proteins, one, a Ca^{2+}-binding protein, leiotonin C, and another

TABLE 1. *Major protein kinases regulating contractility of vascular smooth muscle*

Kinase	Activator	Substrate	Function	Characteristics
MLCK	Ca^{2+} plus calmodulin	20-Kd MLC	Increase rate of actin-myosin interactions and initiate force development	Subject to biochemical regulation by other kinases
Protein kinase C	DAG plus phospholipid Ca^{2+}	Multiple substrates	Maintain developed isometric force	Multiple (at least 7) isozymes
cAMP-dependent protein kinase	cAMP	Multiple membranous and cytosolic substrates	Promote vasorelaxation by cAMP-related vasodilators via multiple mechanisms	Two isozymes in vascular tissue
cGMP-dependent protein kinase	cGMP	Multiple membranous and cytosolic substrates	Mediate vasorelaxation by nitrovasodilators EDRF or ANF	cGMP binding site does not dissociate from the catalytic site during activation (differs from cAMP protein kinase)

that interacts with actin and tropomyosin, leiotonin A−, are important for regulating activity. Another hypothesis (35) suggests that Ca^{2+} binds to aortic thin filaments and stimulates Mg-ATPase activity. Moreover, Ca^{2+} binding is enhanced when a 21,000-dalton protein of the thin filament (which is presumably distinct from the MLC) is phosphorylated. More recent data suggest that caldesmon plays a central role in regulation. Caldesmon can directly inhibit either superprecipitation or Mg-ATPase activity of smooth muscle contractile proteins via high affinity binding to tropomyosin and actin (23,29,36,37). In the presence of Ca^{2+} and calmodulin, Ca^{2+}-calmodulin binding to caldesmon neutralizes inhibition of actin-tropomyosin via a reduction in binding. *In toto,* these data suggest that MLC phosphorylation is the "switch" that turns on Mg-ATPase activity (via increasing actin-myosin interactions) and that caldesmon is a modulator of this system.

Protein kinase C (Table 1) has also been proposed as a regulator of force maintenance in smooth muscle (38). Evidence supporting this hypothesis comes from studies that demonstrate sustained diacylglycerol (DAG) formation by contractile agonists in intact smooth muscle cells or tissue (39,40), the ability of phorbol esters like phorbol dibutyrate and 12-0-tetradecanoyl-phorbol-1B-acetate (which substitute for DAG as activators of protein kinase C) to produce slow, sustained contractions in various vascular smooth muscle preparations (41,42) in the absence of MLC phosphorylation (43), and from experiments that have identified a putative unique phosphoprotein substrate (or substrates) in vascular or tracheal smooth muscle (44,45). Protein kinase C activity has been found in a particulate and soluble fraction of various vascular beds, with 4 to 6 times greater activity present in particulate fractions (46). There is also a twofold increase in vascular reactivity to phorbol esters in vascular smooth muscle isolated from spontaneously hypertensive rats relative to Wistar-Kyoto rats,

although a direct link to altered protein kinase C activity has yet to be established.

Pharmacological Modulation of Contractile Proteins

There are no current antihypertensive agents in clinical use that function solely via inhibition of vascular contractile protein interactions. Thus, this area remains as potential sites of action for the discovery and development of novel antihypertensive agents.

Direct pharmacological regulation of vascular contractile protein interactions can theoretically occur at several sites (Fig. 3). Among these are the aforementioned sites of regulation on the thin filament (caldesmon) or on the thick filament (phosphorylation of the MLC). Most reported efforts to date have focused on developing modulators of MLC phosphorylation as an approach to pharmacologically modulate vascular contractile protein interactions. Direct alteration of MLC phosphorylation can conceivably occur by four distinct modes: inhibition of Ca^{2+} binding to calmodulin; inhibition of Ca^{2+}-calmodulin activation of MLCK; direct inhibition of MLCK catalytic activity; or direct stimulation of MLC phosphatase activity. Organic agents that relax vascular smooth muscle and function exclusively by stimulating phosphatase activity have not been identified. Recent synthesis of peptide analogs of smooth muscle MLC and identification of a 3-Kd internal inhibitory peptide fragment of MLCK that may be shifted during Ca^{2+}-calmodulin binding (47) offer possible avenues for future drug development of specific modulators of MLCK activity. The knowledge that the mechanism of regulation of MLCK, like other protein kinases, involves pseudosubstrate inhibition, may aid in this endeavor (48). Efforts of two pharmaceutical groups during the past few years have resulted in some small peptide

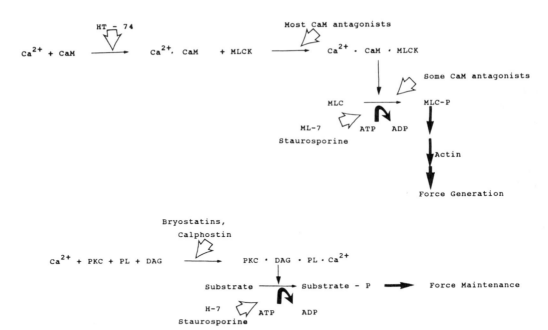

FIG. 3. Major potential sites for pharmacological modulation of Ca^{2+} activation of contraction in vascular smooth muscle. Modulation of Ca^{2+} activation of MLC phosphorylation (MLC-P) can occur at multiple sites, including blocking the binding of Ca^{2+} to calmodulin (CaM) (as occurs with HT-74), blocking the binding of Ca^{2+}. CaM to MLCK, which is the site of action of most CaM antagonists, blocking the phosphorylation of MLC by activated MLCK (some CaM antagonists, such as trifluoperazine, have this activity) or by blocking the binding of ATP to activated MLCK (site of action of staurosporine or the isoquinolinesulfonamide ML-7). Modulation of activation of protein kinase C (PKC) by Ca^{2+}, phospholipids (PL), and DAG can occur by prevention of binding of DAG (as occurs with bryostatins and calphostin) or by inhibition of catalytic activity by blocking the binding of ATP (as with MLCK, the site of action of staurosporine and the isoquinolinesulfonamide H-7).

substrate inhibitors of MLCK, with K_is mostly in the low micromolar or nanomolar range (49,50). However, because of the peptidic nature of these agents and the need for access to intracellular contractile proteins, functional inhibition of vascular force development is not obtained.

A series of nonselective agents that directly inhibit the Ca^{2+}-regulated kinases MLCK and protein kinase C has been described by Hidaka and colleagues (51–54). These agents are isoquinolinesulfonamides and inhibit protein kinase activity by competing for ATP binding (51). Interestingly, other ATP-requiring nonkinase enzymes, such as ATPase, are not inhibited by these agents. Although most of these agents are also effective inhibitors of cAMP- and cGMP-dependent protein kinases, differ-

ences in relative potencies can be obtained by structural modifications (51). In particular, some of these agents, such as ML-7 and ML-9, appear to be relatively potent inhibitors of MLCK ($IC_{50} = 0.3$–4 μM) (54).

Because of this broad spectrum of kinase inhibition, the potential therapeutic usefulness of this class of agents is questioned. However, one of these agents, HA 1004, is an effective inhibitor of vasoconstrictor agents in vascular smooth muscle and has no cardiac depressant effect (53,55). In addition, HA 1004 appears to have *in vivo* pharmacological properties that differ from Ca^{2+} entry blockers. Increases in renal blood flow with HA 1004, but not nicardipine, have been reported in anesthetized dogs (55).

Calmodulin antagonism is currently the

most popular method for inhibiting smooth muscle MLC phosphorylation. By far, the largest group of calmodulin antagonists are those agents that compete with the regulated enzyme for the Ca^{2+}-calmodulin complex. Agents that directly modify Ca^{2+} binding to calmodulin have not been as numerous; HT-74 is one example of this type of agent (56). Many classes of drugs have been shown to bind to calmodulin in a Ca^{2+}-dependent manner and also to inhibit various calmodulin-regulated systems. Among these are phenothiazine, diphenylbutylpiperidine and butyrophenone antipsychotics, tricyclic and nontricylic antidepressants, various neuropeptides (such as β-endorphin) and insect venoms (such as mastoparan and melittin), benzodiazepine antianxiety agents, β-adrenergic antagonists, naphthalene sulfonamide smooth muscle relaxants, the antifungal miconazole analog calmidazolium, class III antiarrhythmic agents such as amiodarone, and certain Ca^{2+} entry blockers (see [57–60] for reviews; also [61–65]). High- (Ca^{2+}-dependent) and low- (Ca^{2+}-independent) affinity binding sites on calmodulin have been identified (66), and separate drug binding sites for these various classes, which appear to exhibit allosteric modulation of binding, have been reported (66,67). The structure-activity relationships for inhibition by these various classes have been reviewed (57–59) and will not be discussed here. However, in general, most organic inhibitors contain a hydrophobic region and a charged amino group separated by an alkyl chain at least 3 atoms long. Original reports linked hydrophobicity with potency of calmodulin antagonism, but it is apparent that other factors, such as electrostatic interactions (57,58), are also important. Unlike Ca^{2+} channel blockers, calmodulin antagonists do not generally exhibit stereoselectivity for binding or inhibition (68).

The potency of calmodulin inhibitors on most biochemical and skinned preparations generally ranges from 1 to 30 μM. Most direct vasodilators (such as nitroprusside and diazoxide) and the Ca^{2+} entry blockers (nifedipine and verapamil) are inactive at concentrations as high as 100 μM (69). Hydralazine also has no effect on Tritox-X 100 purified aortic actomyosin (69) but was shown to inhibit actin-myosin interactions and MLC phosphorylation in carotid arterial actomyosin (70). The reason for this discrepancy is not known. Adenosine can also inhibit MLC and phosphatidylinositol phosphorylation in crude preparations from calf aortic smooth muscle (71). Some dihydropyridine Ca^{2+} blockers, such as felodipine, as well as lipophilic weakly basic Ca^{2+} antagonists, such as cinnarizine, flunarizine, bepridil, and perhexiline, also bind to calmodulin and inhibit calmodulin-regulated MLC phosphorylation and phosphodiesterase activity (63,64,72). It is doubtful that this activity contributes to pharmacological activity, because potency for Ca^{2+} entry blockade is generally several orders of magnitude higher for most of these agents (72).

The pharmacological effects of two novel series of agents that structurally resemble the dihydropyridines or verapamil/W-7 hybrids have been described (73,74). Both series demonstrate Ca^{2+} entry blockade and direct inhibition of aortic actin-myosin interactions at similar concentration ranges (3–30 μM). These agents can be differentiated from standard Ca^{2+} entry blockers in intact muscle or cellular systems (73,74); that is, these agents are more efficacious compared with most mediators (norepinephrine, angiotensin II, histamine, serotonin, leukotrienes, $PGF_{2\alpha}$, thromboxane A_2) of vasoconstriction in rabbit aortic or porcine coronary arterial smooth muscle. These effects are consistent with an intracellular effect at the contractile proteins, because vasoconstrictor agents may mobilize pools of Ca^{2+} (intracellular and/or entry through voltage-independent Ca^{2+} channels) that are not amenable to inhibition by standard Ca^{2+} entry blockers.

Several questions and areas of concern must be addressed in the development of modulators of MLCK activity as antihypertensive agents. Because calmodulin is a ubiquitous Ca^{2+} binding protein that regulates several enzyme systems, the question of selective antagonism of specific calmodulin-regulated systems is important. Much evidence now exists that suggests that different potencies are apparent among the different classes of calmodulin antagonists in different calmodulin-regulated systems (57,59,75,76). Mechanistically, these differences may be partially explained by different binding sites on calmodulin for different antagonists, direct inhibition of the target enzyme by the calmodulin antagonist, or by other mechanisms, such as interference in the enzyme-substrate interaction. This latter possibility has been demonstrated with MLCK, as various calmodulin antagonists appear to inhibit activity through decreased MLC binding to the kinase (77). Other important factors to consider in calmodulin inhibition specificity are the overall importance of each calmodulin-regulated system to normal physiological function, the amount of calmodulin and accessibility of calmodulin to an inhibitor (i.e., membrane-associated or enzyme-associated calmodulin), and possible aberrant function/synthesis of the calmodulin-regulated system in a pathophysiological state. An additional question involves the importance of MLC phosphorylation versus other contractile protein regulatory mechanisms in the chronic regulation of blood pressure. It is difficult to know what the extent of MLC phosphorylation is in arterioles that are ultimately responsible for blood pressure regulation. If MLC phosphorylation is transient and this transience depends on the contractile agonist/vasoconstrictor (as it does in large arteries), then regulatory mechanisms that are more crucial to maintenance of tone may be better targets for antihypertensive therapy. MLCK inhibitors may be a better target for smooth muscle diseases that involve phasic contractions, such as angina or asthma. The answer to this question awaits the development of a potent, selective inhibitor of MLCK.

SECOND MESSENGER SYSTEMS

In vascular smooth muscle, as in most other cells, there are two major second messenger systems that can modulate the activity of either the Ca^{2+} flux and/or the contractile protein regulatory systems. These second messenger systems are the cyclic nucleotides (which are comprised of both the cAMP and cGMP systems) and the phosphatidylinositol cycle (Fig. 4).

Cyclic Nucleotides

Cyclic nucleotide activity is regulated by the actions of three different enzymes. These are the cyclases, which catalyze the formation of cyclic nucleotides from triphosphate precursors, the low K_m cyclic nucleotide phosphodiesterases (PDE), which catalyze the degradation of the cyclic nucleotides, and the protein kinases, which are the effectors of these second messengers. In vascular smooth muscle, increases in either cAMP or cGMP will ultimately produce vasodilation. Thus, any agent that activates or potentiates either cyclase or cyclic nucleotide protein kinase activity, or inhibits PDE activity, will promote vasorelaxation.

Adenylate cyclase is a membrane-bound enzyme whose catalytic activity is modulated by the guanosine triphosphate regulatory proteins. Among the agents that can activate adenylate cyclase and increase cAMP formation in vascular smooth muscle are β-adrenergic agonists, prostaglandin E_2, prostacyclin, and forskolin. Guanylate cyclase is present in both the soluble and particulate fractions in vascular smooth muscle. Among the agents that activate soluble guanylate cyclase activity are the nitrovasodilators and EDRF. The mechanism by which the nitrovasodilators (and possibly EDRF) activates guanylate cyclase involves intracellular biotransformation of the organic nitrates, and possibly oxidation of a sulfhydryl group on guanylate cyclase, formation of nitric oxide, or formation of S-

A. CYCLIC NUCLEOTIDE SYSTEM

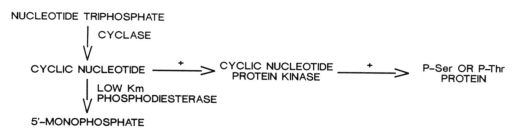

B. PHOSPHATIDYLINOSITOL SYSTEM

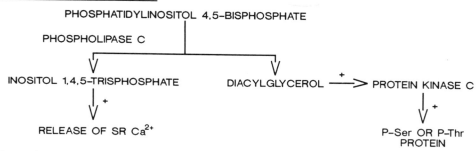

FIG. 4. Second messenger systems in vascular smooth muscle. Two major modulatory second messenger systems are functional in vascular smooth muscle. Activation of the cyclic nucleotide system (either cAMP or cGMP) results in vasorelaxation via ultimate phosphorylation of serine (Ser) or threonine (Thr) sites on key regulatory substrates. Important enzymes in this cascade are the cyclases (formation), low K_m phosphodiesterases (degradation), and protein kinases (effectors). Activation of the phosphatidylinositol system is associated with vasoconstriction. IP_3 can stimulate release of Ca^{2+} from SR, whereas DAG, in the presence of Ca^{2+} and phospholipid, can activate protein kinase C.

nitrosothiols (78–80). Particulate guanylate cyclase activity was discovered largely as a consequence of the discovery of ANF. This cyclase is tightly linked to the ANF receptor and copurifies with it (81,82). To date, the only known activators of particulate guanylate cyclase are the atriopeptins or atriopeptin mimetics.

Low K_m cAMP PDE activity is present in most, if not all, mammalian vascular smooth muscle (Table 2) (see [83–85] for reviews). This enzyme has a low k_m for cAMP (usually 0.2–0.4 μM), and activity can be modulated by cGMP, which can inhibit this PDE at submicromolar concentrations. Thus, this PDE can interact with both cyclic nucleotides at physiologically relevant concentrations of both cyclic nucleotides. Recent data have shown that this vascular PDE isozyme in a variety of species, including primates, can be selectively inhibited by agents such as milrinone, piroximone, imazodan, CI-930, pelrinone, and others. Inhibition of this PDE is accompanied by increases in cAMP content and activation of cAMP protein kinase in a manner analogous to what occurs with other cAMP-related vasodilators (86,87). The subcellular distribution of this isozyme is not known, although it has been identified in particulate fractions of guinea pig aortic smooth muscle (88). Selective inhibitors of this PDE also inhibit the same isozyme(s) in cardiac muscle and ultimately

TABLE 2. *Major cyclic nucleotide PDE isozymes in vascular smooth muscle*

DEAE isozyme elution	Characteristics	
	Substrate	Physiological/pharmacological
Peak I		
1	Low K_m cGMP	cGMP selective; zaprinast-sensitive
2	Low K_m cGMP, low K_m cAMP	V_{max} regulated by Ca^{2+}-calmodulin
Peak III	Low K_m cAMP	cGMP-inhibited; stimulated by cAMP-cAPK phosphorylation; sensitive to inhibition by cardiotonic agents
Peak IV	Low/high K_m cAMP	Non-cGMP inhibitable; sensitive to inhibition by rolipram

increase the rate and force of contraction in the heart. Thus, the hemodynamic benefits of these agents in the acute therapy of heart failure may derive from a single mechanism, low K_m cAMP PDE inhibition, which produces peripheral vasodilation (afterload reduction), coronary vasodilation, and positive inotropy (85). However, as the same isozyme is present in cardiac muscle, this is not a viable target in vascular smooth muscle for antihypertensive therapy, because the accompanying increases in positive inotropy via inhibition of this PDE in the heart would be contraindicated in the therapy of hypertension.

Another PDE isozyme that hydrolyzes cAMP and is not inhibited by cGMP has also been identified in vascular smooth muscle, as well as in tracheal smooth muscle (Table 2) (89,90). This isozyme is sensitive to inhibition by low micromolar concentrations of rolipram and RO 20-1724. Unlike the cGMP-inhibitable low K_m cAMP PDE isozyme previously described, the role of this PDE in regulating vascular relaxation has yet to be determined.

Two forms of low K_m cGMP PDE are present in vascular smooth muscle (Table 2) (85,90–92). Both have K_ms for cGMP in the 0.2- to 1-μM range. One isozyme, which is also present in other tissues including brain and heart, also hydrolyzes cAMP and is activated by Ca^{2+}-calmodulin. Calmodulin serves to increase V_{max} and does not alter the K_m for cGMP. A second isozyme is also present in most, if not all, vascular sources examined. This cGMP PDE is not regulated by calmodulin but is inhibited by a selective inhibitor, zaprinast, at submicromolar concentrations ($IC_{50} = 0.5$–1 μM). Unfortunately, zaprinast is not a very selective inhibitor, because this agent will also inhibit Ca^{2+}-calmodulin PDE at low ($IC_{50} = 5$ μM) micromolar concentrations.

Zaprinast, as well as other selective low K_m cGMP PDE inhibitors, can potentiate the vasorelaxant and hypotensive actions of guanylate cyclase activators, including EDRF, nitrovasodilators, and ANF (92,93). In addition, zaprinast can lower blood pressure and increase natriuresis following intravenous administration to rats or dogs (94; *personal observations*). Both activities are consistent with inhibition of low K_m cGMP PDE. Given the link via guanylate cyclase activation to cGMP formation in the mechanisms of action of EDRF and ANF, a selective agent that could prevent the degradation of cGMP offers a new and exciting approach for the discovery of novel vasodilators that may be useful therapy for hypertension. Certainly, the aspect of identifying an agent that potentiates the activity of endogenous regulators of vascular tone and sodium balance (such as EDRF and ANF) and ultimately produces both vasodilation and accompanying natriuresis is of interest. Further developments in this hypothesis await additional information on the low K_m cGMP PDE(s) in the kidney, as well as the discovery of nanomolar potent/specific inhibitors of the cGMP PDE isozyme present in vascular smooth muscle.

A kinase that mediates the effects of cAMP was first reported by Walsh et al. (95) in skeletal muscle. Subsequently, Kuo and Greengard (96) demonstrated the existence of cAMP-dependent protein kinase in a variety of tissues from a variety of species and suggested that the universal effects of cAMP were mediated through activation of this enzyme. cAMP-dependent protein kinase exists in two major isozymic forms, designated type I and type II (for review, see [97]). The isozymes differ primarily because of differences in the R-subunits and regulation. The distribution of the two isozymes varies according to both tissue and species source. In vascular smooth muscle, there is approximately equal distribution of the isozymes, although vascular bed differences ranging between 40% and 60% of type I are evident (98). No clear teleological or functional reasons are apparent for these different isozymes in vascular muscle.

Activation of cAMP protein kinase has been quantitated by calculating activity ratios in rapidly frozen muscle segments that are undergoing changes in force development (99). Activation of cAMP protein kinase in vascular smooth muscle in response to β-agonists, adenosine, forskolin, papaverine, and milrinone has been demonstrated (98,100–103).

Identification of a protein kinase that is activated by low concentrations of cGMP, but not cAMP, was initially reported by Kuo and Greengard (104). Subsequently, this protein kinase was identified in most tissues (105), with a relatively higher concentration reported in cerebellum, lung, and various smooth muscles. Activation of cGMP-dependent protein kinase as assessed by activity ratio methodology has not been extensively examined, primarily because of a lack of dissociations of the cat-

alytic subunit upon activation. In vascular smooth muscle, activation of cGMP protein kinase has been linked to relaxation produced by atriopeptin II (106).

Selective pharmacological activators of cAMP or cGMP protein kinases have not been identified. Inhibitors of these kinases, however, have been. The previously described isoquinolinesulfonamides are protein kinase inhibitors that compete for ATP binding on the enzyme (51). One of these analogs, H-8, is a micromolar potent inhibitor, although no selectivity for kinase inhibition is evident.

In vascular smooth muscle, the mechanism or mechanisms responsible for cyclic nucleotide-mediated relaxation have not yet been resolved. In fact, it seems likely that multiple mechanisms may be responsible. In contractile proteins, phosphorylation of MLCK catalyzed by cAMP-dependent protein kinase in the absence of bound Ca^{2+}-calmodulin occurs at two distinct sites. When MLCK is phosphorylated, affinity for the Ca^{2+}-calmodulin complex is markedly (15- to 20-fold) reduced, resulting in less Ca^{2+}-calmodulin bound and, ultimately, a lower extent of MLC phosphorylation and subsequent depression of actin-myosin interactions (107–109). cGMP protein kinase (one site, no change in affinity for calmodulin) and protein kinase C (two different sites, similar decrease in affinity for calmodulin) can also phosphorylate MLCK (110,111). It is important to note that phosphorylation of the relevant sites that inhibit MLCK activity only occurs when calmodulin is not already bound to MLCK (in the absence of Ca^{2+}). Thus, it is questionable that relevant phosphorylation could occur after contraction has ensued. Indeed, relaxation of precontracted airway or arterial smooth muscle by cAMP-increasing relaxants can occur with no decrease in MLC phosphorylation (112,113) and no apparent change in calmodulin-binding affinity of MLCK (112).

There are numerous equivocal reports in

the literature in which a role of cAMP- or cGMP-mediated alteration of membranous Ca^{2+} flux and translocation has been proposed. These include increased uptake of Ca^{2+} into microsomal vesicles (114,115), decreased intracellular Ca^{2+} (116,117), decreased IP_3 formation (118), or decreased IP_3-induced release of Ca^{2+} from SR by cGMP (119), decreased influx of Ca^{2+} through potential dependent Ca^{2+} channels (120,121), increased Ca^{2+} efflux (122), activation of sarcolemmal Ca^{2+}-ATPase activity (123), changes in K^+ flux and membrane conductance (124,125), and effects on Na^+-K^+ ATPase activity with subsequent increased Na^+-Ca^{2+} exchange (126). Most of these studies suffer from the lack of identification of phosphoprotein substrates and a link of altered phosphorylation to changes in function of the system. Several other investigators have identified phosphoprotein substrates in vascular membranous preparations for cyclic nucleotide-regulated systems. Among these are the "G-substrate proteins" of 130 and 100 kDa, which were identified by Ives et al. (127) and Casnellie et al. (128) as preferential substrates for cGMP protein kinase. Silver et al. (129) identified proteins of similar molecular weight that were substrates for cAMP and cGMP protein kinase. In the latter study, a single protein of 108 Kda MW was a common substrate for cAMP, cGMP, and high-nanomolar concentrations of ANF. Suematsu et al. (130) identified two low molecular weight proteins (28 and 22 Kda) as substrates for cAMP protein kinase and one 35-Kda protein as a substrate for cGMP protein kinase. Phosphorylation of these substrates was associated with increased Ca^{2+} uptake. In intact vascular smooth muscle, 11 substrates for cGMP-mediated relaxants (seven of which are also substrates for cAMP) with molecular weights ranging from 21 to 49 Kda and isoelectric points of 6.4 to 7.8 have been identified (131,132).

A more recent report suggests that GMP, and not cGMP, may be responsible for va-sorelaxation by cGMP-related agents. Williams et al. (133) demonstrated that high conductance Ca^{2+}-activated K^+ channels in bovine aortic smooth muscle cells can be potentiated by guanine nucleotides. Of note were the more potent and consistent effects of GMP relative to cGMP at enhancing the frequency of opening and percentage of open time for these channels. Of further interest was the lack of activity of adenine nucleotides in this system. These data would suggest that an active low K_m cGMP PDE is necessary for vasorelaxation to occur. It is not consistent, however, with the data previously described that show that inhibitors of low K_m cGMP PDE (such as zaprinast) can potentiate vasorelaxation by ANF or nitrovasodilators. The high concentration of GMP (100 μM) necessary to achieve this effect (133) is not consistent with the submicromolar concentration of cGMP that activate cGMP PDE or cGMP protein kinase.

Phosphatidylinositol Cycle

The role of the phosphatidylinositol cycle in regulating numerous intracellular events is well-established (see [134–136] for reviews). In this regulatory system (Fig. 4), a Ca^{2+}-mediated agonist, such as angiotensin II or norepinephrine, binds to its receptor and as a consequence stimulates the breakdown of phosphatidylinositol-4,5-bisphosphate via phospholipase C to inositol 1,4,5-trisphosphate (IP_3) and DAG. IP_3 stimulates the release of Ca^{2+} from intracellular stores, which are most likely SR. The ability of vasoconstrictors like angiotensin II and norepinephrine to stimulate release of intracellular Ca^{2+} in vascular smooth muscle has been linked to IP_3 formation (137). Thus, IP_3 antagonists may offer a potential target for new antihypertensive agents. However, the questions of tissue specificity (vascular vs others) as well as limited efficacy (i.e., only antagonizing one component of either angiotensin II- or norepinephrine-mediated constriction as opposed to a receptor antagonist) suggest that this would not be a target worthy of pursuit. Several intracellular Ca^{2+} release antagonists have been identified in the literature (see [138] for review). Although the precise mechanism of action has not been elucidated for many of these agents, IP_3 antagonism may be a possibility. One agent in particular, KT-362, may have this property (139). However, it is also evident (138,140) that this agent may possess other properties, such as extracellular Ca^{2+} blockade, at concentrations necessary to achieve intracellular antagonism (10–100 μM).

The important role of protein kinase C in regulating the maintenance of vascular tone has been discussed previously in this review. Since this enyme is an important regulator, it represents a logical target for novel drug discovery. There are several potential sites for the development of pharmacological modulators of protein kinase C (Fig. 3). Substrate inhibitors, either of the ATP or phosphoprotein substrate, offer the potential for development of active site catalytic inhibitors. The previously described isoquinolinesulfonamides are an example of ATP-competitive inhibitors, although there is little specificity for inhibition of kinase activity. More potent inhibitors are two agents obtained in fermentation broths. Staurosporine ($IC_{50} = 7$ nM) and K252A ($IC_{50} = 280$ nM) are also ATP-competitive inhibitors that are roughly equipotent at inhibiting protein kinase C and cAMP protein kinase (65,141; P. Silver, *personal observations*). These agents, as well as other potent protein kinase C inhibitors, are potent and long-acting hypotensive agents in various animal models (142; P. Silver, *personal observations*).

As DAG is the most critical regulator of protein kinase C activity, a logical target would be to discover DAG binding antagonists. This offers the potential to obtain more selective inhibitors than the aforementioned ATP-competitive inhibitors. Moreover, there are now at least seven isozymes

of protein kinase C described in the literature (see [143] for review). Several of these isozymes differ by virtue of a different regulatory domain and thus, to activation by phorbol esters (144), suggesting that selective DAG antagonists of these different isozymes can be designed. Some potent naturally occurring DAG displacers have been identified, including the bryostatins, which are derived from the marine bryozoan *Bugula neritina* (145). As with IP_3, the question of specificity of putative protein kinase C inhibitors looms as the biggest obstacle for efforts directed at this enzyme as a target for novel antihypertensive therapy. Given the high degree of efficacy and low incidence of side effects of current agents on the market (e.g., ACE inhibitors), the potential for side effects is much greater for protein kinase C inhibitors. Additional information on the isozyme(s) present in vascular smooth muscle and their importance in regulation of vascular tone is needed.

Finally, one additional point concerning the phosphatidylinositol system in vascular smooth muscle is worth noting. This system may play an important role as the transducer of smooth muscle mitogens, such as platelet-derived growth factor (PDGF) (146). PDGF and other growth factors have been implicated in vascular smooth muscle cell proliferation and plaque formation in atherosclerosis (147). Thus, the primary role of the phosphatidylinositol system in vascular smooth muscle may reside in regulating growth or migration, and not vasoconstriction. Alternatively, this may also indicate that DAG and/or IP_3 antagonists may possess both antihypertensive and antiatherosclerotic activities in vascular smooth muscle.

ENDOTHELIUM-SMOOTH MUSCLE CELL INTERFACE

For years the vascular endothelium was regarded simply as a diffusion barrier to circulating substances and as the site of exchange of nutrients and waste in the micro-circulation. A critical step in demonstrating the importance of the vascular endothelium in modulating pharmacological responses of the underlying smooth muscle was the discovery that acetylcholine relaxed isolated vascular preparations only when the integrity of the endothelial cell layer was preserved (148). This discovery resolved the apparent discrepancy that had existed between the effective *in vivo* vasodilatory actions of cholinergic agonists and the *in vitro* vasoconstrictor responses usually recorded with these agents. The contractile responses *in vitro* to acetylcholine and carbachol were well documented in such preparations as the rabbit aortic strip, a preparation widely used for bioassays in cardiovascular laboratories, but one in which the endothelial cell layer is usually destroyed during dissection and handling of the helical strip.

When experiments were performed in aortic ring segments (preparations in which the intimal surface is not as subjected to inadvertent damage during handling), cholinergic agonists produced a relaxation response (148). Subsequent experiments (148,149) documented that preservation of the endothelial lining, in ring segments or with careful handling of helical strips of vessels, was an obligatory step in obtaining relaxation responses to cholinergic agonists *in vitro*. This important discovery of endothelium-dependent relaxation led to several subsequent experimental directions including characterization of the endothelium-dependent relaxation pathway and categorization of endothelium-dependent versus -independent vasodilators (Table 3).

Endothelium-Dependent Relaxation Pathway

Several lines of evidence showed that the relaxation of vascular tissue by acetylcholine involved the release of an EDRF or factors. Perfused vascular segments, challenged with acetylcholine, released a nonprostanoid factor that relaxed endothelium-denuded vascular segments aligned downstream in a perfusion (cascade) system (149). Release of an EDRF could also be elicited from cultured endothelial cells placed upstream in a perfusion system (150), although other endothelium-dependent vasodilators (Tables 3 and 4) are utilized for such an experiment because cholinergic receptors are not easily maintained on these cells during passage. Finally, "sandwiching" an endothelium-intact vascular segment to a denuded vascular strip rendered the latter responsive to the relaxant effects of acetylcholine (148).

Although the relaxation response to the nitrovasodilators has been shown to be due to a direct effect on vascular smooth muscle (148,151,152), the relaxation response to these compounds shares several similarities to the EDRF response including (a) an association with elevated levels of cGMP in the smooth muscle cells (151) and (b) an inhibition by methylene blue and hemoglobin (152). The antagonism of EDRF by methylene blue, an inhibitor of soluble guanylate cyclase, was consistent with the observation that EDRF activates the same enzyme (151) that had previously been associated with the nitrovasodilators (153). EDRF is quite labile, having a half-life on the order of seconds (149,150), and is rapidly inactivated by superoxide anions (154). Taken together, these observations led to the proposal that EDRF is nitric oxide (155,156), believed to be the reactive intermediate of organic nitrovasodilators. Nitric oxide can

TABLE 3. *Locus of action for vasodilators*

Smooth muscle	Endothelium
Adenosine	Acetylcholine
ANF	Vasodilator peptides
Calcium channel blockers	Bradykinin
K$^+$ channel openers	CGRP
Nitrovasodilators	VIP
PDE inhibitors	

TABLE 4. *Drugs acting on the endothelium to release an EDRF*

Drug	Tissue	Ref.
A23187	Rat and rabbit aorta	164,165
Acetylcholine	Rabbit aorta	148
Adenosine	Porcine and SHR aorta	179,194
ADP, ATP	Rabbit aorta, canine femoral	167,193
Bradykinin	Several species except rabbit and cat	178,179
CGRP	Rat aorta, human coronary	187,188
Histamine	Rat aorta	198
Norepinephrine	Canine and porcine coronary	195
Serotonin	Canine and porcine coronary	195,197
Substance P and related kinins	Rabbit aorta	180
Thrombin	Canine coronary	191
VIP	Rat aorta, human splenic	183,184
Vasopressin and oxytocin	Canine basilar	181,182

account for many of the pharmacological actions of EDRF (157). The precursor (L-arginine) for its production has been identified (158) and release from endothelial cells has been demonstrated (159). N-monomethyl-L-arginine (L-NMMA), a specific inhibitor of the formation of nitric oxide from L-arginine, blocks the endothelium-dependent relaxation to acetylcholine both *in vitro* (160) and *in vivo* (161) without affecting the relaxation response to a nitrovasodilator. Therefore, several lines of evidence support the idea that EDRF could be nitric oxide. However, it has become clear that acetylcholine can release an endothelium-derived hyperpolarizing factor (EDHF) that is distinct from EDRF (162). The importance of EDHF in the control of vascular tone has yet to be established, but it appears that several relaxant factors from the endothelium may likely exist.

The production and/or release of EDRF requires ATP (163) and is a calcium-dependent phenomenon (164,165). Removal of calcium from the bathing medium inhibited the response to acetylcholine, whereas the relaxation to an endothelium-independent vasodilator was not necessarily affected (165). This calcium-dependent excitation-secretion coupling is diminished during endothelial cell membrane depolarization presumably due to the diminished driving force for transmembrane calcium influx (166). This would explain the depressed efficacy of EDRF against high K^+ depolarized contractions versus agonist-induced contractile events (167).

There is recent evidence that release of EDRF, evoked by some but not all agents, occurs through a G protein-dependent mechanism (168). Relaxations induced by an α_2-adrenergic agonist (UK 14304) and serotonin, but not those elicited with bradykinin, were blocked by pertussis toxin in porcine coronary arteries. Therefore, different release pathways, possibly associated with production of different EDRFs may be operant in endothelial cells.

Endothelium-Dependent Vasodilators

Table 4 lists vasodilators that have been shown to act via release of an EDRF. It has become rare to find a compound that exerts an effect on vascular smooth muscle that is not influenced in some manner by endothelium removal. A paradoxical example is the nitrovasodilators that elicit an enhanced relaxation response in the absence of the endothelium (169).

Acetylcholine

Most of the work compiled on EDRF has been with acetylcholine. The cholinergic receptor is of the M_2 muscarinic subtype, whereas the receptor on the smooth muscle may be of the M_1 or M_2 subtype (170,171). The heterogeneity in the acetylcholine response, seen with some veins (typically contraction [172]) and arteries such as the bovine coronary artery (no response [171]), is attributed to a probable lack of cholinergic receptors on the endothelial cell membrane, although the posterior auricular artery of the cat exhibits an endothelium-independent relaxation response to acetylcholine (173). The physiological relevance of the release of EDRF by acetylcholine has often been questioned because this agent does not circulate. The existence of choline acetyltransferase in endothelial cells (174) suggests the possibility of a paracrine function for acetylcholine *in vivo*.

Agents Effecting Calcium Translocation

Relaxation responses observed with the calcium ionophore A23187 indicate that the release of EDRF requires an influx of calcium (164,165). Because of the heterogeneity to acetylcholine mentioned above, A23187 is often used to establish an EDRF response in particular vessels that lack a cholinergic relaxation response such as venous preparations. Moreover, A23187 serves as a useful "receptor-independent" control response when assessing endothelium responsiveness in such disease states as hypertension and atherosclerosis (175).

The predominant relaxation (versus a contractile) response to A23187 in most preparations suggests an interesting preferential ability of this compound to translocate calcium across the endothelium compared with the vascular smooth muscle cell membrane. Conversely, the dihydropyridine calcium channel "agonist" Bay K 8644 does not appear to release EDRF in most vascular preparations (176). This may reflect the absence of voltage-gated calcium channels in endothelial cells. However, Bay K 8644 has been found to release EDRF in some vascular preparations such as the canine femoral artery (177).

Peptides

The vasodilator response to peptides varies as widely among tissues as does the endothelium-dependent versus -independent component of the response. Bradykinin fails to relax rabbit aortic tissue but can relax other rabbit vessels via the release of vasodilatory prostaglandins (178). In canine and porcine preparations, bradykinin appears to release the same EDRF as acetylcholine (150,178,179). Substance P and related tachykinins (e.g., kassanin, physalemin, and eledoisin) relax rabbit aortic segments via the release of EDRF and show cross-desensitization with repeated exposure (180). Vasopressin and oxytocin, well-known constrictors of peripheral vascular and nonvascular smooth muscle, elicit endothelium-dependent relaxation in the canine basilar artery, which is mediated by the V_1 subtype of vasopressin receptor (181,182). This qualitative difference between peripheral (constriction) and central (dilation) vessels may be of physiological importance during certain states (e.g., hemorrhage) in which plasma vasopressin levels are elevated and both cerebral blood flow and peripheral resistance need to be sustained.

Vasoactive intestinal polypeptide (VIP) has been shown to be an endothelium-dependent vasodilator in rat aorta (183) and human splenic (184) preparations but in most vascular tissues, including human pulmonary artery, VIP relaxes via an endothelium-independent mechanism (184–186). Similar to VIP, calcitonin gene-related peptide (CGRP) can be classified as eliciting both endothelium-dependent (rabbit aorta [187], human coronary [188]) and endothelium-independent (pial arteries from several species [189]) relaxations. Some peptides such as parathyroid hormone may have both an endothelium-dependent and -independent component in the vasodilatory response (190). Thrombin can produce an initial relaxation response in coronary vessels that is due to the release of an EDRF (191). This is followed by a constrictor response via a direct effect on the smooth muscle. ANF appears unique among peptides in relaxing vascular preparations solely by an endothelium-independent process (186). This is evident, although high-affinity receptors exist for ANF on vascular endothelial cells (192).

Adenosine and Related Nucleotides

Adenosine has been identified as an endothelium-independent vasodilator (165,193), although this compound elicits relaxation via an endothelium-dependent component in some preparations such as the porcine aorta (179) and the aorta from the hypertensive rat (194). Adenosine monophosphate (AMP) appears to have the same profile as adenosine (i.e., largely endothelium-independent), whereas adenosine diphosphate (ADP) and adenosine triphosphate (ATP) have been shown to be endothelium-dependent vasodilators (165,193). Taken together, ATP and ADP may elicit relaxation responses having both endothelium-dependent and -independent components due to metabolic breakdown to AMP and adenosine.

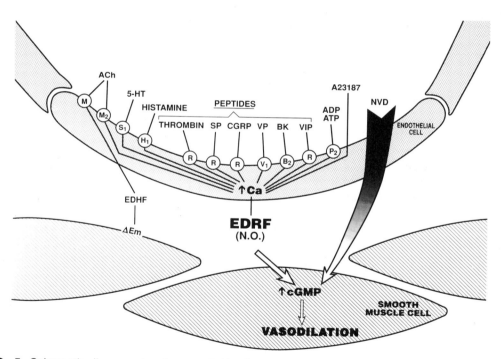

FIG. 5. Schematic diagram showing agents that have been shown to release an EDRF in vascular preparations. Acetylcholine (ACh) has been shown to release both an EDRF and a separate factor that can hyperpolarize smooth muscle (EDHF). Serotonin (5-HT), norepinephrine (not shown), thrombin, histamine, and vasopressin (VP) are vasoconstrictors as well as agents that can release an EDRF under certain conditions in vascular tissue. Several peptides including substance P (SP), CGRP, bradykinin (BK), and VIP have been shown to be endothelium-dependent vasodilators in some (but not necessarily all) vascular preparations. ADP and ATP release an EDRF as does the calcium ionophore A23187, the latter emphasizing the role of intracellular calcium in the excitation-secretion coupling of EDRF. Conversely, nitrovasodilators (NVD) tend to be more effective in the absence of an intact endothelium. Several lines of evidence point to an EDRF being nitric oxide (NO), which relaxes vascular smooth muscle via the same pathway (elevation of cGMP) as with the nitrovasodilators.

Release of EDRF by Vasoconstrictor Agents

Many vasoconstrictor agonists can cause a concomitant receptor-mediated release of EDRF because the increase in force elicited by these agents is enhanced when the endothelium is damaged or EDRF is antagonized. Norepinephrine releases EDRF via an α_2-mediated event in bovine and porcine coronary arteries (195) and canine femoral and pulmonary vessels (196). Serotonin can elicit the release of EDRF via an action on S_1 receptors in coronary arteries (195,197), and histamine can release EDRF in rat vessels as a result of binding to H_1 receptors on the endothelium (198). Therefore, several autacoids, including those often regarded as primarily vasoconstrictor in action, harbor the capacity to release an EDRF under certain circumstances in particular vascular beds (Fig. 5).

VASODILATORS

In the previous (second) edition of *Cardiovascular Pharmacology,* actions of five agents were discussed under the heading of "directly acting smooth muscle relaxants." Four of these agents (sodium nitroprusside, diazoxide, minoxidil, and hydralazine) were considered vasodilators with specific mechanisms of action yet to be defined. The fifth agent was a newer agent, the Ca^{2+} channel blocker, nifedipine. In the preceding sections of this chapter, more recent information about this class of agents has been summarized. Diazoxide and minoxidil can now be classified as the initial members of a newly defined and potentially diverse group of vasodilators, the K^+ channel openers (5). Nifedipine along with verapamil and diltiazem are the initial members of a class of agents of major current therapeutic significance. Considerable information about the mechanisms and physiological significance of the action of nitroprusside has accumulated, whereas the mechanism of action of the less widely employed hydralazine is still not precisely defined.

Detailed review of the pharmacology of each of these agents is beyond the scope of this chapter. However, in the following portions of this section, relevant aspects of some of the actions of these vasodilators are considered.

K^+ Channel Openers

The initial suggestion that the inhibitory effects of chromakalim were due to an opening of membrane K^+ channels in such smooth muscles as rat portal vein (10), and rat aorta (199) was based on experimentally observed membrane hyperpolarization and increased ^{86}Rb efflux. Similar K^+ channel opener experimental profiles have since been described for diazoxide (200), pinacidil (9), and minoxidil (8).

Diazoxide

Diazoxide (7-chloro-1,2,4-benzothiadiazine-3-methyl-1, 1-dioxide) (Fig. 6A) is chemically related to the thiazide diuretics but has no diuretic activity (201). Orally administered diazoxide has antihypertensive efficacy in hypertensive dogs and rats (202). Although diazoxide is much less potent than chromakalim, it can cause profound hypotension accompanied by retention of sodium and water (201).

The hyperglycemia reported during diazoxide therapy has been correlated with such K^+ channel-opening effects as a hyperpolarization of the pancreatic β-cell membrane and an increase in ^{86}Rb efflux rate (5,6). This relative lack of specificity of action has contributed to the restriction of use of diazoxide to such acute therapy as hypertensive emergencies.

Minoxidil

Minoxidil (2,4-diamino-6-piperidinopyrimidine-3-oxide) (Fig. 6B) is an orally effective agent that effectively lowers blood pressure in normotensive animals as well as

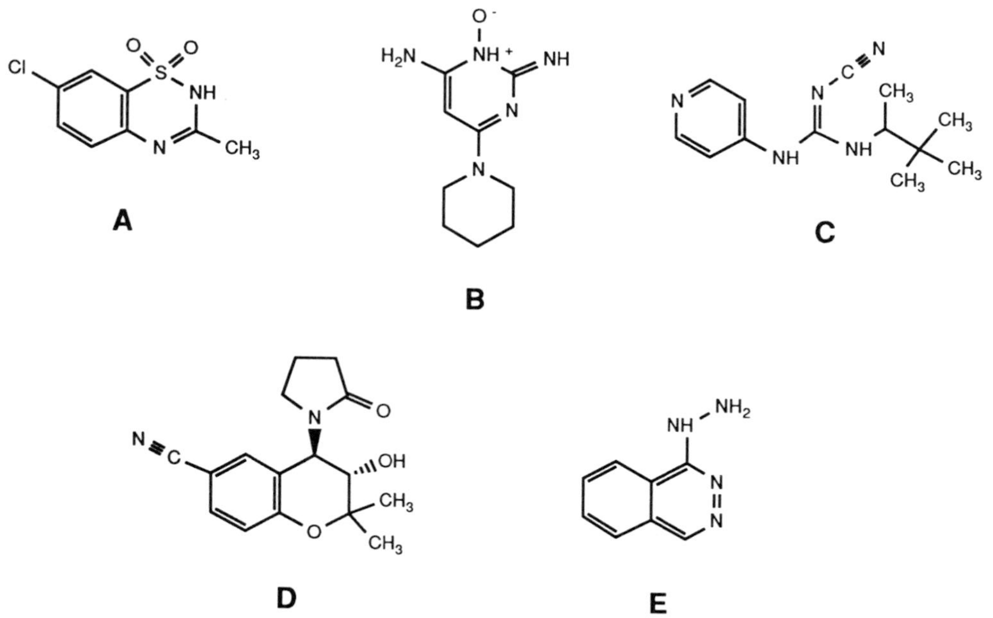

FIG. 6. Chemical structures of four K$^+$ channel openers (A–D) and hydralazine (E). The specific K$^+$ channel openers illustrated are diazoxide (A), minoxidil (B), pinacidil (C), and chromakalim (D).

in hypertensive animal models (203). Investigations on the mechanisms of action of minoxidil were impeded by the lack of *in vitro* activity of this agent until the relatively recent discovery that the compound was transformed *in vivo* to the active minoxidil sulfate form (see [8]). Minoxidil sulfate has been shown to increase ^{42}K efflux in rabbit aorta (8) and to have other cellular actions typical of a K$^+$ channel opener in vascular smooth muscle (7).

In addition to the fluid retention and reflex activation observed with vasodilators such as minoxidil (203), another side effect of this agent, hypertrichosis, has attracted considerable attention. The resulting use of minoxidil topically for male-pattern baldness has overshadowed its use in moderate-to-severe hypertension.

Pinacidil

Pinacidil (*N''*-cyano-*N*-4-pyridyl-*N'*-1,2,2-trimethylpropylguanidine) (Fig. 6C) is a clinically effective vasodilator when used as monotherapy or in combination with a diuretic to alleviate fluid retention (204,205). The pharmacology of pinacidil has been reviewed recently (206), and considerable evidence for a K$^+$ channel-opener mechanism of action for this agent has accumulated (5,9).

Chromakalim

Chromakalim (BRL 34915; 6-cyano-3,4-dihydro-2, 2-dimethyl-trans-4-(2-oxo-1-pyrrolidyl)-2H-benzo (b) pyran-3-ol) (Fig. 6D) is a K$^+$ channel opener currently in clinical development as an antihypertensive vasodilator and a bronchodilator (5). This agent shows a high degree of specificity for vascular and respiratory smooth muscle. The initial demonstration of the K$^+$ channel-opener mechanism for chromakalim (10,199) has been rapidly followed by numerous studies of all aspects of *in vitro* and *in vivo* activities. Both chromakalim and pinacidil show stereospecificity in their activity as K$^+$ channel openers with the (−) enantiomer exhibiting greater potency (9,207).

Nicorandil

Nicorandil (2-nicotinamidoethyl nitrate), a coronary vasodilator, should also be included with this group even though it has a mixed mechanism of action consisting of nitrate-like increases in cGMP (208) and K^+ channel-opening activity (209). This combination of vasodilator mechanisms results in a therapeutically useful agent.

Calcium Channel Blockers

The vasodilator properties of this group of agents have been discussed in detail elsewhere in this volume as well as in many reviews (e.g. [13,210]). The three agents most extensively studied as vasodilators and generally considered to be the "first generation" of calcium channel blockers are verapamil, nifedipine, and diltiazem. Many additional agents of the class are now in development. These "second-generation" compounds ideally would have longer durations of action with fewer side effects than the initial three agents. Among the currently most promising are nicardipine (211), nitrendipine (212,213), felodipine (214), and amlodipine (215).

Nitroprusside

Sodium nitroprusside (sodium nitroferricyanide) is a direct-acting vasodilator that, in contrast to other vasodilators, relaxes both arteriolar and venous smooth muscle. It is not absorbed orally, and systemic administration produces a readily reversible fall in systolic and diastolic blood pressure with decreases in total peripheral vascular resistance (216).

The mechanisms believed to account for the actions of nitroprusside have been discussed in several preceding sections. Briefly, multiple mechanisms of action include membrane hyperpolarization resulting from either activation of electrogenic pumping (217) or increased K^+ permeability (218), inhibition of Ca^{2+} influx through receptor-operated channels (12,14), and increased cellular concentrations of cGMP (79,153). The manner in which cGMP activation could be coupled to inhibition of Ca^{2+} mobilization is not clear, but this interaction could provide a biochemical and cellular basis for the observed actions of nitroprusside in vascular smooth muscle.

Hydralazine

Hydralazine (1-hydrazinophthalazine) (Fig. 6E) acts specifically on arteriolar resistance vessels, producing local increases in blood flow (219). Studies in sensitive peripheral arteries such as the rabbit renal artery (220) and the rat tail artery (221) indicate that the major portion of the activity of hydralazine results from direct activation of the arterial smooth muscle, although additional indirect effects on sympathetic neuronal transmission also have been reported (222).

The presence of vasodilation-induced side effects (sodium and water retention, tachycardia) and enhanced sympathetic tone with hydralazine have led to concurrent use of adrenergic antagonists and diuretics. There is no evidence that hydralazine affects membrane channels or cGMP, as has been reported for other vasodilators.

SUMMARY AND CONCLUSIONS

A considerable number of membrane and intracellular mechanisms important for the sequence of events leading to contraction can be identified in the vascular smooth muscle cell. Specific blockage or activation of a particular cell membrane mechanism has been clearly linked to clinical efficacy for a number of currently employed vasodilators. The ability to increase the open-state probability of the vascular K^+ channel (minoxidil, pinacidil, chromakalim), to block the slow-inactivating, voltage-dependent Ca^{2+} channel (verapamil, diltiazem, nifedipine, and their analogs), and to activate cGMP and inhibit the associated receptor-linked Ca^{2+} mobilization (nitroprusside) can, for each mechanism, elicit vasodilation and decreased blood pressure.

Thus, potent and efficacious vasodilators currently available act by opening vascular K^+ channels or blocking voltage sensitive Ca^{2+} channels. The focus of further efforts in both of these areas is to develop second- and third-generation compounds that have similar activity as vasodilators but with increased bioavailability, duration, and vascular selectivity as well as fewer side effects of the type (e.g., fluid retention, tachycardia) that has decreased the clinical attractiveness of current vasodilators. Activity in these research areas is extensive, and numerous new agents can be anticipated within the next several years.

Increased understanding of the biochemical and cellular basis of the action of nitroprusside and other organic nitrates has attracted increasing interest as it has become apparent that such potentially significant physiological regulatory substances as ANF and EDRF may exert their potent vasodilatory actions at similar loci. In particular, the critical role of the endothelium in the genesis and course of vascular hypertension is the focus of extensive current research, and the implications of changes in endothelial function are only beginning to be elucidated. It has become evident that most vasodilators are influenced in some manner by the endothelium. Those vasodilators that act on the endothelium (i.e., release an EDRF) may have altered efficacy in disease states associated with endothelial damage. In preclinical models of hypertension, both structural and functional alterations in the vascular endothelium have been documented and, at least *in vitro*, endothelium-dependent vasodilators exhibit a diminished efficacy (175). Endothelium-independent vasodilators such as the nitrovasodilators are equally efficacious in vessels from hypertensive and normotensive animals (175).

Because several vasoconstrictor autacoids can also release an EDRF, endothelium damage in hypertension (or atherosclerosis) could explain, in part, the heightened vascular reactivity observed in those disease states (223). A corollary is that vasodilator agents that act on the endothelium (i.e., release an EDRF) would be less effective in hypertensive patients when compared with compounds with direct actions on vascular smooth muscle. Normalization of blood pressure, in preclinical models of hypertension, can restore full efficacy to endothelium-dependent vasodilators (224), although it is not clear if this restoration can occur following chronic, sustained hypertension.

As was discussed previously, no current antihypertensive agents in clinical use act primarily by inhibition of vascular contractile protein interactions. In recent years, a remarkable amplification of our knowledge of smooth muscle contractile regulation has occurred, and a number of intracellular systems have been identified as potential targets for drug discovery. The most attractive initial areas include direct modulation of MLC activity, protein kinase C inhibition, and calmodulin antagonism. The appropriateness of modulation of such general physiological regulatory systems to elicit specific vasodilation without deleterious side effects remains to be verified. However, similar reservations were expressed at early stages in the development of voltage-sensitive Ca^{2+} blockers and, as differences in Ca^{2+} mobilization mechanisms between smooth muscle and other excitable cells and among different types of smooth muscle emerged, increased understanding of the diversity of membrane-associated mechanisms has moderated these reservations. As increased knowledge of the diversity of cellular biochemical mechanisms becomes available and potent selective inhibitors emerge, development of new types of selective vasodilators may well also assume increased attractiveness.

Similar questions of specificity as well as efficacy are currently of concern in considering agents with activity on second messenger systems (e.g., selective PDE inhibitors, phosphatidylinositol cycle modulators, inhibitors of intracellular Ca^{2+} release). Because different systems may well have varied importance in regulation of specific types of smooth muscle, the potential emergence of an agent with an advantageous vasodilator profile remains a distinct possibility.

REFERENCES

1. Jones AW. Content and fluxes of electrolytes. In: Bohr D, Somlyo AP, Sparks, Jr HV, eds. *Handbook of physiology, section 2: the cardiovascular system, vol II, vascular smooth muscle.* Bethesda: American Physiological Society, 1980;253–299.
2. Johansson B, Somlyo AP. Electrophysiology and excitation-contraction coupling. In: Bohn D, Somlyo AP, Sparks Jr HV, eds. *Handbook of physiology, section 2: the cardiovascular system, vol II, vascular smooth muscle.* Bethesda: American Physiological Society, 1980;301–323.
3. Hille B. Potassium channels and chloride channels. In: Hille B, *Ionic channels of excitable membranes.* Sunderland, MA: Sinauer Association, 1984;99–116.
4. Weiss GB. Stimulation with high potassium. In: Daniel EE, Paton DM, eds. *Methods in pharmacology, vol 3: smooth muscle.* New York: Plenum, 1975;339–345.
5. Cook NS. The pharmacology of potassium channels and their therapeutic potential. *Trends Pharmacol Sci* 1988;9:21–28.
6. Trube G, Rorsman P, Ohno-Shosaku T. Opposite effects of tolbutamide and diazoxide on the ATP-dependent K^+ channel in mouse pancreatic β-cells. *Pflugers Arch* 1986;407:493–499.
7. Winquist RJ, Heaney LA, Wallace AA, et al. Glyburide blocks the relaxation response to BRL 34915 (chromakalim), minoxidil sulfate and diazoxide in vascular smooth muscle. *J Pharmacol Exp Ther* 1989;248:149–156.
8. Meisheri KD, Cipkus LA, Taylor CJ. Mechanism of action of minoxidil sulfate-induced vasodilation: a role for increased K^+ permeability. *J Pharmacol Exp Ther* 1988;245:751–760.
9. Southerton JS, Weston AH, Bray KM, Newgreen DT, Taylor SG. The potassium channel opening action of pinacidil: studies using biochemical, ion flux and microelectrode techniques. *Naunyn Schmiedebergs Arch Pharmacol* 1988;338:310–318.
10. Hamilton TC, Weir SW, Weston AH. Comparison of the effects of BRL 34915 and verapamil on electrical and mechanical activity in rat portal vein. *Br J Pharmacol* 1986;88:103–111.
11. Karaki H, Weiss GB. Calcium release in smooth muscle. *Life Sci* 1988;42:111–122.
12. Karaki H, Weiss GB. Calcium channels in smooth muscle. *Gastroenterology* 1984;87:960–970.
13. Fleckenstein A. Calcium antagonism, a basic principle of drug-induced smooth muscle relaxation. In: Fleckenstein A, *Calcium antagonism in heart and smooth muscle.* New York: Wiley, 1983;209–285.
14. Karaki H, Weiss GB. Effects of stimulatory agents on mobilization of high and low affinity site ^{45}Ca in rabbit aortic smooth muscle. *J Pharmacol Exp Ther* 1980;231:450–455.
15. Karaki H, Nakagawa H, Urakawa N. Comparative effects of verapamil and sodium nitroprusside on contraction and ^{45}Ca uptake in the smooth muscle of rabbit aorta, rat aorta and guinea pig taenia coli. *Br J Pharmacol* 1984;81:393–400.
16. Godfraind T. EDRF and cyclic GMP control gating of receptor-operated calcium channels in vascular smooth muscle. *Eur J Pharmacol* 1986;126:341–343.
17. Winquist RJ, Faison EP, Nutt RF. Vasodilator profile of synthetic atrial natriuretic factor. *Eur J Pharmacol* 1984;102:169–173.
18. Taylor CJ, Meisheri KD. Inhibitory effects of a synthetic atrial peptide on contractions and ^{45}Ca fluxes in vascular smooth muscle. *J Pharmacol Exp Ther* 1986;237:803–808.
19. Murad F. Cyclic guanosine monophosphate as a mediator of vasodilation. *J Clin Invest* 1986;78:1–5.
20. Collins P, Griffith TM, Henderson AH, Lewis MJ. Endothelium-derived relaxing factor alters calcium fluxes in rabbit aorta: a cyclic guanosine monophosphate-mediated effect. *J Physiol (Lond)* 1986;381:427–437.
21. Collins P, Henderson AH, Lang D, Lewis MJ. Endothelium-derived relaxing factor and nitroprusside compared in noradrenaline- and K^+-contracted rabbit and rat aortae. *J Physiol (Lond)* 1988;400:395–404.
22. Minneman KP. α_1-Adrenergic receptor subtypes, inositol phosphates, and sources of cell Ca^{2+}. *Pharmacol Rev* 1988;40:87–119.
23. Smith CWJ, Pritchard K, Marston SB. The mechanism of Ca^{2+} regulation of vascular smooth muscle thin filaments by caldesmon and calmodulin. *J Biol Chem* 1987;262:116–122.
24. Small JV, Sobieszek A. The contractile apparatus of smooth muscle. *Int Rev Cytol* 1980;64:241–306.
25. Somlyo AV. Ultrastructure of vascular smooth muscle. In: Bohr DF, Somlyo AP, Sparks Jr HV, eds. *Handbook of physiology, section 2: the cardiovascular system, vol II: vascular smooth muscle.* Bethesda: American Physiological Society, 1980;33–67.
26. Persechini A, Kamm KE, Stull JT. Different phosphorylated forms of myosin in contracting tracheal smooth muscle. *Biophys J* 1986;49:389a.

27. Kamm KE, Stull JT. The function of myosin and myosin light chain kinase phosphorylation in smooth muscle. *Annu Rev Pharmacol Toxicol* 1985;25:593–620.

28. Walsh MP. Calcium regulation of smooth muscle contraction. In: Marme D, ed. *Calcium and cell physiology*. Berlin: Springer-Verlag, 1985;170–203.

29. Silver PJ. Regulation of contractile activity in vascular smooth muscle by protein kinases. *Rev Basic Clinical Pharmacol* 1985;5:341–396.

30. Silver PJ, Stull JT. Phosphorylation of myosin light chain and phosphorylase in tracheal smooth muscle in response to KCl and carbachol. *Mol Pharmacol* 1984;25:267–274.

31. Morgan JP, Morgan KG. Stimulus-specific patterns of intracellular calcium levels in smooth muscle of ferret portal vein. *J Physiol (Lond)* 1984;351:155–167.

32. Dillon PF, Aksoy MO, Driska SP, Murphy RA. Myosin phosphorylation and the cross-bridge cycle in arterial smooth muscle. *Science* 1981;211:495–497.

33. Aksoy MO, Murphy RA, Kamm KE. Role of Ca^{2+} and myosin light chain phosphorylation in regulation of smooth muscle. *Am J Physiol* 1982;242:C109–C116.

34. Nonomura Y, Ebashi S. Calcium regulatory mechanism in vertebrate smooth muscle. *Biomed Res* 1980;1:1–14.

35. Marston SB. The regulation of smooth muscle contractile proteins. *Prog Biophys Mol Biol* 1982;41:1–41.

36. Sobue K, Muramoto Y, Fujita M, Kakiuchi S. Purification of a calmodulin-binding protein from chicken gizzard that interacts with F-actin. *Proc Natl Acad Sci USA* 1981;78:5652–5655.

37. Ngai PK, Walsh MP. Inhibition of smooth muscle actin-activated myosin Mg^{2+}-ATPase by caldesmon. *J Biol Chem* 1984;259:13656–13659.

38. Rasmussen H, Takuwa Y, Park S. Protein kinase C in the regulation of smooth muscle contraction. *FASEB J* 1987;1:177–185.

39. Griendling KK, Rittenhouse SE, Brock TA, et al. Sustained diacylglycerol formation from inositol phospholipids in angiotensin II-stimulated vascular smooth muscle cells. *J Biol Chem* 1986;261:5901–5906.

40. Takuwa Y, Takuwa N, Rasmussen H. Carbachol induces a rapid and sustained hydrolysis of polyphosphoinositides in bovine tracheal muscle. *J Biol Chem* 1986;261:14670–14675.

41. Forder J, Scriabine A, Rasmussen H. Plasma membrane calcium flux, protein kinase C activation and smooth muscle contraction. *J Pharmacol Exp Ther* 1985;235:267–273.

42. Danthuluri NR, Deth RC. Phorbol ester-induced contraction of arterial smooth muscle and inhibition of α-adrenergic response. *Biochem Biophys Res Commun* 1984;125:1103–1109.

43. Chatterjee M, Tejada M. Phorbol ester-induced contraction in chemically-skinned vascular smooth muscle. *Am J Physiol* 1986;251:C356–C361.

44. Parks S, Rasmussen H. Carbachol-induced protein phosphorylation changes in bovine tracheal smooth muscle. *J Biol Chem* 1986;261:15734–15739.

45. Chatterjee M, Foster CJ. Activation of protein kinase C and contraction in skinned vascular smooth muscle. In: Siegman MJ, Somlyo SP, Stephens NL, eds. *Regulation and contraction of smooth muscle (Prog Clin Biol Res)*. New York, AR Liss, 1987;219–231.

46. Silver PJ, Lepore RE, Cumiskey WR, Kiefer D, Harris AL. Protein kinase C activity and reactivity to phorbol ester in vascular smooth muscle from spontaneously hypertensive rats (SHR) and normotensive Wistar Kyoto rats (WKY). *Biochem Biophys Res Commun* 1988; 154:272–277.

47. Strebinska M, Ikebe M, Hartshorne DJ. Trypic hydrolysis of myosin light chain kinase: conversion of calmodulin-dependent to calmodulin-independent forms. *Biophys J* 1986;49:66a.

48. Kemp BE, Pearson RB, Guerriero V, Bagchi IC, Means AR. The calmodulin binding domain of chicken smooth muscle myosin light chain kinase contains a pseudosubstrate sequence. *J Biol Chem* 1987;262:2542–2548.

49. Moreland S, Hunt JT. Analogs of the calmodulin binding site of myosin light chain (MLC) kinase. *FASEB J* 1987;46:1098.

50. Foster CJ, Gaeta FCA. The calmodulin binding domain of chicken gizzard myosin light-chain kinase contains two non-overlapping active site directed inhibitory sequences. *Biophys J* 1988;53:182a.

51. Hidaka H, Inagaki M, Kawamoto S, Sasaki Y. Isoquinolinesulfonamides, novel and potent inhibitors of cyclic nucleotide dependent protein kinase and protein kinase C. *Biochemistry* 1984;23:5036–5041.

52. Kawamoto S, Hidaka H. 1-(5-isoquinolinesulfonyl)-2-methyl-piperazine (H-7) is a selective inhibitor of protein kinase C in rabbit platelets. *Biochem Biophys Res Commun* 1984;125:258–264.

53. Asano T, Hidaka H. Vasodilatory action of HA 1004 [N-(2-guanidinoethyl)-5-isoquinolinesulfonamide], a novel calcium antagonist with no effect on cardiac function. *J Pharmacol Exp Ther* 1984;231:141–145.

54. Saitoh M, Ishikawa T, Matsushima S, Naka M, Hidaka H. Selective inhibition of catalytic activity of smooth muscle myosin light chain kinase. *J Biol Chem* 1987;262:7796–7803.

55. Asano T, Hidaka H. Intracellular Ca^{2+} antagonist, HA 1004: pharmacological properties different from those of nicardipine. *J Pharmacol Exp Ther* 1985;233:454–458.

56. Tanaka T, Umekuwa H, Saitoh M, et al. Modulation of calmodulin function and of Ca^{2+}-induced smooth muscle contraction by the calmodulin antagonist, HT-74. *Mol Pharmacol* 1986;29:264–269.

57. Prozialeck WC. Structure-activity relationships of calmodulin antagonists. *Annu Rep Med Chem* 1983;18:203–212.

58. Hidaka H, Tanaka T. Naphthalenesulfonam-

ides as calmodulin antagonists. In: Means AR, O'Malley BW, eds. *Methods in enzymology, vol 102. Calmodulin and calcium-binding proteins.* New York: Academic Press, 1983;185–194.

59. Roufogalis BD. Calmodulin antagonism. In: Marme D, ed. *Calcium and cell physiology.* Berlin: Springer-Verlag, 1985;148–168.

60. Mannold R. Calmodulin—structure, function and drug action. *Drugs of the Future* 1984;9:677–690.

61. Van Belle H. R24571: a potent inhibitor of calmodulin-activated enzymes. *Cell Calcium* 1981;2:483–494.

62. DeLorenzo RJ, Burdette S, Holderness J. Benzodiazepine inhibition of the calcium-calmodulin protein kinase system in brain membrane. *Science* 1981;213:546–549.

63. Johnson JD, Fugman DA. Calcium and calmodulin antagonists binding to calmodulin and relaxation of coronary segments. *J Pharmacol Exp Ther* 1983;226:330–334.

64. Silver PJ, Dachiw J, Ambrose JM, Pinto PB. Effects of the calcium antagonists perhexiline and cinnarizine on vascular and cardiac contractile protein function. *J Pharmacol Exp Ther* 1985;234:629–635.

65. Silver PJ, Connell ML, Dillon KM, Cumiskey WR, Volberg WA, Ezrin AM. Inhibition of calmodulin and protein kinase C by amiodarone and other class III antiarrhythmic agents. *Cardiovasc Drug Ther* 1989;3:675–682.

66. Johnson JD. Allosteric interactions among drug binding sites on calmodulin. *Biochem Biophys Res Commun* 1983;112:787–793.

67. Inagaki M, Hidaka H. Two types of calmodulin antagonists: a structure related interaction. *Pharmacology* 1984;29:75–84.

68. Norman JA, Drummond AH, Moser P. Inhibition of calcium-dependent regulator-stimulated phosphodiesterase activity by neuroleptic drugs is unrelated to their clinical efficacy. *Mol Pharmacol* 1979;16:1089–1094.

69. Silver PJ, Dachiw J, Ambrose JA. Effects of calcium antagonists and vasodilators on arterial myosin phosphorylation and actin-myosin interactions. *J Pharmacol Exp Ther* 1984; 230:141–148.

70. Jacobs M. Mechanism of action of hydralazine on vascular smooth muscle. *Biochem Pharmacol* 1984;33:2915–2919.

71. Doctrow SR, Lowenstein M. Adenosine and 5'-chloro-5'-deoxyadenosine inhibit the phosphorylation of phosphatidylinositol and myosin light chain of calf aorta smooth muscle. *J Biol Chem* 1985;260:3469–3476.

72. Silver PJ, Ambrose JM, Michalak J, Dachiw J. Effects of felodipine, nitrendipine and W-7 on arterial myosin phosphorylation, actin-myosin interactions and contraction. *Eur J Pharmacol* 1984;104:417–424.

73. Silver PJ, Sulkowski T, Lappe RW, Wendt RL. Wy-46,300 and Wy-46,531: vascular smooth muscle relaxant/antihypertensive agents with combined Ca^{2+} antagonist/myosin phosphorylation inhibitory mechanisms. *J Cardiovasc Pharmacol* 1986;8:1168–1175.

74. Silver PJ, Fenichel R, Wendt RL. Structural variants of verapamil and W-7 with combined Ca^{2+} entry blockade/myosin phosphorylation inhibitory mechanisms. *J Cardiovasc Pharmacol* 1988;11:299–307.

75. Gietzen K, Sadorf I, Bader J. A model for the regulation of the calmodulin-dependent enzymes erythrocyte Ca^{2+}-transport ATPase and brain phosphodiesterase by activators and inhibitors. *Biochem J* 1982;207:541–548.

76. Nakajima T, Katoh A. Selective calmodulin inhibition toward myosin light chain kinase by a new cerebral circulation improver, Ro 22-4839. *Mol Pharmacol* 1987;32:140–146.

77. Zimmer M, Hofmann F. Calmodulin antagonists inhibit activity of myosin light-chain kinase independent of calmodulin. *Eur J Biochem* 1984;142:393–397.

78. Katsuki S, Arnold WP, Mittal C, Murad F. Stimulation of guanylate cyclase activity by sodium nitroprusside, nitroglycerin and nitric oxide in various tissue preparations and comparison to the effects of sodium azide and hydroxylamine. *J Cyc Nuc Res* 1977;3:23–35.

79. Ignarro LJ, Lipton H, Edwards JC, et al. Mechanism of vascular smooth muscle relaxation by organic nitrates, nitrites, nitroprusside and nitric oxide: evidence for the involvement of S-nitrosothiols as active intermediates. *J Pharmacol Exp Ther* 1981;218:739–749.

80. Brien JF, McLaughlin BE, Breedon TH, Bennett BM, Nakatsu K, Marks GS. Biotransformation of glyceryl trinitrate occurs concurrently with relaxation of rabbit aorta. *J Pharmacol Exp Ther* 1986;237:608–614.

81. Tremblay J, Gerzer R, Pang SC, Cantin M, Genest J, Hamet P. ANF stimulation of detergent-dispersed particulate guanylate cyclase from bovine adrenal cortex. *FEBS Lett* 1985;194:210–214.

82. Kuno T, Andersen JW, Kamisaki U, et al. Copurification of an atrial naturiuretic factor receptor and particulate guanylate cyclase from rat lung. *J Biol Chem* 1986;261:5817–5823.

83. Beavo JA. Multiple isozymes of cyclic nucleotide phosphodiesterase. *Adv Second Messenger Phosphoprotein Res* 1988;22:1–38.

84. Weishaar RE, Cain MH, Bristol JA. A new generation of phosphodiesterase inhibitors: multiple molecular forms of phosphodiesterases and the potential for drug selectivity. *J Med Chem* 1985;28:537–545.

85. Silver PJ, Harris AL. Phosphodiesterase isozyme inhibitors and vascular smooth muscle. In: Halpern W, Brayden J, McLaughlin N, et al, eds. *Proceedings of the Second International Symposium on Resistance Vessels.* Ithaca, NY: Perinatology Press, 1988;284–291.

86. Kauffman RF, Schenck KM, Utterback BG, Crowe VG, Cohen MC. *In vitro* vascular relaxation by new inotropic agents: relationship to phosphodiesterase inhibition and cyclic nucleotides. *J Pharmacol Exp Ther* 1987;242:864–872.

87. Silver PJ, Lepore RE, O'Connor B, et al. Inhi-

bition of the low K_m cAMP phosphodiesterase and activation of the cyclic AMP system in vascular smooth muscle by milrinone. *J Pharmacol Exp Ther* 1988;247:34–42.

88. O'Connor B, Silver PJ. Inhibition of guinea pig aortic sarcolemmal Ca^{2+}-Mg^{2+} ATPase and cAMP phosphodiesterase activity by milrinone. *Drug Dev Res* 1990;19:435–442.

89. Prigent AF, Fougier S, Nemoz G, et al. Comparison of cyclic nucleotide phosphodiesterase isoforms from rat heart and bovine aorta. Separation and inhibition by selective reference phosphodiesterase inhibitors. *Biochem Pharmacol* 1988;37:3671–3681.

90. Silver PJ, Hamel LT, Perrone MH, Bentley RG, Bushover CR, Evans DB. Differential pharmacologic sensitivity of cyclic nucleotide phosphodiesterase isozymes isolated from cardiac muscle, arterial and airway smooth muscle. *Eur J Pharmacol* 1988;150:85–94.

91. Lugnier C, Schoeffter P, LeBec A, Strouthou E, Stoclet JC. Selective inhibition of cyclic nucleotide phosphodiesterases of human, bovine and rat aorta. *Biochem Pharmacol* 1986;35:1743–1751.

92. Martin W, Furchgott RF, Villani GM, Jothianandan D. Phosphodiesterase inhibitors induce endothelium-dependent relaxation of rat and rabbit aorta by spontaneously released endothelium-derived relaxing factor. *J Pharmacol Exp Ther* 1986;237:539–547.

93. Harris AL, Lemp BM, Bentley RG, Perrone MH, Hamel LT, Silver PJ. Phosphodiesterase isozyme inhibition and the potentiation by zaprinast of endothelium-derived relaxing factor and guanylate cyclase stimulatory agents in vascular smooth muscle. *J Pharmacol Exp Ther* 1989;249:394–400.

94. Buchholz RA, Dundore RL, Pratt PF, Hallenbeck WD, Wassey ML, Silver PJ. The selective phosphodiesterase I inhibitor zaprinast (ZAP) potentiates the hypotensive effect of sodium nitroprusside (SNP) in conscious SHR. *FASEB J* 1989;3:1186.

95. Walsh DA, Perkins JP, Krebs EG. An adenosine 3′,5′monophosphate-dependent protein kinase from rabbit skeletal muscle. *J Biol Chem* 1968;243:3763–3774.

96. Kuo JF, Greengard P. Cyclic nucleotide-dependent protein kinases. IV. Widespread occurrence of adenosine 3′,5′-monophosphate-dependent protein kinase in various tissues and phyla of the animal kingdom. *Proc Natl Acad Sci USA* 1969;64:1349–1355.

97. Walsh DA, Cooper RH. The physiological regulation and function of cAMP-dependent protein kinases. *Biochem Actions Hormones* 1979;6:1–75.

98. Silver PJ, Michalak RJ, Kocmund SM. Role of cyclic AMP protein kinase in decreased arterial cyclic AMP responsiveness in hypertension. *J Pharmacol Exp Ther* 1986;232:595–601.

99. Corbin JD, Keely SL, Soderling TR, Park CR. Hormonal regulation of adenosine 3′,5′-monophosphate-dependent protein kinase. *Adv Cyclic Nucleotide Protein Phosphorylation Res* 1975;5:265–279.

100. Silver PJ, Schmidt-Silver CJ, DiSalvo J. β-adrenergic relaxation and cAMP kinase activation in coronary arterial smooth muscle. *Am J Physiol* 1982;242:H177–H184.

101. Silver PJ, Walus K, DiSalvo J. Adenosine-mediated relaxation and activation of cyclic AMP-dependent protein kinase in coronary arterial smooth muscle. *J Pharmacol Exp Ther* 1984;228:342–347.

102. Vegesna RV, Diamond J. Effects of isoproterenol and forskolin on tension, cyclic AMP levels, and cyclic AMP dependent protein kinase activity in bovine coronary artery. *Can J Physiol Pharmacol* 1984;62:1116–1123.

103. Kikkawawa F, Furuta T, Ishikawa N, Shigei T. Different types of relationships between β-adrenergic relaxation and activation of cyclic AMP-dependent protein kinase in canine saphenous and portal veins. *Eur J Pharmacol* 1986;128:187–194.

104. Kuo JF, Greengard P. Cyclic nucleotide-dependent protein kinases. VI. Isolation and partial purification of a protein kinase activated by guanosine 3′,5′-monophosphate. *J Biol Chem* 1970;245:2493–2498.

105. Kuo JF. Guanosine 3′,5′-monophosphate-dependent protein kinases in mammalian tissues. *Proc Natl Acad Sci USA* 1974;71:4037–4041.

106. Fiscus RR, Rapoport RM, Waldman SA, Murad F. Atriopeptin II elevates cyclic GMP, activates cyclic GMP-dependent protein kinase and causes relaxation in rat thoracic aorta. *Biochem Biophys Acta* 1985;846:179–184.

107. Adelstein RS, Conti MA, Hathaway DR, Klee CB. Phosphorylation of smooth muscle myosin light chain kinase by the catalytic subunit of adenosine 3′,5′-monophosphate-dependent protein kinase. *J Biol Chem* 1978;253:8347–8350.

108. Silver PJ, DiSalvo J. Adenosine 3′,5-monophosphate-mediated inhibition of myosin light chain phosphorylation in bovine aortic actomyosin. *J Biol Chem* 1979;254:9951–9954.

109. Vallet B, Molla A, Demaille JG. Cyclic adenosine 3′,5′-monophosphate-dependent regulation of purified bovine aortic calcium/calmodulin-dependent myosin light chain kinase. *Biochim Biophys Acta* 1981;674:256–264.

110. Nishikawa M, deLanerolle P, Lincoln TM, Adelstein RS. Phosphorylation of mammalian myosin chain kinase by the catalytic subunit of cyclic AMP-dependent protein kinase and by cyclic GMP-dependent protein kinase. *J Biol Chem* 1984;259:8429–8436.

111. Ikebe M, Inagaki M, Kanamaru K, Hidaka H. Phosphorylation of smooth muscle light chain kinase by Ca^{2+}-activated, phospholipid-dependent protein kinase. *J Biol Chem* 1985;260:4547–4550.

112. Miller JR, Silver PJ, Stull JT. The role of myosin light chain kinase phosphorylation in beta-adrenergic relaxation of tracheal smooth muscle. *Mol Pharmacol* 1983;24:235–242.

113. Gerthoffer WT, Trevethick MA, Murphy RA. Myosin phosphorylation and cyclic adenosine

3′,5-monophosphate in relaxation of arterial smooth muscle by vasodilators. *Circ Res* 1984; 54:83–89.

114. Webb RC, Bhalla RC. Calcium sequestration by subcellular fractions isolated from vascular smooth muscle. Effect of cyclic nucleotides and prostaglandins. *J Mol Cell Cardiol* 1976;8: 145–157.

115. Kattenburg DM, Daniel EE. Effect of an endogenous cyclic AMP-dependent protein kinase catalytic subunit on Ca-uptake by plasma membrane vesicles from rat mesenteric artery. *Blood Vessels* 1984;21:257–266.

116. Rashatwar SS, Cornwell TL, Lincoln TM. Effects of 8-bromo cGMP on Ca^{2+} levels in vascular smooth muscle cells. Possible regulation of Ca^{2+}-ATPase by cGMP-dependent protein kinase. *Proc Natl Acad Sci USA* 1987;84: 5685–5689.

117. Cornwell TL, Lincoln TM. Regulation of phosphorylase A formation and calcium content in aortic smooth muscle and muscle cells: effects of atrial natriuretic peptide II. *J Pharmacol Exp Ther* 1988;247:524–530.

118. Rapoport RM. Cyclic guanosine monophosphate inhibition of contraction may be mediated through inhibition of phosphatidylinositol hydrolysis in rat aorta. *Circ Res* 1986; 58:407–410.

119. Meisheri KD, Taylor CJ, Saneii H. Synthetic atrial natriuretic peptide inhibits intracellular calcium release in smooth muscle. *Am J Physiol* 1986;250:C171–C174.

120. Meisheri KD, Van Breeman C. Effects of β-adrenergic stimulation on calcium movements in rabbit aortic smooth muscle: relationship with cyclic AMP. *J Physiol (Lond)* 1982;331: 429–441.

121. Collins P, Griffith TM, Henderson HH, Lewis MJ. Endothelium-derived relaxing factor alters calcium fluxes in rabbit aorta: a cyclic guanosine monophosphate-mediated effect. *J Physiol (Lond)* 1986;381:427–437.

122. Scheid CR, Fay FS. β-Adrenergic effects on transmembrane ^{45}Ca fluxes in isolated smooth muscle cells. *Am J Physiol* 1984;246:C431–C438.

123. Popescu LM, Panoiu C, Hinescu M, Nutu O. The mechanism of cGMP-induced relaxation in vascular smooth muscle. *Eur J Pharmacol* 1985;107:393–394.

124. Jones AW, Bylund DB, Forte LR. cAMP-dependent reduction in membrane fluxes during relaxation of arterial smooth muscle. *Am J Physiol* 1984;246:H306–H311.

125. Scheid CR, Fay FS. β-Adrenergic stimulation of ^{42}K influx in isolated smooth muscle cells. *Am J Physiol* 1984;246:C415–C421.

126. Scheid CR, Honeyman TW, Fay FS. Mechanism of β-adrenergic relaxation of smooth muscle. *Nature* 1979;277:32–36.

127. Ives HE, Casnellie JE, Greengard P, Jamieson JD. Subcellular localization of cyclic GMP-dependent protein kinase and its substrates in vascular smooth muscle. *J Biol Chem* 1980; 255:3777–3785.

128. Casnellie JE, Ives HE, Jamieson JD, Greengard P. Cyclic cGMP-dependent protein phosphorylation in intact medial tissue and isolated cells from vascular smooth muscle. *J Biol Chem* 1986;255:3770–3776.

129. Silver PJ, Kocmund SM, Pinto PB. Enhanced phosphorylation of arterial particulate proteins by cyclic nucleotides and human atrial natriuretic factor. *Eur J Pharmacol* 1986;122:385–386.

130. Suematsu H, Hirata M, Kuriyama H. Effects of cAMP- and cGMP-dependent protein kinases, and calmodulin on Ca^{2+} uptake by highly purified sarcolemmal vesicles of vascular smooth muscle. *Biochim Biophys Acta* 1984;773:83–90.

131. Rapoport RM, Draznin MB, Murad F. Sodium nitroprusside-induced protein phosphorylation in intact rat aorta is mimicked by 8-bromo cyclic GMP. *Proc Natl Acad Sci USA* 1982;79: 6470–6474.

132. Rapoport RM, Draznin MB, Murad F. Endothelium-dependent relaxation in rat aorta may be mediated through cGMP-dependent protein phosphorylation. *Nature* 1983;306:174–176.

133. Williams DL, Katz GM, Roy-Contancin L, Reuben JP. Guanosine 5′-monophosphate modulates gating of high conductance Ca^{2+}-activated K^+ channels in vascular smooth muscle cells. *Proc Natl Acad Sci USA* 1988;85:9360–9364.

134. Rasmussen H, Barrett PQ. Calcium messenger system: an integrated view. *Physiol Rev* 1984; 64:938–984.

135. Exton JH. Role of calcium and phosphoinositides in the action of certain hormones and neurotransmitters. *J Clin Invest* 1985;75:1753–1757.

136. Berridge MJ. Inositol triphosphate and diacylglyerol as second messengers. *Biochem J* 1984;220:345–360.

137. Alexander RW, Brock TA, Gimbrone MA, Rittenhouse SE. Angiotensin increases inositol triphosphate and calcium in vascular smooth muscle. *Hypertension* 1985;7:447–451.

138. Janis RA, Silver PJ, Triggle DT. Drug action and cellular calcium regulation. *Adv Drug Res* 1987;16:311–591.

139. Hillard CJ, Hrug PW, Gross GJ. Comparison of the vasodilation and inhibition of phosphatidylinositol hydrolysis produced by KT-362 and TMB-8 in canine femoral artery. *Circulation (in press)*.

140. Shibata S, Wakabayashi S, Satake N, Hester RK, Ueda S, Tomiyama A. Mode of vasorelaxing action of 5-[3-[[2-(3,4-dimethoxyphenyl)-ethyl] amino]-1-oxopropyl]-2,3,4,5-tetrahydro-1,5-benzothiazepine fumarate (KT-363), a new intracellular calcium antagonist. *J Pharmacol Exp Ther* 1987;240:16–22.

141. Kase H, Iwahashi K, Matsuda Y. K252a, potent inhibitor of protein kinase C from microbial origin. *J Antibiotics* 1986;39:1059–1065.

142. Hachisu M, Hiranuma T, Sagawa S, Koyama M, Nishio M. Antihypertensive activity of SF 2370 derivatives, a potent protein kinase C inhibitor. *Jpn J Pharmacol* 1987;43(suppl): 295P.

143. Nishizuka Y. The molecular heterogeneity of

protein kinase C and its implications for cellular regulation. *Nature* 1988;334:661–665.

144. Cabot MC, Jaken S. Structural and chemical specificity of diacylglycerols for protein kinase C activation. *Biochem Biophys Res Commun* 1984;125:163–169.

145. Kraft AS, Reeves JA, Ashendel CL. Differing modulation of protein kinase C by bryostatin 1 and phorbol esters in JB6 mouse epidermal cells. *J Biol Chem* 1988;263:8437–8442.

146. Kariya K, Kawahara Y, Tsuda T, Fukuzaki H, Takai Y. Possible involvement of protein kinase C in platelet-derived growth factor-stimulated DNA synthesis in vascular smooth muscle cells. *Atherosclerosis* 1987;63:251–255.

147. Bowen-Pope DF, Ross R, Seifert RA. Logically acting growth factors for vascular smooth muscle cells: endogenous synthesis and release from platelets. *Circulation* 1985;72:735–740.

148. Furchgott RF, Zawadzki JV. The obligatory role of endothelial cells in the relaxation of arterial smooth muscle by acetylcholine. *Nature* 1980;288:373–376.

149. Griffith TM, Edwards DH, Lewis MJ, Newby AC, Henderson AH. The nature of the endothelium-derived vascular relaxant factor. *Nature* 1984;308:645–647.

150. Cocks TM, Angus JA, Campbell HJ, Campbell GR. Release and properties of endothelium-derived relaxing factor (EDRF) from endothelial cells in culture. *J Cell Physiol* 1985;123:310–320.

151. Rapoport RM, Murad F. Agonist-induced endothelium-dependent relaxations in rat thoracic aorta may be mediated through cGMP. *Circ Res* 1983;52:352–357.

152. Martin W, Villani GM, Jothianandan D, Furchgott RF. Selective blockade of endothelium-dependent and glyceryl trinitrate-induced relaxation by hemoglobin and by methylene blue in the rabbit aorta. *J Pharmacol Exp Ther* 1985;232:708–716.

153. Katsuki S, Arnold WP, Murad F. Effects of sodium nitroprusside, nitroglycerin, and sodium azide on levels of cyclic nucleotides and mechanical activity of various tissues. *J Cyclic Nucleotide Res* 1977;3:239–247.

154. Rubanyi GM, Vanhoutte PM. Superoxide anions and hyperoxia inactivate endothelium-derived relaxing factor. *Am J Physiol* 1986;250:H822-H827.

155. Furchgott RF. Studies on relaxation of rabbit aorta by sodium nitrite: the basis for the proposal that the acid-activatable inhibitory factor from bovine retractor penis is inorganic nitrite and the endothelium-derived relaxing factor is nitric oxide. In: Vanhoutte PM, ed. *Mechanisms of vasodilators*. New York: Raven Press, 1988;401–414.

156. Ignarro LJ, Buga GM, Wood KS, Byrns RE, Chaudhuri G. Endothelium-derived relaxing factor produced and released from artery and vein is nitric oxide. *Proc Natl Acad Sci USA* 1987;84:9265–9269.

157. Palmer RMJ, Ferrige AG, Moncada S. Nitric oxide release accounts for the biological activity of endothelium derived relaxing factor. *Nature* 1987;327:524–526.

158. Palmer RMJ, Rees DD, Ashton DS, Moncada S. L-arginine is the physiological precursor for the formation of nitric oxide in endothelium-dependent relaxation. *Biochem Biophys Res Commun* 1988;153:1251–1256.

159. Kelm M, Feelisch M, Spahr R, Piper H-M, Noack E, Schrader J. Quantitative and kinetic characterization of nitric oxide and EDRF released from cultured endothelial cells. *Biochem Biophys Res Commun* 1988;154:236–244.

160. Sakuma I, Stuehr DJ, Gross SS, Nathan C, Levi R. Identification of arginine as a precursor of endothelium-derived relaxing factor. *Proc Natl Acad Sci USA* 1988;85:8664–8667.

161. Rees DD, Palmer RMJ, Moncada S. Role of endothelium-derived nitric oxide in the regulation of blood pressure. *Proc Natl Acad Sci USA* 1989;86:3375–3378.

162. Chen G, Suzuki H, Weston AH. Acetylcholine releases endothelium-derived hyperpolarizing factor and EDRF from rat blood vessels. *Br J Pharmacol* 1988;95:1165–1174.

163. Griffith TM, Edwards DH, Newby AC, Lewis MJ, Henderson AH. Production of endothelium-derived relaxant factor is dependent on oxidative phosphorylation and extracellular calcium. *Cardiovasc Res* 1986;20:7–12.

164. Singer HA, Peach MJ. Calcium and endothelial-mediated vascular smooth muscle relaxation in rabbit aorta. *Hypertension* 1982;4(suppl II):19–25.

165. Winquist RJ, Bunting PB, Baskin EP, Wallace AA. Decreased endothelium-dependent relaxation in New Zealand genetic hypertensive rats. *J Hypertens* 1984;2:541–545.

166. Busse R, Luckhoff A, Pohl U. Bimodal role of endothelial membrane hyperpolarization in endothelium-dependent vasodilation? *J Vasc Med Biol* 1989;1:80.

167. Furchgott RF. The requirement for endothelial cells in the relaxation of arteries by acetylcholine and some other vasodilators. *Trends Pharmacol Sci* 1981;2:173–176.

168. Flavahan NA, Shimokawa H, Vanhoutte PM. Pertussis toxin inhibits endothelium-dependent relaxations to certain agonists in porcine coronary arteries. *J Physiol (Lond)* 1989;408:549–560.

169. Shirasaki Y, Su C. Endothelium removal augments vasodilation by sodium nitroprusside and sodium nitrite. *Eur J Pharmacol* 1985;141:93–96.

170. Eglen RM, Whiting RL. Determination of the muscarinic receptor subtype mediating vasodilatation. *Br J Pharmacol* 1985;84:3–5.

171. Duckles SP. Vascular muscarinic receptors: pharmacological characterization in the bovine coronary artery. *J Pharmacol Exp Ther* 1988;246:929–935.

172. De Mey JG, Vanhoutte PM. Heterogeneous behaviour of the canine arterial and venous wall. Importance of the endothelium. *Circ Res* 1982;51:439–447.

173. Brayden JE, Bevan JA. Neurogenic muscarinic vasodilation in the cat. An example of endothelial cell independent cholinergic relaxation. *Circ Res* 1985;56:205–211.

174. Parnavelas JG, Kelly W, Burnstock G. Ultrastructural localisation of choline acetyltransferase in vascular endothelial cells. *Nature* 1985;316:724–725.

175. Winquist RJ. Endothelium-dependent relaxations in hypertensive blood vessels. In: Vanhoutte PM, ed. *The endothelium. Relaxing and contracting factors.* Clifton, NJ: Humana Press, 1988;473–494.

176. Spedding M, Schini V. Schoeffter P, Miller RC. Calcium channel activation does not increase release of endothelial-derived relaxant factors (EDRF) in rat aorta although tonic release of EDRF may modulate calcium channel activity in smooth muscle. *J Cardiovasc Pharmacol* 1986;8:113–137.

177. Rubanyi GM, Schwartz A, Vanhoutte PM. The calcium agonists Bay K 8644 and (+)202,791 stimulate the release of endothelial relaxing factor from canine femoral arteries. *Eur J Pharmacol* 1985;117:143–144.

178. Cherry PD, Furchgott RF, Zawadzki JV, Jothianandan D. The role of endothelial cells in the relaxation of isolated arteries by bradykinin. *Proc Natl Acad Sci USA* 1982;79:2105–2110.

179. Gordon JL, Martin W. Endothelium-dependent relaxation of the pig aorta: relationship to stimulation of Rb efflux from isolated endothelial cells. *Br J Pharmacol* 1983;79:531–541.

180. Zawadzki JV, Furchgott RF, Cherry PD. Endothelium-dependent relaxation of arteries by acta-substance P, kassinin and octa-cholecystokinin. *Fed Proc* 1983;42:619.

181. Katusic ZS, Shepherd JT, Vanhoutte PM. Vasopressin causes endothelium-dependent relaxations of the canine basilar artery. *Circ Res* 1984;55:575–579.

182. Katusic ZS, Shepherd JT, Vanhoutte PM. Oxytocin causes endothelium-dependent relaxations of canine basilar arteries by activating V1-vasopressinergic receptors. *J Pharmacol Exp Ther* 1986;236:166–170.

183. Davies JM, Williams KI. Relaxation of the rat aorta by vasoactive intestinal polypeptide is endothelial cell dependent. *J Physiol (Lond)* 1983;343:65P.

184. Thom SM, Hughes AD, Goldberg P, Martin G, Schachter M, Sever PS. The actions of calcitonin gene-related peptide and vasoactive intestinal peptide as vasodilators in man in vivo and in vitro. *Br J Clin Pharmacol* 1987;24:139–144.

185. D'Orleans-Juste P, Dion S, Mizrahi J, Regoli D. Effects of peptides and non-peptides on isolated arterial smooth muscles. *Eur J Pharmacol* 1985;114:9–21.

186. Winquist RJ, Faison EP, Waldman SA, Schwartz K, Murad F, Rapoport RM. Atrial natriuretic factor elicits an endothelium-independent relaxation and activates particulate guanylate cyclase in vascular smooth muscle. *Proc Natl Acad Sci USA* 1984;81:7661–7664.

187. Brain SD, Williams TJ, Tippins JR, Morris HR, MacIntyre I. Calcitonin gene-related peptide is a potent vasodilator. *Nature* 1985;313:54–56.

188. Thom S, Hughes A, Sever PS. Endothelium-dependent responses in human arteries. In: Vanhoutte PM, ed. *The endothelium. Relaxing and contracting factors.* Clifton, NJ: Humana Press, 1988;511–528.

189. Hardebo JE, Hanko J, Kahrstrom J, Owman C. Endothelium-dependent relaxation in cerebral arteries. *J Cereb Blood Flow Metab* 1985;5:S533–S534.

190. Wallace A, Vlasuk, G, Faison E, Winquist R. Vasodilation of renal arteries by bovine parathyroid hormone. *Pharmacologist* 1986;28:161.

191. Ku DD. Coronary vascular reactivity after acute myocardial ischemia. *Science* 1982;218:576–578.

192. Vlasuk GP, Babilon R, Nutt RF, Ciccarone TM, Winquist RJ. The actions of atrial natriuretic factor on the vascular wall. *Can J Physiol Pharmacol* 1987;65:1684–1689.

193. De Mey JG, Vanhoutte PM. Role of the intima in cholinergic and purinergic relaxation of isolated canine femoral arteries. *J Physiol (Lond)* 1981;316:347–355.

194. Konishi M, Su C. Role of endothelium in dilator responses of spontaneously hypertensive rat arteries. *Hypertension* 1983;5:881–886.

195. Cocks TM, Angus JA. Endothelium-dependent relaxation of coronary arteries by noradrenaline and serotonin. *Nature* 1983;305:627–630.

196. Miller VM, Vanhoutte PM. Endothelial alpha-2 adrenoceptors in canine pulmonary and systemic blood vessels. *Eur J Pharmacol* 1985;118:123–129.

197. Cohen RA, Shepherd JT, Vanhoutte PM. 5-Hydroxytryptamine can mediate endothelium-dependent relaxation of coronary arteries. *Am J Physiol* 1983;245:H1077–H1080.

198. Van der Voorde J, Leusen I. Role of the endothelium in the vasodilator responses of rat thoracic aorta to histamine. *Eur J Pharmacol* 1983;87:113–120.

199. Weir SW, Weston AH. The effects of BRL 34915 and nicorandil on electrical and mechanical activity and on ^{86}Rb efflux in rat blood vessels. *Br J Pharmacol* 1986;88:121–128.

200. Trieschmann U, Pichlmaier M, Klöckner U, Isenberg G. Vasorelaxation due to K-agonists. Single channel recordings from isolated human vascular myocytes. *Pflugers Arch* 1988;411:R199.

201. Thomson EA, Nickerson M, Gaskell PI, Grahame GR. Clinical observations on an antihypertensive chlorothiazide analogue devoid of diuretic activity. *Can Med Assoc J* 1962;87:1306–1310.

202. Rubin AA, Roth FE, Taylor RM, Rosenkilde H. Pharmacology of diazoxide, an antihypertensive, nondiuretic benzothiadiazine. *J Pharmacol Exp Ther* 1962;136:344–352.

203. DuCharme DW, Freyburger WA, Graham BE, Carlson RE. Pharmacologic properties of minoxidil: a new hypertensive agent. *J Pharmacol Exp Ther* 1973;1984:662–670.

204. Goldberg MR, Sushak MS, Rockhold FW,

Thompson WL, and the Pinacidil vs Prazosin Multicenter Investigator Group. Vasodilator monotherapy in the treatment of hypertension: comparative efficacy and safety of pinacidil, a potassium channel opener, and prazosin. *Clin Pharmacol Ther* 1988;44:78–92.

205. Ward JW. Pinacidil monotherapy for hypertension. *Br J Clin Pharmacol* 1984;18:223–225.

206. Cohen ML. Pinacidil monohydrate—a novel vasodilator: review of preclinical pharmacology and mechanism of action. *Drug Dev Res* 1986;9:249–258.

207. Hof RP, Quast U, Cook NS, Blarer S. Mechanism of action, systemic and regional haemodynamics of the potassium channel activator BRL 34915 and its enantiomers. *Circ Res* 1988;62:679–686.

208. Holzmann S. Cyclic GMP as a possible mediator of coronary arterial relaxation by nicorandil (SG-75). *J Cardiovasc Pharmacol* 1983;5:364–370.

209. Furukawa K, Itoh T, Kajiwara M, et al. Vasodilating actions of 2-nicotinamidoethyl nitrate on porcine and guinea-pig coronary arteries. *J Pharmacol Exp Ther* 1981;218:248–259.

210. Smith RD, Wolf PS, Regan JR, Jolly SR. *The emergence of drugs which block calcium entry.* New York: Springer-Verlag, 1988;1–152.

211. Baker SH. Nicardipine hydrochloride. In: Scriabine A, ed. *New Drugs Annual: cardiovascular drugs* 1983;3:153–172.

212. Stoepel K, Heise A, Kazda S. Pharmacological studies of the antihypertensive effect of nitrendipine. *Arzneimittelforschung* 1981;31:2056–2061.

213. Scriabine A, Vanov S, Deck K. *Nitrendipine.* Baltimore: Urban and Schwarzenberg, 1984.

214. Ljung B. Vascular selectivity of felodipine. *Drugs* 1985;29(suppl 2):46–58.

215. Buhler FR, Mancia G, Reid JL, eds. Calcium antagonists in cardiovascular disease: rationale for 24 hour action. *J Cardiovasc Pharmacol* 1988;12(suppl 7).

216. Pagani M, Vatner SF, Braunwald E. Hemodynamic effects of intravenous sodium nitroprusside in the conscious dog. *Circulation* 1978;57:144–151.

217. Rapoport RM, Murad F. Effects of ouabain and alterations in potassium concentration on relaxation induced by sodium nitroprusside. *Blood Vessels* 1983;20:255–264.

218. Ito Y, Suzuki H, Kuriyama H. Effects of sodium nitroprusside on smooth muscle cells of rabbit pulmonary artery and portal vein. *J Pharmacol Exp Ther* 1978;207:1022–1031.

219. Chevillard C, Saiag B, Worcel M. Hydralazine. In: Vanhoutte PM, Leusen I, eds. *Vasodilation.* New York: Raven, 1981;477–489.

220. Khayyal M, Gross F, Kreye VAW. Studies on the direct vasodilator effect of hydralazine in the isolated rabbit renal artery. *J Pharmacol Exp Ther* 1981;216:390–394.

221. Worcel M. Relationship between the direct inhibitory effects of hydralazine and propildazine on arterial smooth muscle contractility and sympathetic innervation. *J Pharmacol Exp Ther* 1978;207:320–330.

222. Chevillard, C, Mathieu MN, Saiag B, Worcel M. Hydralazine: effect on the outflow of noradrenaline and mechanical responses evoked by sympathetic nerve stimulation of the rat tail artery. *Br J Pharmacol* 1980;69:415–420.

223. Winquist RJ, Webb RC, Bohr DF. Vascular smooth muscle in hypertension. *Fed Proc* 1982;41:2387–2393.

224. Lockette W, Otsuka Y, Carretero O. The loss of endothelium-dependent vascular relaxation in hypertension. *Hypertension* 1986;8(suppl II):61–66.

Cardiovascular Pharmacology, Third Edition,
edited by Michael Antonaccio.
Raven Press, Ltd., New York © 1990.

Calcium Antagonists

David J. Triggle

School of Pharmacy, State University of New York, Buffalo, New York 14260

The calcium antagonists, including the clinically available verapamil, nifedipine, and diltiazem, are a chemically heterogeneous group of agents with the common property of selective antagonism of Ca^{2+} movements through one type of Ca^{2+} channel. They are usually referred to as calcium antagonists, calcium channel antagonists, or calcium channel blockers. The term "calcium channel antagonist" will be used throughout this chapter. These drugs are of major significance in the control of a number of cardiovascular disorders including angina, hypertension, peripheral vascular disorders, and some types of cardiac arrhythmias (Table 1). Sales in the United States are expected to reach almost $3 billion in 1992 from the 1987 level of some $700 million (1). Anticipated developments, including the availability of second- and third-generation agents, and the development of new structures active against different classes of channels, will likely increase the therapeutic roles of these agents and expand their uses beyond the cardiovascular system (Tables 2 and 3). Simultaneously, these agents have proved to be valuable molecular tools with which to determine the localization, properties, and structures of voltage-dependent Ca^{2+} channels.

The development of the Ca^{2+} channel antagonists owes much to the pioneering work of Albrecht Fleckenstein and colleagues in the early 1960s (2–5). Flecken-stein observed that prenylamine and verapamil (Fig. 1) both mimicked the effects of Ca^{2+} withdrawal on the heart and blocked excitation-contraction coupling without major changes in the shape of the cardiac action potential (Fig. 2). Furthermore, the depressant effects of these agents on cardiac contractile activity could be overcome by agents that increased the supply of Ca^{2+} to the cell, including β-adrenoceptor activators, cardiac glycosides, and Ca^{2+} itself. Subsequent work showed that these cardiodepressant properties were shared by other agents including D600, an analog of verapamil, the 1,4-dihydropyridine nifedipine, and the benzothiazepine diltiazem (Fig. 1). Accordingly, it was proposed that these agents represented a new class of drug, the calcium antagonists, that blocked excitation-contraction coupling by interfering directly with the mobilization of extracellular Ca^{2+}. Moreover, these properties were not confined to cardiac muscle, and the agents proved to be highly effective relaxants of smooth muscle, including vascular smooth muscle, functioning by interference with depolarization-induced mobilization of extracellular Ca^{2+}. The principle of Ca^{2+} antagonism was thus established to be quite general to the cardiovascular system. Much subsequent work has delineated the widespread role of Ca^{2+} channels in a multiplicity of cell and tissue types.

TABLE 1. *Therapeutic uses of Ca²⁺ channel antagonists*

	Antagonists		
Use	Verapamil (I)[a]	Nifedipine (II)[a]	Diltiazem (III)[a]
Angina			
Exertional	+++ [b]	+++	+++
Prinzmetal's	+++	+++	+++
Variant	+++	+++	+++
Arrhythmias			
Paroxysmal supraventricular tachyarrhythmias	+++	−	++
Atrial fibrillation and flutter	++	−	++
Hypertension	++	+++	+
Hypertrophic cardiomyopathy	+	−	−
Raynaud's phenomenon	++	++	+
Cardioplegia	+	+	+
Cerebral vasospasm (posthemorrhage)	−	+	−

[a]Classes I, II, and III as defined by WHO (Tables 6 and 7; ref. 150).
[b]Number of plus signs indicates extent of use: +++, very common; −, not used.

REGULATION OF Ca²⁺

The importance of Ca²⁺ to cellular excitability was first realized by the English physician and physiologist Sidney Ringer (1836–1910) who observed in 1883 the critical role of extracellular Ca²⁺ in the maintenance of cardiac contractility (55,56). Subsequent investigations have amply documented the fundamental role of Ca²⁺ in stimulus-response coupling processes and in the maintenance of cellular integrity.

Calcium is an abundant element, making up some 3% of the earth's crust: the average human contains approximately 1 kg of Ca²⁺, the majority of which is immobilized as the mineral hydroxyapatite in bones and teeth. Approximately 1% to 2% of the total body Ca²⁺ is found in the intra- and extracellular fluids, but this fraction controls the critical processes, including excitation-contraction and stimulus-secretion coupling, on which cellular excitability and responsiveness depend.

The role of Ca²⁺ as a critical cellular messenger is probably dictated by several factors. In particular, the high, inwardly directed concentration and electrical gradients are appropriate for current-carrying and messenger functions, the latter role being made possible by the presence of in-

tracellular Ca²⁺ binding proteins. These proteins, including calmodulin and troponin C, serve as receptors that mediate the func-

TABLE 2. *Additional and potential uses of Ca²⁺ channel antagonists (6,7)*

Cardiovascular	
Atherosclerosis	(8,9)
Cardioplegia	(10,11)
Cerebral ischemia, focal	(12,13)
Cerebral ischemia, global	(14,15)
Congestive heart failure	(16,17)
Hypertrophic cardiomyopathy	(18,19)
Migraine	(20,21)
Myocardial infarction	(22,23)
Peripheral vascular diseases	(24,25)
Pulmonary hypertension	(26,27)
Subarachnoid hemorrhage	(28,29)
Nonvascular smooth muscle	
Achalasia	(30,31)
Asthma	(32,33)
Dysmenorrhea	(34)
Eclampsia	(35)
Esophageal spasm	(36)
Intestinal hypermotility	(37)
Obstructive lung disease	(38)
Premature labor	(34,39)
Urinary incontinence	(40,41)
Other	
Aldosteronism	(42)
Cancer chemotherapy	(43,44)
Epilepsy	(45,46)
Glaucoma	(47)
Manic syndrome	(48,49)
Motion sickness	(50)
Spinal cord injury	(51)
Tinnitus	(52)
Tourette's disorder	(53)
Vertigo	(54)

TABLE 3. *Current and potential uses of Ca²⁺ channel antagonists*[a]

Current use	Drug	Potential use	Drug
Myocardial ischemia		Cardiovascular	
Exertional, Prinzmetal's, unstable angina	D,N,V	Migraine	V,N
		Raynaud's disease	N
Hypertension	D,N,V	Cardioprotection	V,N
Hypertensive emergencies	N	Subarachnoid hemorrhage	Nimod
Cardiac arrhythmias		Cerebral insufficiency	N
Supraventricular tachycardia	V		Nimod
Atrial fibrillation and flutter	V,D	Pulmonary hypertension	
Hypertrophic cardiomyopathy	V	Congestive heart failure	
		Noncardiovascular	
		Asthma (exercise induced)	V,N
		Esophageal motor disorders	N
		Premature labor	N
		Urinary incontinence	N
		Intestinal hypermotility	V

D, diltiazem; N, nifedipine; V, verapamil; Nimod, nimodipine.

[a]Only a partial listing of potential uses is provided here. The Ca²⁺ channel antagonists have been suggested to be of potential use in virtually all cases in which hyper- or excessive activity of smooth muscle is involved.

tions of messenger Ca^{2+}. In concert, the coordination chemistry of Ca^{2+} makes possible the formation of tight complexes of flexible geometry with polyanionic ligands thus permitting a cellular distinction from Mg^{2+} (57). The multiple roles of Ca^{2+} in cellular function require that it be a regulated species. Regulation is, in fact, exerted at two major levels: the organismic and the cellular.

At the organismic level, Ca^{2+} absorption and excretion are actively regulated in the gastrointestinal tract and the kidney, respectively. The skeleton serves as the major body reservoir for withdrawal or deposit of Ca^{2+} according to the balance of supply and demand. The balance between absorption, excretion, and deposition serves to maintain the plasma concentrations of Ca^{2+} at approximately 2.5×10^{-3} M (5.0 mEq/liter). This level is controlled by the cooperative actions of three hormones: parathy-

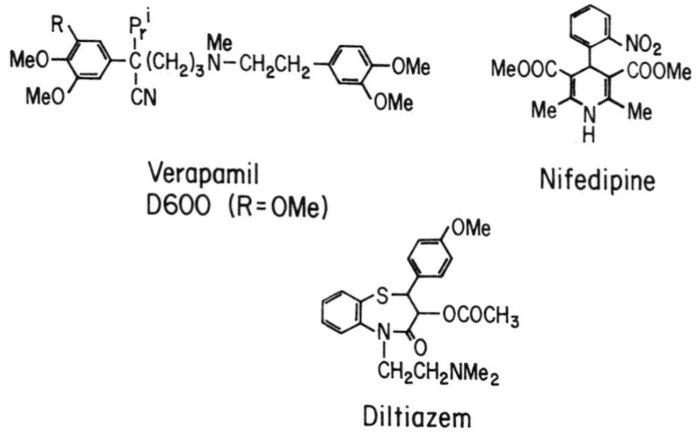

FIG. 1. Chemical structures of Ca²⁺ channel antagonists.

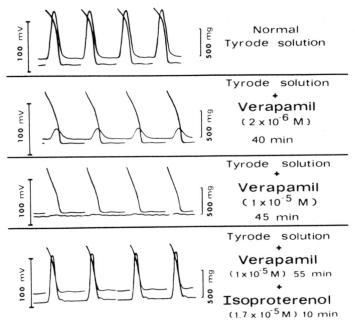

FIG. 2. Uncoupling of cardiac electrical and mechanical activities in guinea pig papillary muscle by high concentrations of verapamil. (From ref. 3.)

roid hormone (PTH), calcitonin, and vitamin D (calcitriol). In turn, the levels and activities of these hormones are regulated by the concentration of Ca^{2+} itself. Thus, a decrease in the plasma concentration of Ca^{2+} is accompanied by an increased PTH level leading to restoration of plasma Ca^{2+} levels by increased absorption from the gut, increased reabsorption in the kidney, and enhanced mobilization from bone. The reciprocal relationships between these hormones and Ca^{2+} and phosphate metabolism are depicted in Table 4.

At the cellular level, Ca^{2+} is regulated at both plasmalemmal and intracellular loci (56,58,59). The concentration of free ionized Ca^{2+} within the cell is normally maintained at very low levels, approximately 10^{-8} M. However, the total cellular concentration may be 10^{-3} M or higher, most of which is stored within intracellular organelles or tightly bound to intracellular pro-

TABLE 4. *Relationship between serum calcium and PTH, calcitonin, and calcitriol*

	Hormone response		
	PTH	Calcitonin	Calcitriol
Plasma signal			
Ca^{2+}	↑	↓	↑
Ca^{2+}	↓	↑	
		Plasma Ca^{2+} change	
Hormone signal			
PTH	↑↓	↑↓	
Calcitonin	↑↓	↓↑	
Calcitriol	↑↓	↑↓	

↑, increases; ↓, decreases.

teins. The Ca^{2+} required to satisfy the requirements of stimulus-response coupling may thus be derived from intracellular sources, extracellular sources, or both; the relative degree of mobilization from these sources is stimulus, tissue, and time dependent (60).

Ca^{2+} control at the plasmalemma is mediated through Ca^{2+} channels, Ca^{2+} pumps, and a Na^+-Ca^{2+} exchange process. Ca^{2+} channels are frequently referred to as potential dependent and receptor operated, designating their primary control by voltage or chemical signals, respectively. These major channel categories may be further subdivided according to electrophysiologic and pharmacologic characteristics. An electrogenic Na^+-Ca^{2+} exchanger (3 Na^+-Ca^{2+}) operates in the plasma membrane and can move Ca^{2+} into or out of the cell according to membrane potential and the ionic gradients for Na^+ and Ca^{2+}. Under depolarizing conditions the exchanger serves as a Ca^{2+} source, but under polarized conditions the exchanger probably operates to extrude Ca^{2+} coupled to Na^+ influx. In the heart the Na^+-Ca^{2+} exchanger probably contributes to setting the amount of Ca^{2+} releasable from intracellular stores, maintains a high intracellular Ca^{2+} during the plateau phase of the action potential, and serves as an efflux pathway during repolarization (61,62). This role, of maintaining a low intracellular ionized Ca^{2+} concentration, is shared by the calmodulin-dependent Ca^{2+}-ATPase (58,63). The latter is a high-capacity, but low-affinity, system and it is likely that in both heart and vascular smooth muscle the Na^+-Ca^{2+} exchanger is quantitatively more important to intracellular Ca^{2+} removal.

At the intracellular level, the major sources and depots for Ca^{2+} mobilization and sequestration are the sarcoplasmic/endoplasmic reticulum and the mitochondria. The Ca^{2+}-ATPases of sarcoplasmic and endoplasmic reticulum are presumed to be very similar in their structure and function, although that of sarcoplasmic reticulum is more abundant, both in heart and skeletal muscle, and is better characterized (58,63). The role of this system in skeletal, cardiac, and smooth muscle in reducing cytosolic Ca^{2+} concentrations to relaxant levels is clearly established, although the release processes are less well understood. Sarcoplasmic reticulum contains large amounts of the extrinsic, hydrophilic Ca^{2+} binding protein calsequestrin, which is presumed, in its internal location, to complex with moderate affinity large amounts of Ca^{2+} to be available for subsequent release.

Ca^{2+} release from the sarcoplasmic reticulum is mediated through the Ca^{2+} release channel, which has been isolated and characterized to have similar properties from both skeletal and cardiac muscle (64). This large protein, Mr 400 to 450 kD, appears to assemble as a tetrameric complex to form the feet of the sarcoplasmic reticulum and to link the transverse t-tubules and the cisternae of the sarcoplasmic reticulum. In this role the protein serves to couple the voltage sensor of the transverse tubules with the Ca^{2+} stores of the sarcoplasmic reticulum. Of considerable interest, the voltage sensor is the 1,4-dihydropyridine-binding subunit of the L class of potential-dependent Ca^{2+} channel, which may thus play a dual role in the excitation-contraction coupling process. Although there are differences between the Ca^{2+} channel release proteins of skeletal and cardiac muscle, both are characterized by their affinity for ryanodine and ruthenium red. In nonmuscle cells, it has been assumed that the endoplasmic reticulum represents the intracellular Ca^{2+} storage/release site. However, the "calciosome," a calsequestrin-containing discrete organelle, may represent the inositol-1,4,5-triphosphate- (IP3) sensitive Ca^{2+}-release system in these cells (65,66).

Both Ca^{2+} uptake and efflux mechanisms operate in the mitochondrial inner membrane. The uptake process is via a uniporter, driven electrophoretically by the membrane potential set up by the proton extrusion process of the respiratory chain. Efflux mechanisms appear to be of two types: an electroneutral Na^+-Ca^{2+} exchange and a less well characterized Na^+-independent pathway (67). Although it has been proposed that mitochondria serve as a Ca^{2+} sink or buffer, it is likely that under physiologic conditions this is not of major importance. Rather, these transport systems relay changes in cytosolic Ca^{2+} concentration to the mitochondrial matrix, thus permitting Ca^{2+}-mediated control of oxidative metabolism via intramitochondrial pyruvate, NAD^+-isocitrate, and 2-oxoglutarate dehydrogenases. Such regulation provides a link between the intracellular concentrations of Ca^{2+} and the availability of ATP.

Accordingly, cellular Ca^{2+} regulation may be viewed as a set of Ca^2-mobilizing and -sequestration processes arranged in both series and parallel manner (Fig. 3). The relative importance of these discrete mobilizing processes, including the several types of receptor-operated and potential-dependent Ca^{2+} channels of the plasma membrane and the release channel of the sarcoplasmic reticulum, will depend on the cell type, the stimulus, and the time course of the response. These mobilization pathways, in conjunction with the several sequestration processes, will determine both the equilibrium levels of intracellular Ca^{2+} and the nonhomogeneous spatial and temporal characteristics of the Ca^{2+} response (68).

Ca^{2+} metabolism is typically discussed at the separate levels of cell and body regula-

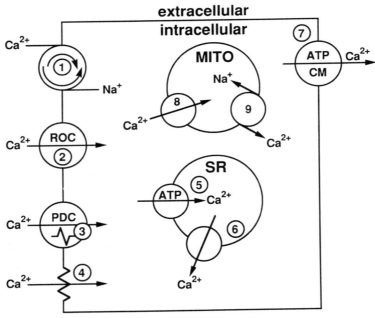

FIG. 3. The regulation of cellular Ca^{2+}. Depicted are events at both plasmalemmal and intracellular surfaces including receptor-operated (ROC) and potential-dependent (PDC) Ca^{2+} channels, a Na^+-Ca^{2+} exchange process (1), Ca^{2+} entry through nonspecific or "leak" pathways, a mitochondrial Ca^{2+} uniporter (8), and Na^+-Ca^{2+} exchange process (9), a Ca^{2+} release channel (6), and ATP-dependent Ca^{2+} uptake (5) in sarcoplasmic/endoplasmic reticulum and a plasmalemmal calmodulin-dependent Ca^{2+}-ATPase.

tion. Increasingly, it is realized that these processes are intimately linked both because of the relationships between serum and cellular Ca^{2+} and linkages to other ions, notably Mg^{2+} and Na^+, and because agents may be involved directly in both cellular and organ Ca^{2+} regulation. Thus, receptors for vitamin D exist in skeletal, smooth, and cardiac muscle cells (69–71), and vitamin D produces a rapid increase in Ca^{2+} uptake in skeletal muscle apparently through voltage-dependent Ca^{2+} channels (72). Furthermore, voltage-dependent Ca^{2+} channels are found also in osteoblasts (73).

Interrelationships between the several pathways of Ca^{2+} regulation are apparent in essential hypertension where an ionic and metabolic classification is becoming available. This classification is based on the apparently paradoxical sets of observations that hypertension may be linked both to elevated and reduced levels of Ca^{2+} (74–77). Thus, hypertension is associated with elevated levels of intracellular Ca^{2+} and high serum levels of Ca^{2+}, and both hyperparathyroidism and vitamin D intoxication are associated with hypertension. In contrast, hypertensive patients may have a dietary Ca^{2+} deficiency, serum Ca^{2+} levels may be low with hypercalciuria, and oral Ca^{2+} supplementation may lower blood pressure in both experimental and clinical situations. Serum Ca^{2+} concentrations are associated with changes in renin and Ca^{2+}-regulating hormone levels such that serum Ca^{2+} levels increase directly with increasing renin levels, and calcitonin levels and inversely with PTH and vitamin D levels (Table 4).

Implicit in this ionic and biochemical classification of hypertension is the thesis that intracellular Ca^{2+} is abnormally elevated in the hypertensive state regardless of the extracellular ionic levels. According to this conceptual framework, the low-renin, low-serum Ca^{2+} hypertensive state will be the more sensitive to dietary Na^+ intake and to Ca^{2+} channel antagonists, whereas the high-renin hypertensive state responds

better to other antihypertensive therapies, including β-blockers and angiotensin-converting enzyme inhibitors. It is important to realize that the small changes in serum Ca^{2+} observed between normotensive and hypertensive states (Fig. 4) may be less important than are the corresponding changes in hormone levels of both the renin-angiotensin-aldosterone and parathyroid-calcitonin-vitamin D systems. A connection between dietary Ca^{2+}, cellular Ca^{2+} regulation, and the vitamin D axis is suggested by the observations that the integral membrane calcium binding protein (IMCAL), ubiquitously distributed in tissues and closely correlated with intestinal mucosal cation transport ability (78,79), is substantially decreased in experimental hypertension (80).

Intracellular Ca^{2+} both regulates the cell and is regulated by the cell. Ca^{2+} out of control is a lethal cell signal (81–90). The destructive effects of aberrantly elevated intracellular Ca^{2+} have long been recognized in the "calcium paradox" whereby

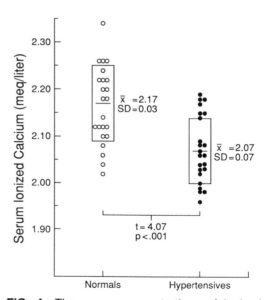

FIG. 4. The serum concentrations of ionized Ca^{2+} in 23 normotensive and 23 hypertensive subjects. (From ref. 77a.)

reperfusion of the heart with a Ca^{2+}-containing medium after a period of Ca^{2+}-free perfusion or ischemia produces irreversible cell damage or death (81,82). The characteristics of this process including a loss of electrical and mechanical excitability, loss of cellular contents, changes in mitochondrial morphology, a fall in high-energy phosphate levels, and a massive accumulation of cell Ca^{2+} are shared by many cell types exposed to such noxious stimuli as ischemia, halogenated hydrocarbons, cell tearing, catecholamine overload, and energy depletion. Because both the presence of extracellular Ca^{2+} and the elevation of intracellular Ca^{2+} are common features of the resultant cellular damage, it is generally assumed that the basic defect is the loss of control of intracellular Ca^{2+}. It is not, however, necessary to assume that the pathways leading to elevation of intracellular Ca^{2+} are identical for every cell insult or for every cell type. Nonetheless, a generalized flow sheet of events leading to Ca^{2+} overload and the consequences of this overload are outlined (Fig. 5).

Of particular importance to this general scheme of cell damage is the loss of cellular

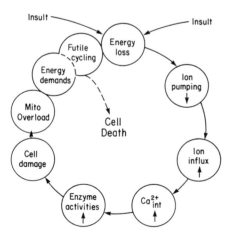

FIG. 5. Schematic representation of a sequence of events leading to cellular Ca^{2+} overload and cell death.

ionic homeostasis, initially for Na^+ and K^+, leading to membrane depolarization and the entry of Ca^{2+} through potential-dependent channels and the Na^+-Ca^{2+} exchanger, the loss of ATP, and the resultant inability to maintain ion-pumping activity at both plasmalemmal and intracellular membranes. This leads to a further elevation of intracellular Ca^{2+}, the overloading of mitochondria by the elevated Ca^{2+}, a continuing depletion of ATP levels, and a decrease in intracellular pH. The detrimental effect of the reduced ATP levels will be further exacerbated in mechanically working tissues such as myocardium. Activation of Ca^{2+}-dependent proteases and phospholipases (83,84) leads to further cell destruction including membrane perturbation and destruction and the production of lysophospholipids and arachidonic acid metabolites. Additionally, oxygen lack decreases the β-oxidation of fatty acids and permits the concentrations of acylcarnitines and acylCoA to rise. These amphipathic species have a variety of actions, including increased expression of myocardial $α_1$-adrenoceptors (85), which likely contribute to membrane dysfunction and electrophysiologic derangements (86,87).

Concomitantly with the elevation of intracellular Ca^{2+}, the cell is exposed to oxygen-derived free radicals contributed from purine catabolism by xanthine oxidase, the mitochondrial electron transport system, and infiltration of neutrophils and monocytes (88). The cell changes and damage caused by radicals and by elevated Ca^{2+} are not independent but rather are mutually reinforcing. Thus, compromised cells are in double jeopardy from both Ca^{2+} and radical attack.

Agents that block the appropriate Ca^{2+} mobilization pathway thus have the potential to modulate both cell function and cell survival (Fig. 6). Their therapeutic significance, although not to be underestimated, must be considered in terms of the pathways thus affected.

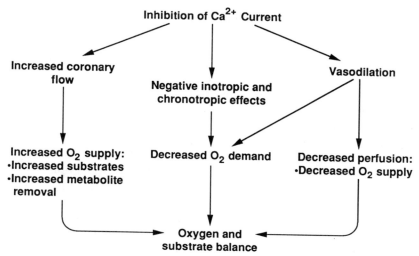

FIG. 6. Flow sheet depicting the consequences of inhibition of Ca^{2+} current by Ca^{2+} channel antagonists in the cardiovascular system.

CALCIUM MODULATORS AND THE CONTROL OF CALCIUM MOBILIZATION

From the preceding discussion it is clear that the mobilization of Ca^{2+} is regulated by several distinct processes at discrete loci (6). Three major foci emerge for consideration: Where are the control points of Ca^{2+} mobilization? Do these control points differ in disease or pathologic states? What are the definitions for drug action at these control points?

In principle, there should exist both activators and antagonists operating through the following systems:

1. potential-dependent Ca^{2+} channels
2. receptor-operated Ca^{2+} channels
3. plasmalemmal Na^{+}-Ca^{2+} exchange
4. plasmalemmal Ca^{2+}-ATPase
5. plasmalemmal Ca^{2+} binding (intra- and extracellular)
6. mitochondrial Ca^{2+} uptake/release
7. sarcoplasmic reticulum Ca^{2+}-ATPase
8. sarcoplasmic reticulum Ca^{2+} release
9. "undefined" Ca^{2+} leak pathways.

In practice, therapeutically useful agents are far more limited in scope and are principally those—the Ca^{2+} channel antagonists—that affect one class of potential-dependent Ca^{2+} channels. The role of these agents will be confined primarily to the inhibition of Ca^{2+} movements through this one pathway. Other Ca^{2+} pathways will be unaffected or largely unaffected, and it is not, therefore, to be expected that the available Ca^{2+} channel antagonists will be effective in all cell or tissue types or against all Ca^{2+}-mobilizing stimuli. This is a particularly important consideration during reperfusion and ischemia where multiple Ca^{2+}-mobilizing pathways are likely to be activated. However, there are agents under pharmacologic investigation that interact with varying degrees of specificity at one or more of the other sites of Ca^{2+} regulation and from which it is likely that new classes of therapeutically useful agents will be generated (6,89).

CALCIUM CHANNELS

The Ca^{2+} channels of the plasmalemmal and intracellular membranes represent major control points for Ca^{2+} mobilization. Ca^{2+} channels may be considered as regulated solely by either electrical or chemical signals. Such exclusivity is, however, unlikely and it is probable that all Ca^{2+} channels are subject to chemical modulation either by direct drug binding or through second messengers generated by specific receptor activation processes (6,90–92).

In principle, several regulatory schemes may be considered (6,93). The receptor and the ion channel may be part of the same protein or oligomeric complex and thus communicate directly. Alternatively, communication may be indirect and the channel is regulated through one or more second messengers, diffusible in the cytosol or membrane, including cAMP, IP3, 1,2-diacylglycerol, and related metabolites. Additionally, channels may be modulated through guanine nucleotide binding (G) proteins and thus share similarities with other chemically liganded receptors (94–96). Finally, channels may be chemically regulated through drug binding sites that are components of the channel itself but that are not receptors for defined neurotransmitters or hormones (97). Independent of chemical sensitivity, Ca^{2+} channels may be regulated by membrane potential being activated and inactivated by changes in electrical signals (98–100). Modulation of the

potential dependence may occur through the action of specific chemical signals (90–92).

Ca^{2+} channels may thus be classified according to a variety of criteria including their specific electrical and chemical properties, permeation selectivity, conductances, and pharmacologic sensitivities. Despite these differences in properties, it is very probable that different types of Ca^{2+} channels share some fundamentally similar characteristics including ion-translocation mechanisms and chemical sensitivity (6, 93). Thus, the 1,4-dihydropyridine-sensitive, voltage-dependent Ca^{2+} channels of skeletal muscle are also sensitive to IP3 (101), indicating a link between two apparently dissimilar channel types.

Potential-dependent Ca^{2+} channels have been classified into three major types (6,93,102) (Table 5). The L channels are of large conductance, inactivate slowly, are widespread in the cardiovascular system, and are likely to be important where relatively large and sustained Ca^{2+} fluxes are required. The T channels activate at more negative potentials, inactivate rapidly, and give rise to transient currents. They are likely to be involved in the generation of rhythmic and pacemaker activities and to serve as a trigger for the initiation of other ionic events. N channels have been de-

TABLE 5. *Properties of plasmalemmal Ca^{2+} channels[a]*

	Channel class		
	L	T	N
Activation range, mV	−10 mV	−70 mV	−30 mV
Inactivation range, mV	−60 to −10 mV	−100 to −60 mV	−120 to −30 mV
Inactivation rate	Very slow	Rapid	Moderate
Conductance	25 pS	8 pS	13 pS
Kinetics	Little activation	Brief burst, inactivation	Long burst
Permeation	$Ba^{2+} > Ca^{2+}$	$Ba^{2+} = Ca^{2+}$	$Ba^{2+} > Ca^{2+}$
Cd^{2+} sensitivity	Sensitive	Insensitive	Sensitive
1,4-DHP sensitivity	Sensitive	Insensitive	Insensitive
w-Conotoxin sensitivity	Sensitive (neurons), insensitive (muscle)	Insensitive	Sensitive

1,4-DHP, 1,4-dihydropyridine.
[a]Data are computed from a variety of sources and are not intended to suggest that these properties are singularly characteristic of each channel class.

scribed thus far only in neurons; this selective localization may explain the apparent insensitivity of many neuronal Ca^{2+}-dependent events to the existing Ca^{2+} channel antagonists.

Whether differences in channel characteristics extend also to permeation mechanisms remains to be resolved. Certainly, the L-, T-, and N-channel classes exhibit different permeation sequences. The L channel appears to generate its permeation sequence through a process of selective ion binding rather than by ion exclusion (102). This view finds support from several sources (reviewed in 102), including saturation of divalent currents with increasing ion concentration consistent with the presence of a cation binding site associated with the channel. That more than one binding site may be present is suggested by the occurrence of widely differing estimates of Ca^{2+} affinity according to whether the channel permeates Ca^{2+} or, in the absence of Ca^{2+}, monovalent ions, and the generation of an anomalous mole fraction effect, whereby current passage by a mixture of ions exhibits minima rather than being a simple monotonic function predicted for a single one site pore. Whether this model applies to other Ca^{2+}-channel types remains to be established.

It is becoming increasingly clear from the contributions of molecular biology that receptors and ion channels form a number of classes and that there is substantial homology between members of any one class. Thus, the sequence of a major component, the α_1 subunit, of the L-type channel shows considerable homology to the Na^+ channel (103), and it is likely that the several subclasses of Ca^{2+} channel themselves constitute one class in the potential-dependent Ca^{2+} channel family (104). This homology likely extends also to cross-interactions between ligands of different primary channel specificity (93).

A major component of the classification of potential-dependent Ca^{2+} channels is provided by pharmacologic agents. The L channel is sensitive to the Ca^{2+} channel antagonists and activators of the 1,4-dihydropyridine, phenylalkylamine, and benzothiazepine classes (Fig. 1) that are the major topic of this chapter. In contrast to the rich pharmacology available for the L channel, few agents are available with actions at T channels and these lack specificity. These agents (Fig. 7) include amiloride (105), diphenylhydantoin (106), tetramethrin (107), and higher alcohols including octan-1-ol (108). Selective ligands for the T channel await discovery.

Polypeptide toxins from the molluscs of the *Conus* genus are highly effective at N channels (109,110). However, the pharmacology appears complex and the N chan-

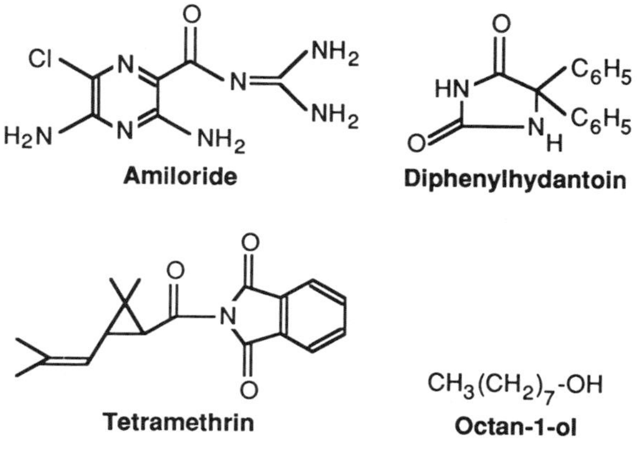

Amiloride

Diphenylhydantoin

Tetramethrin

$CH_3(CH_2)_7\text{-OH}$

Octan-1-ol

FIG. 7. Chemical structures of agents with activities at the T class of potential-dependent Ca^{2+} channel.

nels are likely heterogeneous. Studies with w-conotoxins GVIIA and MVIIA suggest that they interact with a subset of L channels found in nerve cells and that they may, according to species, interact with at least two types of N channels found in nerve terminals and which are involved in neurotransmitter release (110). The actions of other drugs at neuronal N channels are poorly defined; however, it must be recalled that many of the pharmacologic studies on neuronal Ca^{2+} channels were done before a classification had been achieved. Toxin binding is sensitive to the aminoglycoside antibiotics in the sequence neomycin > gentamycin > streptomycin > kanamycin, a property probably underlying their neurotoxic effects (111).

Thus, Ca^{2+} channels may be regarded as pharmacologic receptors (112). Accordingly, they may be expected to exhibit a number of properties including the presence of discrete sites at which activator and antagonist ligands interact. These sites will be characterized by the existence of structure-activity relationships: at present, such relationships have been fairly extensively reported only for the L category of voltage-dependent Ca^{2+} channel (6,93). These sites may represent the loci of interaction of one or more endogenous ligands: none has yet been characterized unambiguously for the Ca^{2+} channel but several putative factors have been reported (97). In common with other receptor systems, Ca^{2+} channels should be regulated species, subject to both homologous and heterologous influences and alterations in disease and pathologic states. This has been realized (113). Finally, the association of Ca^{2+} channels with G proteins strengthens their formal resemblance to other excitable proteins (94–96).

Structural studies on the L channel have revealed the existence of several subunits of different size and properties (114). The α_1 subunit carries the drug binding sites, but it is not yet clear whether this subunit alone comprises the functional channel. The majority of structural studies have been carried out with the 1,4-dihydropyridine binding subunit from skeletal muscle (114). This has the dual function of channel and voltage sensor and the structure of the corresponding subunit from cardiac and other excitable tissues is different (115). Additional differentiation is provided by antibody specificity (116–118). Thus, Lambert-Eaton myasthenic antibody recognizes neuronal L, but not cardiac L, channels, and there are antigenic differences revealed between the 1,4-dihydropyridine binding subunits of cardiac and skeletal muscle. It is therefore evident that several distinct subclasses of L channel exist and that this may contribute to the tissue selectivity of some Ca^{2+} channel antagonists.

CALCIUM CHANNELS IN THE CARDIOVASCULAR SYSTEM

Both L and T Ca^{2+} channel types occur in the cardiovascular system. The L channel, contributing to the plateau component and to the slowly rising currents of the sinoatrial (SA) and atrioventricular (AV) nodes (Fig. 8), has long been recognized as a major contributor of Ca^{2+} current to the cardiac action potential, serving inotropic, pacemaking, and conducting functions (119, 120).

The role of a T channel was observed in guinea pig ventricular cells (121). A small, transient conductance activating and inactivating at relatively negative membrane potentials, equally permeant to Ca^{2+} and Ba^{2+} and insensitive to 1,4-dihydropyridines is clearly distinguishable from the larger and longer lasting L currents (Table 5). This T-channel current is further distinguished from the L current by its relative stability in excised membrane patches under conditions in which the L current is lost. Similar observations have been made by other workers (122). T currents have been reported in other cardiac preparations including canine atrial cells (123). Both L and T channels have also been reported

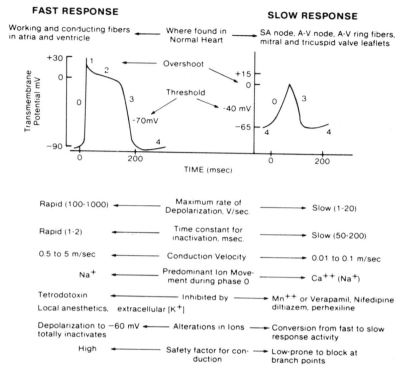

FIG. 8. Schematic representation of differences between the fast and slow inward currents of cardiac action potential. (From ref. 118a.)

in visceral and vascular smooth muscle (124,125). In vascular smooth muscle, tissues studied include azygous vein (126), mesenteric artery (127,128), an aortic cell line (129), ear artery (130,131), saphenous vein (132), and portal vein (133). L-channel activity in mesenteric artery requires ATP, but T-channel activity is present in ATP-free and metabolically depleted conditions (128).

Although the currents observed in both cardiac and vascular smooth muscle conform generally to the L and T classification described previously, it is likely that there exist differences both between cardiac and vascular smooth muscle and between different smooth muscles. Of particular interest are differences in pharmacologic sensitivity.

Cardiac L channels are activated through β-adrenoceptor stimulation. This is achieved through a cAMP-dependent phosphorylation process, mimicked through the intracellular application of cAMP analogs or the catalytic unit of protein kinase A and blocked by the presence of the regulatory subunit or protein phosphatase (134), that serves to enhance the probability of channel opening at a given membrane potential (135). The channel is available for permeation even in the nonphosphorylated state. *In vivo*, phosphorylation of the cardiac L channel is stimulated by all hormones that activate adenylate cyclase and agents, including acetylcholine acting at muscarinic receptors, that activate the inhibitory G protein, G_i, decrease Ca^{2+} current. In contrast, L-channel activation by catecholamines in vascular smooth muscle is independent of adenylate cyclase activation (136,137), which is involved rather in the relaxation process (138). In mesenteric arteries norepinephrine increases the probability of L-channel opening at a given membrane potential (139). L channels in smooth muscle may be regulated by inositol phosphates and 1,2-diacylglycerol, products of the G protein-coupled, receptor-linked, phospholipase-C system (140,141). Phorbol esters modulate Ca^{2+} currents in vascular smooth muscle cells. In an aortic cell line, L-type Ca^{2+} channels, insensitive to cAMP and its derivatives, are activated by phorbol esters, but the T channels present in the same cells are insensitive (142). Cardiac L-type Ca^{2+} channels are also modulated by protein kinase C with initial activation and subsequent depression of activity (143,144). Thus, the L channels of cardiac and vascular smooth muscle are distinguished by their phosphorylation control mechanisms. Although the complete details of the differentiation await resolution, they are likely to have important consequences.

The organic Ca^{2+} channel antagonists, particularly the 1,4-dihydropyridines, are frequently used to distinguish L- and T-channel categories. It is likely that the sensitivity of cardiac and smooth muscle L channels to these agents is different, although quantitative comparative studies are not readily available. Additionally, there are some indications that the pharmacologic distinctions between L- and T-type channels in the cardiovascular system may not be absolute. In atrial cells the 1,4-dihydropyridine felodipine blocks both T and L channels in voltage-dependent fashion, consistent with selective interactions with the inactivated states of the channels (145). Although the affinity of felodipine or the inactivated state of the L channel, 0.67 nM, is much lower than for the T channel, 13 nM, the effective binding constants will not be very different over the physiologically significant voltage range. Several studies in vascular smooth muscle indicate the anticipated sensitivity of the L currents to 1,4-dihydropyridines (127–130,132,133), but in mesenteric artery both channel types were reported to be sensitive to nisoldipine

(146), and in rabbit ear artery the actions of nifedipine were not simply consistent with blockade only of L channels (131).

It is likely that different subpopulations of L and T channels operate in cardiac and vascular smooth muscle. These channels are distinguished electrophysiologically and pharmacologically. These distinctions are of great importance because they likely underlie, at least in part, the observed tissue selectivity of action of the Ca^{2+} channel antagonists.

THE CALCIUM CHANNEL ANTAGONISTS

It is likely that the calcium channels in nodal tissue, myocardial tissue, and vascular smooth muscle differ both from one another and from calcium channels in other excitable tissues including brain and skeletal muscle. These differences may be recognized by the Ca^{2+} antagonists and underlie the several classification schemes advanced for these drugs.

Classification of Ca^{2+} Antagonists

The original classification advanced by Fleckenstein recognized two major groups of agents. Group A included the potent and selective verapamil, diltiazem, and nifedipine, whereas less selective agents, prenylamine, perhexiline, caroverine, and fendiline, that also affected other processes including the Na^+ current, comprised group B. More detailed and modified schemes (147) have been subsequently advanced by Godfraind and colleagues (148), the International Society and Federation of Cardiology (147,149) and by the World Health Organization (WHO) (150). A brief summary of these schemes is presented in Table 6.

The WHO classification recognizes a variety of criteria to distinguish specific and nonspecific Ca^{2+} channel antagonists and by which the specific agents themselves

TABLE 6. *Comparison of classifications of Ca²⁺ channel antagonists*

ISFC[a]	Godfraind[b]	WHO[c]
Highly specific for potential-dependent Ca²⁺ channels (verapamil, nifedipine, diltiazem). All interact at the dihydropyridine site.	Selective for cardiac Ca²⁺ channel: verapamil, nifedipine, diltiazem	Selective for Ca²⁺ channels: verapamil, nifedipine, diltiazem
Less specific agents, bepridil, tiapamil, lidoflazine (interact with Na⁺ channels); flunarizine, cinnarizine	Selective for vascular tissue with no cardiac effects: flunarizine, cinnarizine	Nonselective for Ca²⁺ channels: cinnarizine, flunarizine, prenylamine, others
Other agents: prenylamine, perhexiline	Nonselective agents that also block Na⁺ channels: prenylamine, perhexiline	
Nonspecific agents: primary site of action elsewhere	Site of action elsewhere	

[a]Ref. 149.
[b]Ref. 148.
[c]Ref. 150.
Modified from ref. 147.

could be classified into three primary types: verapamil-like, nifedipine-like, and diltiazem-like (Table 7). These divisions are based on both functional and mechanistic studies and provide a broad parallel to the clinical subdivisions.

Sites of Action of Ca²⁺ Channel Antagonists

That the specific Ca²⁺ channel antagonists, including verapamil, nifedipine, diltiazem, and their analogs, interact at specific binding sites associated with the potential-dependent Ca²⁺ channel is quite evident. The demonstration of structure-activity relationships, including stereoselectivity, is consistent with the existence of specific sites of interaction (reviewed in [6, 151,152]). These sites have been demonstrated directly by radioligand-binding techniques (reviewed in [6,153–155]). Functional demonstrations of Ca²⁺ channel antagonism have included inhibition of stimulus-evoked Ca²⁺ uptake (reviewed in [6]) and the more direct electrophysiologic evidence for selective antagonism of current through the L class of Ca²⁺ channel (reviewed in [6,99,100,102]). Correlations between the properties of the antagonists de-

termined from different procedures adds considerable confidence that a common site of interaction is involved.

Structure-activity relationships are most widely available for the 1,4-dihydropyridines (6,93). Early *in vivo* studies on the hypotensive effects of nifedipine and related compounds (156) defined basic structural features for optimum antagonist activity including (15):

1. The presence of the 1,4-dihydropyridine ring with a free N1-H group. The oxidized pyridine derivatives are completely inactive.
2. The presence of a 4-phenyl ring substituted in the ortho and meta positions by electron-withdrawing substituents.
3. Ester groups at C3 and C5 of the 1,4-dihydropyridine ring. Other electron-withdrawing groups including -CN and -COMe were less effective.

Subsequent structural modifications have shown that the ester groups at C3 and C5 can vary considerably and that activity may be maintained or even increased relative to nifedipine (reviewed in [6,93]). When the ester groups are different, C4 becomes chiral and stereoselective interactions are

TABLE 7. *Pharmacologic profile of Ca^{2+} channel antagonists*

	Selective for slow Ca^{2+} channels			Nonselective for slow Ca^{2+} channels		
	I Verapamil-like	II Nifedipine-like	III Diltiazem	IV Flunarizine-like*	V Prenylamine-like	VI Others (caroverine, perhexiline)
Selective inhibition of myocardial slow Ca^{2+} channels	+	+	+	−	−	−
Additional inhibitory effects on fast Na$^+$ channels	−	−	−	0	+	+
Damping effects on Ca^{2+}-dependent electric activity of pacemaker cells sinus and AV node	+	+	+	0	+	+ (perhexiline)
Inhibition of cardiac inotropism	+	+↑	−	−	0	0
Inhibition of potential-operated Ca^{2+} channels of arterial smooth muscle	+	+	+	+	+	+
Inhibition of receptor-operated Ca^{2+} channels of arterial smooth muscle	+	+	+	+	+	+
Inhibition of myogenic activity on vascular smooth muscle	+	+	+	−	0	0
Antihypertensive effects	+	+	+	−	0	0
Inhibition of [^{3}H]nitrendipine binding	+	+	Facilitation of binding	+	0	0
Antagonism to Ca^{2+} channel agonists of the Bay K 8644 type	+	+	+	−	−	−
Protection against structural damage resulting from cellular Ca^{2+} overload						
In myocardium	+	+	+	+	+	+
In vascular walls	+	+	+	+	+	+
In brain	0	0	0	+	0	0
In kidneys	+	+	+	0	0	0
Inhibition of Ca^{2+}-induced stiffness of blood cells	+	+	0	+	0	0

+, experimentally proven effect; −, no effect; 0, experimental data not available; *, the lack of effect of flunarizine in certain *in vitro* tests may be related to its poor solubility in water; ↑, in the intact organism reflex adjustments overcome the direct inhibitory effect.
From ref. 150.

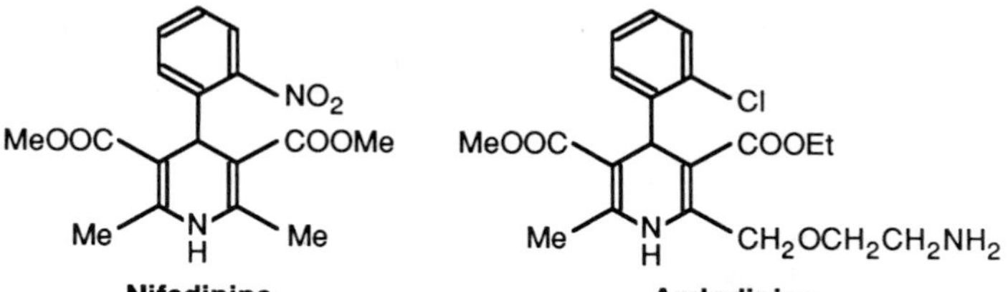

FIG. 9. The chemical structures of a neutral 1,4-dihydropyridine, nifedipine, and a charged derivative, amlodipine.

observed consistent with interaction at a specific site (6,93). Relatively little effort has been devoted to systematic structural modification at other positions of the 1,4-dihydropyridine ring. However, the presence of basic side chains at the 2-position as in amlodipine with a 2-aminoethoxymethyl substituent (Fig. 9), maintains activity but with a stereoselectivity index higher than that observed for other enantiomeric pairs of 1,4-dihydropyridines (158). Additionally, amlodipine and related agents have a duration of action considerably prolonged relative to that of neutral or uncharged analogs (158,159). This suggests that these agents may interact with the receptor site in a manner distinct from that adopted by other 1,4-dihydropyridines (159).

The higher activity of 1,4-dihydropyridines in smooth relative to cardiac muscle has long been recognized and distinguishes nifedipine therapeutically from verapamil and diltiazem (3,4,7,147–150). However, where quantitative data are available very similar structure activity relationships are available for both smooth and cardiac muscle, although the correlation of pharmacologic activities reveals the consistently higher sensitivity of the former (157,160).

The 1,4-dihydropyridine structure embraces both antagonist and activator (stimulant) properties. Few data are yet available to permit resolution of those structural features that determine opposing pharmacologic activities (6,93,151,152). Quite generally the most potent activators (Fig. 10)

have a NO_2 group at the C5 position of the 1,4-dihydropyridine ring. However, there is a remarkable stereochemical discrimination whereby activator and antagonist properties are associated with opposite enantiomers (161–163). It has been suggested that separate 1,4-dihydropyridine sites may be linked to activator and antagonist properties (reviewed in 93). However, interpretation of the structural distinction between activator and antagonist 1,4-dihydropyridines is complicated by observations that activator properties can be observed, although often transiently, with many 1,4-dihydropyridines including potent antagonists and that the expression of activity depends, in any event, qualitatively and quantitatively on membrane potential. Few structure-activity studies are available for the phenylalkylamine series and almost none for the benzothiazepines (6,151,152).

The structure-activity relationships derived from pharmacologic studies have been complemented by data from radioli-

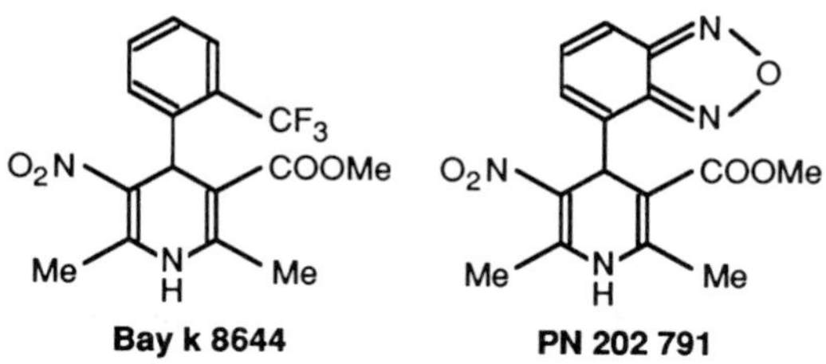

Bay k 8644   **PN 202 791**

FIG. 10. Chemical structures of 1,4-dihydropyridine Ca^{2+} channel activators.

TABLE 8. *Binding characteristics of [³H]1,4-dihydropyridines in cardiac and vascular smooth muscle*

Tissue	Radioligand	K_D ($\times 10^{-9}$ M)	B_{max} (f moles/mg protein)	Ref.
Cardiac				
Ventricle, rat	[³H]Nitrendipine	0.18	400	164
Ventricle, dog	[³H]Nitrendipine	0.11	230	165
Ventricle, rabbit	[³H]Nitrendipine	0.14	335	166
Ventricle, rat	[³H]PN 200 110	0.06	150	166
Vascular				
Aorta, dog	[³H]Nitrendipine	0.25	20	168
Mesenteric, dog	[³H]Nitrendipine	0.31	25	168
Tail, rat	[³H]Nitrendipine	0.36	550	163
Cerebral, rat	[³H]PN 200 110	0.06	45	169

For more extensive data computations, see refs. 6,155,170,171.

gand-binding analyses. Radioligand-binding data (reviewed in [6,93,153–155]) are available for both cardiac and vascular tissues, primarily for [³H]1,4-dihydropyridine interactions with crude microsomal membranes. High-affinity binding sites found for (+)-[³H]nitrendipine and (+)[³H]PN 200 110 (Table 8) are generally sensitive to interaction with agents that serve as Ca²⁺ channel modulators and show similar properties in both cardiac and vascular smooth muscle. The most comprehensive and detailed studies of the binding and biochemical properties of the Ca²⁺ channel are available for the t-tubule membranes of skeletal muscle (114). The binding sites are on the α_1 subunit of the protein complex, which may serve in skeletal muscle the dual role of Ca²⁺ channel and voltage sensor (172,173).

Radioligand-binding and biochemical data indicate the discrete nature of the binding sites for the three principal classes of Ca²⁺ channel ligands (6,151,152,167,174). The schematic representation of Fig. 11 shows the sites linked one to the other and to the permeation and gating machinery of the channel by a set of allosteric interactions. Thus, interaction of verapamil, nifedipine, or diltiazem at these binding sites blocks channel function in voltage- and frequency-dependent fashion. The 1,4-dihydropyridine site, and possibly other sites, can also

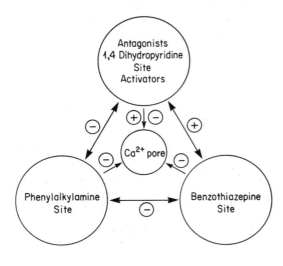

FIG. 11. Schematic representation of three primary ligand binding sites on the L class of voltage-dependent Ca²⁺ channel. Depicted are three allosterically linked sites where the + and − symbols denote positive and negative heterotropic interactions, respectively.

accommodate activator species that stabilize an open channel state. Radioligand-binding studies indicate that positive heterotropic interactions exist between the benzothiazepine and 1,4-dihydropyridine sites, whereby mutual potentiation of binding occurs through increased binding site affinities achieved by reductions in ligand dissociation rates (6,153,155,157). In contrast, the 1,4-dihydropyridine and phenylalkylamine sites serve as mutual inhibitors of drug interactions. These interactions seen in binding studies can also be observed in functional preparations. Diltiazem potentiates the negative inotropic activity of the nifedipine analog, nimodipine (175) and in mesenteric artery strips D600 and nifedipine, and diltiazem and nifedipine showed mutual antagonism and potentiation, respectively, of relaxation of depolarization-induced responses (176).

It is likely that sites of drug interaction at the L class of Ca^{2+} channel exist in addition to those depicted in Fig. 11. Neuroleptics of the diphenylbutylpiperidine series, including pimozide (Fig. 12), penfluridol, fluspirilene, and clopimozide, interact with affinities of 10 to 100 nM to receptors in heart and smooth muscle and with approximately 100-fold higher affinity to skeletal muscle receptors (177,178). These binding sites are distinct from those occupied by verapamil, nifedipine, or diltiazem. Discrete binding sites appear to exist also for ethynylbenzenalkanamines including McN 6186 (179) (Fig. 12), the benzothiazinone HOE 166 (180) (Fig. 12), and the azacyclotridecan-2-imine, MDL 12,330A (181) (Fig. 12). It is likely also that other agents whose primary interactions are at non-Ca^{2+} channel sites and including benzodiazepines, barbiturates, antidepressants, α-adrenoceptor antagonists, 5-hydroxytryptamine antagonists, and antidiarrheal opiates may also exert some part of their pharmacologic activities through interaction at one of the many drug binding sites associated with the Ca^{2+} channel (6).

The association of binding sites, identified largely in membrane fragments, with functional Ca^{2+} channels is based, in part, on the correlations between structure-activity relationships derived from binding and from pharmacologic studies (reviewed in [6,152,155]). Comprehensive studies in cardiac and intestinal smooth muscle dem-

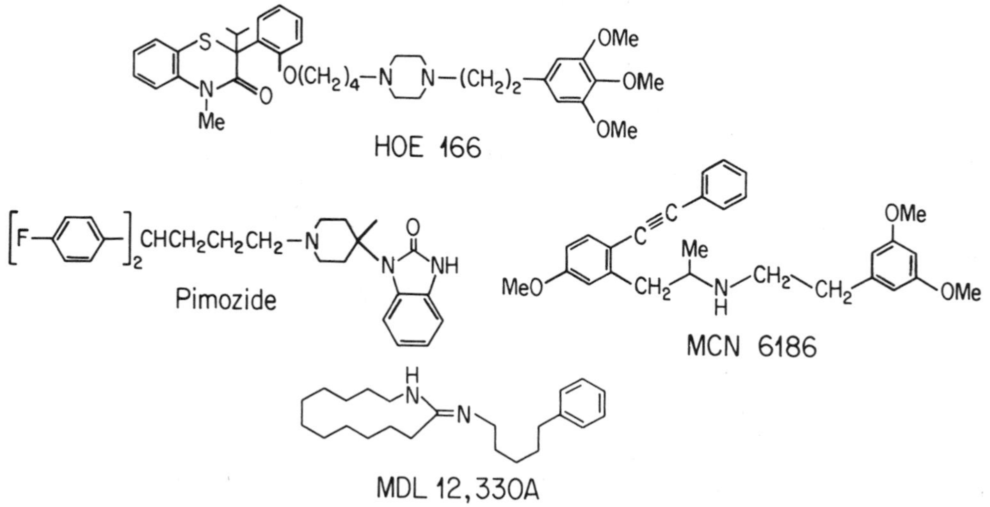

FIG. 12. Chemical structures of agents with Ca^{2+} channel blocking properties that may be exerted at sites distinct from those occupied by the classic agents.

onstrate for a series of 1,4-dihydropyridines the excellent and essentially 1:1 accord between pharmacologic and binding affinities in smooth muscle (6,157,182) (Fig. 13) and, despite the approximately 100-fold lower pharmacologic activities in cardiac muscle, the same rank order of expression of activity. The properties of the binding sites for 1,4-dihydropyridines appear to be very similar in smooth and cardiac muscle (Fig. 13). Comparatively few data are available for vascular smooth muscle (170,171). However, in tail artery (163), coronary artery,

and aorta (183), there exists very good accord between binding and pharmacologic affinities.

Limited studies only are available for binding-pharmacology correlations for other structural classes of Ca^{2+} antagonists. For a series of verapamil analogs in cat heart, the correlation shows, analogously to the 1,4-dihydropyridines, that binding affinities are higher, by one to two orders of magnitude, than negative inotropic potencies (184). These discrepancies are likely due, at least in part, to state-dependent drug inter-

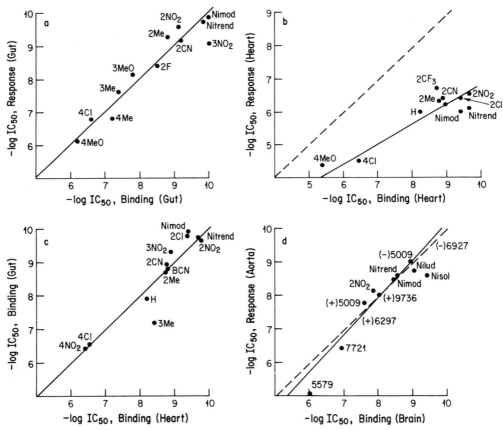

FIG. 13. Correlations between radioligand binding (competition with [³H]1,4-dihydropyridine in microsomal membranes) and pharmacologic affinities of a series of 1,4-dihydropyridines in smooth, cardiac, and neuronal preparations. **a:** K^+ depolarized guinea pig intestinal smooth muscle (ref. 157). **b:** Paced canine papillary muscle (ref. 202). **c:** Correlation between binding affinities in intestinal and cardiac membrane preparations of data shown in panels a and b. **d:** Rat brain membranes and K^+ depolarized rabbit aortic smooth muscle. (Data from ref. 182a.) The *solid lines* represent the correlations and the *dashed lines* the 1:1 relationships. (From ref. 6.)

actions at Ca^{2+} channels, whereby binding and pharmacologic affinities reflect interactions at different populations of channel states.

MECHANISMS OF ACTION

The major categories of Ca^{2+} channel antagonists have been shown to act at an allosterically linked set of sites on a major protein of the L class of voltage-dependent Ca^{2+} channel. Occupancy of these sites, particularly for 1,4-dihydropyridines, promotes both channel activation and antagonism, indicating that these binding sites are associated with the functional machinery of the channel and do not serve merely as sites through which drugs can physically occlude the channel.

Although the relationship of the drug binding sites to channel components mediating permeation, gating, voltage sensitivity, and other functions has yet to be determined, it is clear that these sites are linked to channel functions. This is revealed by the voltage-dependent interactions that have been described for these agents (6, 185). Drug affinity for Ca^{2+} channels may vary dramatically between the open, resting, and inactivated states, the equilibrium between which is determined by stimulus frequency and membrane potential. According to this modulated-receptor hypothesis (186,187), use- or frequency-dependent blockade, whereby inhibitory activity increases with increasing frequency of stimulation, may reflect a preferential interaction of drug with or access to an open or inactivated state of the channel. Potential-dependent interactions by which drug affinity changes with the level of membrane potential represent the selectivity of interaction with channel states, the populations of which depend on the level of membrane potential (Fig. 14). The Ca^{2+} channel antagonists and activators show both frequency- and voltage-dependent interactions according to the preparation employed and the drug category.

It was recognized early that verapamil, D600, and diltiazem showed frequency- and voltage-dependent interactions in cardiac tissue whereby drug potency increased with increasing frequency of stimulation and with increasing levels of depolarization (188,189): this has been confirmed in much subsequent work (190–196). These data indicate that these drugs do not bind, or bind with low affinity, to the resting channel state and that inhibition occurs only after the channel has opened by a depolarizing pulse. The characteristics of block are very similar to those exhibited by local anesthetics at the Na^+ channel, because block accumulates with repetitive pulsing, with increasing frequency amplitude and duration of the pulse, and recovery from block is slow relative to the normal recovery from inactivation. Block and unblock of the channels are favored by depolarization and hyperpolarization, respectively, and the

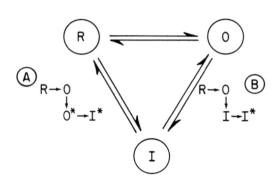

FIG. 14. A schematic representation of an ion channel existing in an equilibrium of resting, open, and inactivated states. Those states marked * indicate stabilization by drug interaction.

rate of drug dissociation depends on membrane potential, increasing with increasing membrane potential (191,196). Additionally, block by verapamil in cardiac preparations does not develop at moderate levels of depolarization (-45 mV) unless repetitive depolarization to more positive potentials is also present (197). These data suggest that verapamil, D600, and diltiazem exhibit frequency-dependent block because they have increased access to the receptor sites through the open-channel state and because they have an enhanced affinity for the open or inactivated state of the Ca^{2+} channel promoted by depolarization (Fig. 14). The extent to which preferential drug interaction with open or inactivated states occurs has not been fully resolved. It is likely, however, that diltiazem interacts primarily with inactivated channels (193,197), whereas verapamil and D600 also interact with open channels.

Although the 1,4-dihydropyridines were originally assumed not to exhibit state-dependent interactions, it is now clear that the properties of the 1,4-dihydropyridines depend, both qualitatively and quantitatively, on membrane potential. Ca^{2+} channel block by the neutral, uncharged, 1,4-dihydropyridine antagonists including nifedipine, nitrendipine, and nisoldipine is independent of stimulus frequency except at 1 Hz and higher, but greatly depends on membrane potential. This voltage dependence of inhibition of Ca^{2+} current has been demonstrated in a number of cardiac (198–204) and vascular smooth muscle preparations (205–207). Estimates of affinity differences for 1,4-dihydropyridines for different channel states are summarized for some vascular smooth muscle and cardiac preparations in Table 9.

The voltage dependence of 1,4-dihydropyridine interactions with vascular smooth muscle has also been established in functional and radioligand-binding measurements (170,207,210–212). That the slow or tonic component of depolarization-induced response in smooth muscle is significantly more sensitive to the Ca^{2+} channel antagonists than the initial or phasic component of response is consistent with a selective interaction with channel states favored by prolonged depolarization (157,170). In mesenteric artery, the K_D values for binding of $(+)[^3H]PN$ 200 110 under polarized and de-

TABLE 9. *Interactions of 1,4-dihydropyridines with Ca^{2+} channels in cardiac and vascular muscle preparations*

Tissue	Drug	IC_{50}, K_I (conc. $\times 10^{-9}$ M)	% Inhibition	Channel/state	Ref.
Vascular smooth muscle					
Mesenteric	Nitrendipine	0.5	50	L, inactivated	205
		222	50	L, resting	205
Mesenteric	Nisoldipine	0.07		L, inactivated	207
		2–15		L, resting	207
Saphenous	Nitrendipine	10		L, resting	206
Cardiac					
Ventricular	Nitrendipine	0.4	50	L, inactivated	199
		700	50	L, resting	
Atrial	Nifedipine	30	50	L, inactivated	200
		300	50	L, resting	
Purkinje	Nisoldipine	1	50	L, inactivated	198
		1,340	50	L, resting	198
Myocytes	Nifedipine	39		L, inactivated	201
		450		L, resting	201
Myocytes	R 202791	9	50	L, inactivated	208
		200	50	L, resting	208

polarized conditions are in good accord with the pharmacologic affinities determined from tension responses, and the binding affinities in the depolarized tissue and the membrane preparation are also in accord (Table 10). Similarly, radioligand-binding studies in cardiac preparations, vesicles, and intact myocytes have established the voltage dependence of Ca^{2+} channel antagonist interactions, whereby depolarization increases the affinity of 1,4-dihydropyridine interactions (209,215–218). In marked contrast, binding of the activator enantiomers of 1,4-dihydropyridines, including S Bay K 8644 and S 202 791, is independent of membrane potential (209, 219,220). Accordingly, the affinities of these activator species may differ little between open- and inactivated-channel states. This may underlie observations that the single enantiomer S Bay K 8644 may exert activator and antagonist effects at polarized and depolarized membrane potentials, respectively, in cardiac and vascular smooth muscle preparations (163,221).

The neutral 1,4-dihydropyridines appear to access their receptor sites via the hydrophobic pathway (Fig. 14). This is consistent with their hydrophobic nature and their high membrane:water partition coefficients, suggesting that they may use a membrane diffusion approach to access the receptor (222). However, 1,4-dihydropyridines possessing charged groups, including nicardipine and amlodipine (198,223), behave differently, exhibiting both frequency- and voltage-dependent interactions when they are in the ionized form, suggesting that they may access receptor sites by the dual pathways of the modulated receptor model (Fig. 14). The behavior of amlodipine bears a striking resemblance to the situation with the local anesthetics because recovery from block by the ionized species is much slower than by the neutral species. These data suggest a binding location for 1,4-dihydropyridines that is not directly accessible to the aqueous environment but which is accessible by protons.

It is usually assumed that 1,4-dihydropyridine activators and antagonists interact at a common site. However, some studies suggest discrete sites at which activator and antagonist species may exhibit cooperative interactions (216,224).

Similarities exist between Ca^{2+} channel-ligand interactions at Ca^{2+} channels and drug-receptor interactions (97,225). These similarities are further strengthened by observations that Ca^{2+} channels (and other ion channels) are regulated by G proteins (226,227) and that the interactions of drugs with the Ca^{2+} channel are influenced by G-protein state. Thus, in cardiac cells the stimulatory G_s protein of adenyl cyclase can activate directly the Ca^{2+} channel independent of the activation mediated through the cAMP-protein kinase A pathway (228). In neuronal cells, D600, nifedipine, and diltiazem potentiate Ca^{2+} current in the presence of activated G_o/G_i proteins and the actions of the activator Bay K 8644

TABLE 10. *Comparison of binding and pharmacologic affinities of (+)PN 200 110 in mesenteric artery (212)*

	Dissociation constant (+)PN 200 110	
	Radioligand binding K_D (M)	Pharmacology IC_{50} (M)
Polarized		
5 mM KCl	200×10^{-12}	—
2 min contraction	—	270×10^{-12}
Depolarized		
100 mM KCl	44×10^{-12}	—
30 min contraction	—	33×10^{-12}

are enhanced (229). Thus G-protein activation may promote activator actions of Ca^{2+} channel ligands, whereas antagonist actions may dominate in their absence. Accordingly, both membrane potential and G-protein state are determinants of the activities of these drugs.

ACTIONS AT NON-Ca^{2+} CHANNEL SYSTEMS

The available data suggest that the L category of voltage-dependent Ca^{2+} channels in the cardiovascular system represents the major therapeutic target of the Ca^{2+} channel antagonists. However, all of the available agents do have effects on other systems including a variety of neurotransmitter and hormone receptors, other categories of ion channel, and a number of membrane transport systems. The clinical significance of these interactions remains to

be defined. However, high concentrations of the Ca^{2+} channel antagonist may be achieved in membranes, both plasmalemmal and intracellular, reflecting the very high membrane:water partition coefficients of these agents (230,231). Thus, nimodipine with a partition coefficient of 5,000 will, at plasma concentrations of 10^{-9} M achieve greater than micromolar concentrations in the membrane (232). The membrane concentrations of other agents may be even higher. The ratio of concentrations at which Ca^{2+} channel antagonism is exerted to the concentration at which other nonspecific effects are exerted is clearly an important consideration; this ratio, quite generally, is lower for agents of the verapamil and diltiazem classes than for the 1,4-dihydropyridines.

Interactions of verapamil and D600 with a number of receptor systems have been described (6,233,234,244) (Table 11). The ability to interact at micromolar concentrations

TABLE 11. Ca^{2+} *channel antagonist interactions at neurotransmitter receptors*

Antagonist	Receptor	K_i or IC_{50} (M)	Ref.
α_1-Adrenoceptor			
D600	Brain	1.1	235
(−)D600	Vas deferens	1.5	236
(+)D600	Vas deferens	1.7	236
(−)Verapamil	Heart	4.8	237
(+)Verapamil	Heart	6.8	237
Verapamil	Aorta	8.7	238
Diltiazem	Aorta	9.8	238
α_2-Adrenoceptor			
D600	Heart	14.4	237
(−)Verapamil	Heart	2.2	237
(+)Verapamil	Heart	14.8	237
Diltiazem	Heart	15.2	237
Verapamil	Aorta	6.8	239
Diltiazem	Aorta	70	239
Muscarinic			
Verapamil	Heart	7.0	240
β-Adrenoceptor			
Verapamil	Heart(β_1)	115	241
Diltiazem	Heart(β_1)	131	241
Verapamil	Lymphocyte(β_2)	32	241
Diltiazem	Lymphocyte(β_2)	137	241
Serotonin			
Verapamil	Brain (5HT2)	0.3	242
D600	Brain (5HT2)	0.7	242
(−)Verapamil	Brain (5HT1)	3.9	243
(+)Verapamil	Brain	13	243

suggests that these effects could contribute to their total pharmacologic profile. In contrast, the 1,4-dihydropyridines are generally ineffective against these receptor systems even at concentrations of 10^{-4} M. An exception is provided by nicardipine, which is a relatively potent inhibitor of several receptor systems including α-adrenergic and muscarinic with K_I values of approximately 10^{-7} M (239,245).

1,4-Dihydropyridines are, however, effective against several other receptor systems including the platelet-activating factor receptor where nifedipine is some 10 to 20 times less effective than verapamil or diltiazem (246), the adenosine receptor where nifedipine has a K_I of 4×10^{-6} M (247), and at the thromboxane A_2 receptor where nifedipine has a K_I value of 3.8×10^{-5} M (248).

Interactions at other categories of ion channels have been described, notably for the Na^+ channel, where verapamil and D600 are effective inhibitors of the fast Na^+ current at concentrations between 10^{-6} and 10^{-5} M (249,250). Recent reports indicate that 1,4-dihydropyridines can also serve both as activators and antagonists at Na^+ channels (251). These interactions are not surprising in view of the homologies that exist between voltage-dependent channel types.

Several enzyme and transport systems are also sensitive to the Ca^{2+} channel antagonists. Calmodulin-dependent cyclic nucleotide phosphodiesterase is inhibited by nicardipine and other 1,4-dihydropyridines (252,253). Both stimulant and inhibitory effects have been observed on membrane transport systems. Nimodipine and nitrendipine at submicromolar concentrations stimulate the Na^+,K^+-ATPase from vascular smooth muscle; however, other antagonists including nifedipine are ineffective (254). Ca^{2+} uptake by sarcoplasmic reticulum is stimulated by 1,4-dihydropyridines and blocked by verapamil, albeit at the high concentrations of 10^{-4} to 10^{-3} M (255,256). The mitochondrial Na^+-Ca^{2+} exchanger is inhibited by the several types of Ca^{2+} channel antagonist (257). However, diltiazem is the most potent of the clinically available agents, with effective concentrations of approximately 10^{-5} M, although the structural requirements for inhibition of the exchanger and the Ca^{2+} channel are quite different (258).

Ca^{2+} channel antagonists bind to the nucleoside transporter of a number of cell types and also inhibit adenosine influx and efflux from erythrocytes. This system is most sensitive to the 1,4-dihydropyridines, which are effective at concentrations from 10^{-7} to 10^{-6} M, whereas verapamil and diltiazem are approximately 100-fold less effective (259,260). The structural requirements for Ca^{2+} antagonist interaction at the Ca^{2+} channel and the transporter are quite distinct, including opposing stereoselectivity. However, it is likely that the transporter provides, in at least some tissues, the low affinity 1,4-dihydropyridine binding sites.

The extent to which the several processes outlined contribute to the total therapeutic profile of the Ca^{2+} channel antagonists is not established. It is clearly possible to envisage that the receptor-blocking properties of verapamil may contribute to its cardiodepressant effects and that some of the tissue-protecting effects of the Ca^{2+} antagonists stem from their actions on other ion-transport and sequestering systems. It is also possible that these effects contribute to the efficacy of these agents in processes such as inhibition of platelet aggregation and antiatherogenic activity, which may not be mediated through voltage-dependent Ca^{2+} channels.

SELECTIVITY OF ACTION OF THE Ca^{2+} CHANNEL ANTAGONISTS

The Ca^{2+} channel antagonists are a therapeutically and pharmacologically selective group of agents. Their actions are mostly confined to the cardiovascular system, although their target, the L class of voltage-dependent Ca^{2+} channel, is widespread in excitable cells including skeletal muscle and neurons. They do not have obvious therapeutic actions in the central nervous system, in most nonvascular smooth muscles or in secretory cells. However, under experimental conditions their actions may be very obvious in such systems.

Within the cardiovascular system, considerable selectivity of action occurs. Although verapamil, nifedipine, and diltiazem, as representatives of the three major categories of agent, are all vasodilating species, not all vascular beds are equally sensitive to Ca^{2+} channel antagonist action and a major distinction is found between the relative cardiac and vascular effects of these agents. Nifedipine and other 1,4-dihydropyridines are selective vasodilating species and significantly less effective in depressing cardiac pacemaker and tension responses: indeed, a modest initial tachycardia is frequently seen after nifedipine administration *in vivo* due to reflex sympathetic stimulation. In marked contrast, verapamil and diltiazem show prominent cardiac effects, particularly on nodal function, underlying the use, notably of verapamil, in the control of supraventricular tachycardia (Tables 1 and 12).

Selectivity of action is also exhibited between different vascular tissues both *in vivo* and *in vitro*. Several descriptions have appeared of the regional hemodynamic effects of the Ca^{2+} channel antagonists in a number of species (264–266). Thus, in anesthetized cats all Ca^{2+} channel antagonists dilated coronary and cerebral vascular beds dose dependently, and blood flow to skeletal muscle was increased markedly by the

1,4-dihydropyridines, only somewhat by diltiazem, and not at all by verapamil (267). Mechanistic interpretation of such *in vivo* observations is complex due to the large number of hemodynamic variables simultaneously affected. However, it is of interest that vascular differences can also be observed *in vitro*.

It was recognized early that the small blood vessels are more sensitive than the large vessels to the Ca^{2+} channel antagonists (264–268). In a comparison of the responses of several vascular smooth muscles to a common stimulus, K^+ depolarization, with a series of Ca^{2+} channel antagonists including verapamil, diltiazem, nifedipine, and several related 1,4-dihydropyridines, differential sensitivity was observed between several vascular and nonvascular smooth muscles (269). Notably, tracheal smooth muscle was the least sensitive of the nonvascular smooth muscles and mesenteric artery was significantly more sensitive than aorta (Fig. 15). Comparison of sensitivities of K^+-depolarized peripheral and cerebral arteries of the rat revealed the latter to be the more sensitive, particularly to verapamil and nifedipine (Table 13) (270).

Selectivity may also occur as a consequence of disease states. Thus, hypertensive vascular smooth muscle is more sensitive to the Ca^{2+} channel antagonists than is normotensive tissue (271–274), and verapamil and diltiazem, but not nifedipine, become more effective negative inotropes under ischemic conditions (275).

It is likely that a variety of factors contribute to the observed tissue selectivity of the Ca^{2+} channel antagonists. Several in-

TABLE 12. *Cardiac and vascular selectivity of Ca^{2+} channel antagonists*

Preparation	Verapamil	Nifedipine IC_{50} (M)	Diltiazem	Ref.
Vascular smooth muscle + depolarized	$\sim 10^{-7}$	$\sim 5 \times 10^{-9}$	$\sim 5 \times 10^{-7}$	261
Canine trabeculae, negative inotropic	2×10^{-7}	1×19^{-7}	4×10^{-7}	262
Rabbit atrium AV node	2×10^{-7}	3×10^{-7}	2×10^{-7}	263
Rabbit atrium SA node	4×10^{-6}	3×10^{-6}	2×10^{-6}	264

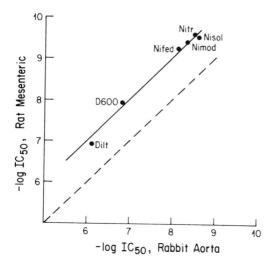

FIG. 15. Correlation of activities of a series of Ca^{2+} channel antagonists including diltiazem (Dilt), D600, nifedipine (Nifed), nitrendipine (Nitr), nimodipine (Nimod), and nisoldipine (Nisol) in K^+ depolarized rat mesenteric artery and rabbit aortic tissues. The *solid line* indicates the correlation and the *dashed line* represents the 1:1 relationship.

vestigations have pursued the concept that subtypes of Ca^{2+} antagonist receptors may exist in different cardiovascular tissues. Comparative studies of [³H]1,4-dihydropyridine-binding characteristics in vascular and cardiac tissues have, however, failed to find differences other than the higher density of binding sites in cardiac tissue (153,154,276). Similarly, a comparative survey of [³H]1,4-dihydropyridine binding to membranes from different vascular tissues found differences only in the densities of binding sites and no observable differences in ligand affinity were observed (277).

With some justification it may be argued that simple measurement of ligand binding to crude membrane preparations is inappropriate to the search for receptor subtypes. In fact, it is likely that the tissue selectivity

of the Ca^{2+} channel antagonists depends on a number of factors that operate alone or in combination. These factors include (6,151)

1. Pharmacokinetic factors: tissue and cellular distribution, metabolism, and clearance.
2. Ca^{2+} source mobilized: the relative use of intracellular and extracellular pools. Mobilization of intracellular Ca^{2+} is expected to be an insensitive process.
3. Hemodynamic effects: reflex cardiovascular pathways in intact animals.
4. Class of Ca^{2+} channel: each class has its own discrete pharmacology. Quite generally the L-class antagonists are ineffective at the T and N classes of Ca^{2+} channel.
5. State-dependent interaction: voltage- and frequency-dependence of interactions. Drug actions will depend on the structure of the drug, charged, hydrophobic or hydrophilic, on membrane potential, and on the frequency of stimulation.
6. Kinetics of channel opening: a drug may not have an opportunity to access a preferred state if channel open time is brief.
7. Activator-antagonist properties of drug: extent to which a drug is a pure antagonist or activator or has mixed properties. This will be determined both by drug structure and membrane potential.

TABLE 13. *IC_{50} values of Ca^{2+} channel antagonists on peripheral and cerebral vasculature of rat (270)*

	K^+ depolarization response IC_{50} (M)	
	Mesenteric	Middle cerebral
Verapamil	2.0×10^{-8}	1.3×10^{-7}
Diltiazem	1.2×10^{-7}	3.0×10^{-7}
Nifedipine	4.0×10^{-10}	4.5×10^{-9}
Nicardipine	1.0×10^{-9}	3.0×10^{-9}

8. Pathologic state of tissue: altered expression of receptors by number, influence of pH, or membrane potential.
9. Nonspecific effects: extent to which drugs may interact with other receptor or channel systems.

Thus, it is quite likely that modest depolarization of vascular smooth muscle in hypertension will lead to an enhanced sensitivity to Ca^{2+} channel antagonists through state-dependent processes (278). Similarly, channels that open only transiently may not permit adequate time for drug equilibration with a high-affinity binding state. The insensitivity of neuronal processes dependent on L-channel activation may be due to this effect. The disentanglement of these and other factors are the clues to the rational definition of the therapeutic applications of the existing and future generations of Ca^{2+} channel antagonists.

THERAPEUTIC APPLICATIONS

Currently available Ca^{2+} channel antagonists are mainly used in the area of cardiovascular disorders including angina, some cardiac arrhythmias, hypertension, and peripheral vascular diseases. Extensions to other areas of use are under active clinical investigation. The extent to which each agent is used in these areas depends on the origin and basis of the pathologic defect, mechanism of action, any contraindications, and incidence of side effects.

Angina

It is likely that several underlying mechanisms contribute to the antianginal actions of the Ca^{2+} channel antagonists. These include coronary vasodilation, decreased myocardial work as a consequence of reduced afterload, negative inotropic and chronotropic effects, redistribution of coronary flow to ischemic areas, and protection against Ca^{2+} overload (3,81,279). The relative contributions made are both drug and disorder specific, although verapamil, nifedipine, and diltiazem all find use in several forms of angina: exertional, variant, and unstable. However, comprehensive comparisons of the several antagonists are generally lacking.

In chronic stable angina associated with exertion, the β-adrenoceptor antagonists exert their beneficial effect principally through reduction of oxygen demand. This effect may be shared by verapamil through its negative inotropic effect (Tables 1 and 12), but nifedipine functions primarily through its vasodilating properties as an afterload reducer. Diltiazem probably functions both through reduction of heart rate and blood pressure to yield a reduced double product. A reduced double product is also seen with verapamil, but it is likely that other actions may also contribute, including selective effects in ischemic regions. These different underlying mechanisms may contribute to the different patient response. Additionally, nifedipine may provoke angina presumably through the reflex tachycardia that may be observed during acute dosing. The extent of the reflex tachycardia is patient dependent, varying with age and the patency of the baroreceptor reflex mechanisms, and is usually not observed during chronic dosing. The agents are approximately equieffective in stable angina with daily dose levels of 400 mg verapamil, 60 mg nifedipine, and 360 mg diltiazem, but nifedipine may be marginally less preferred unless in combination with a β-adrenoceptor antagonist.

In variant, Prinzmetal's, or vasospastic angina, the underlying defect is associated with coronary spasm, particularly of the larger arteries. The etiology of the spasm is complex and variable and includes endothelial damage that alters the vasodilator:vasoconstrictor balance of a number of agents, the actions of platelet vasoconstrictors and neurogenic mechanisms, and the effects of diurnal rhythms controlling sympathetic:parasympathetic balance. Verapamil, nifedipine, and diltiazem appear to be approximately equally and highly effective in variant angina.

Unstable angina has several components of origin including the presence of an atherosclerotic plaque, the rupture or instability of which may lead to increasing and more prolonged anginal episodes (280,281). The role of Ca^{2+} channel antagonists in this complex syndrome may well depend on the dynamic status and the proneness to infarction of the heart. Verapamil and diltiazem are both effective, but nifedipine is probably contraindicated unless associated with β-blockade.

Thus, the role of the Ca^{2+} channel antagonists in anginal therapy is complex. Considerable interpatient variation and a spectrum of indication for Ca^{2+} channel antagonists and β-adrenoceptor antagonists will exist, determined by the balance between angina and infarction (279,282). The Ca^{2+} channel antagonists do not appear to be effective and may well be contraindicated in acute myocardial infarction (283).

Cardiac Arrhythmias

Both SA and AV nodes include prominent roles for Ca^{2+} currents in depolarizing and pacemaking functions. The sinus node is inhibited by all three major Ca^{2+} antagonists, but the extent to which this translates into decreased heart rate depends in part, on any reflex sympathetic stimulation.

Such stimulation is normally most prominent with nifedipine and least prominent with diltiazem. At the AV node both nodal conduction time and nodal refractoriness are increased by verapamil and diltiazem (Table 14).

Both verapamil and diltiazem are used in the control of chronic atrial fibrillation, verapamil being used in both intravenous and oral forms (284–286). Verapamil and diltiazem may be used together with digoxin for more effective treatment. Verapamil and diltiazem are not effective against atrial flutter, but because they both decrease AV conduction they reduce the response rate of the ventricles.

Both verapamil and diltiazem, in oral or intravenous forms, are effective against paroxysmal supraventricular tachycardia, conversion to sinus rhythm being achieved in the majority of cases (287–290). Maintenance can be accomplished through combination with propranolol (288,290).

Both verapamil and diltiazem inhibit reentry tachycardias at the AV node in Wolff-Parkinson-White arrhythmias, but there is a risk of enhanced conduction along the anterograde pathway leading to ventricular fibrillation.

Hypertension

Verapamil, diltiazem, and nifedipine are all effective antihypertensive agents, primarily because of their vasodilating prop-

TABLE 14. *Electrophysiologic properties of Ca^{2+} channel antagonists*

	Verapamil	Nifedipine	Diltiazem
AV node conduction	↓↓	↓	0
AV node ERP	↑↑	↑	0
AV node ERP	0	0	0
His-Purkinje-ERP	0	0	0
RR interval	↑↓	↑↓	0
QRS interval	0	0	↓
PR interval	↑	↑	0
AH interval	↑	↑	0
HV interval	0	0	0

↑, increases; ↓, decreases, 0, no change.
Adapted from ref. 283a.

erties. Much, however, remains to be established concerning their relative usefulness in severe to mild hypertension, their roles in single or combined therapy, and the relative importance of compensating factors in the hypotensive response (279).

Nifedipine enjoys established use in the control of severe hypertension and is probably more efficacious than verapamil or diltiazem. The actions of nifedipine are not accompanied by significant reflex tachycardia, indicating the blunted baroreceptor reflexes of severe hypertension, and the absence of postural hypotension indicates that compensatory supine to erect vasoconstriction still exists (279,291–293). Failure or blunted responses to the acute hypotensive effects of nifedipine may be attributed to high renin status.

All three agents, verapamil, nifedipine, and diltiazem, are effective in the treatment of mild to moderate hypertension (291–293). They are used either alone or in combination with β-blockers or angiotensin-converting enzyme (ACE) inhibitors. Whereas their antihypertensive actions appear to be generally comparable, there are several differences of action particularly with respect to nifedipine versus diltiazem and verapamil. Cardiac depression is not usually found with nifedipine, with which a modest initial tachycardia is often seen, but is more common with verapamil and diltiazem. It is assumed that the basis of the antihypertensive actions stems from inhibition of Ca^{2+} entry into vascular smooth muscle through the voltage-dependent Ca^{2+} channels. However, other actions may also be operative. Thus, centrally mediated hypotensive mechanisms have been suggested for 1,4-dihydropyridines (296), and diltiazem has been suggested to inhibit also the release of intracellular Ca^{2+} (297).

Nifedipine is the more potent vasodilator eliciting greater compensating reflex activation. All three agents increase plasma catecholamine levels, reflecting sympathetic activation, but the effect is larger and more consistent with nifedipine than with verapamil or diltiazem (298). Catecholamine levels return to normal following chronic administration. The agents do not have, in contrast to other vasodilating species, significant effects on the renin-angiotensin-aldosterone axis, and there are usually only modest increases in plasma renin levels during the acute phase of treatment (279,299,300). However, the activity of the Ca^{2+} channel antagonists in hypertension may well depend on the hormonal and ionic status of the population. The Ca^{2+} channel antagonists may be more effective in low-renin, low-serum Ca^{2+}, salt-sensitive states (83,84,303). These observations may underlie the relative sensitivities of patient subgroups including the elderly, blacks, and other low-renin individuals to the Ca^{2+} channel antagonists relative to β-blockers (304).

The renal effects of the Ca^{2+} channel antagonists also contrast with other vasodilators because they increase acutely, and possibly also on longer term administration, the excretion of sodium and water (299,301). This diuretic effect may be more prolonged with second generation Ca^{2+} channel antagonists and may arise both from increased renal plasma flow and from direct stimulatory effects on renal tubular Na^+ excretion. The antihypertensive effects of the Ca^{2+} channel antagonists also appear to be unaccompanied by adverse effects on other regulatory processes including insulin secretion or response in diabetic or nondiabetic individuals after chronic administration or plasma lipoprotein levels (300,302). This presents a further contrast to other antihypertensive agents.

Cerebral and Peripheral Vascular Disorders

The vasodilating properties of the Ca^{2+} channel antagonists find application in the control of a number of vasoconstrictive vascular disorders (20,279,293,305,306).

Flunarizine, verapamil, and nifedipine have all been reported to be effective in migraine prophylaxis, but comparisons to the effects of other agents are, for the most part, lacking. It is assumed that the mechanism of action is an underlying vasodilation of cerebral blood vessels contracted by mediator or neurogenic stimuli. It is likely, however, that other effects operate. Verapamil is a potent serotonin antagonist and may also prevent platelet aggregation and release. The 1,4-dihydropyridine nimodipine, with enhanced lipid solubility relative to nifedipine, is also effective against migraine. Cerebral vasospasm subsequent to subarachnoid hemorrhage responds to nimodipine (28,307) at concentrations exerting minimal peripheral side effects. Similarly, nimodipine is reported to reduce the cerebral neurologic defects subsequent to acute ischemic stroke (29,308).

The vasospasm induced by cold and emotion in Raynaud's disease responds to the Ca^{2+} channel antagonists (24,25,305). The 1,4-dihydropyridines, including nimodipine, appear to be the more effective species (309) against the spastic form of the disorder. The Ca^{2+} channel antagonists are markedly less effective against the obstructive form of the disorder.

Congestive Heart Failure

The Ca^{2+} channel antagonists, particularly nifedipine, have been employed in congestive heart failure (16,17,279,310,311). Their role relative to the ACE inhibitors remains to be established. The reduction in afterload produced, together with its modest diuretic properties, may offer an advantage to nifedipine. The more marked negative inotropic properties of verapamil suggest that greater caution should be taken with this agent. The reduced or absent sympathetic drive seen in congestive heart failure may, however, also generate cardiodepressant properties with nifedipine. However, Ca^{2+} antagonists are employed for congestive heart failure with coexisting angina or hypertension and the presence of

tachycardia or bradycardia should select for diltiazem or nifedipine, respectively.

Cardiomyopathy

Hypertrophic cardiomyopathy responds to the Ca^{2+} channel antagonists because they improve diastolic function (279,311, 312). Verapamil has been shown to be the most effective and the most widely used of the antagonists, but nifedipine and diltiazem are also employed. However, nifedipine is contraindicated in hypertrophic obstructive cardiomyopathy.

Atherosclerosis

Ca^{2+} plays a critical role in the atherogenic process and the Ca^{2+} channel antagonists slow the development of atherosclerosis in experimental models (313–316). However, these experimental models have not demonstrated unequivocally whether the antiatherogenic properties stem from Ca^{2+} channel antagonism. It is known, however, that Ca^{2+} chelating agents and inorganic cations (La^{3+}) can slow atherogenic development presumably by impeding the development of the calcification process at the atheromatous plaque. Processes of greater relevance to the sites of action of the Ca^{2+} channel antagonists include the medial to intimal migration of smooth muscle cells and their subsequent proliferation (317), endothelium-mediated relaxation processes, and the enhanced reactivity to vasoconstrictor stimuli seen in atherosclerotic smooth muscle (318) and platelet aggregation (319). Of particular interest, LDL-receptor-mediated events including the proliferation of LDL receptors and LDL endocytosis both appear to be stimulated by Ca^{2+} channel antagonists (320,321). The relationship of these processes to the progression and modification by Ca^{2+} channel antagonists of experimental and human atherosclerosis remains to be established. It is entirely possible that these actions are not related to Ca^{2+} channel antagonism.

A number of other therapeutic and potential therapeutic areas of the Ca^{2+} channel antagonists from achalasia to vertigo have been indicated briefly in a previous section. Possible future developments will be discussed later.

PHARMACOKINETIC CONSIDERATIONS

Despite their chemical heterogeneity, the major Ca^{2+} channel antagonists have a number of pharmacokinetic considerations in common. In particular, verapamil, nifedipine, and diltiazem are all well absorbed after oral administration, extensively protein bound, and subject to extensive metabolism (322–326) (Table 15). The metabolites of nifedipine are inactive, but both verapamil and diltiazem give rise to active metabolic products (Fig. 16).

Nifedipine is rapidly absorbed and relatively highly bioavailable following oral dosing. The cardiovascular effects are related to serum concentrations (327). In one study (328), systolic and diastolic blood pressures and heart rate were linearly related to the logarithm of the serum nifedipine concentration following oral administration in normal volunteers. More limited data are available for other 1,4-dihydropyridines (329–331).

Verapamil is administered as the racemic mixture and rapidly and well absorbed after oral administration, but its bioavailability is low because of extensive first-pass metabolism (326). Variations in hepatic blood flow may account for variations in measured plasma levels (332). Metabolism of verapamil via N-demethylation yields norverapamil, an active metabolite, in addition to inactive metabolites produced by cleavage of the 3,4-dimethoxyphenethyl group and O-demethylation (332). Verapamil is metabolized stereoselectively, the more active (–)-enantiomer being more rapidly metabolized. There are important consequences to this selective metabolism with respect to differences in intravenous and oral administration routes. After intravenous administration of racemic verapamil, the enantiomer plasma ratio is 0.56 ± 0.10 compared with 0.23 ± 0.05 after oral administration. Thus, higher plasma concentrations of verapamil are required after oral

TABLE 15. *Pharmacokinetics of Ca^{2+} channel antagonists*

	Diltiazem	Nifedipine	Verapamil
Absorption			
Oral (%)	>90	>90	>90
Bioavailability (%)	~20	60–70	10–20
Onset of action			
Sublingual (min)	—	3	—
Oral (min)	<30	<20	<30
Peak effect			
Oral	30 min	1–2 hr	3–5 hr
Intravenous	—	—	10–15 min
Protein binding (%)	90	90	90
Elimination half-life (hr)	5	5[a]	8
Metabolism	Active[b] metabolites	Inactive metabolites	Active[b] metabolites
Volume of distribution (single dose)	5.3 liter/kg	1.3 liter/kg	6.1 liter/kg
Excretion (%)			
Renal	30	90%, 24 hr	70
Fecal	60	~10%	15

[a]6–11 hr after oral tablets rather than capsules.
[b]Less active than parent, but longer elimination half-life.

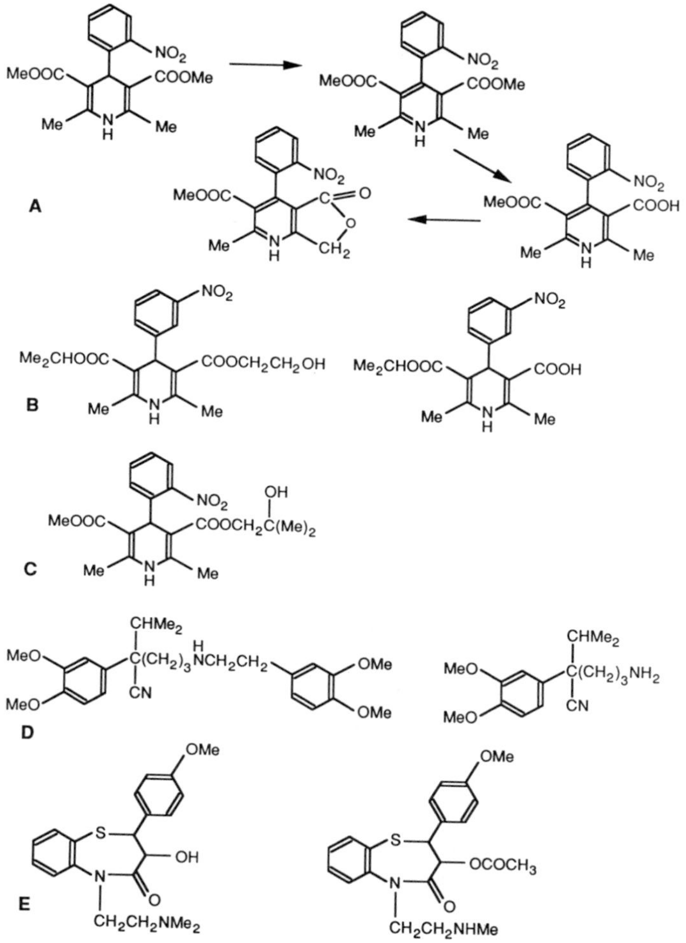

FIG. 16. Metabolites of Ca^{2+} channel antagonists. **A**, nifedipine; **B**, nimodipine; **C**, nisoldipine; **D**, verapamil; **E**, diltiazem.

administration to compensate for this preferential metabolism (333,334).

Diltiazem (325,335) is administered as a single enantiomer and has a higher bioavailability than nifedipine and verapamil. The mean half-life is approximately 4.5 hr, but this may be delayed in the elderly patient. Desdeacetyldiltiazem is a major active metabolite of diltiazem, the disposition of which appears to be significantly slower than that of diltiazem itself.

Tiapamil, an achiral analog of verapamil with generally lower potency, is similar to verapamil, subject to significant first-pass

metabolism, and has a mean half-life of 2.5 hr (336,337). Its bioavailability of approximately 20% is also similar to that of verapamil. The major metabolites, via loss of the N-methyl and N-dimethoxyphenethyl groups, are inactive. Very little unchanged drug is excreted, but the major metabolic route of excretion (fecal) differs from that of verapamil, which is via urinary excretion.

A number of 1,4-dihydropyridine analogs of nifedipine have been studied. These include nicardipine (338), nitrendipine (331), nimodipine (330), and nisoldipine (341,342).

They are all subject to first-pass metabolism, all bioavailable to the extent of 5% to 25%, and all extensively protein bound. The mean half-lives are between 90 and 120 min. Their metabolic pathways are similar to that employed by nifedipine and involve ring oxidation to inactive pyridine metabolites; nimodipine gives rise initially to 1,4-dihydropyridine metabolites that may be active and side-chain hydroxylation of nisoldipine may also yield an active metabolite (Fig. 16).

SIDE EFFECTS AND CONTRAINDICATIONS OF Ca²⁺ CHANNEL ANTAGONISTS

It has been remarked that, despite the powerful cardiovascular effects of the Ca^{2+} channel antagonists, the side effects reported are relatively modest (341). The three major agents have a variety of individual side effects, but common to all are facial flushing, headaches, dizziness, and ankle edema, albeit in varying proportions according to the agent (Table 16) (341,342). The ankle edema likely arises from precapillary vasodilation rather than from general salt or water retention (343). Quite generally, the incidence of reported side effects appears to be least for diltiazem and greater for verapamil and nifedipine.

For verapamil, constipation is the most frequent and troubling of the minor side effects. Why this should occur with verapamil and not occur, or occur only infrequently, with nifedipine and diltiazem is not established. Conceivably, the constipating effect of verapamil is unrelated to Ca^{2+} channel antagonism but rather is due to the multiple-receptor inhibitory effects of the agent. The more severe side effects of verapamil are derived from its cardiodepressant actions, which can lead to contraindications. However, unlike β-adrenoceptor antagonists, bronchospasm and peripheral vasoconstriction are not side effects.

Most of the side effects of nifedipine are minor and include vasodilation-induced events. However, tachycardia and orthostatic hypotension are generally absent. These effects are dose dependent, the frequency increasing with increasing dose. Major side effects of nifedipine appear to be uncommon, presumably because of the clinical absence of direct cardiac depressant effects (342–344).

Diltiazem appears to be quite free of side effects at the lower doses. However, at higher doses a number of more obvious side effects including constipation, edema, headaches, and rash do occur (7,279).

Contraindications to the Ca^{2+} channel antagonists stem from the relative cardiodepressant-vasodilator profile of the agents (Table 1), but all agents are contraindicated in obstructive conditions, including aortic stenosis and cardiomyopathy. The relative cardiodepressant properties of verapamil and, to a lesser extent, diltiazem, indicate considerable caution or absolute contrain-

TABLE 16. *Side effects of Ca²⁺ channel antagonists*

	Diltiazem	Nifedipine	Verapamil[a]
Ankle edema	++	++	++
Constipation	+	0	++++
Dizziness	++	+ or ++	++
Facial flushing	+	+++	++
Headaches	+	++	+
Ischemia	0	+	0
Rash	+	0	+
Tachycardia	0	++	0

[a]0, 0%; +, 0%–5%; ++, 5%–10%; +++, 10%–20%; ++++, >20%.

TABLE 17. Contraindications of Ca^{2+} channel antagonists

	Diltiazem	Nifedipine	Verapamil
Aortic stenosis	++	++	++
AV conduction defects	++	0	++
Cardiac failure	+	0	+
Hypotension	+	++	+
Obstructive cardiomyopathy	++	++	++
Sick sinus syndrome	+	0	+
Sinus bradycardia	0, +	0	0, +

Data adapted from ref. 10.

dication in patients with AV conduction defects, sick sinus syndrome, and impaired left ventricular function. Considerable caution or contraindication is needed with all three agents in hypotensive situations (Table 17).

DRUG INTERACTIONS

A number of drug interactions, both pharmacologic and pharmacodynamic, exist for the Ca^{2+} channel antagonists. These interactions are seen with major classes of drugs including those used in ischemic heart disease, hypertension, and cardiac failure. Interactions also occur with other specific agents (342,345,347). A summary is presented in Table 18.

Interactions of the Ca^{2+} channel antago- nists with β-receptor antagonists differ according to their cardiodepressant-vasodilator profile. The combination could be assumed to be favorable because the Ca^{2+} antagonists increase blood supply and the β-antagonists decrease the work of the ischemic myocardium. However, the potential also exists for unwanted cardiodepressant actions. Attention has thus focused on the combinations of verapamil with β-blockers because, of the Ca^{2+} channel antagonists, verapamil has the most potent negative dromotropic and inotropic effects. However, several studies have reported the enhanced benefit of a β-blocker-verapamil combination (348–350), although careful monitoring is desired. In contrast, less concern has been expressed about the combination of nifedipine with β-blockers, reflecting the reduced cardiodepressant po-

TABLE 18. Drug interactions of Ca^{2+} channel antagonists

	Diltiazem	Nifedipine	Verapamil
Antihypertensives	—	—	—
Antiarrhythmic drugs			
Disopyramide	—	0	—
Quinidine	—	0	—
β-Adrenergic blockers	+	++	—
Cardiac glycosides	ND	0	—
H₂-receptor antagonists			
Cimetidine	ND	—	ND
Ranitidine	ND	0	ND
General anesthetics			
Halothane	ND	—	—
Isoflurane	ND	ND	—
Nitrates	++	++	++

0, no interaction; +, generally positive; ++, positive; —, negative; ND, insufficient data.

tency of nifedipine. However, it should be noted that the presence of β-blockers will reduce or eliminate the reflex sympathetic activation seen acutely with nifedipine alone and may reveal its cardiodepressant properties. Nonetheless, the combination of nifedipine and β-blockers is generally more desirable than other combinations (353).

Although the Ca^{2+} channel antagonists are known from both radioligand and pharmacologic studies to interact allosterically, little is known of any interaction in clinical circumstances. However, high-dose combinations of nifedipine and verapamil produced an unacceptably high level of side effects (345). The available but limited studies have been reviewed by Piepho et al. (347). Combinations of Ca^{2+} channel antagonists and organic nitrates are employed in the control of angina. This combination may reduce the incidence of tolerance seen with the nitrates alone. Combinations of Ca^{2+} channel antagonists and ACE inhibitors seem to be appropriate and useful because these agents alone attack low- and high-renin hypertension, respectively. Whether the combination of Ca^{2+} channel antagonists and diuretics will be useful remains to be established, because the Ca^{2+} channel antagonists, unlike other vasodilators, do not activate significantly the renin-angiotensin-aldosterone system (351). Additionally, nifedipine and other 1,4-dihydropyridines are themselves modest natriuretic agents.

A number of other pharmacodynamic interactions have also been observed with the Ca^{2+} channel antagonists (342,345–347). These include the antiarrythmics quinidine, disopyramide, procainamide, and others that should be used in combination with the Ca^{2+} channel blockers, particularly verapamil, with extreme caution. Interactions of Ca^{2+} channel antagonists and the general anesthetics halothane and isoflurane have been noted to produce excessive hypotension and increased bradycardia with nifedipine and verapamil, respectively (347).

Completely unrelated to Ca^{2+} channel antagonist properties are the abilities of the antagonists, particularly verapamil, to overcome the multiple drug resistance exhibited to many chemotherapeutic agents (352). This interaction arises from the ability of these agents to interact at a specific glycoprotein that is expressed in large amounts of resistant cells and that serves to enhance the cellular efflux of chemotherapeutic agents. A similar phenomenon is involved in the development of resistance to antimalarial agents (353).

Pharmacokinetic interactions have been observed with digoxin and digitoxin with all three Ca^{2+} channel antagonists (347). However, only the interactions with verapamil are of clinical significance because plasma levels of digoxin may rise as much as 70%, probably through impairment of renal clearance. Combinations of Ca^{2+} channel antagonists, particularly verapamil, and digoxin or digitoxin should probably be avoided in the renally impaired patient. Interactions have also been found with the H_2 antagonist cimetidine, which elevated Ca^{2+} channel antagonist bioavailability. Cimetidine inhibits hepatic drug-metabolizing enzymes and reduces hepatic blood flow. Interactions between nifedipine and the anticonvulsant phenytoin have also been reported, presumably reflecting displacement of protein-bound anticonvulsant by nifedipine. Other interactions are reviewed by Piepho et al. (347).

REGULATION OF CALCIUM CHANNELS

That cell membrane receptors for hormones and neurotransmitters are regulated is well recognized. Changes in number and function occur during cell development and growth, during homologous and heterologous drug action, and in disease states (354–356). Potential-dependent Ca^{2+} channels are also subject to regulatory influence, and this phenomenon may underlie tolerance or withdrawal processes as well as a number of disease states.

It is probable that ion channels and cell surface receptors are regulated in similar fashion. Both are membrane proteins and enjoy common processing via protein synthesis, glycosylation, Golgi modification, and membrane insertion (355–357). There may, however, also be significant differences because receptors for hormones and neurotransmitters have defined physiologic ligands, whereas an endogenous ligand for the Ca^{2+} channel remains to be identified (97). Little is yet known concerning Ca^{2+} channel regulation, but several processes may be considered. The specific drug binding sites associated with the channel may serve, under conditions of chronic occupancy, to regulate in a manner similar to that employed by hormones and neurotransmitters. Heterologous regulation may occur through hormone or another receptor activation process that may regulate directly or indirectly Ca^{2+} channels. Roles may also exist in Ca^{2+} channel regulation for Ca^{2+} and membrane potential, which may be regarded as a channel substrate and signal, respectively (113).

Withdrawal from Ca^{2+} Channel Antagonists

The withdrawal phenomenon from Ca^{2+} channel antagonist therapy has been reviewed (6,151,279,358). However, few objective studies have been documented. Reports, limited to one or a few patients, of possible withdrawal phenomena are available for nifedipine (359–362), verapamil, and diltiazem (363). Enhanced human vascular reactivity to norepinephrine and K^+ depolarization-induced responses have been reported in patients withdrawn from nifedipine and verapamil (364). However, other studies have not revealed an objective withdrawal phenomenon (365–367). A number of reasons may underlie these discrepancies. Withdrawal to Ca^{2+} channel antag-

onists, in common with that observed for other cardiovascular drugs, probably does not occur in all individuals, and the appearance of the phenomenon likely depends on the protocols and time course of the withdrawal process.

A number of mechanisms may, in principle, underlie any withdrawal process (113). Up- and down-regulation of Ca^{2+} channel numbers and function following chronic antagonist and activator administration have been reported (368,369). The reduction in membrane potential during vascular relaxation and in intracellular Ca^{2+} may regulate Ca^{2+} channels (6,113,151), and any reduction in sympathetic drive during antagonist administration may serve to regulate the activities of α- and β-adrenoceptors of vascular and cardiac muscle (369,370).

Heterologous Regulation of Ca^{2+} Channels

Ca^{2+} channels are subject to hormonal regulation (113). Channel numbers in cultured human skeletal muscle increase following insulin treatment (371) and thyroid hormone treatment of cultured chick cardiac cells produces an increase in channel density (372). Chronic alcohol treatment increases channel density in the central nervous system of the rat (373), and channel density is reported to be increased *in utero* from estrogen-dominated rats (374). A number of neurochemical lesions, both peripheral and central, have been shown to regulate both channels and other receptors (113).

Regulation of Channels in Disease States

Hypertrophic obstructive cardiomyopathy responds to Ca^{2+} channel antagonists, as discussed earlier. The Syrian cardiomyopathic hamster serves as a model for this disease, and Ca^{2+} overload of myocytes has been implicated. This Ca^{2+} overload may arise from an increased number of potential-dependent Ca^{2+} channels and, consistent with this assumption, increased channel numbers and function have been reported by some, but not all, workers (375,376). However, an increase in channel density is reported in human cardiomyopathic tissue (377). Increased Ca^{2+} channel numbers are reported to occur in rat heart hypertrophied in response to pressure overload (378), but the role of channel changes in the initiation of pathology remains to be established.

Ca^{2+} channel numbers have been reported to be increased in both heart and brain of spontaneously hypertensive rats relative to controls (379,380). The significance of these findings to the etiology of this disease is uncertain. The ratio of L- to T-channel types in vascular smooth muscles from neonatal rats is different from that in spontaneously hypertensive rats, showing an increase in the relative amount of L-channel current (381).

Changes in Ca^{2+} channel numbers have been described in experimental ischemic states with reductions in both verapamil and 1,4-dihydropyridine sites (382,383). After short ischemic periods these changes are reversible, but more prolonged ischemia produces irreversible reduction in channel numbers.

FUTURE Ca^{2+} ANTAGONISTS

New representatives of the Ca^{2+} channel antagonist class are becoming available. Particularly numerous are 1,4-dihydropyridines of which amlodipine, felodipine, isradipine, nicardipine, nimodipine, nisoldipine, and nitrendipine are available or are under active development (Fig. 17) (384,385). A number of other 1,4-dihydropyridines including flordipine, mesudipine, oxodipine, niludipine, and ryodipine have also been discussed in the preclinical literature and are currently less well developed. Several phenylalkylamines including anipamil, gallopamil, and tiapamil are also available (Fig. 18), but no analogs of diltiazem.

The large number of 1,4-dihydropyridine structures available probably represents both the clinical usefulness of the parent compound, nifedipine, its observed limita-

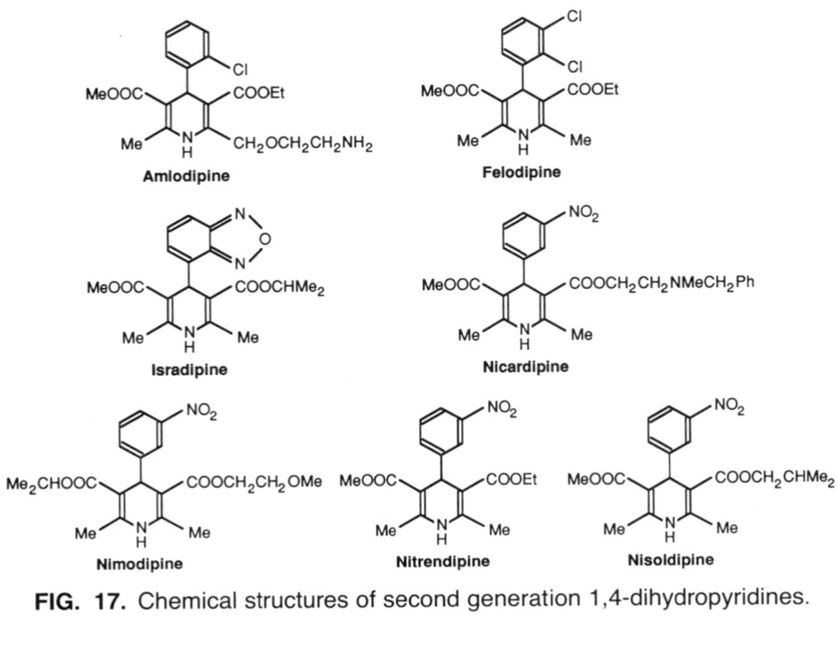

FIG. 17. Chemical structures of second generation 1,4-dihydropyridines.

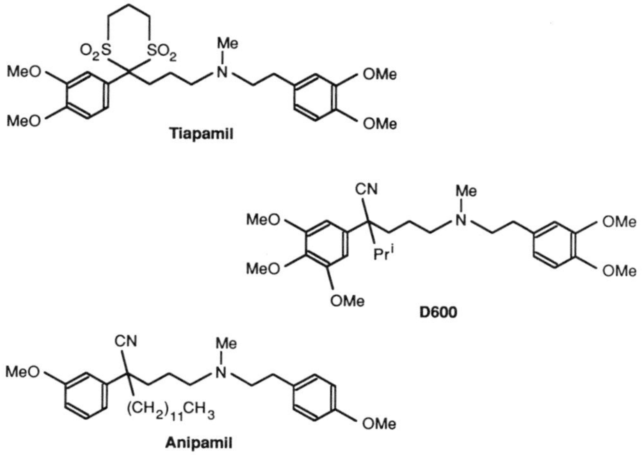

FIG. 18. Chemical structures of analogs of verapamil.

tions, and the realization that small changes in chemical structure may change the cardiovascular selectivity profile and produce regional vascular selectivity. Thus, both pharmacodynamic and pharmacokinetic profiles may be altered in second generation 1,4-dihydropyridines. A summary of some properties of 1,4-dihydropyridines that are clinically available or are close to clinical availability is presented in Table 19.

Although differences are outlined between these several 1,4-dihydropyridine Ca^{2+} channel antagonists, it should be emphasized that few truly comparative pharmacologic or clinical studies have been performed. Furthermore, where differences are indicated it remains to be established to what extent these may be attributable to differences in interaction at Ca^{2+} channel receptors or to differences in pharmacokinetic aspects.

Amlodipine represents an agent of extremely prolonged duration of action. This represents both a slow access to and egress from receptor sites (223) as well as reduced clearance and metabolism (158). These differences may contribute to fewer vasodilator side effects with amlodipine than with nifedipine (386,387). Felodipine is reported to be substantially more vascular selective than nifedipine (388,389), and this may underlie its reported utility in congestive heart failure relative to nifedipine (390).

Among the other 1,4-dihydropyridines, nimodipine has attracted particular interest because of its apparent selectivity for cerebral over peripheral vasculature (391). It is this selectivity that underlies its use and potential uses in cerebral vascular disorders, as discussed previously. It remains to be determined whether its apparent memory-enhancing effects are to be attributed to central neuronal or ventral vascular effects (392). Isradipine (393,394) appears to be similar to nifedipine in both angina and hypertension. Nicardipine is very similar to nifedipine in many respects including duration of action and cardiovascular profile, although it has been suggested to be more vascular selective (395–397). Nisoldipine is reported to be a more selective vasodilator than nifedipine (398) and is effective in both angina of effort and hypertension (399,400). Nitrendipine is a widely employed experimental agent (6,401) with a generally similar profile to nifedipine, except that it is of longer duration and is more vascular selective. It has been widely investigated clinically, and its more prolonged duration of action will establish it as an antihypertensive agent (402,403).

Tiapamil is a nonchiral analog of verap-

TABLE 19. *Characteristics and clinical indications for 1,4-dihydropyridines*

	Amlodipine	Felodipine	Isradipine	Nicardipine	Nifedipine	Nimodipine	Nisoldipine	Nitrendipine
Duration of action (approximate)	24	20	4	8	4	4	8–10	12
Daily dose (mg/times daily)	2.5–10/1	5–10/3	5/3	5–30/3	10–20/3	30–40/3	10/1–2	10–20/1–2
Vascular selectivity	Coronary, peripheral	Coronary, peripheral	Coronary, peripheral	Coronary, peripheral	Coronary, peripheral	Cerebral	Coronary, peripheral	Peripheral
Myocardial contractility	?	Low	?	Low	↓	?	?	↓
Heart rate (initial)	↑	↑	↑	↑	↑	?	↑	↑
Indications	Reflex Angina, hypertension	Reflex Angina, hypertension, congestive heart failure	Reflex Angina, hypertension	Reflex Angina, hypertension	Reflex Angina, hypertension	Migraine, subarachnoid hemorrhage, stroke?	Reflex Angina, hypertension	Reflex Hypertension

amil with antihypertensive, antianginal, and antiarrhythmic properties (336). It is no longer in development. Compared with verapamil, it is a less potent Ca^{2+} channel but a more potent Na^+ channel antagonist (404), features that probably contribute to its antiarrhythmic properties with which, in contrast to verapamil, it is effective against ventricular tachycardia.

Gallopamil (D600) is a pharmacologically well-characterized agent, generally acknowledged to be a more potent Ca^{2+} channel antagonist than verapamil. However, clinical comparisons are not available although the two agents generally seem to be similar (405). Anipamil has an apparently prolonged duration of action, but unlike verapamil has little effect on nodal tissue (385).

REFERENCES

1. Stinson SC. Drug industry steps up fight against heart disease. *Chem Eng News* Oct. 3, 1987;35–70.
2. Fleckenstein A, Kammermeier H, Doring H, Freund HJ. Zum Wirkungs-mechanismus neuartiger koronardilatoren mit gleichzetig Sauerstoff-einsparenden Myokard-Effekten, Prenylamin und Iproveratril. *Z Kreislasufforsch* 1967; 56:716–744, 839–853.
3. Fleckenstein A. *Calcium antagonism in heart and smooth muscle. Experimental facts and therapeutic prospects.* New York: Wiley, 1983.
4. Fleckenstein A. History of calcium antagonists. *Circ Res* 1983;52(Suppl I):3–16.
5. Fleckenstein A. Specific pharmacology of calcium in myocardium, cardiac pacemakers and vascular smooth muscle. *Annu Rev Pharmacol Toxicol* 1977;17:149–166.
6. Janis RA, Silver P, Triggle DJ. Drug action and cellular calcium regulation. *Adv Drug Res* 1987;16:309–591.
7. Opie LH. Calcium channel antagonists. III: Use and comparative efficacy in hypertension and supraventricular arrhythmias. Minor indications. *Cardiovasc Drugs Ther* 1988;1:625–656.
8. Weinstein DB, Heider JG. Antiatherogenic properties of calcium antagonists. *Am J Cardiol* 1987;59:163B–172B.
9. Triggle DJ. Calcium antagonists in atherosclerosis: a review and commentary. *Cardiovasc Drug Rev* 1989;6:320–335.
10. deJong JW. Cardioplegia and calcium antagonists: a review. *Ann Thorac Surg* 1986;42: 593–598.
11. Nayler WG. Calcium antagonists and the ischemic myocardium. *Int J Cardiol* 1987;15: 267–285.
12. Gelmers HJ. Effect of nimodipine on the clinical source of patients with acute ischemic stroke. In: Betz E, Deck K, Hoffmeister F, eds. *Nimodipine. Pharmacological and clinical properties.* New York: Schattauer-Verlag, 1985; 421–429.
13. Kirsch JR, Dean JM, Rogers MC. Current concepts in brain resuscitation. *Arch Intern Med* 1986;146:1413–1419.
14. Steen PA, Gisvold SE, Milde JH, et al. Nimodipine improves outcome when given after complete cerebral ischemia in primates. *Anesthesiology* 1985;62:406–414.
15. Grotta JC, Pettigrew LC, Rosenbaum D, Reid C, Rhoades H, McCandlers D. Efficacy and mechanism of action of a calcium channel blocker after global cerebral ischemia in rats. *Stroke* 1988;19:447–454.
16. Walsh RW, Porter CB, Starling MR. Beneficial hemodynamic effects of intravenous and oral diltiazem in severe congestive heart failure. *J Am Coll Cardiol* 1984;3:1044–1049.
17. Parmley WW. Medical treatment of congestive heart failure: where are we now? *Circulation* 1987;75(Suppl IV):4–10.
18. Kaltenbach M, Hopf R. Treatment of cardiomyopathic hypertrophy: relation to pathological mechanisms. *J Mol Cell Cardiol* 1985; 17(Suppl):59–68.
19. Landmark K, Sire S, Thaulow E. Hemodynamic effects of nifedipine and propranolol in patients with hypertrophic obstructive cardiomyopathy. *Heart J* 1982;48:19–26.
20. Solomon GD, Steel G, Spaccavento LJ. Verapamil prophylaxis of migraine. A double-blind, placebo-controlled study. *JAMA* 1983;250:2500–2502.
21. Steardo L, Marano E, Barone P, Denman DW, Monteleone P, Cardine G. Prophylaxis of migraine attacks with a calcium channel blocker: flunarizine versus methysergide. *J Clin Pharmacol* 1986;26:524–528.
22. Hugenholtz P, Serruys P, Fleckenstein A. Why Ca^{2+} antagonists will be most useful before or during early myocardial ischemia and not after infarction has been established. *Eur Heart J* 1986;7:270–278.
23. Depelchin P, Sobolski J, Jottrand M, Flament C. Secondary prevention after myocardial infarction: effects of beta blocking agents and calcium antagonists. *Cardiovasc Drugs Ther* 1988;2:139–148.
24. Kahan A, Foult JM, Weber S. Nifedipine and l-adrenergic blockade in Raynaud's phenomenon. *Eur Heart J* 1985;6:702–705.
25. Smith CR, Rodeheffer RJ. Raynaud's phenomenon. Pathophysiologic features and treatment with calcium channel blockers. *Am J Cardiol* 1985;55:154B–157B.
26. Simonneau G, Escourrou P, Duroux P. Inhibition of hypoxic pulmonary vasoconstriction by nifedipine. *New Engl J Med* 1981;304: 1582–1585.

27. Rich S, Brindage BH. High-dose calcium channel blocking therapy for primary hypertension: evidence for long term reduction in pulmonary arterial pressure and regression of right ventricular hypertrophy. *Circulation* 1987;76:135–141.

28. Allen GS, Ahn HS, Preziosi T, et al. Cerebral arterial spasm—a controlled trial of nimodipine in patients with subarachnoid hemorrhage. *New Engl J Med* 1983;308:619–624.

29. Faluer LM. Acute operation and preventive nimodipine impose outcome in patients with explained cerebral aneurysms. *Neurosurgery* 1984;15:57–66.

30. Hongo M, Traube M, McCallister RG, Jr, McCallum RW. Effects of nifedipine on esophageal motor function in humans: correlation with plasma nifedipine concentration. *Gastroenterology* 1985;86:8–12.

31. Richter JE, Spurling TJ, Cordova, CM, Castell DO. Effects of oral calcium blocker, diltiazem, on esophageal contractions. Studies in volunteers or patients with nutcracker esophagus. *Dig Dis Sci* 1984;29:649–656.

32. Barnes P, Rudolph M, Tattersfield A, Towart R, Yang K, eds. *Br J Clin Pharmacol* 1985;87:487–494.

33. Ahmed T, D'Brot J, Abraham W. The role of calcium antagonists in bronchial reactivity. *J Allergy Clin Immunol* 1988;81:133–134.

34. Forman A, Andersson K-E, Maigaard S. Effect of calcium channel blockers on the female genital tract. *Acta Pharmacol Toxicol* 1986;58(Suppl 2):183–191.

35. Ebeigbe AB, Ezimokhai M. Vascular smooth muscle responses in pregnancy-induced hypertension. *Trends Pharmacol Sci* 1988;9:455–457.

36. Traube M, Hongo M, Magyar L, McCallum RW. Effects of nifedipine in achalasia and in patients with high-amplitude peristaltic esophageal contractions. *JAMA* 1984;252:1733–1736.

37. Goetsch RA, Fink S, Chaudhuri TK. Effect of nifedipine on gastric emptying. *Milit Med Res* 1986;151:438–439.

38. Nair N, Townley RG, Againdra B, Nair CK. Safety of nifedipine in subjects with bronchial asthma and COPD. *Chest* 1984;86:515–518.

39. Ulmsten V, Andersson KE, Wingerup L. Treatment of premature labor with the calcium antagonist nifedipine. *Arch Gynecol* 1980;229:1–5.

40. Elmer M. Terodiline in children with diurnal enuresis. *Scand J Urol Nephrol* 1984;87:59–61.

41. Klarskov P, Gerstenber TC, Hald T. Bladder training and terodiline in females with iodiopathic urge incontinence and stable detrusor function. *J Urol Nephrol* 1986;20:41–46.

42. Nadler JL, Hsueh W, Horton R. Therapeutic effect of calcium channel blockade in primary aldosteronism. *J Clin Endocrinol Metab* 1985;60:896–899.

43. Tsuruo T, Iida H, Tsukagoshi S, Sakurai Y. Cure of mice bearing P 388 leukemia by vincristine in combination with a calcium channel blocker. *Cancer Treat Rep* 1985;69:523–525.

44. Benson AB, Trump DL, Koeller JM. Phase I study of vinblastine and verapamil given by concurrent iv infusion. *Cancer Treat Rep* 1985;69:795–799.

45. Overweg J, Ashton D, deBeukelaar F, Binnie CD, Wauquier A, Van Wieringen A. Add on therapy in epilepsy with calcium entry blockers. *Eur Neurol* 1986;25(Suppl 1):93–101.

46. Raeburn D, Gonzales RA. CNS disorders and calcium antagonists. *Trends Pharmacol Sci* 1988;9:117–119.

47. Abelson MB, Gilbert CM, Smith LM. Sustained reduction of intraocular pressure in humans with the calcium channel blocker verapamil. *Am J Ophthalmol* 1988;105:155–159.

48. Dubovsky SL, Franks RD, Allen S, Murphy J. Calcium antagonists in mania; a double-blind study of verapamil. *Psychiatry Res* 1986;18:309–320.

49. Giannini AJ, Loiselle RH, Price WA, Giannini MC. Comparison of antimanic efficacy of clonidine and verapamil. *J Clin Pharmacol* 1985;25:307–308.

50. Lee JA, Watson LA, Boothby G. Calcium antagonists in the prevention of motion sickness. *Aviat Space Environ Med* 1986;57:45–48.

51. Black P, Markowitz RS, Finkelstein SD, McMonagle-Strucko K, Gillespie JA. Experimental spinal cord injury: effect of a calcium channel antagonist (nicardipine). *Neurosurgery* 1988;22:61–66.

52. Theopold HM. *Laryngol Rhinol Otol (Stuttg)* 1988;64:609–613.

53. Walsh TL, Lavenstein B, Liacmele WL, Bronheim S, O'Leary J. Calcium antagonists in the treatment of Tourette's disorder. *Am J Psychol* 1986;143:1467–1469.

54. Hofferberth B. Calcium entry blockers in the treatment of vertebrobasilar insufficiency. *Eur Neurol* 1986;25(Suppl 1):80–85.

55. Ringer S. A further contribution regarding the influence of different constituents on the blood on the contraction of the heart. *J Physiol (Lond)* 1883;4:29–42.

56. Campbell AK. *Intracellular calcium: its universal role as regulator.* New York: John Wiley, 1983.

57. Dalgarno D, Klevit RE, Levine BA, Williams R-JP. The calcium receptor and trigger. *Trends Pharmacol Sci* 1984;5:266–269.

58. Carafoli E. Intracellular calcium homeostasis. *Annu Rev Biochem* 1987;56:395–433.

59. Buhler FR, Ernie P, Carafoli E, Van Breemen C. Cellular calcium control mechanisms. *J Cardiovasc Pharmacol* 1988;12(Suppl 5):1–138.

60. Rasmussen H. The calcium messenger system. *New Engl J Med* 1986;314:1094–1102.

61. Kaczorowski GJ, Garcia ML, King VF, Slaughter RS. Development of inhibitors of sodium, calcium exchange. In: Baker PF, ed. *Calcium in drug actions.* Heidelberg: Springer-Verlag, 1988;163–183.

62. Blaustein MP. Sodium/calcium exchange and the control of contractility in cardiac muscle and vascular smooth muscle. *J Cardiovasc Pharmacol* 1988;12(Suppl 5):56–68.

63. MacLennan DH, Brandl CJ, Korczak B, Green

NM. Amino-acid sequence of Ca^{2+} + Mg^{2+}-dependent ATPase from rabbit muscle sarcoplasmic reticulum deduced from its complementary DNA sequence. *Nature* 1985;316: 696–700.

64. Smith JS, Imagawa T, Ma J, Fill M, Campbell KP, Coronado R. Purified ryanodine receptor from rabbit skeletal muscle is the calcium-release channel of sarcoplasmic reticulum. *J Gen Physiol* 1988;92:1–26.

65. Berridge MP. Inositol trisphosphate and diacylglycerol: two interacting second messengers. *Annu Rev Biochem* 1987;56:159–193.

66. Volpe P, Krause K-H, Hashimoto S, et al. "Calciosome," a cytoplasmic organelle: the inositol 1,4-5-trisphosphate-sensitive Ca^{2+} store of nonmuscle cells. *Proc Natl Acad Sci USA* 1988;85:1091–1095.

67. McCormack JG, Denton RM. Ca^{2+} as a second messenger within mitochondria. *Trends Biochem Sci* 1986;11:258–262.

68. Berridge MJ, Galione A. Cytosolic calcium oscillators. *FASEB J* 1988;2:3074–3082.

69. Simpson RV, Thomas GA, Arnold AJ. Identification of 1,25-dihydroxyvitamin D3 receptors and activities in muscle. *J Biol Chem* 1985; 260:8882–8891.

70. Watters MR, Cuneo DM, Jamison AP. Possible significance of new target tissues for 1,25-dihydroxyvitamin D3. *J Steroid Biochem* 1983; 19:913–920.

71. Kawashima H. Receptor for 1,25-dihydroxyvitamin D3 in a vascular smooth muscle cell line derived from rat aorta. *Biochem Biophys Res Commun* 1987;146:1–6.

72. DeBoland AR, Boland RL. Rapid changes in skeletal muscle calcium uptake induced in vitro by 1,25-dihydroxyvitamin D3 are suppressed by calcium channel blockers. *Endocrinology* 1987;120:1858–1864.

73. Guggino SE, Wagner JA, Snowman AM, Hester LD, Sacktor B, Snyder SH. Phenylalkylamine-sensitive calcium channels in osteoblast-like sarcoma cells. *J Biol Chem* 1988;265: 10155–10161.

74. Lau K, Eby B. The role of calcium in genetic hypertension. *Hypertension* 1985;7:657–667.

75. Resnick LM, Laragh JH. Renin, calcium metabolism and the physiologic basis of antihypertensive therapy. *Am J Cardiol* 1985;56: 68H–74H.

76. Resnick LM. Uniformity and diversity of calcium metabolism in hypertension. A conceptual framework. *Am J Med* 1987;82(Suppl 1B):16–26.

77. Bukoski RD, McCarron DA. Calcium and hypertension. In: Baker PF, ed. *Calcium in drug action*. Heidelberg: Springer-Verlag, 1988; 467–487.

77a. McCarron DA. Low serum concentrations of ionized calcium in patients with hypertension. *New Engl J Med* 1982;307:226–228.

78. Kowarski S, Schachter D. Intestinal membrane calcium-binding protein. Vitamin D-dependent membrane component of the intestinal calcium transport mechanism. *J Biol Chem* 1980;255: 10834–10840.

79. Kowarski S, Cowen LA, Takahashi MT, Schachter D. Tissue distribution and vitamin D-dependence of IMCAL in the rat. *Am J Physiol* 1987;16:G411–419.

80. Kowarski S, Cowen LA, Schachter D. Decreased contrast of integral membrane calcium-binding protein (IMCAL) in tissues of the spontaneously hypertensive rat. *Proc Natl Acad Sci USA* 1987;83:1097–1100.

81. Orrenius S, McConkey DJ, Jones DP, Nicofera P. Ca^{2+}-activated mechanisms in toxicity and programmed cell death. *ISI Atlas Sci Pharmacol* 1988;2:389–391.

82. Chapman RA, Tunstall J. The calcium paradox of the heart. *Prog Biophys Mol Biol* 1987;50: 67–96.

83. Mellgren RL. Calcium dependent proteases: an enzyme system active at cellular membranes? *FASEB J* 1987;1:110–115.

84. Glende EA, Jr, Pushpendran KC. Activation of phospholipase A2 by carbon tetrachloride in isolated rat hepatocytes. *Biochem Pharmacol* 1986;35:3301–3307.

85. Heathers GP, Yamada KA, Kanter EM, Corr PB. Long-chain acylcarnitines mediate the hypoxia-induced increase in α_1-adrenergic receptors on adult canine myocytes. *Circ Res* 1987;61:735–746.

86. Corr PB, Gross RW, Sobel BE. Amphipathic metabolites and membrane dysfunction in ischemic myocardium. *Circ Res* 1984;55:135–154.

87. Liedtke AJ. Lipid burden in ischemic myocardium. *J Mol Cell Cardiol* 1988;20(Suppl II): 65–74.

88. Halliwell B, ed. *Oxygen radicals and tissue injury*. Bethesda, MD: FASEB, 1988.

89. Triggle DJ. New approaches to calcium modulation based-receptor pharmacology. In: Machleidt H, ed. *Contributions of chemistry to health, proceedings of the Fifth Chemrawn Conference*. Weinheim, Federal Republic of Germany: VCH Verlagsgesellschaft, 1987;201–214.

90. Siegelbaum SA, Tsien RW. Modulation of gated ion channels as a mode of transmitter action. *Trends Neurosci* 1983;6:307–313.

91. Rosenthal W, Schultz G. Modulations of voltage-dependent ion channels by extracellular signals. *Trends Pharmacol Sci* 1987;8:351–354.

92. Hofmann F, Nastainczyk W, Rohrkasten A, Schneider T, Sieber M. *Trends Pharmacol Sci* 1987;8:393–398.

93. Triggle DJ, Langs DA, Janis RA. Ca^{2+} channel ligands: structure-activity relationships of 1,4-dihydropyridines. *Med Res Rev* 1989;9: 123–180.

94. Dunlap K, Holz GG, Rane SG. G proteins as regulators of ion channel function. *Trends Neurosci* 1987;10:241–244.

95. Yatani A, Imoto Y, Codina J, Hamilton SL, Brown AM, Birnbaumer L. The stimulating G protein of adenylyl cyclase Gs, also stimulates

dihydropyridine-sensitive Ca^{2+} channels. *J Biol Chem* 1988;263:9887–9895.

96. Scott RH, Dolphin AC. Activation of a G protein promotes agonist responses to calcium channel ligands. *Nature* 1987;330:760–762.

97. Triggle DJ. Endogenous ligands for the calcium channel: myths and realities. In: Morad M, Nayler W, Kazda S, Schramm M, eds. *The calcium channel: structure, function and implications.* Berlin: Springer-Verlag, 1988;549–563.

98. Hagiwara S, Byerly L. Calcium channel. *Annu Rev Neurosci* 1981;4:69–125.

99. Tsien RW. Calcium channels in excitable cell membranes. *Annu Rev Physiol* 1983;45:341–358.

100. Morad M, Nayler W, Kazda S, Schramm M, ed. *The calcium channel: structure, function and implications.* Berlin: Springer-Verlag, 1988.

101. Vilven J, Coronado R. Opening of dihydropyridine calcium channels in skeletal muscle membranes by inositol trisphosphate. *Nature* 1988; 356:587–589.

102. Tsien RW, Hess P, McCleskey EW, Rosenberg RL. Calcium channels: mechanisms of selectivity, permeation and block. *Annu Rev Biophys Biophys Chem* 1987;16:265–290.

103. Tanabe T, Takashima H, Mikami A, et al. Primary structure of the receptor for calcium channel blockers from skeletal muscle. *Nature* 1987;328:313–318.

104. Stevens CF. Channel families in the brain. *Nature* 1987;328:198–199.

105. Tang C-M, Presser F, Morad M. Amiloride selectively blocks the low threshold (T) calcium channel. *Science* 1988;240:213–215.

106. Twombly DA, Yoshii M, Narahashi T. Mechanisms of calcium channel block by phenytoin. *J Pharmacol Exp Ther* 1988;246:189–195.

107. Yoshii M, Tsunoo A, Narahashi T. Effects of pyrethroids and veratridine on two types of Ca channels in neuroblastoma cells. *Soc Neurosci Abstr* 1985;11:518.

108. Llinas R, Yaron Y. Specific blockage of the low threshold calcium channel by high molecular weight alcohols. *Soc Neurosci Abst* 1986;12: 49.3.

109. Feigenbaum P, Garcia ML, Kazczorowski GJ. Evidence for distinct sites coupled to high affinity ω-conotoxin receptors in rat brain synaptic plasma membrane vesicles. *Biochem Biophys Res Commun* 1988;154:298–305.

110. Gray WR, Olivera BM, Cruz LJ. Peptide toxins from venomous Conus snails. *Annu Rev Biochem* 1988;57:665–700.

111. Knauss HG, Striessnig J, Koza A, Glossmann H. Neurotoxic aminoglycoside antibiotics are potent inhibitors of [125I]omega conotoxin GVIA binding to guinea pig cerebral cortex membranes. *Naunyn Schmiedebergs Arch Pharmacol* 1987;336:583–586.

112. Janis RA, Triggle DJ. The 1,4-dihydropyridine receptor—a regulatory component of the Ca^{2+} channel. *J Cardiovasc Pharmacol* 1984;6:S949–S953.

113. Ferrante J, Triggle DJ. Homologous and heterologous regulation of voltage-dependent Ca^{2+} channels. *Biochem Pharmacol* 1990;39:1267–1270.

114. Vaghy PL, McKenna E, Itagaki K, Schwartz A. Resolution of the identity of the Ca^{2+} antagonist receptor in skeletal muscle. *Trends Pharmacol Sci* 1988;9:398–402.

115. Takahashi M, Catterall WA. Dihydropyridine-sensitive calcium channels in cardiac and skeletal muscle membranes: studies with antibodies against the subunits. *Biochemistry* 1987;26: 5518–5526.

116. Lang B, Newsom-Davis J, Wray DW. The effect of Lambert-Eaton myasthenic syndrome antibody on slow action potentials in mouse cardiac ventricle. *Proc R Soc Lond [Biol]* 1988;235:B103–B110.

117. Takahashi M, Catterall WA. Dihydropyridine-sensitive calcium channels in cardiac and skeletal muscle membranes. Studies with antibodies against the alpha-subunits. *Biochemistry* 1987;26:5518–5526.

118. Chang FC, Hosey MM. Dihydropyridine and phenylalkylamine receptors associated with cardiac and skeletal muscle calcium channels are structurally different. *J Biol Chem* 1988; 263:18929–18937.

118a. Saini RK. Calcium antagonists. In: Antonaccio M, ed. *Cardiovascular Pharmacology,* 2nd ed. New York: Raven Press, 1984;415–452.

119. Reuter H. Ion channels in cardiac cell membranes. *Annu Rev Physiol* 1984;46:473–484.

120. Noble D. The surprising heart: a review of recent progress in cardiac electrophysiology. *J Physiol (Lond)* 1984;353:1–50.

121. Nilus B, Hess P, Lansman JB, Tsien RW. A novel type of cardiac calcium in ventricular cells. *Nature* 1985;316:443–446.

122. Mitra R, Morad M. Two types of calcium channels in guinea pig ventricular myocytes. *Proc Natl Acad Sci USA* 1986;83:5340–5344.

123. Bean BP. Two kinds of calcium channels in canine atrial cells. Differences in kinetics, selectivity and pharmacology. *J Gen Physiol* 1985; 86:1–30.

124. Hess P, Fox AP, Lansman JB, Nowycky MC, Tsien RW. Calcium channel types in differences in gating, permeation and pharmacology. In: Ritchie JM, Keynes RD, Bolis L, eds. *Ion channels in neural membranes.* New York: Alan R. Liss, 1986;227–252.

125. Bolton TB, MacKenzie I, Aaronson PI, Lin SP. Calcium channels in smooth muscle cells. *Biochem Soc Trans* 1988;16:492–493.

126. Sturek M, Hermsmeyer K. Calcium and sodium channels in spontaneously contracting vascular smooth muscle cells. *Science* 1986; 233:475–478.

127. Bean BP, Sturek M, Puga A, Hermsmeyer K. Calcium channels in muscle cells isolated from rat mesenteric arteries: modulation by dihydropyridine drugs. *Circ Res* 1986;59:229–235.

128. Ohya Y, Sperelakis N. ATP regulation of the slow calcium channels in vascular smooth muscle cells of guinea pig mesenteric artery. *Circ Res* 1989;64:145–154.

129. Friedman ME, Suarez-Kurtz G, Kaczorowski

GJ, Katz GM, Reuben JP. Two calcium currents in a smooth muscle cell line. *Am J Physiol* 1986;250:H699–H703.

130. Benham CD, Hess P, Tsien RW. Two types of calcium channels in single smooth muscle cells from rabbit ear artery studied with whole-cell and single-channel recordings. *Circ Res* 1987; 61(Suppl I):I-10–I-16.

131. Aaronson PI, Bolton TB, Lang RJ, Mackenzie I. Calcium currents in single isolated smooth muscle cells from the rabbit ear artery in normal-calcium and high-barium solutions. *J Physiol (Lond)* 1988;405:57–75.

132. Yatani A, Seidel CL, Allen J, Brown AM. Whole-cell and single-channel calcium currents of isolated smooth muscle cells from saphenous vein. *Circ Res* 1987;60:523–533.

133. Loirand G, Pacaud P, Mironneau C, Mironneau J. Evidence for two distinct calcium channels in rat vascular smooth muscle cells in short-term primary culture. *Pflugers Arch* 1986;407: 566–568.

134. Hescheler J, Kameyama M, Trautwein W, Miesks G, Soling H-D. Regulation of the cardiac calcium channel by protein phosphatases. *Eur J Biochem* 1987;165:261–266.

135. Kameyama M, Hescheler J, Hofmann F, Trautwein W. Modulation of Ca current during the phosphorylation cycle in the guinea pig heart. *Pflugers Arch* 1986;407:123–128.

136. Droogmans G, Dederck I, Casteels R. Effect of adrenergic agents on Ca^{2+}-channel currents in single vascular smooth muscle cells. *Pflugers Arch* 1987;409:7–12.

137. Benham CD, Tsien RW. Noradrenaline modulation of calcium channels in single smooth muscle cells from rabbit ear artery. *J Physiol (Lond)* 1988;404:767–784.

138. Kamm KE, Stull JT. The function of myosin light chain kinase phosphorylation in smooth muscle. *Annu Rev Pharmacol Toxicol* 1985;25: 593–620.

139. Nelson MT, Standen NB, Brayden JE, Worley JF, III. Noradrenaline contracts arteries by activating voltage-dependent calcium channels. *Nature* 1988;326:382–385.

140. Berridge MJ. Inositol trisphosphate and diacylglycerol: two interacting second messengers. *Annu Rev Biochem* 1987;56:159–193.

141. Berridge MJ. Inositol trisphosphate and diacylglycerol: two interacting second messengers. *ISI Atlas of Science* 1987;1:91–97.

142. Fish RD, Sperti G, Colucci WS, Clapham DE. Phorbol ester increases the dihydropyridine-sensitive calcium conductance in a vascular smooth muscle cell line. *Circ Res* 1988;62: 1049–1054.

143. Dosemeci A, Dhallan RS, Cohen NM, Lederer WJ, Rogers TB. Phorbol ester increases calcium current and stimulates the effects of angiotensin II on cultured neonatal rat heart myocytes. *Circ Res* 1988;62:347–357.

144. Lacerda AE, Rampe D, Brown AM. Effects of protein kinase C activators on cardiac Ca^{2+} channels. *Nature* 1988;335:249–251.

145. Cohen CJ, Spires S, Van Skiver D. Modulation

of L- and T-type calcium channels in guinea pig atrial cells by 1,4-dihydropyridines. In: Hondeghem L, Katzung BG, eds. *Molecular and cellular mechanisms of antiarrhythmic agents.* Futura Press (*in press*).

146. Worley JF, III, Deitmer JW, Nelson MT. Single nisoldipine-sensitive calcium channels in smooth muscle cells isolated from rabbit mesenteric artery. *Proc Natl Acad Sci USA* 1986;83:5746–5750.

147. Opie LH. Calcium channel antagonists. Part I: fundamental properties; mechanisms, classification, sites of action. *Cardiovasc Drugs Ther* 1987;1:411–430.

148. Godfraind T, Miller R, Wibo M. Calcium antagonism and calcium entry blockade. *Pharmacol Rev* 1986;38:321–416.

149. Opie LH. Calcium ions, drug action and the heart—with special reference to calcium channel blockers (calcium antagonist drugs). In: Denborough MA, ed. *The role of calcium in drug action.* Oxford: Pergamon Press, 1987; 103–138.

150. Vanhoutte PM. The expert committee of the World Health Organization on classification of calcium antagonists. The viewpoint of the Raporteur. *Am J Cardiol* 1987;59:3A–8A.

151. Triggle DJ, Janis RA. Calcium channel ligands. *Annu Rev Pharmacol Toxicol* 1987;27:347–369.

152. Triggle DJ, Janis RA. Calcium channel ligands: structure-function relationships. In: Venter JC, Triggle DJ, eds. *Structure and physiology of the slow inward calcium channel.* New York: Alan R. Liss, 1987;29–50.

153. Triggle DJ, Janis RA. Calcium channel antagonists. New perspectives from the radioligand binding assay. In: Back N, Spector S, eds. *Modern methods in pharmacology,* vol 2. New York: Alan R. Liss, 1984;1–28.

154. Janis RA, Triggle DJ. 1,4-Dihydropyridine Ca^{2+} channel activators: a comparison of binding characteristics with pharmacology. *Drug Rev Res* 1984;4:257–274.

155. Triggle DJ, Janis RA. Calcium channels and calcium channel ligands. In: Williams M, Glennon RA, Timmermans PBMW, eds. *Receptor pharmacology and function.* New York: Marcel Dekker, 1988;665–693.

156. Loev B, Goodman MM, Snader KM, Tedeschi R, Macko E. "Hantzsch-type" dihydropyridine hypotensive agents. *J Med Chem* 1974; 17:956–965.

157. Bolger GT, Gengo PJ, Luchowski EM, et al. Characterization of the binding of the Ca^{2+} channel antagonist, [3H]nitrendipine to guinea pig ileal smooth muscle. *J Pharmacol Exp Ther* 1983;225:291–309.

158. Arrowsmith JE, Campbell SF, Cross PE, et al. Long-acting dihydropyridine calcium antagonists. I. 2-Alkoxymethyl derivatives incorporating basic substituents. *J Med Chem* 1986; 29:1696–1702.

159. Kass RS, Arena JP, Chin S. Cellular electrophysiology of amlodipine: probing the L-type calcium channel. *Am J Cardiol* 1989;64:35I–42I.

160. Rodenkirchen R, Bayer R, Steiner R, Bossert

F, Meyer H, Moller E. Structure-activity studies on nifedipine in isolated cardiac muscle. *Naunyn Schmiedebergs Arch Pharmacol* 1979; 310:69–78.

161. Hof P, Ruegg PR, Hoff UT, Vogel A. Stereoselectivity at the Ca^{2+} channel: opposite action of the enantiomers of a 1,4-dihydropyridine. *J Cardiovasc Pharmacol* 1985;7:689–693.

162. Franckowiak G, Bectem M, Schramm M, Thomas G. The optical isomers of the 1,4-dihydropyridines Bay K 8644 show opposite effects on Ca^{2+} channels. *Eur J Pharmacol* 1985;114:223–226.

163. Wei X-Y, Luchowski EM, Rutledge A, Su CM, Triggle DJ. Pharmacologic and radioligand binding analysis of the actions of 1,4-dihydropyridine activator-antagonist pairs in smooth muscle. *J Pharmacol Exp Ther* 1986;239: 144–153.

164. Janis RA, Maurer SC, Sarmiento JG, Bolger GT, Triggle DJ. Binding of [3H] nimodipine to cardiac and smooth muscle membranes. *Eur J Pharmacol* 1982;82:191–194.

165. DePover A, Lee SW, Matlib MA, et al. Specific binding of [3H]nitrendipine to membranes from coronary arteries and heart in relation to pharmacological effects. Parodoxical stimulation by diltiazem. *Biochem Biophys Res Commun* 1982; 108:110–117.

166. Janis RA, Sarmiento JG, Maurer SC, Bolger GT, Triggle DJ. Characterization of the binding of [3H]nitrendipine to rabbit ventricular membranes: modification of other Ca^{++} channel antagonist and by the Ca^{2+} channel against Bay K 8644. *J Pharmacol Exp Ther* 1984;231:8–15.

167. Ptasienski JM, McMahon KK, Hosey MM. High and low affinity states of the dihydropyridines and the phenylalkylamine receptors on the cardiac calcium channel and their interconversion by divalent cations. *Biochem Biophys Res Commun* 1985;129:910–917.

168. Triggle CR, Agrawal DK, Bolger GT, et al. Calcium channel antagonist binding to isolated vascular smooth muscle membranes. *Can J Physiol Pharmacol* 1982;60:1738–1741.

169. Godfraind T, Morel N. Identification of Ca channels in microvessels isolated from rat brain. *Br J Pharmacol* 1986;89:507P.

170. Triggle DJ, Zheng W, Hawthorn M, et al. Calcium channels in smooth muscle. Properties and regulation. *Ann NY Acad Sci* 1989; 560:215–229.

171. Wei X-Y, Triggle DJ. The binding of calcium channel antagonists and activators in vascular smooth muscle. In: Aoki K, Frohlich ED, eds. *Calcium in central hypertension.* Tokyo: Academic Press, 1988;258–272.

172. Rios E, Brum G. Involvement of dihydropyridine receptors in excitation-contraction coupling in skeletal muscle. *Nature* 1987;325:717–720.

173. Brum G, Fitts R, Pizzaro G, Rios E. Voltage sensors of the frog skeletal muscle membrane require calcium to function in excitation-con-

traction coupling. *J Physiol (Lond)* 1987;398: 473–505.

174. Hosey MM, Lazdunski M. Calcium channels: molecular pharmacology, structure and regulation. *J Membr Biol* 1988;104:81–105.

175. DePover A, Grupp IL, Grupp G, Schwartz A. Diltiazem potentiates the negative inotropic action of nimodipine in heart. *Biochem Biophys Res Commun* 1983;114:922–929.

176. Yousif F, Triggle DJ. Functional interactions between organic calcium channel antagonists. *Can J Physiol Pharmacol* 1983;63:193–195.

177. Gould RJ, Murphy KMM, Reynolds IJ, Snyder SH. Antischizophrenic drugs of the diphenylbutylpiperidine type act as calcium channel antagonists. *Proc Natl Acad Sci USA* 1983;80: 5122–5125.

178. Qar J, Galizzi J-P, Fosset M, Lazdunski M. Receptors for diphenylbutylpiperidine neuroleptics in brain, cardiac and smooth muscle membranes. Relationship with receptors for 1,4-dihydropyridines and phenylalkylamines and with Ca^{2+} channel blockade. *Eur J Pharmacol* 1987;141:261–268.

179. Rampe D, Skattebol A, Triggle DJ, Brown AM. Effects of McN-6186 on voltage-dependent Ca^{++} channels in heart and pituitary cells. *J Pharmacol Exp Ther* 1989;248:164–170.

180. Striessnig J, Moosburger E, Grabner M, et al. Evidence for a distinct Ca^{2+} antagonist receptor for the novel benzothiazinone compound HOE 166. *Naunyn Schmiedebergs Arch Pharmacol* 1988;337:331–340.

181. Rampe D, Triggle DJ, Brown AM. Electrophysiological and biochemical studies on the putative Ca^{++} channel blocker MDL 12,330A in an endocrine cell. *J Pharmacol Exp Ther* 1987;243:402–407.

182. Boyd RA, Giacomini JC, Wong FM, Nelson WL, Giacomini KM. Comparison of binding affinities and negative inotropic potencies of the 1,4-dihydropyridine calcium channel blockers in rabbit myocardium. *J Pharmacol Exp Ther* 1987;243:118–125.

182a. Belleman P, Schade A, Towart R. Dihydropyridine receptor in rat brain labeled with [3H]nimodipine. *Proc Natl Acad Sci* 1983;80: 2356–2360.

183. Yamada S, Harada Y, Nakayama K. Characterization of calcium channel antagonist binding sites labelled with [3H]nitrendipine in porcine coronary artery and aorta. *J Pharmacol Exp Ther* 1988;154:203–205.

184. Goll A, Glossmann H, Mannhold R. Correlation between the negative inotropic potencies and binding parameters of 1,4-dihydropyridine and phenylalkylamine calcium channel blockers in rat heart. *Naunyn Schmiedebergs Arch Pharmacol* 1986;334:303–312.

185. Hondeghem LM, Katzung BG. Antiarrhythmic agents: the modulated receptor mechanism of action of sodium and calcium channel-blocking drugs. *Annu Rev Pharmacol Toxicol* 1984;24: 387–423.

186. Hille B. Local anesthetics: hydrophilic and hy-

drophobic pathways for the drug-receptor reaction. *J Gen Physiol* 1977;69:497–515.

187. Hondeghem L, Katzung BG. Time- and voltage-dependent interactions of antiarrhythmic drugs with cardiac sodium channels. *Biochim Biophys Acta* 1977;472:373–390.

188. Bayer R, Henneckes R, Kaufmann R, Mannhold R. Inotropic and electro-physiological actions of verapamil and D600 in mammalian myocardium. I. Pattern of inotropic effects of the racemic compounds. *Naunyn Schmiedebergs Arch Pharmacol* 1975;290:49–68.

189. Ehara T, Kaufmann R. The voltage- and time-dependent effects of (-)verapamil on the slow inward current in isolated cat ventricular myocardium. *J Pharmacol Exp Ther* 1978;207:49–55.

190. Linden J, Brooker G. The influence of resting membrane potential on the effect of verapamil on atria. *J Mol Cell Cardiol* 1980;12:325–331.

191. Pelzer D, Trautwein W, McDonald TF. Calcium channel blockers and recovery from block in mammalian ventricular muscle treated with organic channel inhibitors. *Pflugers Arch* 1982; 394:97–105.

192. Trautwein W, Pelzer D, McDonald TF. Interval- and voltage-dependent effects of the calcium channel-blocking agents D600 and AQA 39 on mammalian ventricular muscle. *Circ Res* 1983;52(Suppl 1):60–68.

193. Lee KS, Tsien RW. Mechanism of calcium channel blockade by verapamil, D600 diltiazem and nitrendipine in single dialysed heart cells. *Nature* 1983;302:790–794.

194. Kohlhardt M. Saturation characteristics, Ca^{2+} and drug-induced block of cardiac Isi-mediated action potentials. *Naunyn Schmiedebergs Arch Pharmacol* 1983;323:251–260.

195. Tung L, Morad M. Voltage- and frequency-dependent block of diltiazem on the slow inward current and generation of tension in frog ventricular muscle. *Pflugers Arch* 1983;398:189–198.

196. McDonald TF, Pelzer D, Trautwein W. Cat ventricular muscle treated with D600: characteristics of calcium channel block and unblock. *J Physiol (Lond)* 1984;352:217–244.

197. Kanaya S, Arlock P, Katzung BG, Hondeghem LM. Diltiazem and verapamil preferentially block inactivated calcium channels. *J Mol Cell Cardiol* 1983;15:145–148.

198. Sanguinetti MC, Kass RS. Voltage dependent block of calcium channel current in calf cardiac Purkinje fiber by dihydropyridine calcium channel antagonists. *Circ Res* 1984;55:336–348.

199. Bean BP. Nitrendipine block of cardiac calcium channels: high affinity binding to the inactivated state. *Proc Natl Acad Sci USA* 1984;81: 6388–6392.

200. Uehara A, Hume JR. Interactions of organic calcium channel antagonists with calcium channels in single frog atrial cells. *J Gen Physiol* 1985;85:621–647.

201. Gurney AM, Nerbonne JM, Lester HA. Photoinduced removal of nifedipine reveals mechanisms of calcium antagonist actions on single heart cells. *J Gen Physiol* 1985;86:353–379.

202. Hamilton SL, Yatani A, Brush K, Schwartz A, Brown AM. A comparison between the binding and electrophysiological effects of dihydropyridines on cardiac membranes. *Mol Pharmacol* 1987;31:221–231.

203. Kass RS, Krafte DS. Negative surface charge density near heart calcium channels. *J Gen Physiol* 1987;89:629–644.

204. Kawashima Y, Ochi R. Voltage-dependent decrease in the availability of single calcium channels by nitrendipine in guinea pig ventricular cells. *J Physiol* 1988;402:219–235.

205. Bean BP, Sturek M, Puga A, Hermsmeyer K. Calcium channels in muscle cells isolated from rat mesenteric arteries: modulation by dihydropyridine drugs. *Circ Res* 1986;59:229–235.

206. Yatani A, Seidel CL, Allen J, Brown AM. Whole cell and single channel calcium currents of isolated smooth muscle cells from saphenous vein. *Circ Res* 1987;60:523–533.

207. Nelson MT, Worley JF III. Dihydropyridine inhibition of single calcium channels and contraction in rabbit mesenteric artery depends on voltage. *Ann NY Acad Sci (in press)*.

208. Yatani A, Hamilton SL, Brown AM. Diphenylhydantoin blocks cardiac calcium channels and binds to the dihydropyridine receptor. *Circ Res* 1986;59:356–361.

209. Wei X-Y, Rutledge A, Triggle DJ. Voltage-dependent binding of 1,4-dihydro-pyridine Ca^{2+} channel antagonists and activators in cultured neonatal rat ventricular myocytes. *Mol Pharmacol* 1989;35:541–552.

210. Hondeghem LM, Ayad MJ, Robertson RM. Verapamil, diltiazem and nifedipine block the depolarization-induced potentiation of norepinephrine contractions in rabbit aorta and porcine coronary arteries. *J Pharmacol Exp Ther* 1986;239:808–813.

211. Wibo M, DeRoth L, Godfraind T. Pharmacologic relevance of dihydropyridine binding sites in membranes from rat aorta: kinetic and equilibrium studies. *Circ Res* 1988;62:91–96.

212. Morel N, Godfraind T. Prolonged depolarization increases the pharmacological effects of dihydropyridines and their binding affinity for calcium channels of vascular smooth muscle. *J Pharmacol Exp Ther* 1987;243:711–715.

213. Morel N, Godfraind T. Selective modulation by membrane potential of the interaction of some calcium entry blockers with calcium channels in rat mesenteric artery. *Br J Pharmacol* 1988;95:252–258.

214. Hering S, Beech DJ, Bolton TB, Lim SP. Action of nifedipine or Bay K 8644 is dependent on calcium channel state in single smooth muscle cells from rabbit ear artery. *Pflugers Arch* 1988;411:590–592.

215. Schilling WP, Drewe JA. Voltage-sensitive nitrendipine binding in an isolated cardiac sarcolemma preparation. *J Biol Chem* 1986;261: 2750–2758.

216. Kokubun S, Prod'hom B, Becker C, Porzig H,

Reuter H. Studies on Ca channels in intact cardiac cells: voltage-dependent effects and cooperative interactions of dihydropyridine enantiomers. *Mol Phramacol* 1987;30:571–584.

217. Porzig H, Becker C. Potential-dependent allosteric modulations of 1,4-dihydropyridine binding by d-(cis)-diltiazem and (+)verapamil in living cardiac cells. *Mol Pharmacol* 1988;34:172–179.

218. Kamp TJ, Sanguinetti MC, Miller RJ. Voltage-dependent binding of dihydropyridine calcium channel blockers to guinea pig ventricular myocytes. *J Pharmacol Exp Ther* 1988;247:1240–1247.

219. Ferrante J, Luchowski E, Rutledge A, Triggle DJ. Binding of the 1,4-dihydropyridine calcium channel activator, (−) S Bay K 8644, to cardiac preparations. *Biochem Biophys Res Commun* 1989;158:149–154.

220. Williams JS, Grupp IL, Grupp G, Vaghy PL, Dumont L, Schwartz A. Profile of the oppositely acting enantiomers of the dihydropyridine 202 791 in cardiac preparations: receptor binding, electrophysiological and pharmacological studies. *Biochem Biophys Res Commun* 1985;131:13–21.

221. Kass RS. Voltage-dependent modulation of cardiac calcium channel current by optical isomers of Bay K 8644: implications for channel gating. *Circ Res* 1987;61(Suppl I):I-1–5.

222. Chester DW, Herbette LG, Mason RP, Joslyn AF, Triggle DJ, Koppel DE. Diffusion of dihydropyridine calcium channel antagonists in cardiac sarcolemmal lipid multilayers. *Biophys J* 1987;52:1021–1030.

223. Kass RS, Arena JP. Influence of pHo on calcium channel block by amlodipine: a charged dihydropyridine compound: implications for location of the dihydropyridine receptor. *J Gen Physiol (in press)*.

224. Lee RT, Smith TW, Marsh JD. Evidence for distinct calcium channel agonist and antagonist binding sites in intact cultured embryonic chick ventricular cells. *Circ Res* 1987;60:683–691.

225. Triggle DJ, Janis RA. The 1,4-dihydropyridine receptor—a regulatory component of the Ca^{2+} channel. *J Cardiovasc Pharmacol* 1984;6:S949–S953.

226. Dunlap K, Holz GG, Rane SG. G proteins as regulators of ion channel function. *Trends Neurosci* 1987;10:241–244.

227. Brown AM, Birnbaumer L. Direct G protein gating of ion channels. *Am J Physiol* 1988;254:H401–H410.

228. Yatani A, Imoto Y, Codina J, Hamilton SL, Brown AM, Birnbaumer L. The stimulating G protein of adenylyl cyclase, Gs, also stimulates dihydropyridine-sensitive Ca^{2+} channels. *J Biol Chem* 1988;265:9887–9895.

229. Scott RH, Dolphin AC. The agonist effect of Bay K 8644 on neuronal calcium channel currents is promoted by G protein activation. *Neurosci Lett* 1988;89:170–175.

230. Herbette LG, Chester DW, Rhodes DG. Structural analysis of drug molecules in biological membranes. *Biophys J* 1986;49:91–94.

231. Pang DC, Sperelakis N. Uptake of calcium antagonist drugs into muscles as related to their lipid solubilities. *Biochem Pharmacol* 1984;33:821–826.

232. Herbette LG, Katz AM. Molecular model for the binding of 1,4-dihydropyridine calcium channel antagonists to their receptors in the heart: drug imaging in membranes and considerations for drug design. In: Venter JC, Triggle DJ, eds. *Structure and physiology of the slow inward calcium channel*. New York: Alan R. Liss, 1987;89–108.

233. Triggle DJ, Swamy VC. Calcium antagonists. Some chemical-pharmacologic aspects. *Circ Res* 1983;52(Suppl I):17–28.

234. DeFeudis FW. Further promiscuity of phenylalkylamine Ca^{2+} antagonists. *Trends Pharmacol Sci* 1988;9:352–353.

235. Fairhurst AS, Whittaker ML, Ehlert FJ. Interaction of D600 (methoxyverapamil) and local anesthetics with rat brain—adrenergic and muscarinic receptors. *Biochem Pharmacol* 1980;29:155–162.

236. Jim K, Harris A, Rosenberger LB, Triggle DJ. Stereoselective and nonstereoselective effects of D600 (methoxyverapamil) in smooth muscle preparations. *Eur J Pharmacol* 1981;76:67–72.

237. Nayler WG, Thompson JE, Jarrott B. The interaction of calcium antagonists (slow channel blockers) with myocardial alpha-adrenoceptors. *J Mol Cell Cardiol* 1982;14:185–188.

238. Nishimura M, Kanaide H, Nakamura M. Binding of [3H]prazosin to porcine aortic membranes: interaction of calcium antagonists with vascular alpha1-adrenoceptors. *J Pharmacol Exp Ther* 1986;236:789–793.

239. Descombes JJ, Stoclet JC. Diphenylalkylamine calcium antagonists interact with α-adrenoceptor binding sites in aortic membranes. *Eur J Pharmacol* 1985;115:313–318.

240. Karliner JS, Motulsky HJ, Dunlap J, Brown JH, Insel PA. Verapamil competitively inhibits α1-adrenergic and muscarinic but not α-adrenergic receptors in rat myocardium. *J Cardiovasc Pharmacol* 1982;4:515–520.

241. Feldman RD, Park GD, Lai CYC. The interaction of verapamil and norverapamil with β-adrenergic receptors. *Circulation* 1985;72:547–554.

242. Taylor JE, DeFeudis FV. Inhibition of [3H]spiperine binding to 5-HT2 receptors of rat cerebral cortex by the calcium antagonists verapamil and D600. *Eur J Pharmacol* 1985;106:215–216.

243. Adachi H, Shoji T. Characteristics of the inhibition of ligand binding to serotonin receptors in rat brain membranes by verapamil. *Jpn J Pharmacol* 1986;41:431–435.

244. DeFeudis FV. Interactions of Ca^{2+} antagonists at 5-HT2 and H2 receptors and GABA uptake sites. *Trends Pharmacol Sci* 1987;8:200–201.

245. Thayer SA, Welcome M, Chhabra A, Fairhurst

AS. Effects of dihydropyridine calcium channel blocking drugs on rat brain muscarinic and α-adrenergic receptors. *Biochem Pharmacol* 1980;34:170–185.

246. Wade PJ, Lad N, Tiffin DP. Interaction of the human platelet PAF-ACETHER binding site with calcium and calcium channel antagonists. *Prog Lipid Res* 1986;25:163–165.

247. Hu PS, Lindgren E, Jacobson KA, Fredholm BB. Interaction of dihydropyridine calcium channel agonists and antagonists with adenosine receptors. *Pharmacol Toxicol* 1987;61: 121–125.

248. Johnson GJ, Dunlop PC, Leis LA, Fron AHL. Dihydropyridine agonist Bay K 8644 inhibits platelet activation by competitive antagonism of thromboxane A2 prostaglandin H2 receptor. *Circ Res* 1988;62:494–505.

249. Bayer R, Kalusche D, Kaufmann R, Mannhold R. Inotropic and electrophysiological action of verapamil and D600 in mammalian myocardium. III. Effects of the optical isomers on transmembrane action potentials. *Naunyn Schmiedebergs Arch Pharmacol* 1975;290:81–97.

250. Galper JB, Catterall WA. Inhibition of sodium channels by D600. *Mol Pharmacol* 1979;15: 174–178.

251. Yatani A, Kunze DL, Brown AM. Effects of dihydropyridine calcium channel modulators on cardiac sodium channels. *Am J Physiol* 1985:254:H140–H147.

252. Sakamoto N, Terai M, Takenaka T, Maeno H. Inhibition of cyclic AMP phosphodiesterase by YC-93,2,6-dimethyl-4-(3-nitrophenyl)-1,4-dihydropyridine-3,-5-dicarboxylic acid-5[-(N-benzyl-N-methylamino)ethyl ester 5-methyl ester hydrochloride, a potent vasodilator. *Biochem Pharmacol* 1978;27:1269–1274.

253. Matsushima S, Tanaka T, Saitoh M, Watanabe M, Hikada H. Different sensitivities of Ca^{2+} calmodulin-dependent cyclic nucleotide phosphodiesterases from rabbit aorta and brain to dihydropyridine calcium channel blockers. *Biochem Biophys Res Commun* 1987;148:1468–1474.

254. Pan M, Janis RA. Stimulation of Na^+, K^+-ATPase of isolated smooth muscle membrane by the Ca^{2+} channel inhibitors, nimodipine and nitrendipine. *Biochem Pharmacol* 1984;33:787–791.

255. Colvin RA, Pearson N, Messineo FC, Katz AM. Effects of Ca channel blockers on Ca transport and Ca ATPase in skeletal and cardiac sarcoplasmic reticulum vesicles. *J Cardiovasc Pharmacol* 1982;4:935–941.

256. Movsesian MA, Ambudkar IS, Adelstein RS, Shamoo AE. Stimulation of canine cardiac sarcoplasmic reticulum Ca^{2+} uptake by dihydropyridine Ca^{2+} antagonists. *Biochem Pharmacol* 1985;34:195–201.

257. Vaghy PL, Johnson JD, Matlib, MA, Wang T, Schwartz A. Selective inhibition of $Na+$-induced Ca^{2+} release from heart mitochondria by diltiazem and certain other Ca^{2+} antagonist drugs. *J Biol Chem* 1982;257:6000–6002.

258. Chiesi M, Rogg H, Eichenberger K, Gazzotti P, Carafoli E. Stereospecific action of diltiazem on the mitochondrial Na-Ca exchange system and on sarcolemmal Ca-channels. *Biochem Pharmacol* 1987;36:2735–2740.

259. Marangos PJ, Finkel MS, Verma A, Maturi MF, Patel J, Patterson RE. Adenosine uptake sites in dog heart and brain; interaction with calcium antagonists. *Life Sci* 1984;35:1109–1116.

260. Striessnig J, Zernig G, Glossmann H. Human red-blood cell Ca^{2+} antagonist binding sites: evidence for an unusual receptor coupled to the nucleoside transporter. *Eur J Biochem* 1985; 150:67–77.

261. Godfraind T, Miller R, Wibo M. Calcium antagonism and calcium entry blockade. *Pharmacol Rev* 1986;38:321–416.

262. Millard RW, Lathrop DA, Grupp G. Differential cardiovascular effects of calcium channel blocking agents: potential mechanisms. *Am J Cardiol* 1982;49:499–506.

263. Kawai C, Konishi T, Matsuyama E. Comparative effects of three calcium antagonists, diltiazem, verapamil and nifedipine, on the sinoatrial and atrioventricular nodes. *Circulation* 1981;63:1035–1042.

264. Flaim SF, Zelis R. Effect of diltiazem on total cardiac output distribution in conscious rats. *J Pharmacol Exp Ther* 1982;222:359–366.

265. Hof RP. Calcium antagonists and the peripheral circulation: differences and similarities between PY 108–068, nicardipine, verapamil and diltiazem. *Br J Pharmacol* 1983;78:375–394.

266. O'Hara N, Ono H, Oguro K, Hashimoto K. Vasodilatory effects of perhexiline, glycerol trinitrate and verapamil on the coronary, femural, renal and mesenteric vascilative of the dog. *J Cardiovasc Pharmacol* 1981;3:251–268.

267. Hof RP. Selective effects of different calcium antagonists in the peripheral circulation. *Trends Pharmacol Sci* 1984;5:100–102.

268. Godfraind T, Kaba A, Polster P. Differences in sensitivity of arterial smooth muscle to inhibition of their contractile responses to depolarization by potassium. *Arch Int Pharmacodyn Ther* 1968;172:235–239.

269. Yousif FB, Triggle DJ. Inhibitory action of a series of Ca^{2+} channel antagonists against agonist and K^+ depolarization induced responses in smooth muscle: an assessment of selectivity of action. *Can J Physiol Pharmacol* 1986;64:273–283.

270. Julou-Schaeffer G, Freslon JL. Compared effects of calcium entry blockers on calcium-induced tension in rat isolated cerebral and peripheral resistance vessels. *Naunyn Schmiedebergs Arch Pharmacol* 1987;337:670–676.

271. Robinson BF, Dobbs RJ, Bayley S. Response of forearm resistance vessels to verapamil and sodium nitroprusside in normotensive and hypertensive men: evidence for a functional ab-

normality of vascular smooth muscles in primary hypertension. *Clin Sci* 1982;63:33–42.

272. Sharma JN, Fernandez PG, Laher I, Triggle CR. Differential sensitivity of Dahla salt-sensitive and Dahl salt-resistant rats to the hypotensive action of acute nifedipine administration. *Can J Physiol Pharmacol* 1984;62:241–243.

273. Aoki K, Frohlich E, eds. *Calcium in essential hypertension.* Tokyo: Academic Press, 1988.

274. Atkinson J, Sautel M, Sonnay M, et al. Greater vasodepressor sensitivity to nicardipine in spontaneously hypertensive rat (SAR) compared to normotensive rats. *Naunyn Schmiedebergs Arch Pharmacol* 1988;337:471–476.

275. Smith HJ, Briscoe MG. The relative sensitization by acidosis of five calcium blockers in cat papillary muscle. *J Mol Cell Cardiol* 1985;17:710–716.

276. Bristow MR, Ginsburg R, Laser JA, McAutey BJ, Minobe W. Tissue response selectivity of calcium antagonists in rat due to heterogeneity of [3H]nitrendipine binding sites. *Br J Pharmacol* 1984;82:309–320.

277. Pinquier J-L, Urien S, Chaumet-Riffaud P, Comte A, Tillement J-P. Binding of [3H]isradipine (PN 200 110) on smooth muscle cell membranes from different bovine arteries. *J Cardiovasc Pharmacol* 1988;11:402–406.

278. Nelson MT, Worley JF III. Dihydropyridine inhibition of single calcium channels and contraction in rabbit mesenteric artery depends on voltage. *J Physiol (Lond)* 1989;412:65–91.

279. Opie LH. Calcium channel antagonists. II. Use and comparative properties of the three prototypical calcium antagonists in ischemic heart disease, disease, including recommendations based on an analysis of 41 trials. *Cardiovasc Drug Ther* 1988;1:461–491.

280. Rashimtoola SH, Nunley D, Grunkemeier G, Tepley J, Lambert L, Starr A. Ten year survival for unstable angina. *New Engl J Med* 1983;308:676–681.

281. Forrester JS, Litvack F, Grindfest W. A perspective of coronary disease seen through the arteries of living man. *Circulation* 1987;75:505–513.

282. Hugenholtz PG. Unstable angina pectoris. In: Krebs R, ed. *Treatment of cardiovascular diseases by Adalat (R) (Nifedipine).* Stuttgart: Schattauer, 1986;187–229.

283. Lauie CJ, Murphy JG, Gersh BJ. The role of beta-receptor and calcium entry-blocking agents in acute myocardial infarction in the thrombolytic era. *Cardiovasc Drug Ther* 1988; 2:601–608.

283a. Singh BN, Nademannee K, Feld G. Calcium blockers in the treatment of cardiac arrhythmias. In: Flaim SF, Zelis R, eds. *Calcium blockers. Mechanisms of action and clinical applications.* Baltimore: Urban and Schwarzenberg, 1982.

284. Klein HO, Kaplinsky E. Digitalis and verapamil in atrial fibrillation and flutter. Is verapamil now the preferred agent? *Drugs* 1986;31:185–197.

285. Lewis R, Lakhani M, Moreland TA. A comparison of verapamil and digoxin in the treatment of atrial fibrillation. *Eur Heart J* 1987;8:148–153.

286. Roth A, Harrison E, Mitani G, Cohen J, Rahimtoola SH, Elkayam U. Efficacy and safety of medium- and high-do diltiazem alone and in combination with digoxin for control of heart rate at rest and during exercise in patients with chronic atrial fibrillation. *Circulation* 1986;73:316–324.

287. Mauritson DR, Winniford MD, Walker WS, Rude RE, Cary JR, Hillis LD. Oral verapamil for paroxysmal supraventricular tachycardia. A long-term, double-blind randomized trial. *Ann Intern Med* 1982;96:409–412.

288. Yee R, Gulamhusein SS, Klein GJ. Combined verapamil and propranolol for supra-ventricular tachycardia. *Am J Cardiol* 1984;53:757–763.

289. Yeh S-J, Kou H-W, Lin F-C, Hung J-S, Wu D. Effects of oral diltiazem in paroxysmal supraventricular tachycardia. *Am J Cardiol* 1983;52:271–278.

290. Yeh S-J, Lin F-C, Chou Y-Y, Hung J-S, Wu D. Termination of paroxysmal supra-ventricular tachycardia with a single oral dose of diltiazem and propranolol. *Circulation* 1985;71:104–109.

291. Sorkin EM, Clissold SP, Brogden RN. Nifedipine. A review of its pharmacodynamic and pharmacokinetic properties, and therapeutic efficacy in schemic heart disease, hypertension and related cardiovascular disorders. *Drugs* 1985;30:182–274.

292. Besch M, Corea L, Muiesan G, et al. Similarities and differences in the antihypertensive effects of two calcium antagonist drugs, verapamil and nifedipine. *J Am Coll Cardiol* 1986;7:916–924.

293. Katz AM, Leach NM. Differential effects of 1,4-dihydropyridine calcium channel blockers: therapeutic implications. *J Clin Pharmacol* 1987;27:825–834.

294. Moser A. Calcium entry blockers for systemic hypertension. *Am J Cardiol* 1987;59:115A–125A.

295. Fitzsimmons TJ. Calcium antagonists: a review of the recent comparative trials. *J Hypertension* 1987;5(Suppl 3):511–515.

296. Brand V, Laurent S, Tscoucaris-Kupfer L, Legrand M, Brisac AM, Schmitt H. Central and peripheral cardiovascular effects of the enantiomers of the calcium antagonist PN 200 110. *Eur J Pharmacol* 1988;150:43–50.

297. St John Sutton M, Morad M. Mechanisms of action of diltiazem in isolated human atrial and ventricular myocardium. *J Mol Cell Cardiol* 1987;19:497–508.

298. Kwioski W, Erne P, Bertol O. Acute and chronic sympathetic reflex activation and antihypertensive response to nifedipine. *J Am Cell Cardiol* 1986;7:344–348.

299. Bauer JH, Sunderrajan S, Reams G. Effects of

calcium entry blockers on renin-angiotensin-aldosterone system, renal function and hemodynamics, salt and acute excretion and body fluid composition. *Am J Cardiol* 1985;56:62H-67H.

300. Schoen RE, Frishman WH, Shamoon H. Hormonal and metabolic effects of calcium channel antagonists in man. *Am J Med* 1988;84:492–504.

301. Bauer JH, Reams G. Short- and long-term effects of calcium entry blockers on the kidney. *Am J Cardiol* 1987;59:66A–71A.

302. Collins WCJ, Cullen MJ, Feely J. Calcium channel blocker drugs and diabetic control. *Clin Pharmacol Ther* 1987;42:420–423.

303. Laragh JH, ed. Calcium metabolism and calcium channel blockers for treating and understanding hypertension. *Am J Med* 1984; 77(Suppl 6B):1–23.

304. Kiowski W, Buhler F, Fadayomi MO, et al. Age, race, blood pressure and renin predictors for antihypertensive treatment with calcium antagonists. *Am J Cardiol* 1985;56:81H–85H.

305. Tietze KJ, Schwartz ML, Vlasses PH. Calcium antagonists in cerebral/peripheral vascular disorders. Current status. *Drugs* 1987;32:531–538.

306. Greenberg DA. Calcium channel antagonists and the treatment of migraine. *Clin Neuropharmacol* 1986;9:311–328.

307. Allen GS. Role of calcium antagonists in cerebral arterial spasm. *Am J Cardiol* 1985;55: 149B–153B.

308. Gelmers H. Effects of nimodipine on the clinical course of patients with acute ischemic stroke. *Acta Neurol Scand* 1984;64:232–239.

309. Van Heereveld H, Wollersheim H, Gough K, Tiltien H. Intravenous nicardipine in Reynaud's phenomenon: a controlled trial. *J Cardiovasc Pharmacol* 1988;11:68–74.

310. Baughmann KL. Calcium channel blocking agents in congestive heart failure. *Am J Med* 1986;80(Suppl 2B):46–50.

311. Kaltenbach M, Hopf R. Treatment of hypertrophic cardiomyopathy: relation to pathological mechanisms. *J Mol Cell Cardiol* 1985; 71(Suppl 2):59–68.

312. Nayler WG. *Calcium antagonists.* New York: Academic Press, 1988.

313. Henry PD. Atherosclerosis, calcium and calcium antagonists. *Circulation* 1985;72:456–459.

314. Kramsch DM. Calcium antagonists and atherosclerosis. *Adv Exp Biol Med* 1985;183:323–348.

315. Weinstein DB, Heider JG. Antiatherogenic properties of calcium antagonists. *Am J Cardiol* 1987;59:163B–172B.

316. Triggle DJ. Calcium antagonists in atherosclerosis: a review and commentary. *Cardiovasc Drug Rev* 1989;6:320–335.

317. Jackson CL, Bush RC, Bowyer DE. Inhibitory effect of calcium antagonists on balloon catheter-induced arterial smooth muscle cell proliferation and lesion size. *Atherosclerosis* 1988; 69:115–122.

318. Verbeuren TJ, Jordaens FH, Zonnekeyn LL, Van Hove CE, Coene M-C, Herman AG. Effect of hypercholesterolemia on vascular reactivity in the rabbit. I. Endothelium-dependent and endothelium-independent contractions and relaxations in isolated arteries of control and hypercholesterolemic rabbits. *Circ Res* 1986;58: 552–564.

319. Ware JA, Johnson PC, Smith M, Salzman EW. Inhibition of human platelet aggregation and cytoplasmic calcium response by calcium antagonists. Studies with aequorin and Qin 2. *Circ Res* 1986;59:39–42.

320. Filpovic I, Buddecke G. Calcium channel blockers stimulate LDL receptor synthesis in human skin fibroblasts. *Biochem Biophys Res Commun* 1986;136:845–850.

321. Stein O, Leitersdorf E, Stein Y. Verapamil enhances receptor-mediated endocytosis of low density lipoproteins by aortic cells in culture. *Arteriosclerosis* 1985;5:35–44.

322. Henry PD. Comparative pharmacology of calcium antagonists; nifedipine, verapamil and diltiazem. *Am J Cardiol* 1980;46:1047–1058.

323. Kates RE. Calcium antagonists. Pharmacokinetic properties. *Drugs* 1983;25:113–124.

324. Sorkin EM, Clissold SP, Brogden RN. Nifedipine. A review of its pharmacodynamic and pharmacokinetic properties, and therapeutic efficacy in ischaemic heart disease, hypertension and related cardiovascular disorders. *Drugs* 1985;30:182–274.

325. Chaffman M, Brogden RN. Diltiazem. A review of its pharmacological properties and therapeutic efficacy. *Drugs* 1985;29:387–454.

326. Baker SH. Verapamil. In: Scriabine A, ed. *New drugs annual: cardiovascular drugs,* vol 2. New York: Raven Press, 1984;71–102.

327. Kuhlmann J, Graefe KH, Ramsch KD, Ziegler R. Clinical pharmacology of nifedipine. In: Krebs R, ed. *Treatment of cardiovascular diseases by Adalat (nifedipine).* Stuttgart: Schattauer, 1986;93–144.

328. Traube M, Hongo M, McCallister RG, McCallum RW. Correlations of plasma levels of nifedipine and cardiovascular effects after sublingual dosing in normal subjects. *J Clin Pharmacol* 1985;25:125–129.

329. Baker SH. Nicardipine hydrochloride. In: Scriabine A, ed. *New drugs annual: cardiovascular drugs,* vol 1. New York: Raven Press, 1983;153–172.

330. Scriabine A, Battye R, Hoffmeister F, et al. Nimodipine. In: Scriabine A, ed. *New cardiovascular drugs, 1985.* New York: Raven Press, 1985;197–218.

331. Scriabine A, Garthoff B, Kazda S, Ramsch K-D, Schluter G., Stoepel K. Nitrendipine. In: Scriabine A, ed. *New drugs annual: cardiovascular drugs,* vol 2. New York: Raven Press, 1984;37–50.

332. Woodcock BG, Schulz W, Kober G, Rietbrock N. Direct determination of hepatic extraction of verapamil in cardiac patients. *Clin Pharmacol Ther* 1981;30:52–56.

333. Echizen H, Vogelgesang B, Eichelbaum M. Effects of d,1-verapamil on atrioventricular conduction in relation to its stereoselective first pass metabolism. *Clin Pharmacol Ther* 1985; 38:71–76.

334. Vogelgesang B, Echizen H, Schmidt E, Eichelbaum M. Stereoselective first-pass metabolism of highly cleared drugs: studies on the bioavailability of l- and d-verapamil examined with a stable isotope technique. *Br J Clin Pharmacol* 1984;18:733–740.

335. Flaim SF. Diltiazem. In: Scriabine A, ed. *New drugs annual: cardiovascular drugs,* vol. 2. New York: Raven Press, 1984;123–156.

336. Holck M, Osterreider W. Tiapamil. In: Scriabine A, ed. *New cardiovascular drugs, 1987.* New York: Raven Press, 1987;77–94.

337. Wendt G. Pharmacokinetics and metabolism of tiapamil. *Cardiology* 1982;69(Suppl 1):68–78.

338. Baker SH. Nicardipine hydrochloride. *New drugs annual: cardiovascular drugs,* vol. 1. New York: Raven Press, 1983;153–172.

339. Jahr H, Krause HP, Siefert HM, Suwelack D, Weber H. Pharmacokinetics of nisoldipine. I. Absorption, concentration in plasma and excretion after single administration of [14C]nisoldipine in rats, dogs, monkey and swine. *Arzneimittelforschung* 1986;38:1093–1098.

340. Scherling D, Karl W, Ahr HJ, Wehinger E. Pharmacokinetics of nisoldipine. III. Biotransformation of nisoldipine in rat, monkey and man. *Arzneimittelforschung* 1984;38:1105–1110.

341. Opie LH. Calcium channel antagonists. Part IV: Side effects and contraindications, drug interactions and combinations. *Cardiovasc Drug Ther* 1988;2:177–189.

342. Reicher-Reiss H, Neufeld HN, Ebner EX. Calcium antagonists-adverse drug interactions. *Cardiovasc Drug Ther* 1987;1:403–409.

343. Gustafsson D. Microvascular mechanisms involved in calcium antagonist edema formation. *J Cardiovasc Pharmacol* 1987;10(Suppl 1): S121–131.

344. Leisten L, Kuhlmann J, Ebner F. Side effects and pharmacodynamic interactions. In: Krebs R, ed. *Treatment of cardiovascular diseases by Adalat (nifedipine).* Stuttgart: Schattauer, 1986; 270–314.

345. Prida XE, Gelman JS, Feldman RL. Comparison of diltiazem and nifedipine alone and in combination in patients with coronary artery spasm. *J Am Coll Cardiol* 1987;9:412–419.

346. Reicher-Reiss H, Neufeld HN, Ebner FX. Calcium antagonists—adverse drug interactions. *Cardiovasc Drug Ther* 1987;1:403–409.

347. Piepho RW, Culbertson VL, Rhodes RS. Drug interactions with the calcium-entry blockers. *Circulation* 1987;75(Suppl V):181–194.

348. Winniford MD, Huxley RL, Hillis DL. Randomized, double-blind comparison of propranolol alone and a propranolol-verapamil combination in patients with severe angina of effort. *J Am Coll Cardiol* 1983;1:492.

349. Johnston DL, Gebhardt VA, Donald A, Kostuk WJ. Comparative effects of propranolol and verapamil alone and in combination on left ventricular function and volume in patients with chronic exertional angina: a double-blind, placebo controlled, randomized, cross-over study with radionuclide ventriculography. *Circulation* 1987;68:1280–1289.

350. Darzie H, Cleland J, Findlay I, Murry G, McInnes G. Continuation of verapamil and beta blockers in systemic hypertension. *Am J Cardiol* 1986;57:80D.

351. Johnston DL, Lesoway R, Humen DP. Clinical and hemodynamic evaluation of propranolol in combination with verapamil, nifedipine and diltiazem in exertional angina pectoris: a placebo-controlled double blind randomized, cross-over study. *Am J Cardiol* 1985;55:680–687.

352. Gottesman MM, Pastan I. Resistance to multiple chemotherapeutic agents in human cancer cells. *Trends Pharmacol Sci* 1988;9:54–58.

353. Krogstad DJ, Gluzman IY, Kyle DE, et al. Efflux of chloroquine from Plasmodium falciparium: mechanisms of chloroquine resistance. *Science* 1987;238:1283–1284.

354. Hollenberg MD. Examples of homospecific and heterospecific receptor regulation. *Trends Pharmacol Sci* 1985;6:242–245.

355. Goldstein JL, Brown MS, Anderson RGW, Russell DW, Schneider WJ. Receptor-mediated endocytosis: concepts emerging from the LDL receptor system. *Annu Rev Cell Biol* 1985;1:1–89.

356. Benovic JL, Bouvier M, Caron MG, Lefkowitz RJ. Regulation of adenylyl cyclase-coupled β-adrenergic receptors. *Annu Rev Cell Biol* 1988;4:405–428.

357. Verner K, Schatz G. Protein translocation across membranes. *Science* 1988;241:1307–1313.

358. Raftery EB. Cardiovascular drug withdrawal syndromes. A potential problem with calcium antagonists. *Drugs* 1984;28:371–374.

359. Kaye R, Blake J, Rubin D. Possible coronary spasm rebound to abrupt nifedipine withdrawal. *Am Heart J* 1982;103:308.

360. Moses JW, Wertheimer JH, Bodenheimer MM, Banka VS, Teldman M, Helfant RH. Efficacy of nifedipine in rat angina refractory to propranolol and nitrates in patients with obstructive coronary artery disease. *Ann Intern Med* 1981;94:425–429.

361. Schick EC, Liang C-S, Heupler FA, et al. Randomized withdrawal from nifedipine: placebo-controlled study in patients with coronary artery spasm. *Am Heart J* 1982;104:690–697.

362. Lette J, Gagnon R-M, Lemire JG, Morisette M. Rebound of vasospastic angina after cessation of long-term treatment with nifedipine. *Can Med Assoc J* 1984;130:1169–1171.

363. Subramanian VB. Calcium antagonist withdrawal syndrome: objective demonstration with frequency-modulated ambulatory ST-segment monitoring. *Br Med J* 1983;286:520–521.

364. Nelson DO, Mangel AW, Graham CA, et al. Al-

tered human vascular activity following withdrawal from calcium channel blockers. *J Cardiovasc Pharmacol* 1984;6:1249–1250.

365. Freedman SB, Richmond DR, Kelly DT. Long-term follow-up of verapamil and nitrate treatment for coronary artery spasm. *Am J Cardiol* 1982;50:711–715.

366. Gottlieb SO, Gerstenblith G. Safety of acute calcium antagonist withdrawal: studies in patients from unstable angina withdrawn from nifedipine. *Am J Cardiol* 1985;55:27E–30E.

367. Schroeder JS, Walker SD, Skalland ML, Hemberger JA. Absence of rebound from diltiazem therapy in Prinzmetal's variant angina. *J Am Coll Cardiol* 1985;6:174–178.

368. Skattebol A, Brown AM, Triggle DJ. Homologous regulation of voltage-dependent calcium channels by 1,4-dihydropyridines. *Biochem Biophys Res Commun* 1989;160:929–936.

369. Gengo P, Skattebol A, Moran JF, Gallant S, Triggle DJ. Regulation by chronic drug administration of neuronal and cardiac calcium channel, beta-adrenoceptor and muscarinic receptor levels. *Biochem Pharmacol* 1988;37:627–633.

370. Mehta J, Lopez LM. Calcium blocker withdrawal phenomenon: increase in affinity of alpha2 adrenoceptors for agonist as a potential mechanism. *Am J Cardiol* 1986;58:242–246.

371. Desnuelle C, Askanao V, Engel WK. Insulin increases voltage-dependent Ca^{2+} channels in membranes of aneurally cultured human muscle. *Neurology* 1986;36(Suppl 1):171–172.

372. Kim D, Smith TW, Marsh JD. Effect of thyroid hormone on slow calcium channel function in cultured chick ventricular cells. *J Clin Invest* 1987;80:88–94.

373. Dolin S, Little H, Hudspith M, Pagonis C, Littleton J. Increased dihydropyridine-sensitive calcium channels in rat brain may underlie ethanol physical dependence. *Neuropharmacology* 1987;26:275–279.

374. Batra S. Increase by estrogen of calcium entry and calcium channel density in uterine smooth muscle. *Br J Pharmacol* 1987;92:389–392.

375. Wagner JA, Reynolds IJ, Weisman HF, Dudeck P, Weisfeldt ML, Snyder SH. Calcium antagonist receptors in cardiomyopathic hamster: selective increases in heart, muscle, brain. *Science* 1986;232:515–518.

376. Howlett SE, Rafuse VF, Gordon T. [3H]Nifedipine binding sites in normal and cardiomyopathic hamsters: absence of a selective increase in putative calcium channels in cardiomyopathic hearts. *Cardiovasc Res* 1988;22:840–846.

377. Finkel MS, Patterson RE, Roberts WC, Smith TD, Keiser HR. Calcium channel binding characteristics in the human heart. *Am J Cardiol* 1988;62:1281–1284.

378. Mayoux E, Callens F, Swynghedauw B, Charlemagne D. Adaptational process of the cardiac Ca^{2+} channels to produce overload, biochemical and physiological properties of the dihydropyridine receptors in normal and hypertrophic

rat hearts. *J Cardiovasc Pharmacol* 1988;12:390–396.

379. Chatelain P, Demol D, Roba J. Comparison of [3H]nitrendipine binding to heart membranes of normotensive and spontaneously hypertensive rats. *J Cardiovasc Pharmacol* 1984;6:220–223.

380. Huguet F, Huchet A-M, Gerard P, Narcisse G. Characterization of dihydropyridine binding sites in the rat brain: hypertension and age-dependent modulation of [^{3}H](H)PN 200 110 binding. *Brain Res* 1987;412:125–130.

381. Rusch NJ, Hernsmeyer K. Calcium currents are altered in the vascular muscle cell membrane of spontaneously hypertensive rats. *Circ Res* 1988;63:997–1002.

382. Dillon JS, Nayler WG. [3H]Verapamil binding to rat cardiac sarcolemmal membrane fragments: an effect of ischemia. *Br J Pharmacol* 1987;90:99–109.

383. Gu XH, Dillon JS, Nayler WG. Dihydropyridine binding sites in aerobically perfused, ischemic, and reperfused rat hearts: effect of temperature and time. *J Cardiovasc Pharmacol* 1988;12:272–278.

384. Freedman DD, Waters DD. Second generation dihydropyridine calcium anagonists. Greater vascular selectivity and some unique applications. *Drugs* 1987;34:578–598.

385. Opie LH. Calcium channel antagonists. V. Second-generation agents. *Cardiovasc Drug Ther* 1988;2:191–203.

386. Buhler FR, Mancia G, Reid JL, eds. Calcium antagonists in cardiovascular disease: rationale for 24 hour action. *J Cardiovasc Pharmacol* 1988;12(Suppl 7).

387. Julius S. Amlodipine in hypertension: an overview of the clinical dossier. *J Cardiovasc Pharmacol* 1988;12(Suppl 7):S27–S33.

388. Ljung B. Vascular selectivity of felodipine. *Drugs* 1985;29(Suppl 2):46–58.

389. Johansson B, Hansson L, eds. Emerging concepts in calcium antagonism with special reference to felodipine. *J Cardiovasc Pharmacol* 1987;10(Suppl 1).

390. Tweddel AG, Hutton I. Felodipine in ventricular dysfunction. *Eur Heart J* 1986;7:54–60.

391. Towart R. The selective inhibition of serotonin-induced contractions of rabbit cerebral vascular smooth muscle by calcium antagonist 1,4-dihydropyridines. An investigation of the mechanism of action of nimodipine. *Circ Res* 1981;48:650–657.

392. Deyo RA, Straube KT, Disterhoft JF. Nimodipine facilitates associative learning in aged rabbits. *Science* 1989;243:809–811.

393. Taylor SH, Jackson NC, Allen J, Tool P. Efficacy of a new calcium antagonist PN 200 110 (Isradipine) in angina pectoris. *Am J Cardiovasc* 1987;59:123B–129B.

394. Parker JO, Enjalbert M, Bernstein V. Efficacy of the calcium antagonist isradipine in angina pectoris. *Cardiovasc Drugs Ther (in press)*.

395. Scheidt S, LeWinter MM, Hermanovich J,

Venkataraman K, Freedman D. Efficacy and safety of nicardipine for chronic stable angina pectoris: a multicenter, randomized trial. *Am J Cardiol* 1986;58:715–721.

396. Sorkin EM, Clissold SP. Nicardipine. A review of its pharmacodynamic and pharmacokinetic properties, and therapeutic efficacy, in the treatment of angina pectoris, hypertension and related cardiovascular disorders. *Drugs* 1987; 33:296–345.

397. Khurmi NS, Raftery EB. Comparative effects of prolonged therapy with four calcium ion antagonists (diltiazem, nicardipine, tiapamil and verapamil) in patients with chronic stable angina pectoris. *Cardiovasc Drug Ther* 1987;1: 81–87.

398. Warltier DC, Zyvoloski MG, Gross GJ, Brooks HG. Comparative actions of dihydropyridine slow calcium channel blocking agents in conscious dogs: systemic and coronary hemodynamics with and without combined beta adrenergic blockade. *J Pharmacol Exp Ther* 1984; 230:367–375.

399. Lopez LM, Rubin MR, Holland JP, Menta JL. Improvement in exercise performance with nisoldipine, a new second generation calcium blocker in stable angina patients, clinical investigations. *Am Heart J* 1985;110:991–996.

400. Daniels AR, Opie LH. Monotherapy with the calcium channel antagonist nisoldipine for systemic hypertension and comparison with diuretic drugs. *Am J Cardiol* 1987;60:703–707.

401. Scriabine A, Vanov V, Deck K, eds. *Nitrendipine*. Baltimore: Urban and Schwarzenberg, 1984.

402. Frohlich ED, Buhler FR, eds. Calcium antagonists: first line partner for antihypertensive care. *J Cardiovasc Pharmacol* 1988;12(Suppl 4).

403. Buhler FR, Rosenthal T, eds. Calcium antagonists in hypertension. 25th anniversary international symposium. *J Cardiovasc Pharmacol* 1988;12(Suppl 6).

404. Osterreider W. Inhibition of the fast inward Na^+ current by the Ca^{2+} channel blocker tiapamil. *J Cardiovasc Pharmacol* 1986;8:1101–1106.

405. Khurmi NS, O'Hara MJ, Bowles MJ, Subramanian VB, Raftery EB. Randomized double-blind comparison of gallopamil and propranolol in stable angina pectoris. *Am J Cardiol* 1984; 53:684–688.

Cardiovascular Pharmacology, Third Edition,
edited by Michael Antonaccio.
Raven Press, Ltd., New York © 1990.

Central Neurotransmitters Involved in Cardiovascular Regulation

Robert B. McCall

Cardiovascular Diseases Research, The Upjohn Company, Kalamazoo, Michigan 49001

Tremendous progress has been made during the past decade in identifying mechanisms that regulate sympathetic outflow from the central nervous system. This chapter reviews recent developments that have had a major influence on our understanding of the central neurotransmitters that regulate sympathetic nerve discharge and therefore blood pressure. A critical factor responsible for advances in this field is the development of neuroanatomical techniques that have allowed the identification of interconnections between areas important in the central regulation of blood pressure. These techniques include the use of fluorescent dyes that exhibit retrograde transport properties and other markers such as the conjugated derivatives of horseradish peroxidase that allow tracing of pathways by both anterograde and retrograde transport. Immunochemical techniques have provided biochemical information indicating a wide variety of putative neurotransmitters contained within these central pathways. A number of more classical physiological techniques have begun to elucidate the role of these pathways in central autonomic regulation and to determine the functional significance of putative neurotransmitters contained within these pathways. Correlative techniques (e.g., single-unit, spike-triggered average of sympathetic nerve activity) (see [1] for review) have been developed to identify neu-rons contained within central sympathetic pathways. The techniques of microiontophoresis and microinjection of putative transmitters or their antagonists are being widely used and have provided valuable information regarding the function of putative neurotransmitters. Similar information has been obtained in studies in which the cardiovascular effects of chemical or electrical microstimulation of central sympathetic pathways are altered by pharmacological manipulations. Thus, the complexity of the central autonomic nervous system has begun to yield to the combined use of the techniques described above. This multidisciplinary approach has provided the most complete understanding of the central sympathetic nervous system summarized in this chapter.

GENERAL ORGANIZATION OF CENTRAL SYMPATHETIC PATHWAYS

Arterial blood pressure is maintained by the tonic vasomotor activity of sympathetic preganglionic neurons (SPN) that are located in the intermediolateral cell column of the thoracic and lumbar spinal cord (see Fig. 1 for general organization of sympathetic nervous system). Transection of the spinal cord markedly attenuates spontaneous sympathetic nerve discharge indicat-

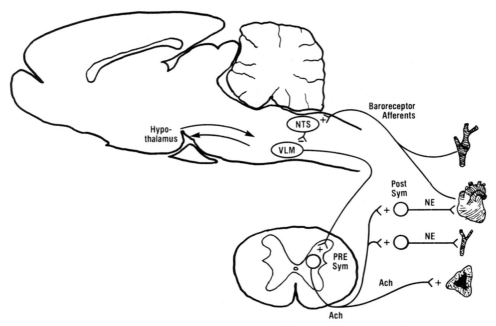

FIG. 1. General organization of the sympathetic nervous system. Sympathetic preganglionic neurons (PRE Sym) located in the intermediolateral cell column of the spinal cord represent the final site of integration of sympathetic information in the central nervous system. SPN project directly to the adrenal gland and to postganglionic sympathetic neurons (Post Sym), which then project to the heart and blood vessels. SPN receive inputs from a variety of brain-stem areas, the most critical being the ventral lateral medulla (VLM). Sympathetic neurons in the ventral lateral medulla receive inputs from many areas of the central nervous system including the hypothalamus and the NTS (i.e., the site of termination of baroreceptor afferent nerves). NE, norepinephrine; Ach, acetycholine.

ing that supraspinal inputs are critical in maintaining the activity of SPN. The medulla and pons have been recognized as essential for maintaining tonic sympathetic activity since the late 1800s when experiments showed that transection of the brain stem caudal to the inferior colliculus failed to lower blood pressure, whereas subsequent transections more caudally produced increasingly greater falls in blood pressure. Reductions in blood pressure reached a maximum with transections at the level of the obex (see [2] for historical review). A major goal of central autonomic research has been to identify the descending neuronal pathways that project to SPN and to determine the neurotransmitters contained within these pathways (see [3–5] for review). Supraspinal structures that project

to the intermediolateral cell column include the rostral ventrolateral medulla, medullary and pontine raphe nuclei (obscurus, pallidus, and magnus), the nucleus interfascicularis hypoglossi, the A5 noradrenergic cell group, the Kölliker-Fuse nucleus located in the lateral portion of the parabrachial nucleus complex, the paraventricular hypothalamic nucleus, and the lateral hypothalamic area (Fig. 2). Indeed, many of these brain-stem structures are interconnected and appear to play a critical role in the elaboration of central sympathetic outflow. Furthermore, medullary and pontine nuclei involved in autonomic control project to hypothalamic structures that are involved in the regulation of fluid balance (e.g., paraventricular hypothalamic nucleus and the organ of the lamina terminalis) and that also

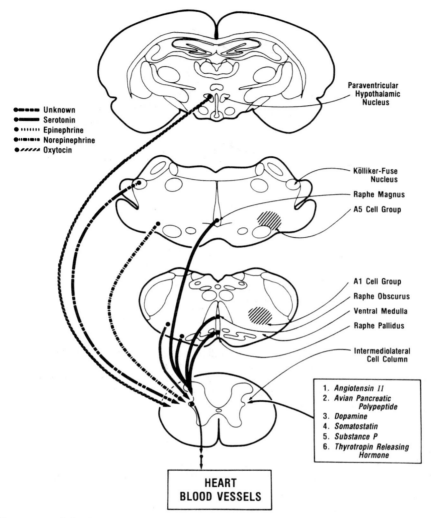

Unknown
Serotonin
Epinephrine
Norepinephrine
Oxytocin

Paraventricular
Hypothalamic
Nucleus

Kölliker-Fuse
Nucleus

Raphe Magnus

A5 Cell Group

A1 Cell Group

Raphe Obscurus

Ventral Medulla

Raphe Pallidus

Intermediolateral
Cell Column

1. *Angiotensin II*
2. *Avian Pancreatic*
   Polypeptide
3. *Dopamine*
4. *Somatostatin*
5. *Substance P*
6. *Thyrotropin Releasing*
   Hormone

HEART
BLOOD VESSELS

FIG. 2. Summary of the inputs to the intermediolateral cell column. The 5-HT inputs arise from the raphe pallidus, raphe obscurus, raphe magnus, and the ventrolateral medulla. The epinephrine input arises from the C1 area of the rostral ventrolateral medulla. The norepinephrine input arises from the A5 cell group. Other inputs come from the Kölliker-Fuse nucleus and paraventricular hypothalamic nucleus. (From ref. 4.)

send descending projects to autonomic areas of the lower brain stem and spinal cord (6–10). Thus, reciprocal innervations exist between the ventrolateral medulla and (a) the parabrachial nucleus, (b) the paraventricular nucleus (PVN), and (c) raphe nuclei. The parabrachial nucleus is also reciprocally innervated by the PVN. The A5 catecholamine cell group projects to all

these areas. Figure 3 illustrates the interconnected areas of the central nervous system that are critical in autonomic control mechanisms.

The baroreceptor reflex is primarily responsible for the homeostasis of arterial blood pressure. Baroreceptors arising in the aortic arch and the carotid sinuses project centrally within the aortic depressor and

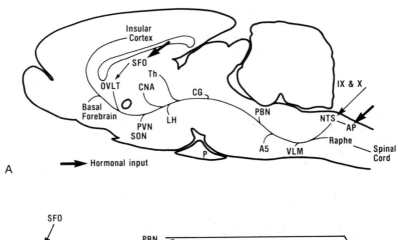

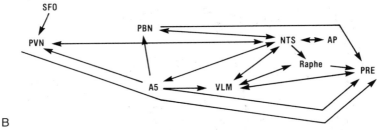

FIG. 3. Brain areas involved in the control of cardiovascular function. **A** illustrates locations of important nuclei involved in cardiovascular regulation. **B** is a wiring diagram depicting connections between these nuclei. CG, central gray area; CNA, central nucleus of the amygdala; LH, lateral hypothalamus; P, pituitary; PBN, parabrachial nucleus; SON, supraoptic nucleus; Th, midline thalamic nuclei, VLM, ventrolateral medulla.

carotid sinus branches of the IXth (glossopharyngeal) and Xth (vagus) cranial nerves. A large body of evidence indicates that the nucleus tractus solitarius (NTS), and in particular its dorsomedial subdivision, is the location of the first synapse in the baroreceptor afferent pathway (see [10] for review). Thus, efferent projections from this area define probable nuclei for participation in the central regulation of the cardiovascular system, whereas afferents into this region may function to modulate baroreceptor reflexes. The NTS has been shown to be reciprocally innervated by the ventrolateral medulla, the A5 catecholamine cell group, the parabrachial nucleus, and the PVN. These projections undoubtedly play an important role in the regulation of the cardiovascular system. In addition, the NTS projects to cardiac vagal motoneurons

located in the dorsal motor nucleus of the vagus and in the nucleus ambiguus complex (10). These pathways represent the neuronal basis for the baroreceptor-mediated control of heart rate.

Finally, an important development in the field of cardiovascular control is the appreciation that certain humoral substances in the blood can influence the central integration of sympathetic nerve activity by a direct action on selected central structures. Sites of potential interaction between circulating substances and central structures include the circumventricular organs (i.e., subfornical organ [SFO], organum vasculosum of the lamina terminalis [OVLT], median eminence, and the area postrema [AP]). Circumventricular organs lack an effective blood-brain barrier and thus provide sites through which humorally derived substances can penetrate into the brain and activate neural and humoral mechanisms. Circumventricular organs have been shown to project to central nuclei that are involved in cardiovascular regulation. For example, the SFO projects to the PVN and the median preoptic area, whereas the AP shares reciprocal projections with the NTS (10,11). These pathways represent the basis by which blood-borne substances can regulate central sympathetic nerve activity.

The above discussion is a brief overview of the areas of the central nervous system that are critical for the generation of sympathetic nerve activity and the regulation of the cardiovascular system. Subsequent sections of this chapter will discuss these areas in greater detail with emphasis on the nature and function of neurotransmitters that help to regulate activity within and between autonomic nuclei in the central nervous system.

ROSTRAL VENTROLATERAL MEDULLA

Function in Cardiovascular Regulation

The observation that transection at the pontomedullary border has little effect on arterial blood pressure whereas transection more caudally at the level of the obex produces levels of blood pressure similar to that observed after spinal cord transection indicates that the medulla is essential in maintaining sympathetic activity and blood pressure. Attempts to more specifically localize the site that is critical in maintaining blood pressure have proved elusive. Indeed, lesions encompassing large areas of the medulla often fail to markedly affect sympathetic activity or blood pressure. Experiments during the past several years, however, indicate that a restricted area in the rostral ventrolateral medulla is necessary for the maintenance of blood pressure. These studies are summarized below and reviewed in more detail elsewhere (1,12,13).

Attention was initially focused on the rostral ventrolateral medulla by the observation that direct application of pentobarbital or glycine to the ventrolateral surface of the medulla reduced blood pressure to levels seen after spinal cord transection (14,15). Electrical stimulation of the rostral ventrolateral area elicits pressor responses that are accompanied by increases in sympathetic activity (16–18). Microinjection of excitatory amino acids into restricted regions of the rostral ventrolateral medulla mimics the pressor effects of electrical stimulation indicating that neuronal cell bodies rather than fiber tracts mediate the increases in blood pressure and sympathetic activity (17–22). Discrete bilateral lesions in the rostral ventrolateral area of the medulla reduce blood pressure to the level observed following spinal cord transection (16,23,24). Neuroanatomical findings (17, 19,25–28) indicate that a population of neurons located in the area described by the microinjection and lesion experiments project to the intermediolateral cell column of the spinal cord (i.e., site of SPN). Electrophysiological studies have identified neurons within this region that exhibit discharges that are correlated to sympathetic nerve activity, receive baroreceptor inputs, and terminate in the intermediolateral cell column (29–35). Analysis of the precise anatomical location within the rostral ventrolateral medulla containing these neurons reveals that they are located in a discrete area extending from the caudal pole of the facial nucleus caudally to include the rostral third of the inferior olive. The region is limited dorsally by the nucleus ambiguus and medially by the inferior olive. Taken together, these observations indicate that this discrete area of the rostral ventrolateral medulla is essential for the maintenance of tonic sympathetic activity and therefore blood pressure.

Neurotransmitters Contained Within the Descending Pathway from the Rostral Ventrolateral Medulla to SPN

Epinephrine

The preceding discussion summarizes a substantial body of evidence indicating that a population of neurons in the rostral ventrolateral medulla provides a tonic excitatory drive to SPN. Reis and co-workers (12,17,18,24) have pointed out the striking similarity between the location of the tonic vasomotor region of the rostral ventrolateral medulla and the distribution of the C1 epinephrine cell group (Fig. 4). Anatomical evidence overwhelmingly indicates that C1

epinephrine neurons project to the intermediolateral cell column (28,36). The magnitude of the pressor response elicited by chemical or electrical stimulation of the rostral ventrolateral medulla correlates with the placement of the electrode in the C1 area. Moreover, stimulation of medullary sites that contain the descending C1 axons also produces pressor responses (18). Localized bilateral lesions coinciding precisely with the C1 area cause a decrease in blood pressure comparable with levels observed after spinal cord transection. These findings led to the hypothesis that descending epinephrine neurons from the C1 area of the rostral ventrolateral medulla provide a tonic excitatory input to SPN that is re-

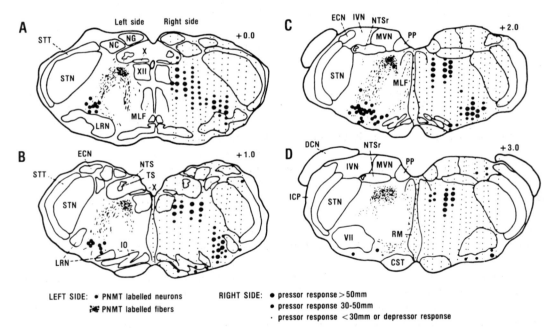

FIG. 4. C1 area of rostral ventrolateral medulla. Locations of the most active medullary pressor regions to constant current electrical stimulation compared with locations of C1 cells and fibers immunocytochemically labeled for phenylethanolamine N-methyltransferase (PNMT). Left side of each section, PNMT-labeled C1 neurons and PNMT-labeled fibers. Right side of each section, pressor responses to electrical stimulation. (From ref. 18.) STT, spinal trigeminal tract; NC, nucleus cuneatus; NG, nucleus gracilis; STN, spinal trigeminal nucleus; LRN, lateral reticular nucleus; MLF, medial longitudinal fasciculus; TS, tractus solitarius; IO, inferior olive; MVN, medial vestibular nucleus; IVN, inferior vestibular nucleus, ICP, inferior cerebellar peduncle; DCN, dorsal cochlear nucleus; NTSr, nucleus tractus solitarius pars rostralis; PP, nucleus prepositus; CST, corticospinal tract; RM, raphe magnus.

sponsible for the maintenance of resting arterial blood pressure.

In direct opposition to this hypothesis, however, is the finding that microiontophoretic application of epinephrine consistently inhibits the firing of SPN (37–39). The epinephrine-induced inhibition of SPN firing is mediated via an α_2-adrenergic receptor because the inhibition can be blocked by the α_2-antagonists yohimbine and piperoxane (38,39). This observation is supported by autoradiographic studies that indicate that α_2-adrenergic receptors are highly concentrated over clusters of SPN (40). Ross et al. (28) pointed out that the results of microiontophoretic studies must be viewed cautiously because epinephrine released from nerve terminals may act on receptors distant from those acted on by iontophoretic epinephrine. Thus, epinephrine may produce inhibition by acting on receptors located on SPN soma and excitation via receptors located on distal dendrites or antecedent interneurons. Indeed, excitatory and inhibitory effects of norepinephrine have been observed, occasionally on the same SPN (41). However, microiontophoresis of α_2-antagonists fail to block the excitation of SPN elicited by stimulation of pressor sites located in the C1 area of the rostral ventrolateral medulla (Morrison, *personal communication*). In addition, Sangdee and Franz (42) found that two selective inhibitors of central epinephrine synthesis (LY 134046 and SKF 64139) gradually, but markedly, enhanced descending intraspinal transmission to SPN. These data suggest that bulbospinal epinephrine pathways depress rather than enhance the excitability of SPN.

The most convincing argument that epinephrine-containing C1 neurons mediate a sympathoexcitatory function is the remarkable correlation between the location of rostral ventrolateral pressor sites and the distribution of the medullospinal epinephrine neurons. However, this is only correlative data and should be viewed with caution, particularly in light of recent anatomical data. Helke et al. (55) identified a group of substance-P immunoreactive neurons in the immediate vicinity of C1 epinephrine neurons that project to the intermediolateral cell column. In fact, recent studies indicate that only approximately 50% of the neurons in the rostral ventrolateral medulla that project to the intermediolateral cell column contain epinephrine (1,36). Electrophysiological investigations in the rat support this contention. The rostral ventrolateral medulla contains reticulospinal neurons that are baroreceptor sensitive. These neurons can be subdivided into two groups based on their axonal conduction velocity, their average discharge rate, and their sensitivity to administration of the α_2-agonist clonidine. The first group is characterized by axonal conduction velocities of 3.5 to 8.0 m/sec, a maximum discharge rate of 15 to 35 spikes/sec and clonidine insensitivity. The second group exhibits axonal conduction velocities of 0.4 to 0.8 m/sec, a slow discharge rate and an extreme sensitivity to the inhibitory effects of clonidine. The characteristics of the latter group are consistent with the idea that these cells are the C1 epinephrine-containing neurons (1,43). Interestingly, two distinct groups of reticulospinal neurons arising in the rostral ventrolateral medulla have not been identified in the cat (29,33,34). The C1 area also contains neurons whose cell bodies are immunoreactive to serotonin (5-HT) (44), acetylcholine (45), met- and leu-enkephalin (46), somatostatin (47), neurotensin (48), neuropeptide Y (49), cholecystokinin (50), vasoactive intestinal peptide (51), and thyrotropin-releasing hormone (TRH) (52). The fact that several nonepinephrine-containing neurons, some of which project to the intermediolateral cell column, coupled with the observation that microiontophoretic epinephrine consistently inhibits SPN, leads to the conclusion that C1 epinephrine neurons have a sympathoinhibitory rather than a sympathoexcitatory function. However, this conclusion must be made tentatively because

C1 epinephrine neurons contain other peptides such as neuropeptide Y (53) and substance P (54), the latter being sympathoexcitatory (see below). It is possible that these neurons are functionally heterogeneous, having different effects of SPN depending on the type and number of receptors found on specific SPN. Clearly, further experiments are required to definitively demonstrate the functional importance of these neurons.

Substance P

Substance P is heavily concentrated in the intermediolateral cell column of the spinal cord (55). Autoradiographic binding studies indicate that the intermediolateral cell column contains a dense distribution of high-affinity substance-P binding sites that are located on SPN (56). The origin of the substance-P input to the intermediolateral cell column remains somewhat controversial. A major source of input appears to arise from substance-P neurons located in the rostral ventrolateral medulla. This was first demonstrated by experiments in which unilateral electrolytic lesions of the rostral ventrolateral medulla bilaterally reduced the content of substance P by 40% in the intermediolateral cell column (55). Subsequent anatomical studies confirm that substance-P neurons located in the rostral ventrolateral medulla project to the intermediolateral cell column. At least some of these neurons also contain epinephrine (54). In addition, substance P is colocalized with 5-HT-containing neurons in medullary raphe nuclei. Although these neurons project to the spinal cord, they have not been shown to innervate the intermediolateral cell column (57). Finally, a portion of the substance-P input to the intermediolateral cell column arises from spinal interneurons (58).

Microiontophoretically applied substance P excites SPN (59,60). The onset of the excitatory response is delayed (i.e., 30 sec) and the increased firing rate of SPN contin-

ues long after the application of substance P is terminated (i.e., 30–320 sec). Similarly, intrathecal administration of substance P or stable agonist analogs of the peptide increase blood pressure, renal sympathetic nerve activity, plasma catecholamines, and total peripheral resistance (61–64).

The studies cited above have led to the generally accepted conclusion that substance P acts to excite SPN. However, the importance of the rostral ventrolateral medullary substance-P neurons in the maintenance of tonic sympathetic activity and therefore blood pressure is much more controversial. Intrathecal administration of substance-P antagonists (e.g., [D-Pro^2, D-Trp^{7,9}]-substance P or [D-Pro^4, D-Trp^{7,9}]-substance P) causes dose-dependent decreases in arterial blood pressure. Higher doses of these antagonists reduce blood pressure to levels observed following spinal cord transection (65). Microinjection of excitatory amino acids into the rostral ventrolateral medulla elicits a pressor response, which is accompanied by an increase in the release of immunoreactive substance P from the spinal cord. Both the pressor response and the release of substance P can be prevented by intrathecal administration of a substance-P antagonist (66). Similarly, microinjection of the gamma-aminobutyric acid (GABA) antagonist bicuculline into the rostral ventrolateral medulla elicits a sympathetically mediated pressor response that can be blocked by intrathecal administration of a substance-P antagonist (67). These and similar studies (for a review, see [68]) led to the hypothesis that substance-P neurons arising in the ventral lateral medulla and descending to the intermediolateral cell column function as a major tonic excitatory pathway to SPN. This hypothesis hinges on the specificity of the substance-P antagonists at the level of the SPN. This issue is critical because the D-amino acid antagonists of substance P have been reported to be nonspecific for substance P in the isolated spinal cord (69) and to have neurotoxic (70) and local anesthetic properties (71). In an attempt to determine the specificity of these antagonists, Yusof and Coote (62) studied the effect of intrathecal administration of a substance-P antagonist on the increase in renal nerve sympathetic activity elicited by intrathecal administration of substance P, 5-HT, and glutamate. They found that the antagonist blocked the sympathoexcitatory effect of all these agents indicating that the antagonist was nonspecific. In contrast, Yashpal et al. (64) reported that intrathecal administration of a substance-P antagonist blocks the pressor effect of intrathecal substance P but not that of intrathecal angiotensin II (Ang). However, the mechanism of the pressor action of Ang was not determined (e.g., sympathoexcitation versus decreased spinal blood flow). In summary, available evidence supports a sympathoexcitatory role of substance P in the spinal cord, although the importance of this system in the tonic maintenance of sympathetic activity requires further study.

5-HT

The most lateral 5-HT cells of the B_1- and B_3-cell groups lie just medial to the pressor area of the rostral ventrolateral medulla and have been postulated to play an important role in maintaining tonic vasomotor activity (72). Indeed, these neurons have been shown to project to the intermediolateral cell column (73). Chemical or electrical stimulation of this area results in a pressor response, and this is attenuated by pretreatment with the 5-HT neurotoxin 5,7-dihydroxytryptamine (5,7-DHT) (72). More recent studies, however, did not confirm these observations (67,74). A recent study by Minson et al. (75) helps to explain these contradictory findings. They found that glutamate microinjections into the area of the epinephrine-containing neurons evoked a pressor response that was not altered by 5,7-DHT. After ablation of the area of the epinephrine-containing neurons by electrolytic lesion, more medial microinjections of glutamate elicited a pressor response that

was presumably mediated by 5-HT. These data indicate that the lateral wings of the B_1 and B_3 5-HT cell groups have a sympathoexcitatory function that is independent of the more laterally positioned sympathoexcitatory neurons in the rostral ventrolateral medulla. The role of 5-HT in the regulation of sympathetic activity is described in more detail below.

Glutamate

Intrathecal administration of the excitatory amino-acid antagonist kynurenic acid eliminates spontaneous sympathetic activity and blocks the sympathoexcitatory effect of electrical stimulation of the rostral ventrolateral medulla. The effects of kynurenic acid are reversed by intrathecal administration of the excitatory amino acid kainic acid. This observation suggests that the depressor effects of kynurenic acid are produced by a specific action on a spinal excitatory amino-acid receptor (76). Similarly, intrathecal injection of a second excitatory amino-acid antagonist, HA-966, also eliminates sympathetic nerve discharge and reduces arterial blood pressure to levels observed following spinal cord transection (3). Microiontophoresis of excitatory amino acids excite SPN (77). In a slice preparation, glutamate depolarizations of presumed SPN are typically associated with a decrease in membrane resistance and are unaffected by tetrodotoxin. Focal electrical stimulation elicits a fast excitatory postsynaptic potential (EPSP) that is identical to the ionic mechanisms involved in the glutamate depolarization and is blocked by glutamate antagonists of the kainate/quisqualate subtype (78). These data are consistent with the hypothesis that medullospinal neurons arising in the rostral ventrolateral medulla utilized an excitatory amino acid as their neurotransmitter. Direct support for this hypothesis comes from the work of Morrison et al. who found that microiontophoresis of kynurenic acid directly onto SPN blocked the excitation produced by stimulation of the rostral ventrolateral medulla (*personal communication*).

CAUDAL VENTROLATERAL MEDULLA

Function in Cardiovascular Regulation

The caudal ventrolateral medulla corresponds with the external formation of the nucleus ambiguus at the level of the obex, overlaps at its most rostral extent with the sympathoexcitatory neurons of the rostral ventrolateral medulla and contains the A1 noradrenergic cell group (1). Electrical or chemical stimulation of this area produces cardiovascular effects opposite those observed in more rostral portions of the ventrolateral medulla. For example, microinjection of glutamate into the caudal ventrolateral medulla results in decreases in arterial blood pressure and peripherally recorded sympathetic nerve discharge (1,12, 13,79,80). Conversely, microinjection of hyperpolarizing agents such as GABA or the GABA agonist muscimol results in increases in blood pressure, heart rate, and sympathetic activity (81,82). This occurs even when blood pressure is maintained below the threshold for arterial baroreceptor activation (83). Electrolytic or kainic-acid lesions of the caudal ventrolateral medulla result in increases in blood pressure, heart rate, sympathetic nerve discharge, and plasma vasopressin levels (1,12,13,84,85). Collectively, these data indicate that the caudal ventrolateral medulla exerts a tonic inhibition of sympathetic activity and arginine vasopressin (AVP) release from the posterior pituitary.

Regulation of Rostral Ventrolateral Medulla

There is increasing evidence to indicate that neurons in the caudal ventrolateral medulla tonically inhibit medullospinal sympathoexcitatory neurons in the rostral ventrolateral medulla. Anatomical studies indicate that neurons arising in the caudal ventrolateral medulla project to the rostral ventrolateral medulla (86). Microinjections of tetrodotoxin into the rostral ventrolateral medulla prevent the increases in arterial blood pressure and sympathetic nerve activity observed following lesions of the caudal ventrolateral medulla (84). Microinjections of muscimol into the rostral ventrolateral medulla block the vasopressor effects of subsequent muscimol microinjections into the caudal ventrolateral medulla (87). Evidence exists to suggest that A1 noradrenergic neurons may tonically inhibit sympathoexcitatory neurons in the rostral ventrolateral medulla. Microinjection of norepinephrine or clonidine into the rostral ventrolateral medulla results in an α_2-receptor-mediated decrease in arterial blood pressure (88,89). In addition, microinjection of tyramine, a catecholamine-releasing agent, into the rostral ventrolateral medulla produces hypotension (84). The effect of tyramine can be blocked by pretreatment with the catecholamine uptake inhibitor imipramine. Destruction of noradrenergic terminals in the rostral ventrolateral medulla by 6-hydroxydopamine (6-OHDA) also abolishes the effect of tyramine and in addition prevents the increase in arterial blood pressure normally seen after lesion of the caudal ventrolateral medulla (84). These data suggest that A1 noradrenergic neurons tonically inhibit sympathoexcitatory neurons in the rostral ventrolateral medulla. This conclusion, however, must be made tentatively. The results obtained with adrenergic agonists and tyramine might be explained by a direct action on rostral ventrolateral epinephrine neurons. In this regard, monoamine neurons possess autoreceptors and regulate their discharge via axon collaterals that project back to their soma (90). In addition, microinjection of 6-OHDA produces local damage that includes noncatecholamine-containing neurons. Furthermore, Day et al. (80) have shown that electrical microstimulation of the A1 area does not elicit vasodepressor responses, whereas stimulation of a slightly more medial region elicits decreases in blood pressure. Finally, nonadrenergic neurons in the caudal ventrolateral medulla project to the spinal cord (17,91). Thus, it is possible that not all vasodepressor effects elicited from the caudal ventrolateral medulla are mediated via the rostral ventrolateral medulla. The role of the A1-noradrenergic neurons in mediating the depressor response remains to be determined.

Evidence exists to indicate that cholinergic mechanisms in the rostral ventrolateral medulla play a role in mediating responses elicited from the caudal ventrolateral medulla. Microinjections of the δ-receptor agonist D-Ala^2-D-Leu^5-enkephalin (DADLE) into the caudal ventrolateral medulla produces a hypertensive response that is reversed by blockade of cholinergic receptors in the rostral ventrolateral medulla (247). Microinjection of the cholinergic agonist carbachol or the acetylcholine esterase inhibitor physostigmine into the rostral ventrolateral medulla elicits a marked increase in arterial blood pressure that is mediated by an increase in sympathetic nerve activity (248). Intravenous administration of physostigmine produces a similar increase in arterial blood pressure that is prevented by microinjections of tetrodotoxin or lidocaine into the rostral ventrolateral medulla (249). Recent anatomical data indicate that cholinergic interneurons in the rostral ventrolateral medulla make synaptic contact with descending sympathoexcitatory neurons (250). These data suggest that cholinergic interneurons in the rostral ventrolateral medulla provide an excitatory input to descending sympathoexcitatory neurons and mediate the pressor effects of intravenous physostigmine and microinjections of DADLE into the caudal ventrolateral medulla.

Regulation of Vasopressin Release

Anatomical studies indicate that a large number of neurons in the caudal ventrolateral medulla project to the regions of the supraoptic and paraventricular nuclei of the hypothalamus that contain the AVP neurosecretory cells. Double-labeling experiments show that more than 80% of these ascending neurons are A1 norepinephrine-containing neurons (92,93). Early evidence suggesting that neurons in the caudal ventrolateral medulla were involved in the ascending control of AVP release was obtained by electrical stimulation of this area, which caused an increase in the release of AVP (94). In addition, topical application of GABA antagonists on the ventrolateral surface of the medulla resulted in an increase in AVP secretion that was not attributable to changes in arterial blood pressure (95). More recently, it has been demonstrated that microinjection of muscimol into the caudal ventrolateral medulla inhibits the release of AVP in response to hemorrhage and to constriction of the inferior vena cava (96). Conversely, microinjections of L-glutamate or the GABA antagonist bicuculline cause dose-dependent increases in plasma AVP (97). Finally, microinjection of norepinephrine into the PVN enhances AVP release (98). These studies suggest that A1 norepinephrine neurons stimulate the release of AVP.

Electrophysiological studies provide more support for this hypothesis. Electrical stimulation of the A1 region elicits an increase in firing of AVP-containing neurons in the PVN and in the supraoptic nucleus. The excitatory effect of A1 stimulation is abolished by local administration of 6-OHDA (99,100). Interestingly, pretreatment with 6-OHDA fails to alter basal levels of plasma AVP (101). In addition, the excitatory effect of A1 stimulation on AVP secretory neurons in the PVN is blocked by microiontophoretic application of the α-adrenergic antagonist phentolamine (102). Norepinephrine enhances the excitability and promotes bursting activity in supraoptic nucleus neurosecretory neurons via an α_1-receptor mechanism *in vitro* (103). Similarly, stimulation of norepinephrine neurons in the locus coeruleus also stimulates AVP release (104). Taken together, these data support the concept that ascending noradrenergic neurons facilitate the release of AVP. The fact that 6-OHDA pretreatment fails to alter basal levels of AVP suggests that norepinephrine may act as a modulator to maintain the sensitivity of neurosecretory neurons to stimuli that normally elicit AVP release (101).

The role of the caudal ventrolateral medulla in regulating AVP release is likely more complicated than is indicated by the above discussion. For example, the data presented suggest that lesions of the caudal ventrolateral medulla would result in a decreased release of AVP. In fact, however, lesion of the caudal ventrolateral medulla results in large increases in plasma AVP (105,106). It has been suggested that these results are likely due to injury discharge in noradrenergic pathways that enhance AVP secretion (48). Moreover, microiontophoretic application of norepinephrine onto AVP secretory neurons inhibits rather than excites the discharges of these neurons. Interestingly, superfusion of norepinephrine in a hypothalamic slice preparation excites AVP secretory neurons in the supraoptic and paraventricular nuclei. The excitatory response is mediated via an α_1-receptor because the response can be blocked by prazosin. Following prazosin, norepinephrine inhibited rather than excited AVP neurons (107). These data suggest that norepinephrine has a dual action on AVP secretory neurons. Similarly, norepinephrine produces both excitation and inhibition of the firing of SPN (see below). The differences between the effects of iontophoretically applied norepinephrine *in vivo* and superfused norepinephrine *in vitro* may be explained if the different techniques expose different populations of receptors to norepinephrine. The story is further complicated by the fact that norepinephrine neurons innervate both AVP-positive and closely adjacent AVP-negative neurons (108). Electrical stimulation of the A1 area inhibits non-AVP neurons in the PVN via a β-receptor (102). Thus, the actual role of the A1 norepinephrine neurons in regulating AVP release requires additional studies.

A5 NORADRENERGIC CELL GROUP

The major noradrenergic input to the SPN in the intermediolateral cell column of the spinal cord arises from the A5 cell group of the ventrolateral pons (109,110). More than 90% of the neurons in the A5 area project to the thoracic spinal cord and at least 90% of the spinally projecting neurons in the A5 area contain norepinephrine (110). The A5 noradrenergic cell group also sends projections to the central nucleus of the amygdala, perifornical area of the hypothalamus, midbrain periaqueductal gray, parabrachial nucleus, and the NTS. The A5 area receives inputs from the PVN, the Kölliker-Fuse nucleus, the parabrachial nucleus, the intermediate and caudal portion of the nucleus of the solitary tract, and the A1 area (111). Thus, virtually all areas that project to, or receive inputs from, the A5 area are involved in cardiovascular regulation.

Electrical and glutamate stimulation of the A5 area results in increases and decreases in blood pressure, respectively (112,113). Intraventricular administration of 6-OHDA abolishes the depressor response to chemical stimulation, but the pressor response to electrical stimulation remains intact (113). These data suggest that the pressor response following electrical stimulation was mediated by noncatecholamine fibers that pass through the A5 area whereas the depressor response is mediated by A5 noradrenergic neurons. The decrease in arterial blood pressure following chemical stimulation of the A5 area is associated with a decrease in cardiac output, decreases in vascular resistance in skeletal muscle, and increases in mesenteric and skin vascular resistance. The hemodynamic effects associated with glutamate stimulation of the A5 area are prevented by pretreatment with 6-OHDA (114). Loewy et al. (113) found that individual A5 catecholamine neurons project to both the intermediolateral cell column and the NTS. Microinjection of 6-OHDA into either of these areas blunted the A5 depressor response, suggesting that both areas contribute to the decrease in blood pressure following chemical stimulation of A5 norepinephrine neurons. Microinjection of 6-OHDA directly into the A5 area produces extensive destruction of norepinephrine neurons but fails to alter arterial blood pressure in conscious animals (115).

Norepinephrine Regulation of SPN Firing

These data suggest that A5 norepinephrine neurons inhibit SPN in the intermediolateral cell column of the spinal cord. However, the exact nature of the interaction between A5 noradrenergic neurons and SPN is likely obscured by the diffuse innervation of A5 neurons to nuclei involved in cardiovascular regulation. More direct information regarding the role of norepinephrine in the regulation of SPN firing comes from microiontophoretic studies. Microiontophoretic application of norepinephrine consistently inhibits the firing rate of SPN (37–39,116,117). The inhibitory effects of microiontophoretically applied norepinephrine are blocked by α_2-adrenergic antagonists (i.e., yohimbine and piperoxane) but not by the α_1-receptor antagonist prazosin or by β-receptor antagonists (37,39). This indicates that the inhibitory effects of norepinephrine are mediated by α_2-adrenergic receptors. Consistent with this view are the observations that (a) microiontophoretic application of the α_2-agonist clonidine inhibits the firing rate of SPN, whereas the α_1-agonist phenylephrine has no effect (37) and (b) α_2-adrenergic receptors are highly concentrated over clusters of SPN in the intermediolateral cell column (40).

Although the above data suggest that noradrenergic neurons inhibit the firing of SPN, there is a substantial body of evidence suggesting the opposite. Administration of α_1-adrenergic receptor antagonists (i.e., prazosin, WB-4101, or ketanserin) inhibit spontaneous sympathetic nerve discharge via an action in the spinal cord (118–120). Because α_1-receptors are thought to

mediate excitatory effects of norepinephrine in the central nervous system (121), these data indirectly support a sympathoexcitatory role of norepinephrine in the spinal cord. Administration of the catecholamine precursor L-dopa increases excitability in spinal sympathetic pathways (122). More direct evidence for an excitatory function of norepinephrine at the level of SPN comes from work done in spinal cord slice preparations. Superfusion of a spinal slice with norepinephrine causes a membrane depolarization in antidromically identified SPN and results in repetitive cell discharges (78,123–125). Pretreating the slices with α_1-receptor antagonists, but not α_2- or β-receptor antagonists, prevent the depolarizing effect of norepinephrine (78).

Thus, data exist to support either an excitatory or an inhibitory role of norepinephrine in regulating SPN discharge. This controversy may be resolved by recent studies in which the spinal slice preparation was employed. Nishi et al. (78,126) found that SPN in a slice preparation exhibit a fast EPSP (or rarely a fast inhibitory postsynaptic potential [IPSP]) in response to single focal stimulation. Trains of repetitive stimuli produced a slow EPSP that was occasionally accompanied by a slow IPSP. The slow EPSP was always associated with an increased input resistance, disappeared at levels of anodal hyperpolarization exceeding −80 mV, and was specifically blocked by the α_1-receptor antagonist prazosin. Norepinephrine superfusion produced a depolarization that shared the same characteristics of the slow EPSP. The slow IPSP was not normally observed until the slow EPSP was eliminated by prazosin. Following the use of prazosin, norepinephrine produced a hyperpolarization. Both the slow IPSP and the norepinephrine-induced hyperpolarization were accompanied by a decreased input resistance, reversed at −90 mV, and abolished by the α_2-adrenergic receptor antagonist yohimbine. These data support the hypothesis that noradrenergic neurons can both excite and inhibit SPN. The inhibitory interaction is mediated by

α_2-receptors located on or near the soma; the excitatory interaction occurs through α_1-receptors located on distal dendrites. Because the recording electrode of large, multibarreled pipettes used in microiontophoretic experiments must be near the soma in order to record action potentials, iontophoresis of norepinephrine appears to have only an inhibitory effect. In contrast, norepinephrine reaches the excitatory receptors located on dendritic trees in a superfused slice preparation. Although the above hypothesis is attractive and fits well with present data, it will be difficult to prove. Alternatively, the effects of noradrenergic neurons are mediated via one subtype of α-receptor, whereas epinephrine-containing neurons selectively interact with the other subclass of α-receptor. In this case, microiontophoretic application of a catecholamine might not give an accurate idea of the physiological function of the neurotransmitter. In either case, the fact that lesions of the A5 area fail to alter arterial blood pressure (115) indicates that this area is not essential in maintaining tonic sympathetic nerve activity and likely functions as a modulatory system (see below).

MEDULLARY RAPHE NUCLEI

Midline medullary raphe nuclei are often referred to as the medullary "depressor area" because numerous studies have shown that electrical stimulation of this area typically produces a marked decrease in blood pressure and sympathetic nerve discharge (127, 128). Microinjection of L-glutamate at sites that elicit a depressor response following electrical stimulation results in a decrease in arterial blood pressure and inhibition of spontaneous sympathetic activity (34). Electrolytic lesion of the midline from the obex to the level of the genu of the facial nerve results in an increase in sympathetic nerve discharge (129). These data indicate that neurons in the medullary raphe nuclei

provide a tonic inhibition of sympathetic nerve activity. In support of this conclusion, electrophysiological studies have identified a group of midline raphe neurons whose tonic discharges are temporally related to sympathetic activity and are increased during baroreceptor reflex activation (130–132), suggesting that they subserve a sympathoinhibitory function. These neurons have been shown to project to the intermediolateral cell column (131,132). Recent studies indicate that the midline medulla is not simply a sympathoinhibitory area, but rather is heterogeneous with respect to autonomic function (see [3,133, 134] for review). Electrical stimulation of the midline medulla results in increases as well as decreases in arterial blood pressure and sympathetic nerve activity (135, 136). The pressor effect of electrical stimulation is mimicked by microinjection of L-glutamate, indicating that neuronal cell bodies rather than fibers of passage mediate the sympathoexcitatory response (133,134). Electrophysiological studies have identified sympathoexcitatory neurons in the midline medulla (i.e., exhibit discharges that are temporally related to sympathetic activity and are inhibited during baroreceptor activation [130–132]). These neurons project to the spinal cord but have not been shown to terminate in the intermediolateral cell column (131).

GABA Mediation of Midline Depressor Response

Available evidence indicates that GABA mediates the depressor response elicited by stimulation of the midline medulla. For example, picrotoxin, an agent that blocks the Cl^- channel associated with GABA-receptor activation, abolishes the decrease in arterial blood pressure and sympathetic nerve activity observed following midline stimulation (127). Similar effects were seen with bicuculline, a direct GABA-receptor antagonist. The blockade of the sympathoinhibitory effect of midline stimulation was not a result of blood pressure changes produced by the antagonists and was specific for inhibition elicited from the midline because other sympathoinhibitory processes were unaffected. These data suggest that the midline medullary depressor response is mediated via a GABAergic inhibition of central sympathetic neurons. This hypothesis is supported by the observation that the benzodiazepine diazepam potentiated the sympathoinhibitory response to midline stimulation (127). In this regard, diazepam potentiates the effects of GABA in the central nervous system.

A recent study suggests that the sympathoinhibition elicited by stimulation of midline medullary depressor sites results from a GABA-mediated inhibition of medullospinal sympathoexcitatory neurons located in the rostral ventrolateral medulla (34). Electrical stimulation of midline depressor sites inhibited the firing of electrophysiologically identified medullospinal sympathoexcitatory neurons in the rostral ventrolateral medulla. Microiontophoresis of bicuculline blocked the inhibition elicited from the midline and increased the firing rate of sympathoexcitatory neurons. In contrast, microiontophoresis of glutamate increased the firing rate of sympathoexcitatory neurons but failed to affect the midline-evoked inhibition of neuronal firing. Stimulation of midline depressor sites excited a second group of spontaneously active neurons in the rostral ventrolateral medulla, which were often located in the same recording field as the sympathoexcitatory neurons. These neurons were excited by midline stimulation with an onset latency of 21 msec, whereas sympathoexcitatory neurons were inhibited with an onset of 23 msec. These data suggest that neuronal elements in medullary raphe nuclei inhibit sympathoexcitatory medullospinal neurons in the rostral ventrolateral medulla by activating closely adjacent GABAergic interneurons. This interpretation fits with recent anatomical studies that indicate that the re-

gion of the rostral ventrolateral medulla containing sympathoexcitatory neurons has a high concentration of GABAergic cell bodies (137). Furthermore, this inhibition is tonically active and of nonbaroreceptor origin. This is indicated by the observations that (a) midline lesions increase sympathetic activity but have no effect on baroreceptor reflexes (129), (b) the putative GABA interneurons fire spontaneously and are not affected by baroreceptor activation (34), and (c) microiontophoretically applied bicuculline increases the discharge rate of sympathoexcitatory neurons (34). A possible role of GABA in mediating baroreceptor inhibition in the ventrolateral medulla is discussed below.

5-HT Mediation of Midline Pressor Response

The midline area of the lower brain stem contains the B1, B2, and B3 5-HT cell groups, which have been demonstrated to project to the intermediolateral cell column of the spinal cord (73,138). Indeed, the intermediolateral cell column contains high concentrations of 5-HT and a recent study combining receptor autoradiography combined with retrograde labeling of SPN indicates that 5-HT receptors are highly concentrated over SPN (139). The area of the midline medulla that contains 5-HT neurons projecting to the intermediolateral cell column corresponds to the medullary depressor region (127,128,140). The close association between 5-HT descending neurons and midline sites that elicit vasodepressor responses when stimulated has led to the conclusion that the descending 5-HT pathway inhibits SPN (141,142). The finding that stimulation of presumed 5-HT-containing axons in the dorsolateral funiculus of the spinal cord inhibits sympathetic activity supports this hypothesis (143). In addition, administration of 5-HT precursors produces a dose-dependent depression of spinal sympathetic reflexes

(122). Finally, a large body of pharmacological evidence involving administration of 5-HT, 5-HT precursors, or 5-HT synthesis inhibitors suggests that 5-HT neurons inhibit sympathetic activity. These data have been summarized in an excellent review (144). The above data are all indirect assessments of the role of 5-HT in regulating the firing of SPN and may in fact be misleading. For example, the depressor response elicited by stimulation of the midline medulla is mediated by GABA rather than by 5-HT (see above). In addition, the 5-HT precursor tryptophan has been used in many studies to suggest that 5-HT neurons function to inhibit sympathetic activity and lower blood pressure (144). Recently, however, it has been demonstrated that the hypotensive effect of tryptophan is mediated via nonserotonergic mechanisms (145).

Microiontophoretic application of 5-HT excites SPN (77,116,117). The excitatory effect of 5-HT on SPN is blocked by microiontophoretic application of the 5-HT antagonists methysergide and metergoline (77). More important, iontophoretic 5-HT antagonists decrease the spontaneous discharge rate of SPN in intact but not in spinal transected animals (77). Similarly, intravenous administration of methysergide and metergoline inhibits spontaneous sympathetic activity in intact animals but not in animals depleted of 5-HT (146). These observations indicate that medullospinal 5-HT neurons provide a tonic excitatory input to SPN. Support for a direct excitatory action of 5-HT on SPN also comes from slice studies in which superfusion of 5-HT depolarizes SPN, with an associated increase in membrane resistance (78,147). The depolarizing action of 5-HT persists in the presence of tetrodotoxin or in the absence of external Ca^{2+}, indicating that 5-HT acts directly on SPN (147).

Recent studies indicate that the pressor response elicited by stimulation of the midline medulla is mediated by medullospinal 5-HT neurons. The pressor response associated with midline stimulation is associated with an increase in sympathetic nerve activity. Intravenous or intrathecal administration of methysergide or metergoline blocks the sympathoexcitatory response elicited from midline medullary raphe nuclei. The specificity of the 5-HT antagonism is demonstrated by the fact that the antagonists fail to block the sympathoexcitatory response to electrical stimulation of pressor sites in the rostral ventrolateral medulla. Sympathoinhibitory responses elicited from the midline medulla are either unaffected or potentiated by 5-HT antagonists (136). The 5-HT uptake inhibitor chlorimipramine potentiates the sympathoexcitatory response elicited from the raphe but not from the rostral ventrolateral medulla (136). Stimulation of the B3 cell group causes an increase in blood pressure that is associated with an increase in 5-HT release in the thoracic spinal cord (148). These data indicate that medullospinal 5-HT neurons provide a tonic excitatory input to SPN (see [133,134] for reviews). The 5-HT receptor subtype that mediates the excitatory effect of 5-HT on SPN is unclear because microiontophoretic application of $5-HT_{1A}$ and $5-HT_2$ agonists fail to affect the firing rate of SPN (*unpublished observations*).

Medullospinal 5-HT neurons have recently been electrophysiologically characterized (132). Medullospinal 5-HT neurons share a number of important physiological and pharmacological characteristics with identified 5-HT neurons in the dorsal raphe nucleus (149) including: (a) an extremely regular discharge rate of approximately 1 spike/sec, (b) spike durations of greater than 2 msec, (c) axonal conduction velocities that are appropriate for transmission through unmyelinated axons, (d) inhibition of neuronal firing produced by microiontophoretic 5-HT, and (e) sensitivity to the inhibitory effect of the $5-HT_{1A}$ agonist 8-OH DPAT. Medullospinal 5-HT neurons were antidromically activated by electrical stimulation of the intermediolateral cell column. Interestingly, the discharges of medullary 5-HT neurons are not temporally related to sympathetic nerve activity and are not affected by baroreceptor reflex activation, indicating that these neurons receive little or no afferent inputs from central baroreceptor or sympathetic pathways (132). In light of the fact that these neurons provide a tonic excitatory input to SPN (see above), this observation suggests that 5-HT acts as a modulator to increase the excitability of SPN (see below). Serotonergic and GABAergic pathways involved in the midline medulla regulation of blood pressure are summarized in Fig. 5.

Substance P and TRH have been demonstrated to coexist with medullary 5-HT neurons that project to the intermediolateral cell column (150,151). In addition, substance P, TRH, and 5-HT coexist in nerve terminals that appear to make contact with SPN (152). The functional significance of colocalization of neurotransmitters within a single neuron is not known and corelease from defined nerve endings has so far not been demonstrated in the central nervous system. Nevertheless, it is worth noting that substance P is thought to excite SPN (see above). Microiontophoretically applied TRH also weakly excites SPN suggesting that this neuropeptide may function in sympathoexcitatory processes (153). Studies also suggest that medullospinal 5-HT neurons also contain enkephalin (150) and GABA (154), although termination in the intermediolateral cell column has not been demonstrated. Intrathecal administration of dynorphin decreases blood pressure, heart rate, and sympathetic activity (155). Enkephalin depresses sympathetic activity in

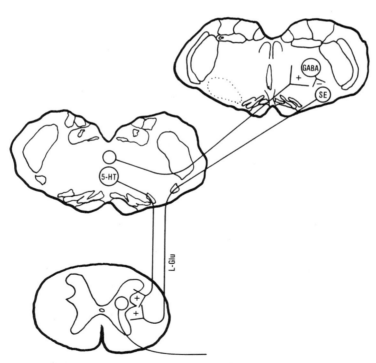

FIG. 5. Summary of the role of the midline medulla in cardiovascular regulation. 5-HT neurons project to sympathetic preganglionic neurons in the intermediolateral cell column and provide a tonic excitatory input to these neurons. Other midline neurons project to GABAergic interneurons in the rostral ventrolateral medulla. GABAergic interneurons provide a tonic nonbaroreceptor inhibition of medullospinal sympathoexcitatory neurons. L-Glu, L-glutamate; SE, sympathoexcitatory neuron.

both an intraspinal excitatory pathway and a spinal reflex pathway (156). Naloxone blocks a portion of the postexcitatory depression following SPN discharge (157). These data suggest that opioids may inhibit activity at the level of the SPN. Finally, GABA-like terminals make synaptic contacts with SPN soma and dendrites (3). GABAergic neurons likely provide a tonic inhibitory input to SPN because iontophoretic GABA inhibits SPN firing whereas iontophoretic bicuculline increases spontaneous SPN discharge (158,159).

DORSAL RAPHE NUCLEUS

Several studies suggest that 5-HT neurons in the dorsal raphe nucleus play a role in the central regulation of blood pressure. For example, electrical stimulation of the dorsal raphe nucleus elicits increases in arterial blood pressure and sympathetic nerve activity (160,161). Depletion of brain 5-HT attenuates the pressor response to raphe stimulation whereas 5-HT uptake inhibition potentiates the response (160). Furthermore, the pressor response is blocked by administration of the 5-HT antagonist metergoline (161). Microinjection of metergoline into the anterior hypothalamus/preoptic area (AH/PO) attenuates the pressor response to dorsal raphe stimulation (162). Microinjection of 5-HT into the AH/PO elicits a pressor response (162). Microinjection of the neurotoxin 5,7-DHT into the dorsal raphe blocks the effects of stimulation of the raphe and results in enhanced pressor responses to microinjections of 5-HT into the AH/PO (163). These studies suggest that 5-HT neurons in the dorsal raphe can facilitate sympathetic blood pressure possibly through an action in the AH/PO. A hypothalamic cholinergic mechanism has been implicated in the dorsal raphe pressor response (162). Additional studies suggest that 5-HT neurons in the dorsal raphe nucleus may play a facilitatory role in the regulation of vasopressin and renin secretion (164,165).

PVN

The peripheral pressor and antidiuretic actions of AVP are well-known (for review see [166]). In recent years, a number of anatomical studies have shown that in addition to the classic neurosecretory pathways to the posterior pituitary, paraventricular neurons project to nuclei in the central nervous system that are involved in central autonomic regulation. These neurons are located in the parvocellular subdivision of the PVN and send descending projections to the medulla and spinal cord (167–169). Approximately 15% of these neurons send collateral axons to both the dorsal medulla (i.e., NTS and dorsal motor nucleus of the vagus) and to the spinal cord (170). The remaining neurons appear to project solely to either the dorsal medulla or the spinal cord. Immunohistochemistry has been used to demonstrate that a portion of the descending neurons contain AVP or oxytocin and neurophysin (167,170,171). However, the majority of the fibers has not been characterized as to neurotransmitter content (172). Electrophysiological studies confirm the existence of PVN pathways to the NTS, the ventrolateral medulla, and the spinal cord (173–175). PVN neurons that send descending projections have been shown to receive baroreceptor inputs (176). Ascending inputs from brain-stem catecholamine cell groups have already been discussed. Thus, the PVN receives afferent input from medullary cardiovascular sites and exerts regulatory effects on the cardiovascular system through release of vasopressin into the peripheral circulation and through efferent signals to the medulla and to the spinal cord.

Immunohistochemical studies show that spinally projecting neurons from the PVN contain oxytocin and vasopressin and that these two putative neurotransmitters are contained in the intermediolateral cell column (168,170,177,178). An early study reports that microiontophoresis of AVP and oxytocin, as well as electrical stimulation of the PVN, inhibited the firing of SPN (179).

More recent studies fail to support these observations. Electrical stimulation of the parvocellular subdivision of the PVN elicits a pressor response that is accompanied by an increase in sympathetic activity and vasoconstriction in the mesenteric, renal, and skeletal muscle vascular beds (172,180). Backman and Henry (181) found that microiontophoretic application of AVP increased the firing of SPN. Superfusion of AVP depolarizes putative SPN in a slice preparation (182). Vasopressin₁ antagonists block the depolarizing effect of AVP, whereas a vasopressin₂ agonist has little effect. AVP-induced depolarizations are partially reduced, but never eliminated, by a low-Ca/high-Mg solution or by tetrodotoxin, which suggests that AVP excites SPN by a direct depolarization and by an indirect effect via the release of an excitatory transmitter (182). The role of AVP in mediating the pressor response to PVN stimulation has been investigated. Intrathecal administration of as little as 1 pmole of AVP elicits a pressor response that is accompanied by vasoconstriction in renal, mesenteric, and hindquarter vascular beds (172,183). The effect is due to an action of vasopressin within the spinal cord because blockade of peripheral vasopressin receptors had no effect on the response. Intrathecal administration of a vasopressin antagonist at doses that had no nonspecific depressant effects blocked the pressor response to intrathecal AVP. Interestingly, the same dose of the AVP antagonist failed to block the pressor response to stimulation of the PVN. Assuming the antagonist had access to the same group of receptors affected by neurally released AVP, these data suggest that the cardiovascular effects produced by stimulation of the PVN do not depend on the release of vasopressin from spinal cord nerve terminals (172). Support for this conclusion is found in studies performed using Brattleboro rats, which lack hypothalamic and spinal AVP (172). Stimulation of the PVN in Brattleboro rats elicits a pressor response that is identical to that observed in Long-Evans control rats

(172). Thus, although AVP appears to depolarize SPN, the role that this transmitter plays in regulating the firing of SPN remains unclear. In addition, the identity of other spinal transmitters arising in the PVN is unknown. The role of AVP in modulating baroreceptor reflexes at the level of the NTS is described below.

NTS

Stretch receptors in the major arteries and cardiac atria and ventricles detect changes in arterial pressure, central venous pressure, and left ventricular pressure, respectively. The cell bodies of these viscerosensory afferent neurons are located in the petrosal and nodose ganglia. Baroreceptor afferent fibers enter the central nervous system in the IXth and Xth cranial nerves and terminate primarily in the dorsomedial subdivision of the NTS (10). The basic function of the baroreceptor reflex in buffering against acute changes in arterial blood pressure is reviewed elsewhere (11,184). The following sections deal with (a) identification of neurotransmitters that convey sensory information to the NTS, (b) neurotransmitters in the NTS that modulate baroreceptor afferent information, and (c) neurotransmitters that mediate baroreceptor inhibition of central sympathetic neurons.

Putative Neurotransmitters in Baroreceptor Afferent Nerves

Two neurotransmitters have been considered as likely candidates for the baroreceptor afferent nerves: L-glutamic acid and substance P. Microinjection of L-glutamate into the NTS mimics baroreceptor reflex activation by eliciting a dose-dependent hypotension, bradycardia, and apnea (185). Microinjection of the glutamate antagonist glutamic acid diethylester (GDEE) into the NTS results in increases in arterial blood pressure and heart rate and blocks the baroreceptor-mediated bradycardia produced by intravenous injection of phenyl-ephrine (186). More recently, it has been shown that NTS microinjections of GDEE or a second glutamate antagonist, HA-966, but not saline block baroreceptor reflexes as judged by (a) inhibition of sympathetic activity elicited by stimulation of barore-ceptor afferent nerves, (b) the barorecep-tor-mediated locking of sympathetic slow waves to the cardiac cycle, and (c) the in-hibition of sympathetic activity associated with an intravenous pressor dose of phen-ylephrine (187). The sympathoinhibitory re-sponse to afferent stimulation was restored after NTS microinjections of GDEE by in-creasing the intensity of afferent stimula-tion or by directly stimulating the NTS. These data suggest that the impairment of baroreceptor reflexes produced by GDEE was independent of mechanical damage or local anesthetic effects (187). Microinjec-tions of a fourth glutamate antagonist, kynurenic acid, also blocks the barorecep-tor-mediated bradycardia associated with phenylephrine pressor responses (83). Bio-chemical studies indicate that the inter-mediate area of the NTS contains a high-affinity uptake system for inactivation of L-glutamate and a high concentration of this excitatory amino acid, which is consistent with this area being richly innervated by glutaminergic neurons (188). Unilateral re-moval of the nodose ganglion results in a 50% reduction in the uptake of L-glutamate bilaterally into homogenates of NTS and a reduction in the content of glutamate in the NTS (188). However, a recent study was unable to confirm these observations (189). Finally, electrical stimulation of barorecep-tor afferent nerves elicits hypotension and bradycardia, which are associated with an increase in release of L-glutamate from the NTS (190). Collectively, these data suggest that L-glutamate may be a neurotransmitter released by baroreceptor afferents in the NTS.

A large body of evidence also suggests that substance P may be released by pri-mary baroreceptor afferents in the NTS.

The area of the NTS that is innervated by primary baroreceptor afferents contains significantly more substance P than do other areas of the nucleus (191). Both the petrosal and nodose ganglia contain sub-stance P (191). Unilateral nodose ganglion-ectomy results in a decline of substance P in the ipsilateral intermediate and caudal areas of the NTS (192). Furthermore, dis-crete varicose nerve fibers containing sub-stance P have been identified in the periph-eral regions known to contain baro- and chemoreceptor afferent nerves (i.e., the tunica adventitia of the aortic arch, the ca-rotid sinus region, and among the glomus cells of the carotid body) as well as in nerve fascicles and trunks in proximity to the aortic arch and the carotid sinus nerve (192,193). Substance P is released in a calcium-dependent manner from NTS tis-sue slices *in vitro* during potassium depo-larization and in the presence of capsaicin (194). The latter observation is significant because capsaicin has been demonstrated to evoke the release of substance P from re-gions receiving sensory afferents but not from other nonsensory regions of the cen-tral nervous system (195). Microinjection of substance P into the NTS has been reported to mimic baroreceptor reflex activation by producing a decrease in arterial blood pres-sure, heart rate, and sympathetic nerve ac-tivity (196). However, other studies have not been able to confirm these observations (197). A recent study showing that small microinjected doses of substance P (0.1– 10 ng) resulted in hypotension, bradycar-dia, and apnea but higher doses (100 ng) had no effect may help to explain these dis-crepant studies (198). Microiontophoretic application of substance P results in an in-crease in firing of NTS neurons (199). Fi-nally, microinjection of capsaicin (which is presumed to cause the release of substance P from nerve terminals) into the NTS pro-duces a cardiovascular response that is identical to baroreceptor reflex activation (196). Thus, data exist to support the hy-pothesis that both L-glutamic acid and substance P are contained within primary baro-receptor afferents that terminate in the NTS.

Putative Neurotransmitters in NTS Modulating Baroreflexes

The NTS is richly innervated by mono-amine-, amino acid-, and peptidergic-con-taining neurons. A large body of work has attempted to identify putative neurotrans-mitters that modulate baroreceptor reflexes within the NTS. Typically, these studies employ the technique of microinjection of agonists and sometimes antagonists into the NTS. Many inconsistencies regarding transmitter effects have been observed due most likely to differences in injection sites within the NTS and to differences in doses and volumes employed. Although most studies have identified pharmacological ef-fects in the NTS, few have attempted to de-fine the physiological relevance of neuro-transmitters contained within the NTS. The following is a very brief review of this lit-erature.

The NTS is heavily innervated by cate-cholamine-containing neurons. Microinjec-tion of either norepinephrine or epinephrine into the NTS consistently produces a de-crease in arterial blood pressure and heart rate (142). Microiontophoretic application of norepinephrine or epinephrine inhibits the firing of NTS neurons regardless of the response of these neurons to barorecep-tor reflex activation (i.e., 40% inhibited, 15% excited during baroreceptor activa-tion) (200). The firing of NTS neurons are also inhibited by microiontophoretic appli-cation of the α_1-receptor agonist methox-amine and the α_2-receptor agonist cloni-dine. Furthermore, the inhibitory effects on iontophoretic catecholamines are reduced by both α_1- and α_2-receptor antagonists (200,201). These data suggest that the inhib-itory effect of catecholamines in the NTS is mediated by both α_1- and α_2-receptors. De-struction of the catecholamine innervation

of the NTS by microinjection of 6-OHDA results in a permanent liability of arterial blood pressure, despite preservation of re-flex bradycardia (202). These data suggest that catecholamines modulate baroreceptor reflexes.

The NTS is heavily innervated by 5-HT-containing neurons. However, microin-jection of 5-HT into the NTS produces variable effects, resulting in both pres-sor (203,204) and depressor (205,206) re-sponses. Both the pressor and depressor ef-fects of microinjected 5-HT can be blocked by the 5-HT antagonist metergoline (203, 205,206). In addition, the magnitude of the 5-HT-induced pressor response is poten-tiated by microinjection of the 5-HT uptake inhibitor fluoxetine (203). The hypotension and bradycardia produced by 5-HT are blocked by NTS microinjection of the 5-HT_2-receptor antagonist ketanserin. Mi-croinjections of 5-HT_1 agonists such as 8-OH DPAT and RU-24969 have no cardio-vascular effects (206). Bilateral NTS mi-croinjections of ketanserin produce an increase in the level and the variability of arterial blood pressure but do not block the baroreceptor reflex arc (206). Similarly, metergoline does not affect baroreceptor reflexes (205). These data suggest that al-though serotonergic mechanisms in the NTS may be involved in the modulation of cardiovascular activity, serotonin is not in-tegral to the baroreceptor reflex arc. Fur-thermore, the variability in the response to microinjections suggests that 5-HT may have multiple actions in the NTS.

Acetylcholine is also found in the NTS. Microinjections of acetylcholine into the NTS elicit a baroreceptor reflex-like re-sponse that includes a decrease in arterial blood pressure and a bradycardia. How-ever, microinjections of cholinergic antag-onists into the NTS fail to block the baro-receptor reflex, suggesting that cholinergic processes are not an integral part of baro-receptor pathways in the NTS (188).

Recent studies indicate that NTS neu-rons involved in cardiovascular regulation are tonically inhibited by GABA. Microinjection of GABA or the GABA agonist muscimol into the NTS elicits an increase in arterial blood pressure (207,208). The increase in arterial blood pressure results from an increase in sympathetic nerve activity and an elevation of plasma AVP levels (207). Similar results are observed following microinjection of the GABA uptake inhibitor nipecotic acid into the NTS (207, 208). In contrast, microinjection of the GABA antagonist bicuculline results in a decrease in arterial blood pressure (207, 208). Finally, microinjections of muscimol or nipecotic acid into the NTS reduce the depressor response to aortic nerve stimulation (209). These data are consistent with the hypothesis that NTS neurons involved in baroreceptor pathways are under tonic GABAergic inhibition.

The NTS contains a large number of neuropeptides that may act to modulate baroreceptor afferent processing. Microinjections of AVP into the NTS consistently increase arterial blood pressure via an increase in spontaneous sympathetic nerve discharge (210,211). Pretreatment with microinjected AVP antagonists blocks the pressor effect of AVP (210). In addition, microinjection of an AVP antagonist into the NTS reduces the increase in arterial blood pressure elicited by electrical stimulation of the PVN (212). Microinjection of AVP antagonists alone has no cardiovascular effects (211), suggesting that the AVP innervation of the NTS is not tonically active. Microinjection of Ang into the NTS has been reported to produce both pressor and depressor effects (213–215). The action of Ang may be a function of the microinjected dose because at least two investigators now report that low doses of microinjected Ang produce depressor responses, whereas higher doses elicit pressor responses (214, 215). Microinjection of the Ang antagonist saralasin has been reported to produce a small increase in arterial blood pressure (215) but also has been shown to enhance baroreceptor reflexes (216). Thus, the role of Ang in the NTS remains unclear. The effects of blood-borne AVP and Ang on central baroreceptor and sympathetic pathways are discussed below.

Microinjection of met- or leu-enkephalin into the NTS produces an increase in blood pressure and heart rate. The opioid antagonist naloxone blocked these actions (217). Microinjection of β-endorphin into the NTS has been reported to produce a depressor response (218). Finally, microinjection of either TRH or somatostatin into the NTS results in a decrease in arterial blood pressure and a bradycardia (204,219).

Neurotransmitters Mediating Baroreceptor Inhibition of Sympathetic Neurons

The importance of the ventrolateral medulla in the regulation of the cardiovascular system has already been described. A large body of evidence indicates that this area is critical in mediating the baroreceptor inhibition of sympathetic nerve discharge. The ventrolateral medulla is heavily innervated by neurons arising in the NTS (19,86). The NTS areas projecting to the ventrolateral medulla correspond to the zones in which baroreceptor afferents contained within the IXth and Xth cranial nerves terminate (10,19). Indeed, electrophysiological studies indicate that medullospinal sympathoexcitatory neurons in the rostral ventrolateral medulla receive a baroreceptor input (29–34). Electrolytic or kainic-acid lesions of the rostral ventrolateral medulla in animals previously receiving a contralateral NTS lesion abolished reflex responses to carotid stretch or vagal stimulation (24). These data suggest that the integrity of the rostral ventrolateral medulla is required to maintain baroreceptor reflexes.

Evidence also suggests that the caudal ventrolateral medulla is necessary to maintain baroreceptor reflexes. Microinjection of the GABA agonist muscimol into the caudal ventrolateral medulla hyperpolarizes the area (i.e., silences neurons without interfering with axonal conduction), increases arterial blood pressure, and blocks baroreceptor reflexes (82). Similarly, microinjection of the glutamate antagonist kynurenic acid into the caudal ventrolateral medulla blocks baroreceptor reflexes (83). These data are compatible with the hypothesis that second-order baroreceptor neurons arising in the NTS project to the caudal ventrolateral medulla where they utilize a glutamate-like transmitter to excite inhibitory neurons that project to the rostral ventrolateral medulla.

Current evidence suggests that the inhibitory interneurons in the caudal ventrolateral medulla, which are excited by NTS inputs, utilize GABA to mediate baroreceptor-induced inhibition of sympathoexcitatory neurons in the rostral ventrolateral medulla. Microinjection of the GABA antagonist bicuculline into the rostral ventrolateral medulla increases arterial blood pressure and produces a 48% reduction in the baroreceptor-mediated depressor response to aortic depressor nerve stimulation (220). Bicuculline applied to the ventral surface of the medulla oblongata in the area of rostral medulla reduces the inhibition of renal sympathetic nerve activity produced by baroreceptor reflex activation (221). However, neither of these studies controlled for the large increase in sympathetic activity produced by bicuculline. Thus, it is possible that the reduction in baroreceptor inhibition is a simple consequence of the dramatic increase in sympathetic activity that might lead to a decrease in the ability to inhibit sympathetic neurons. Recently, however, Sun and Guyenet (35) found that microiontophoresis of bicuculline blocked the baroreceptor-induced inhibition of medullospinal sympathoexcitatory neurons in the rostral ventrolateral medulla. Microiontophoretically applied glutamate produced an increase in neuronal firing comparable with that observed with bicuculline but did not significantly alter the baroreceptor-mediated inhibition of these sympathoexcitatory neurons. These data suggest that

GABA mediates the baroreceptor inhibition of rostral ventrolateral sympathoexcitatory neurons. Whether the GABA cell bodies are located in the caudal ventrolateral medulla or are contained within the rostral ventrolateral medulla remains to be determined. In contrast to the above studies, we found that GABA antagonists given intravenously or microinjected into the rostral ventrolateral medulla failed to block the baroreceptor-mediated inhibition of inferior cardiac sympathetic nerve discharge (33), as well as the baroreceptor-mediated temporal locking of sympathetic slow waves to the cardiac cycle (222). Intravenous picrotoxin also failed to block the baroreceptor-mediated inhibition of medullospinal sympathoexcitatory neurons recorded in the rostral ventrolateral medulla but did antagonize the GABA-mediated inhibition of sympathoexcitatory neurons produced by stimulation of the midline medulla and the inhibitory effect of microiontophoretically applied GABA (33). The discrepancy between this and previous studies has not been resolved. An interesting ancillary observation made in this study was that midcollicular transection of the brain stem did not alter sympathetic activity but prevented the increase in sympathetic activity produced by intravenous picrotoxin. These data suggest that forebrain GABAergic neurons tonically inhibit excitatory pathways projecting to sympathetic neurons in the brain stem (33).

Activation of cardiopulmonary receptors by electrical stimulation of the afferent vagus nerve results in an inhibition of sympathetic nerve discharge. Intravenous administration of picrotoxin blocks vagally induced inhibition of sympathetic activity, suggesting that the inhibition is mediated by GABA (222). More recently, it was demonstrated that the sympathoinhibitory effect of vagal afferent stimulation resulted from inhibition of rostral ventrolateral medullary sympathoexcitatory neurons (223). Furthermore, microiontophoresis of bicuculline blocks the vagally induced inhibi-

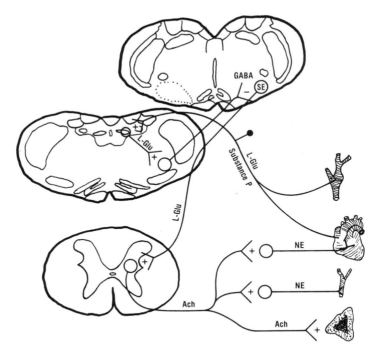

FIG. 6. Model of the neural circuitry involved in the baroreceptor reflex. Baroreceptor afferents arising in the aortic arch and carotid sinus terminate in the NTS. Evidence suggests that L-glutamate (L-Glu) and/or substance P acts as the transmitter in these afferent pathways. A proposed glutaminergic pathway arising in the NTS activates interneurons in the caudal ventrolateral medulla that project to the rostral ventrolateral medulla. This pathway activates GABAergic interneurons, which inhibit glutaminergic medullospinal sympathoexcitatory neurons. The exact location of the GABA interneuron is unknown. The transmitter description is made tentatively and awaits confirmation by further studies. NE, norepinephrine; SE, sympathoexcitatory neuron; Ach, acetylcholine.

tion of these neurons (223). These data indicate that stimulation of cardiopulmonary afferents results in a GABA-mediated inhibition of sympathoexcitatory neurons in the rostral ventrolateral medulla. Putative neurotransmitters contained within medullary baroreceptor reflex pathways are summarized in Fig. 6.

Neurosecretory neurons in the supraoptic and paraventricular nuclei are inhibited during baroreceptor reflex activation. Studies suggest that GABA mediates this inhibition. For example, the baroreceptor-mediated inhibition of firing of AVP-containing neurons in the supraoptic nucleus observed during increases in arterial blood pressure are prevented by microiontophoresis of bicuculline (224). Similarly, mi-

croiontophoresis of bicuculline blocks the baroreceptor-induced inhibition of AVP secretory neurons in the PVN (225). The data suggest that the baroreceptor inhibition of AVP-containing secretory neurons is mediated by GABA.

NEUROHUMORAL CONTROL

Hormones circulating in the blood can influence the activity of central nervous system pathways involved in cardiovascular regulation via an action on blood-brain-barrier deficient circumventricular organs. The role of blood-borne Ang in influencing central autonomic regulation has recently been reviewed (226) and is described only briefly here. Infusion of Ang into the vertebral artery produces a rapid rise in arterial blood pressure. Venous infusion of the same dose of Ang has no effect. The pressor effect of intravenous Ang is blunted by lesion of the AP (i.e., medullary circumventricular organ). Chronic infusions of Ang produce an elevation in arterial blood pressure that is reduced in AP-lesioned animals. Furthermore, AP lesions blunt the development of two-kidney, one clip renal hypertension as well as the increase in arterial blood pressure seen following acute unilateral renal artery stenosis (226,227). Finally, both the OVLT and the SFO have been shown to play a critical role in body fluid homeostasis by integrating information derived from blood-borne Ang with input arising from vascular pressure and volume receptors (228). Thus, Ang gains access to the central nervous system via circumventricular organs where it plays a role in cardiovascular regulation.

Circulating AVP has also been shown to influence cardiovascular regulation by acting within the central nervous system to modify the reflex control of sympathetic nerve discharge (see [229] for review). For example, intravertebral infusion of AVP causes a greater baroreceptor-mediated reduction in heart rate than equivalent doses administered intravenously. In addition, the augmentation of the AVP pressor response following baroreceptor denervation far exceeds that observed with intravenously infused phenylephrine. These data indicate that circulating AVP acts to sensitize baroreceptor reflexes. More recently, studies indicate that at equal intravenous pressor doses, AVP produces a much greater reflex inhibition of renal sympathetic nerve activity than does phenylephrine. The enhanced sympathoinhibitory effect of AVP is not observed in AP-lesioned animals (229). The effects of AVP in the AP appear to be mediated by the V1 AVP receptor (230). Osmotically stimulated AVP also augments baroreceptor-mediated inhibition through an action in the AP (230). Thus, circulating AVP enters the brain via the AP and functions to potentiate baroreceptor-mediated inhibition of sympathetic nerve activity.

CENTRALLY ACTING ANTIHYPERTENSIVE AGENTS

α-Receptor Agonists and Antagonists

The therapeutically useful agents clonidine and α-methyl dopa act in the central nervous system to inhibit spontaneous sympathetic nerve discharge and therefore lower arterial blood pressure (see [231] for review). At the molecular level there is consensus that clonidine acts by virtue of its α_2-adrenergic receptor agonist properties. α-Methyl dopa is metabolized to form α-methyl norepinephrine or α-methyl epinephrine within noradrenergic or adrenergic synaptic terminals, respectively. Like clonidine, the affinity of these false transmitters for α_2-receptors is greater than that of norepinephrine or epinephrine. Thus, potential sites of action of these compounds include any neuron involved in cardiovascular regulation that contains α_2-receptors.

Clonidine is thought to act in the brain stem or spinal cord because midcollicular transection does not affect the drug's hypotensive and sympatholytic actions (231). One possible site of action is at the level of catecholamine neurons. It is thought that α_2-receptors located on the somatodendritic portion of central catecholamine neurons mediate a catecholamine inhibition of neuronal firing (121). Clonidine has been shown to inhibit the firing rate of catecholamine neurons located in the locus coeruleus, A5, A2, and C2 cell groups (1,121). Thus, the consequence of clonidine activation of α_2-receptors on catecholamine neurons is a widespread reduction in catecholamine release in the central nervous system. The net effect of decreased catecholamine release depends on the overall effects of catecholamines on central cardiovascular neurons. Massive depletion of brain catecholamines does not markedly affect the central antihypertensive properties of clonidine. This indicates that an action of clonidine to inhibit central catecholamine neurons is not sufficient to explain the drug's action. Furthermore, the observation suggests that catecholamine neurons both excite and inhibit central sympathetic neurons (see below).

The fact that clonidine is effective in catecholamine-depleted animals suggests that the drug acts on postsynaptic α_2-receptors to produce its sympatholytic effects (232). Studies indicate that the rostral ventrolateral medulla and SPN located in the intermediolateral cell column of the spinal cord are likely sites of action of clonidine. Microinjection of clonidine into the rostral ventrolateral medulla produces a marked hypotensive response that is associated with an inhibition of spontaneous sympathetic nerve discharge (233–235). Granata et al. (234) suggested that the active site of clonidine in the rostral ventrolateral medulla was in the immediate vicinity of the C1 epinephrine cell group. Indeed, microiontophoresis of clonidine inhibits the firing of presumed epinephrine neurons in the rostral ventrolateral medulla (43). However, because epinephrine neurons may inhibit rather than excite SPN (see above), this observation does not necessarily account for the hypotensive activity of clonidine. In a recent study, Gatti et al. (235) found that microinjection of small amounts of clonidine into the nucleus reticularis lateralis of the ventrolateral medulla but not into the nucleus reticularis rostroventrolateralis (i.e., the C1 area) produced a marked hypotension. Microinjection of the α_2-receptor antagonist idazoxan into the nucleus reticularis lateralis reduced the hypotensive effects of systemically administered clonidine by 65% (235). These data suggest that a site in the nucleus reticularis lateralis is responsible for a large portion of the hypotensive action of clonidine. Evidence also supports a spinal site of action of clonidine. For example, clonidine has been shown to

reduce activity in spinal sympathetic pathways (236). In addition, microiontophoresis of clonidine inhibits the firing of SPN via an α_2-adrenergic receptor (37).

The effects of adrenergic agents on sympathetic activity has shed light on the role of catecholamine neurons in the central regulation of blood pressure. In addition to the sympatholytic actions of α_2-receptor agonists, studies have demonstrated that α_1-receptor antagonists inhibit sympathetic activity (118–120), whereas α_2-receptor antagonists increase sympathetic discharge (237). The sympatholytic properties of selective α_1-receptor antagonists explain why these agents fail to produce an expected tachycardia (119). The fact that α_1-receptor antagonists reduce sympathetic activity suggests that noradrenergic neurons excite sympathetic neurons in the central nervous system because it appears that α_1-receptors mediate the excitatory effects of norepinephrine (121). Thus, a portion of clonidine's action may be explained by inhibiting the firing of norepinephrine neurons that normally act to facilitate central sympathetic neurons (possibly at the level of SPN [3,41]). In this regard, clonidine reduces sympathetic activity in catecholamine-depleted animals; however, the dose required for inhibition is at least three times greater than in control animals (232). The α_2-adrenergic antagonists (e.g., piperoxane, yohimbine, and rauwolscine) likely increase sympathetic activity by acting postsynaptically to block the direct inhibitory effects of catecholamines and by acting at α_2-receptors on noradrenergic soma to produce an increase in firing of these cells (237). Figure 7 summarizes possible sites at which adrenergic agents affect sympathetic activity.

5-HT$_{1A}$ Agonists

Medullary 5-HT neurons provide a tonic excitatory input to SPN (see above). Thus, agents that antagonize the effects of 5-HT might be expected to act at the level of the

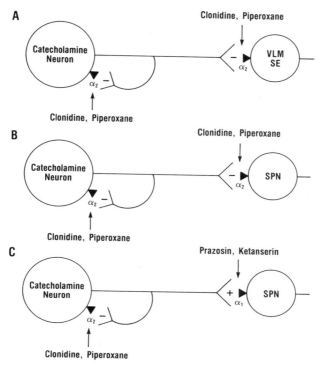

FIG. 7. Three possible mechanisms to explain sympathetic effects of adrenergic receptor agonists and antagonists. Clonidine inhibits sympathetic activity by acting postsynaptically in the ventrolateral medulla (VLM) or on SPN (**A** and **B**). Clonidine may also inhibit sympathetic activity by acting at autoreceptors to inhibit catecholamine neurons which normally excite SPN (**C**). Prazosin and ketanserin act postsynaptically to block the excitatory effect of catecholamines (C). SE, sympathoexcitatory neuron.

SPN to inhibit sympathetic nerve discharge. In the cat, the 5-HT antagonists methysergide and metergoline inhibit spontaneous nerve activity recorded either from SPN (77) or a peripheral sympathetic nerve (146). However, these agents fail to lower arterial blood pressure in rodents or humans perhaps because of their partial agonist properties (3). Recent studies indicate that the 5-HT$_{1A}$ agonist 8-OH DPAT acts in the central nervous system to inhibit spontaneous sympathetic activity and therefore lower arterial blood pressure (238–240). The sympatholytic effects of 8-OH DPAT are likely mediated by a 5-HT$_{1A}$ receptor because (a) other structurally dissimilar 5-HT$_{1A}$ agonists produce similar effects (238, 240) and (b) administration of the 5-HT$_{1A}$ antagonist spiperone prevents or reverses the sympatholytic effects of 8-OH DPAT (238). In an early clinical trial, the 5-HT$_{1A}$ agonist flesinoxan has been shown to lower arterial blood pressure in hypertensive patients, suggesting a therapeutic usefulness for these compounds in the treatment of hypertension (Wouters, *personal communication*).

The mechanism of the sympatholytic action of 8-OH DPAT has begun to be explored. Like catecholaminergic neurons, the soma and dendrites of serotonergic neurons contain 5-HT receptors that mediate a feedback 5-HT inhibition of the firing of 5-HT neurons (i.e., autoreceptor inhibition [149]). Recent studies indicate that the 5-HT "autoreceptor" may be identical to the 5-HT$_{1A}$ receptor in the dorsal raphe nucleus (241) and in medullary raphe nuclei (242).

Microiontophoresis of 8-OH DPAT has been shown to inhibit the firing of electrophysiologically identified 5-HT neurons in the dorsal raphe (245) and in raphe pallidus and obscurus (132). In the latter study these 5-HT neurons were demonstrated to project to the intermediolateral cell column of the spinal cord (132). This observation led to the hypothesis that 8-OH DPAT produces its central sympatholytic effects by inhibiting the firing of medullospinal sympathoexcitatory neurons and thereby disfacilitating sympathetic nerve discharge (132,238). In support of this hypothesis, midcollicular transection does not affect the inhibition of sympathetic activity observed following administration of 8-OH DPAT (*unpublished observations*). However, recent work supports a postsynaptic action of 8-OH DPAT. Large electrolytic lesions encompassing the midline area of the lower brain stem from the level of the obex through the level of the facial nucleus fails to alter the sympatholytic effect of 8-OH DPAT. Because this lesion destroyed the great majority of 5-HT cell bodies that project to the spinal cord, these

data suggest that 8-OH DPAT must act at a postsynaptic site to inhibit sympathetic nerve discharge (243). This hypothesis was critically addressed by determining the inhibitory effects of 8-OH DPAT on activity recorded simultaneously from the inferior cardiac sympathetic nerve and from medullary 5-HT neurons that project to the intermediolateral cell column. Figure 8 illustrates that medullary 5-HT neuronal activity is more sensitive to the inhibitory effect of 8-OH DPAT than is sympathetic nerve activity. Indeed, low doses of 8-OH DPAT (1–3 μg/kg, i.v.) completely suppress the firing of medullary 5-HT neurons but have no effect on sympathetic nerve discharge. Higher doses of 8-OH DPAT (10–100 μg/kg) are required to inhibit sympathetic activity (243). Collectively, these data provide strong evidence that direct inhibition of medullospinal 5-HT neuronal firing is not sufficient to explain the central sympatholytic effects of 8-OH DPAT. A postsynaptic action of 8-OH DPAT has been demonstrated on SPN (*unpublished observations*). As previously noted, mi-

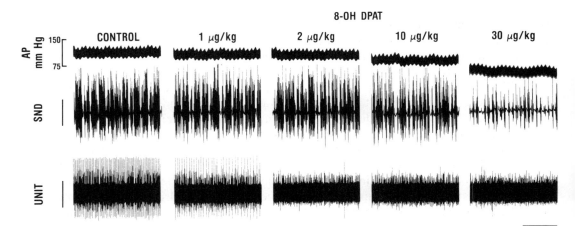

FIG. 8. Effects of 8-OH DPAT on arterial pressure (AP), sympathetic nerve discharge (SND), and medullary 5-HT neuronal firing (unit). Largest amplitude unit in recording field was determined to be a 5-HT neuron (*lower trace*). Low doses of 8-OH DPAT (1–2 μg/kg, i.v.) markedly depressed the firing of the 5-HT neuron but had little effect on blood pressure or SND. Larger doses of 8-OH DPAT (10–30 μg/kg) were required to depress AP and SND. Horizontal calibration is 1 min. Vertical calibration is 70 μV for SND and 50 μV for unit.

croiontophoresis of 5-HT excites SPN (77). Microiontophoresis of 8-OH DPAT has little effect on SPN firing but blocks the excitatory effect of iontophoretic 5-HT. Thus, at the level of the SPN, 8-OH DPAT acts as a 5-HT antagonist. In addition, microinjection of 8-OH DPAT into the ventrolateral area of the medulla produces a marked hypotensive response (244). Thus, in a manner analogous to α_2-adrenergic agonists, 5-HT_{1A} agonists inhibit the firing of 5-HT neurons, but a postsynaptic site of action appears to explain the sympatholytic effects of this class of centrally acting antihypertensive agents.

SUMMARY AND CONCLUSIONS

The past decade has seen tremendous progress in determining the nature of the neurotransmitters that regulate central nervous system pathways involved in the central regulation of blood pressure. Investigations have gone beyond the cataloging of effects observed after intraventricular administration of agents and are now pursuing the identity and functional importance of neurotransmitters contained within pathways shown to be important in cardiovascular regulation. In addition, several key components of the brain-stem networks involved in the control of sympathetic activity have been identified. For example, numerous studies indicate the importance of neurons located in the rostral ventrolateral medulla in the regulation of SPN. Indeed, this area is believed to contain medullospinal sympathoexcitatory neurons that represent the final site of integration of many brain-stem and reflex pathways involved in the regulation of sympathetic nerve activity (1). The neurotransmitter that is utilized by this medullospinal pathway remains unknown. Epinephrine, substance P, and glutamate have all been hypothesized as primary chemical mediators in the descending pathway from the brain stem to SPN (Table 1). Interestingly,

lesions of, or antagonists to, epinephrine, substance P, glutamate, and 5-HT neurons all abolish sympathetic activity and reduce blood pressure to a level similar to that in a spinal animal. Clearly, not all these transmitters are primary mediators of sympathetic information carried from the brain stem to the spinal cord. Rather, it is likely that monoamines and neuropeptides act in the intermediolateral cell column, as in other areas of the central nervous system, as neuromodulators to set the level of excitability of SPN rather than relaying sympathetic information over a functionally specific medullospinal pathway. This conclusion is supported by the observation that midline medullary 5-HT neurons provide a tonic excitatory input to SPN but receive no afferent inputs from other central sympathetic or baroreceptor pathways. However, the firing of 5-HT neurons appears to relate to the state of vigilance of the animal (246), suggesting that 5-HT neurons may lower the threshold of SPN to sympathetic inputs during states of wakefulness (i.e., act as the autonomic nervous system of the sympathetic nervous system). In addition, the time course of the norepinephrine-mediated slow EPSPs and IPSPs in SPN (41) is consistent with a gain-setting function. By analogy, epinephrine is likely to act as a neuromodulator in the intermediolateral cell column rather than to serve as the primary mediator of sympathetic information descending from the rostral ventrolateral medulla. Similarly, it is difficult to imagine that an agent with such a long duration of excitatory action as substance P (59,60) could serve as the primary descending transmitter in a system in which moment-to-moment changes in activity are essential. It seems more likely that substance P functions to set the excitability of SPN. Pharmacological antagonism of any of the excitatory neuromodulators might act to decrease, at least temporarily, the excitability of SPN to the point at which primary sympathetic activity from the brain stem could not excite SPN. This accounts for the

TABLE 1. Summary of effects of putative neurotransmitters at sites in the central nervous system involved in autonomic regulation

	NE	Epi	5-HT	Glu	GABA	Subst P	TRH	Enk	AVP	Ang	Ach
SPN	$E(\alpha_1)$ and $I(\alpha_2)$	E or I[a]	E, perhaps I	E	I	E	E	I	E		E
RVLM	$I(\alpha_2)$	I		E	I			I			
CVLM				E	I						
PVN	$E(\alpha_1)$ and I			E	I						
SON	$E(\alpha_1)$ and $I(\alpha_2)$			E	I						
NTS	E and I	E and I	E or I[a]	E	I	E	E	I	I direct, E indirect	E or I	

E, excitation; I, inhibition; RVLM, rostral ventrolateral medulla; CVLM, caudal ventrolateral medulla; SON, supraoptic nucleus; NE, norepinephrine; Epi, epinephrine; Glu, glutamate; Subst P, substance P; Enk, enkephalin; Ach, acetylcholine.
[a]Controversial.

wide variety of pharmacological agents that act to eliminate sympathetic activity and reduce arterial blood pressure.

On the basis of the above arguments, the most logical candidate for a transmitter-mediating, primary excitatory sympathetic information from the brain stem to SPN would be an excitatory amino acid (Table 1). Fast EPSPs in SPN appear to be mediated by glutamate (41), and excitatory amino-acid antagonists markedly inhibit sympathetic activity (3,76). The rapid time course of glutamate effects is consistent with a system in which activity changes from moment to moment. In more general terms, evidence is beginning to build to suggest that excitatory amino acids are important in mediating activity in sympathetic and baroreceptor pathways throughout the brain stem (Table 1). In addition, it appears that GABA provides a tonic inhibition to most if not all pathways involved in the central regulation of blood pressure (Table 1). GABA inhibition appears to be of both baroreceptor and nonbaroreceptor origin. The role of neuropeptides in regulating central sympathetic pathways is beginning to be recognized. The significance of the co-localization of peptides and monoamines is unknown. Future research will determine the overall importance of these putative transmitters in cardiovascular regulation. In addition, the nature of neurotransmitters mediating cardiovascular responses from many areas of the central nervous system has not been investigated (Table 1). These are but a few of the many unresolved issues in the field of the central regulation of blood pressure.

REFERENCES

1. Guyenet PG. Role of the ventral medulla oblongata in blood pressure regulation. In: Loewy AD, Spyer KM, eds. *Autonomic nervous system: central regulation of autonomic function.* New York: Oxford University Press (*in press*).
2. Gebber GL. Brainstem systems involved in cardiovascular regulation. In: Randall WC, ed. *Nervous control of cardiovascular function.* Oxford: Oxford University Press, 1984;346–368.
3. McCall RB. Effects of putative neurotransmitters on sympathetic preganglionic neurons. In: Berne RM, ed. *Annual reviews of physiology,* vol 50. Palo Alto: Annual Reviews Inc., 1988;553–564.
4. Loewy AD, Neil JJ. The role of descending monoaminergic systems in central control of blood pressure. *Fed Proc* 1981;40:2778–2785.
5. Luiten PGM, Ter Horst GJ, Steffens AB. The hypothalamus, intrinsic connections and outflow pathways to the endocrine system in relation to the control of feeding and metabolism. *Prog Neurobiol* 1987;28:1–54.
6. Fulwiler CE, Saper CB. Subnuclear organization of the efferent connections of the parabrachial nucleus in the rat. *Brain Res Rev* 1984;7:229–259.
7. Saper CB, Levisohn D. Afferent connections of the median preoptic nucleus in the rat: anatomical evidence for a cardiovascular integrative mechanism in the anteroventral third ventricular (AV3V) region. *Brain Res* 1983;288:21–32.
8. Andrezik JA, Chan-Palay V, Palay SL. The nucleus paragigantocellularis lateralis in the rat: demonstration of afferents by the retrograde transport of HRP. *Anat Embryol* 1981;161:373–390.
9. Saper CB. Reciprocal parabrachial-cortical connections in the rat. *Brain Res* 1982;242:33–40.
10. Schwaber JS. Neuroanatomical substrates of cardiovascular and emotional-autonomic regulation. In: Magro A, Osswald W, Reis D, Vanhoutte P, eds. *Central and peripheral mechanisms of cardiovascular regulation.* New York: Plenum Press, 1986;353–384.
11. Brody MJ. Central nervous system mechanisms of arterial pressure regulation. *Fed Proc* 1986;45:2700–2706.
12. Reis DJ, Ross C, Granata AR, Ruggiero DA. Role of C1 area of rostroventrolateral medulla in cardiovascular control. In: Buckley JP, Ferrario CM, eds. *Brain peptides and catecholamines in cardiovascular regulation.* New York: Raven Press, 1987;1–14.
13. Calaresu FR, Yardley CP. Medullary basal sympathetic tone. In: Berne RM, ed. *Annual reviews of physiology,* vol 50. Palo Alto: Annual Reviews Inc., 1988;511–524.
14. Feldberg W, Guertzenstein PG. A vasodepressor effect of pentobarbitone sodium. *J Physiol* 1972;224:83–103.
15. Guertzenstein PG, Silver A. Fall in blood pressure from discrete regions of the ventral surface of the medulla by glycine and lesions. *J Physiol* 1974;242:489–503.
16. Dampney RAL, Moon EA. Role of ventrolateral medulla in vasomotor response to cerebral ischemia. *Am J Physiol* 1980;239:H349–H358.
17. Ross CA, Ruggerio DA, Joh THE, Park DH, Reis DH. Adrenaline synthesizing neurons in the rostral ventrolateral medulla: a possible role in tonic vasomotor control. *Brain Res* 1983;273:356–361.

18. Ross CA, Ruggerio DA, Park DH, et al. Tonic vasomotor control by the rostral ventrolateral medulla: effect of electrical or chemical stimulation of the area containing C1 adrenaline neurons on arterial pressure, heart rate and plasma catecholamines and vasopressin. *J Neurosci* 1984;4:474–494.

19. Dampney RAL, Goodchild AK, Robertson LG, Montgomery W. Role of ventrolateral medulla in vasomotor regulation: a correlative anatomical and physiological study. *Brain Res* 1982; 249:223–235.

20. Gatti PJ, Norman WP, Da Silva AMT, Gillis RA. Cardiorespiratory effects produced by microinjecting L-glutamic acid into medullary nuclei associated with the ventral surface of the feline medulla. *Brain Res* 1986;381:281–288.

21. Willette RN, Barcas PP, Krieger AJ, Sapru HN. Vasopressor and depressor areas in the rat medulla: identification by microinjection of L-glutamate. *Neuropharmacology* 1983;22:1071–1079.

22. Willette RN, Punnen-Grandy S, Krieger AJ, Sapru HN. Differential regulation of regional vascular resistance by the rostral and caudal ventrolateral medulla in the rat. *J Auton Nerv Syst* 1987;18:143–151.

23. Benarroch EE, Granata AR, Ruggiero D, Park DH, Reis DJ. Neurons of the C1 area mediate cardiovascular responses initiated form the ventral medullary surface. *Am J Physiol* 1986; 250:R932–R945.

24. Granata AR, Ruggiero DA, Park DH, Joh THE, Reis DH. Brain stem area with C1 epinephrine neurons mediates baroreflex vasodepressor responses. *Am J Physiol* 1985;248:H547–H567.

25. Amendt K, Czachurski J, Dembowsky K, Seller H. Neurons within the "chemosensitive area" on the ventral surface of the brainstem which project to the intermediolateral column. *Pflugers Arch* 1978;375:289–292.

26. Loewy AD, Wallach JH, McKellar S. Efferent connections of the ventral medulla oblongata in the rat. *Brain Res Rev* 1981;3:63–80.

27. Blessing WW, Goodchild AK, Dampney RAL, Chalmers JP. Cell groups in the lower brainstem of the rabbit projecting to the spinal cord, with special reference to catecholamine-containing neurons. *Brain Res* 1981;221:35–55.

28. Ross CA, Ruggiero DA, Joh THE, Park DH, Reis DJ. Rostral ventrolateral medulla: selective projections to the thoracic autonomic cell column from the region containing C1 adrenaline neurons. *J Comp Neurol* 1984;228:168–185.

29. Barman SM, Gebber GL. Axonal projection patterns of ventrolateral medullospinal sympathoexcitatory neurons. *J Neurophysiol* 1985; 53:1551–1566.

30. Brown DL, Guyenet PG. Cardiovascular neurons of brainstem with projections to spinal cord. *Am J Physiol* 1984;247:R1009–R1016.

31. Guyenet PG, Brown DL. Nucleus paragigantocellularis lateralis and lumbar sympathetic discharge in the rat. *Am J Physiol* 1986;250: R1081–R1094.

32. McAllen RM. Identification and properties of subretrofacial bulbospinal neurones: a descending cardiovascular pathway in the cat. *J Auton Nerv Syst* 1986;17:151–164.

33. McCall RB. Lack of involvement of GABA in baroreceptor-mediated sympathoinhibition. *Am J Physiol* 1986;253:R1065–R1073.

34. McCall RB. GABA-mediated inhibition of sympathoexcitatory neurons by midline medullary stimulation. *Am J Physiol* 1988;255:R605–R615.

35. Sun MK, Guyenet PG. GABA-mediated baroreceptor inhibition of reticulospinal neurons. *Am J Physiol* 1985;249:R672–R680.

36. Tucker DC, Saper CB, Ruggiero DA, Reis DJ. Organization of central adrenergic pathways: I. Relationships of ventrolateral medullary projections to the hypothalamus and spinal cord. *J Comp Neurol* 1987;259:591–603.

37. Guyenet PG, Cabot JB. Inhibition of sympathetic preganglionic neurons by catecholamines and clonidine: mediation by an adrenergic receptor. *J Neurosci* 1981;1:908–917.

38. Guyenet PG, Stornetta RL. Inhibition of sympathetic preganglionic discharges by epinephrine and α-methylepinephrine. *Brain Res* 1982; 235:271–283.

39. Kadzielawa K. Inhibition of the activity of sympathetic preganglionic neurones and neurones activated by visceral afferents, by alpha-methylnoradrenaline and endogenous catecholamines. *Neuropharmacology* 1983;22:3–17.

40. Seybold AV, Elde RP. Receptor autoradiography in thoracic spinal cord: correlation of neurotransmitter binding sites with sympathoadrenal neurons. *J Neurosci* 1984;4:2533–2542.

41. Nishi S, Yoshimura M, Polosa C. Synaptic potentials and putative transmitter actions in sympathetic preganglionic neurons. In: Ciriello J, Calaresu FR, Renaud LP, Polosa C, eds. *Organization of the autonomic nervous system central and peripheral mechanisms.* New York: Alan R. Liss, 1987;15–26.

42. Sangdee C, Franz DN. Evidence for inhibition of sympathetic preganglionic neurons by bulbospinal epinephrine pathways. *Neurosci Lett* 1983;37:167–173.

43. Sun M-K, Guyenet PG. Effect of clonidine and GABA on the discharges of medullospinal sympathoexcitatory neurons in the rat. *Brain Res* 1986;368:1–19.

44. Jacobs BL, Gannon PJ, Azmitia EC. Atlas of serotonergic cell bodies in the cat brainstem: an immunocytochemical analysis. *Brain Res Bull* 1984;13:1–31.

45. Willenberg IM, Dermietzel R, Leibstein AG, Effenberger M. Mapping of cholinoceptive (nicotinoceptive) neurons in the lower brainstem: with special reference to the ventral surface of the medulla. *J Auton Nerv Syst* 1985;14:287–298.

46. Finley JC, Maderdrut JL, Petrusz P. The immunocytochemical localization of enkephalin in the central nervous system of the rat. *J Comp Neurol* 1981;198:541–565.

47. Finley JC, Maderdrut JL, Roger LJ, Petrusz P. The immunocytochemical localization of somatostatin-containing neurons in the rat central nervous system. *Neuroscience* 1981;6:2173–2192.

48. Ciriello J, Caverson MM, Polosa C. Function of the ventrolateral medulla in the control of the circulation. *Brain Res Rev* 1986;111:359–391.

49. Chronwall BM, DiMaggio DA, Massari VJ, et al. The anatomy of neuropeptide-Y-containing neurons in rat brain. *J Neurosci* 1985;15:1159–1181.

50. Mantyh PW, Hunt SP. Evidence for cholecystokinin-like immunoreactive neurons in the rat medulla oblongata which project to the spinal cord. *Brain Res* 1984;291:49–54.

51. Leibstein AG, Dermietzel R, Willenberg IM, Pauschert R. Mapping of different neuropeptides in the lower brainstem of the rat: with special reference to the ventral surface. *J Auton Nerv Syst* 1985;14:299–313.

52. Eskay RL, Long RT, Palkovits M. Localization of immunoreactive thyrotropin releasing hormone in the lower brainstem of the rat. *Brain Res* 1983;277:159–162.

53. Hokfelt T, Lundberg JM, Tatemoto K, et al. Neuropeptide Y (NPY) and FMRFamide neuropeptide-like immunoreactivities in catecholamine neurons of the rat medulla oblongata. *Acta Physiol Scand* 1983;117:315–318.

54. Lorenz RG, Saper CB, Wong DL, Ciaranello RD, Loewy AD. Co-localization of substance P and phenylethanolamine N-methyltransferase-like immunoreactivity in neurons of the ventrolateral medulla that project to the spinal cord: potential role in control of vasomotor tone. *Neurosci Lett* 1985;55:255–260.

55. Helke CJ, Neil JJ, Massari VJ, Loewy AD. Substance P neurons project from the ventral medulla to the intermediolateral cell column in the rat. *Brain Res* 1982;243:147–152.

56. Helke CJ, Charlton CG, Wiley RG. Studies on the cellular localization of spinal cord substance P receptors. *Neuroscience* 1986;19:523–533.

57. Johansson O, Hokfelt T, Pernow B, et al. Immunohistochemical support for three putative transmitters in one neuron: co-existence of 5-hydroxytryptamine, substance P and thyrotropin releasing hormone-like immunoreactivity in medullary neurons projecting to the spinal cord. *J Neurosci* 1981;6:1857–1881.

58. Davis BM, Krause JE, McKelry JF, Cabot JB. Effects of spinal lesions on substance P levels in the rat sympathetic preganglionic cell column: evidence for local spinal regulation. *Neuroscience* 1984;13:1311–1326.

59. Backman SB, Henry JL. Effects of substance P and thyrotropin-releasing hormone on sympathetic preganglionic neurones in the thoracic intermediolateral nucleus of the cat. *Can J Physiol Pharmacol* 1983;62:248–251.

60. Gilbey MP, McKenna KE, Schramm LP. Effects of substance P on sympathetic preganglionic neurones. *Neurosci Lett* 1983;41:157–159.

61. Helke CJ, Phillip ET, O'Neil JT. Regional peripheral and CNS hemodynamic effects of intrathecal administration of a substance P receptor agonist. *J Auton Nerv Syst* 1987;21:1–7.

62. Yusof APM, Coote JH. The action of a substance P antagonist on sympathetic nerve activity in the rat. *Neurosci Lett* 1987;75:329–333.

63. Keeler JR, Charlton CG, Helke CJ. Cardiovascular effects of spinal cord substance P: studies with a stable receptor agonist. *J Pharmacol Exp Ther* 1985;233:755–760.

64. Yashpal K, Gauthier S, Henry JL. Substance P given intrathecally at the spinal T_9 level increases arterial pressure and heart rate in the rat. *J Auton Nerv Syst* 1987;18:93–103.

65. Loewy AD, Sawyer WB. Substance P antagonists inhibit vasomotor responses elicited from ventral medulla in rat. *Brain Res* 1982;245:379–383.

66. Takano Y, Martin JE, Leeman SE, Loewy AD. Substance P immunoreactivity released from spinal cord after kainic acid excitation of the ventral medulla oblongata: a correlation with increases in blood pressure. *Brain Res* 1984;291:168–172.

67. Keeler JR, Helke CJ. Spinal cord substance P mediates bicuculline-induced activation of cardiovascular responses from the ventral medulla. *J Auton Nerv Syst* 1985;13:19–33.

68. Loewy AD. Substance P neurons of the ventral medulla: their role in the control of vasomotor tone. In: Hainsworth R, Linden RJ, McWilliam PN, Mary DASG, eds. *Cardiogenic reflexes*. Oxford: Oxford University Press, 1987;269–285.

69. Salt TE, De Vries GJ, Rodriguez RE, Cahusac PMB, Morris R, Hill RG. Evaluation of (D-Pro^2,D-Trp^{7,9})-substance P as an antagonist of substance P responses in the rat central nervous system. *Neurosci Lett* 1982;30:291–295.

70. Hokfelt T, Vincent S, Hellsten L, et al. Immunohistochemical evidence for a "neurotoxic" action of (D-Pro^2,D-Trp^{7,9}) substance P, an analogue with substance P antagonistic activity. *Acta Physiol Scand* 1981;113:571–573.

71. Post C, Karlsson J-A, Butterworth FG, Persson CGA, Strichartz GR. Local anaesthetic effects of substance P (SP) analogues in vitro. In: Jordan CC, Oehme P, eds. *Substance P: metabolism and biological activity*. London: Taylor and Francis, 1985;227–241.

72. Howe PRC, Kuhn DM, Minson JB, Stead BH, Chalmers JP. Evidence for a bulbospinal serotonergic pressor pathway in the rat brain. *Brain Res* 1983;270:29–36.

73. Loewy AD, McKellar S. Serotonergic projections form the ventral medulla to the intermediolateral cell column in the rat. *Brain Res* 1981;211:146–152.

74. Head GA, Howe PRC. Effects of 6-hydroxydopamine and the PNMT inhibitor LY134046 on pressor responses to stimulation of the subretrofacial nucleus in anaesthetized stroke-

prone spontaneously hypertensive rats. *J Auton Nerv Syst* 1987;18:213–224.

75. Minson JB, Chalmers JP, Caon AC, Renaud B. Separate areas of rat medulla oblongata with populations of serotonin- and adrenaline-containing neurons alter blood pressure after L-glutamate stimulation. *J Auton Nerv Syst* 1987;19:39–50.

76. Guyenet PG, Sun M-K, Brown DL. Role of GABA and excitatory aminoacids in medullary baroreflex pathway. In: Ciriello J, Calaresu FR, Renaud LP, Polosa C, eds. *Organization of the autonomic nervous system: central and peripheral mechanisms.* New York: Alan R. Liss, 1987;215–225.

77. McCall RB. Serotonergic excitation of sympathetic preganglionic neurons: a microiontophoretic study. *Brain Res* 1983;289:121–127.

78. Nishi S, Yoshimura M, Polosa C. Synaptic potentials and putative transmitter actions in sympathetic preganglionic neurons. In: Ciriello J, Calaresu FR, Renaud LP, Polosa C, eds. *Organization of the autonomic nervous system: central and peripheral mechanisms.* New York: Alan R. Liss, 1987;15–26.

79. Blessing WW, Reis DJ. Inhibitory cardiovascular function of neurons in the caudal ventrolateral medulla of the rabbit: relationship to the area containing A1 noradrenergic cells. *Brain Res* 1982;253:161–171.

80. Day TA, Ro A, Renaud LP. Depressor area within caudal ventrolateral medulla of the rat does not correspond to the A1 catecholamine cell group. *Brain Res* 1983;279:299–302.

81. Blessing WW, Reis DJ. Evidence that GABA- and glycine-like inputs inhibit vasodepressor neurons in the caudal ventrolateral medulla of the rabbit. *Neurosci Lett* 1983;37:57–62.

82. Willette RN, Krieger AJ, Barcas PP, Sapru HN. Medullary-aminobutyric acid (GABA) receptors and the regulation of blood pressure in the rat. *J Pharmacol Exp Ther* 1983;226:893–899.

83. Guyenet PG, Filtz TM, Donaldson SR. Role of excitatory aminoacids in rat vagal and sympathetic baroreflexes. *Brain Res* 1987;407:272–284.

84. Granata AR, Kumada M, Reis DJ. Sympathoinhibition by A1-noradrenergic neurons is mediated by neurons in the C1 area of the rostral medulla. *J Auton Nerv Syst* 1985;14:387–395.

85. Elliott JM, Kapoor V, Cain M, West MJ, Chalmers JP. The mechanism of hypertension and bradycardia following lesions of the caudal ventrolateral medulla in the rabbit: the role of sympathetic nerves, circulating adrenaline, vasopressin and renin. *Clin Exp Hypertens* 1985; A7:1059–1082.

86. Ross CA, Ruggiero DA, Reis DJ. Projections from the nucleus tractus solitarii to the rostral ventrolateral medulla. *J Comp Neurol* 1985; 242:511–534.

87. Willette RN, Punnen S, Krieger AJ, Sapru HN. Interdependence of rostral and caudal ventro-lateral medullary areas in the control of blood pressure. *Brain Res* 1984;321:169–174.

88. Bousquet P, Feldman J, Boch R, Schwartz J. Central cardiovascular effects of alpha-adrenergic drugs: differences between catecholamines and imidazolines. *J Pharmacol Exp Ther* 1985;230:232–236.

89. Sinha JN, Gurtu S, Sharma K, Bhargava KP. An analysis of the α-adrenoceptor modulation of vasomotor tone at the level of lateral medullary pressor area (LMPA). *Naunyn Schmiedebergs Arch Pharmacol* 1985;330:163–168.

90. Aghajanian GK. The modulatory role of serotonin at multiple receptors in brain. In: Jacobs BL, Gelperin A, eds. *Serotonin neurotransmission and behavior.* Cambridge: MIT Press, 1981;156–185.

91. McKellar S, Loewy AD. Efferent projections of the A1 catecholamine cell group in the rat: an autoradiographic study. *Brain Res* 1982; 241:11–29.

92. Blessing WW, Jaeger CB, Ruggiero DA, Reis DJ. Hypothalamic projections of medullary catecholamine neurons in the rabbit: a combined catecholamine fluorescence and HRP transport study. *Brain Res Bull* 1982;9:279–286.

93. Sawchenko PE, Swanson LW. The organization of noradrenergic pathways from the brainstem to the paraventricular and supraoptic nuclei in the rat. *Brain Res Rev* 1982;4:275–325.

94. Mills E, Wang SC. Liberation of antidiuretic hormone: location of ascending pathways. *Am J Physiol* 1964;207:1399–1404.

95. Feldberg W, Rocha SM. Vasopressin release produced in anaesthetized cats by antagonists of GABA and glycine. *Br J Pharmacol* 1978; 62:99–106.

96. Blessing WW, Willoughby JO. Inhibiting the rabbit caudal ventrolateral medulla prevents baroreceptor-initiated secretion of vasopressin. *J Physiol (Lond)* 1985;367:253–265.

97. Blessing WW, Willoughby JO. Excitation of neuronal function in rabbit caudal ventrolateral medulla elevates plasma vasopressin. *Neurosci Lett* 1985;58:189–194.

98. Benetos A, Gavras I, Gavras H. Norepinephrine applied in the paraventricular hypothalamic nucleus stimulates vasopressin release. *Brain Res* 1986;381:322–326.

99. Day TA, Ferguson AV, Renaud LP. Facilitatory influence of noradrenergic afferents on the excitability of rat paraventricular nucleus neurosecretory cells. *J Physiol (Lond)* 1984;355: 237–249.

100. Day TA, Renaud LP. Electrophysiological evidence that noradrenergic afferents selectively facilitate the activity of supraoptic vasopressin neurons. *Brain Res* 1984;303:233–240.

101. Davis BJ, Blair ML, Sladek JR, Sladek CD. Effects of lesions of hypothalamic catecholamines on blood pressure, fluid balance, vasopressin and renin in the rat. *Brain Res* 1987; 405:1–15.

102. Tanaka J, Kaba H, Saito H, Seto K. Inputs

from the A1 noradrenergic region to hypothalamic paraventricular neurons in the rat. *Brain Res* 1985;355:368–371.

103. Randle JCR, Bourque CW, Renaud LP. α-Adrenergic activation of rat hypothalamic supraoptic neurons maintained in vitro. *Brain Res* 1984;307:374–378.

104. Sved AF. Pontine pressor sites which release vasopressin. *Brain Res* 1986;369:143–150.

105. Imizumi T, Granata AR, Benarroch EE, Sved AF, Reis DJ. Contributions of arginine vasopressin and the sympathetic nervous system to fulminating hypertension after destruction of neurons of caudal ventrolateral medulla in the rat. *J Hypertens* 1985;3:491–501.

106. Minson J, Chalmers J, Kappor V, Cain M, Caon A. Relative importance of sympathetic nerves and of circulating adrenaline and vasopressin in mediating hypertension after lesions of the caudal ventrolateral medulla in the rat. *J Hypertens* 1986;4:273–281.

107. Yamashita H, Dyball REJ, Inenaga K, Kannan H. The effects of noradrenaline on supraoptic and paraventricular cells of mice in vitro. In: Ciriello J, Calaresu FR, Renaud LP, Polosa C, eds. *Organization of the autonomic nervous system: central and peripheral mechanisms.* New York: Alan R. Liss, 1987;417–423.

108. Silverman AJ, Hou YuA, Oldfield BJ. Ultrastructural identification of noradrenergic nerve terminals and vasopressin-containing neurons of the paraventricular nucleus in the same thin section. *J Histochem Cytochem* 1983;31:1151–1156.

109. Loewy AD, McKellar S, Saper CB. Direct projections from the A5 catecholamine cell group to the intermediolateral cell column. *Brain Res* 1979;174:309–314.

110. Byrum CE, Stornetta R, Guyenet PG. Electrophysiological properties of spinally-projecting A5 noradrenergic neurons. *Brain Res* 1984;303:15–29.

111. Byrum CE, Guyenet PG. Afferent and efferent connections of the A5 noradrenergic cell group in the rat. *J Comp Neurol* 1987;261:529–542.

112. Neil JJ, Loewy AD. Decreases in blood pressure in response to L-glutamate microinjections in the A5 catecholamine cell group. *Brain Res* 1982;241:271–278.

113. Loewy AD, Marson L, Parkinson D, Perry MA, Sawyer WB. Descending noradrenergic pathways involved in the A5 depressor response. *Brain Res* 1986;386:313–324.

114. Stanek KA, Neil JJ, Sawyer WB, Loewy AD. Changes in regional blood flow and cardiac output after L-glutamate stimulation of A5 cell group. *Am J Physiol* 1984;246:H44–H51.

115. Stornetta RL, Guyenet PG, McCarty R. Modulation of autonomic outflow by pontine A5 noradrenergic neurons. In: Nakamura K, ed. *Brain and blood pressure control.* Amsterdam: Elsevier, 1986;23–28.

116. Coote JH, Macleod VH, Fleetwood-Walker S, Gilbey MP. The response of individual sympathetic preganglionic neurones to microelectrophoretically applied endogenous monoamines. *Brain Res* 1981;215:1135–145.

117. DeGroat WC, Ryall RW. An excitatory action of 5-hydroxytryptamine on sympathetic preganglionic neurons. *Exp Brain Res* 1967;3:299–305.

118. McCall RB, Harris LT. Characterization of the central sympathoinhibitory action of ketanserin. *J Pharmacol Exp Ther* 1987;241:736–740.

119. McCall RB, Humphrey SJ. Evidence for a central depressor action of postsynaptic α₁-adrenergic receptor antagonists. *J Auton Nerv Syst* 1981;3:9–23.

120. McCall RB, Schuette MR. Evidence for an alpha-1 receptor-mediated central sympathoinhibitory action of ketanserin. *J Pharmacol Exp Ther* 1984;228:704–710.

121. Aghajanian GK, Rogawski MA. The physiological role of α-adrenoceptors in the CNS: new concepts from single-cell studies. *Trends Pharmacol Sci* 1983;4:315–317.

122. Hare BD, Neumayr RJ, Franz DN. Opposite effects of L-dopa and 5-HTP on spinal sympathetic reflexes. *Nature* 1972;239:336–337.

123. Ma RC, Dun NJ. Norepinephrine depolarizes lateral horn cells of neonatal rat spinal cord in vitro. *Neurosci Lett* 1985;60:163–168.

124. Yoshimura M, Polosa C, Nishi S. Noradrenaline modifies sympathetic preganglionic neuron spike and afterpotential. *Brain Res* 1986;362:370–374.

125. Yoshimura M, Polosa C, Nishi S. Noradrenaline induces rhythmic bursting in sympathetic preganglionic neurons. *Brain Res* 1987;420:147–151.

126. Yoshimura M, Polosa C, Nishi S. Slow IPSP and the noradrenaline-induced inhibition of the cat sympathetic preganglionic neuron in vitro. *Brain Res* 1987;419:383–386.

127. McCall RB, Humphrey SJ. Evidence for GABA mediation of sympathetic inhibition evoked from midline medullary depressor sites. *Brain Res* 1985;339:356–361.

128. Wang SC, Ranson SW. Autonomic responses to electrical stimulation of the lower brain stem. *J Comp Neurol* 1939;71:437–455.

129. McCall RB, Harris LT. Sympathetic alterations after midline medullary raphe lesions. *Am J Physiol* 1987;253:R91–R100.

130. Morrison SF, Gebber GL. Classification of raphe neurons with cardiac-related activity. *Am J Physiol* 1982;243:R49–R59.

131. Morrison SF, Gebber GL. Raphe neurons with sympathetic-related activity: baroreceptor responses and spinal connections. *Am J Physiol* 1984;246:R338–R348.

132. McCall RB, Clement ME. Identification of serotonergic and sympathetic neurons in medullary raphe nuclei. *Brain Res* 1988;477:172–182.

133. McCall RB, Harris LT. Role of serotonin and serotonin receptor subtypes in the central regulation of blood pressure. In: Rech RH, Gudelsky GA, eds. *5-HT agonists as psychoactive drugs.* Ann Arbor: NPP Books, 1988;1433–1462.

134. McCall RB. Role of serotonin in the regulation of sympathetic nerve discharge. In: Saxena P, Bevan P, eds. *Cardiovascular pharmacology of 5-hydroxytryptamine: prospective therapeutic applications* (in press).

135. Adair JR, Hamilton BL, Scappaticci KA, Helke CJ, Gillis RA. Cardiovascular responses to electrical stimulation of the medullary raphe area of the cat. *Brain Res* 1977;128:141–145.

136. McCall RB. Evidence for a serotonergically mediated sympathoexcitatory response to stimulation of medullary raphe nuclei. *Brain Res* 1984;311:131–139.

137. Ruggiero DA, Meeley MP, Anwarand M, Reis DJ. Newly identified GABAergic neurons in regions of the ventrolateral medulla which regulate blood pressure. *Brain Res* 1985;339:171–177.

138. Loewy AD. Raphe pallidus and raphe obscurus projections to the intermediolateral cell column in the rat. *Brain Res* 1981;222:129–132.

139. Seybold AV, Elde RP. Receptor autoradiography in thoracic spinal cord: correlation of neurotransmitter binding sites with sympathoadrenal neurons. *J Neurosci* 1984;4:2533–2542.

140. Jacobs BL, Gannon PJ, Azmitia EC. Atlas of serotonergic cell bodies in the cat brainstem: an immunocytochemical analysis. *Brain Res Bull* 1984;13:1–31.

141. Gilbey MP, Coote JH, Macleod VH, Peterson DF. Inhibition of sympathetic activity by stimulating in the raphe nuclei and the role of 5-hydroxytryptamine in this effect. *Brain Res* 1981;226:131–142.

142. Howe PRC. Blood pressure control by neurotransmitters in the medulla oblongata and spinal cord. *J Auton Nerv Syst* 1985;12:95–115.

143. Coote JH, Macleod VH. The spinal route of sympatho-inhibitory pathways descending from the medulla oblongata. *Pflugers Arch* 1975;359:335–347.

144. Kuhn DM, Wolf WA, Lovenberg W. Review of the central serotonergic neuronal system in blood pressure regulation. *Hypertension* 1980;2:243–255.

145. Wolf WA, Kuhn DM. Antihypertensive effects of L-tryptophan are not mediated by brain serotonin. *Brain Res* 1984;295:356–359.

146. McCall RB, Humphrey SJ. Involvement of serotonin in the central regulation of blood pressure: evidence for a facilitating effect on sympathetic nerve activity. *J Pharmacol Exp Ther* 1982;222:94–102.

147. Ma RC, Dun NJ. Excitation of lateral horn neurons of the neonatal rat spinal cord by 5-hydroxytryptamine. *Dev Brain Res* 1986;24:89–98.

148. Pilowsky PM, Kapoor V, Minson JB, West MJ, Chalmers JP. Spinal cord serotonin release and raised blood pressure after brainstem kainic acid injection. *Brain Res* 1986;366:354–357.

149. Aghajanian GK, Wang RY. Physiology and pharmacology of central serotonergic neurons. In: Lipton MA, DiMascio A, Killam KF, eds. *Psychopharmacology: a generation of progress.* New York: Raven Press, 1978;171–183.

150. Bowker RM, Westlund KN, Sullivan MC, Wilber JF, Coulter JD. Descending serotonergic, peptidergic and cholinergic pathways from the raphe nuclei: a multiple transmitter complex. *Brain Res* 1983;288:33–48.

151. Helke CJ, Sayson SC, Keeler JR, Charlton CG. Thyrotropin releasing hormone-immunoreactive neurons project from the ventral medulla to the intermediolateral cell column: partial coexistence with serotonin. *Brain Res* 1986;381:1–7.

152. Appel NM, Wessendorf MW, Elde RP. Thyrotropin-releasing hormone in spinal cord: coexistence with serotonin and with substance P in fibers and terminals apposing identified preganglionic sympathetic neurons. *Brain Res* 1987;415:137–143.

153. Backman SB, Henry JL. Effect of substance P and thyrotropin-releasing hormone on sympathetic preganglionic neurons in the upper thoracic intermediolateral nucleus of the cat. *Can J Physiol Pharmacol* 1984;62:248–251.

154. Millhorn DE, Hokfelt T, Seroogy K, Oertel W, Verhofstad AAJ, Wu J-Y. Immunohistochemical evidence for colocalization of γ-aminobutyric acid and serotonin in neurons of the ventral medulla oblongata projecting to the spinal cord. *Brain Res* 1987;410:179–185.

155. Xie CW, Tang J, Han JS. Clonidine stimulated the release of dynorphin in the spinal cord of the rat: a possible mechanism for its depressor effects. *Neurosci Lett* 1986;65:224–228.

156. Franz DN, Hare BD, McCloskey KL. Spinal sympathetic neurons: possible sites of opiate-withdrawal suppression by clonidine. *Science* 1982;215:1643–1645.

157. McKenna KE, Schramm LP. Mechanisms mediating the silent period. Studies in the isolated spinal cord of the neonatal rat. *Brain Res* 1985;329:233–240.

158. Backman SB, Henry JL. Effects of GABA and glycine on sympathetic preganglionic neurons in the upper thoracic intermediolateral nucleus of the cat. *Brain Res* 1983;277:365–369.

159. Gordon FJ. Spinal GABA receptors and central cardiovascular control. *Brain Res* 1985;328:165–169.

160. Kuhn DM, Wolf WA, Lovenberg W. Pressor effects of electrical stimulation of the dorsal and median raphe nuclei in anesthetized rats. *J Pharmacol Exp Ther* 1980;214:403–409.

161. Wolf WA, Kuhn DM, Lovenberg W. Pressor effects of dorsal raphe stimulation and intrahypothalamic application of serotonin in the spontaneously hypertensive rat. *Brain Res* 1981;208:192–197.

162. Robinson SE. Serotonergic-cholinergic interactions in blood pressure control in the rat. *Fed Proc* 1984;43:21–24.

163. Robinson SE, Austin MJ, Gibbens DM. The role of serotonergic neurons in dorsal raphe, median raphe and anterior hypothalamic pres-

sor mechanisms. *Neuropharmacology* 1985; 24:51–58.

164. Iovino M, Steardo L. Effect of substances influencing brain serotonergic transmission on plasma vasopressin levels in the rat. *Eur J Pharmacol* 1985;113:99–103.

165. Gotoh E, Murakami K, Bahnson TD, Ganong WF. Role of brain serotonergic pathways and hypothalamus in regulation of renin secretion. *Am J Physiol* 1987;253:R179–R185.

166. Valiquette, G. Posterior pituitary hormones and neurophysins. In: Motta M, ed. *The endocrine functions of the brain*. New York: Raven Press, 1980;385–417.

167. Swanson LW. Immunohistochemical evidence for a neurophysin-containing autonomic pathway arising in the paraventricular nucleus of hypothalamus. *Brain Res* 1977;128:346–353.

168. Swanson LW, McKellar S. The distribution of oxytocin- and neurophysin-stained fibers in the spinal cord of the rat and monkey. *J Comp Neurol* 1979;188:87–106.

169. Armstrong WE, Warach S, Hatton GI, McNeil TH. Subnuclei in the rat hypothalamic paraventricular nucleus: a cytoarchitectural, horseradish peroxidase and immunocytochemical analysis. *Neuroscience* 1980;5:1931–1958.

170. Swanson LW, Kuypers HGJM. The paraventricular nucleus of the hypothalamus: cytoarchitectonic subdivisions and organization of projections to the pituitary, dorsal vagal complex, and spinal cord as demonstrated by retrograde fluorescence double-labeling methods. *J Comp Neurol* 1980;194:555–570.

171. Sofroniew MV. Vasopressin and oxytocin in the mammalian brain and spinal cord. *Trends Neurosci* 1983;5:467–472.

172. Brody MJ, O'Neill TP, Porter JP. Role of paraventricular and arcuate nuclei in cardiovascular regulation. In: Magro A, Osswald W, Reis D, Vanhoutte P, eds. *Central and peripheral mechanisms of cardiovascular regulation*. New York: Plenum Press, 1986;443–464.

173. Kannan H, Yamashita H. Connections of neurons in the region of the nucleus tractus solitarius with the hypothalamic paraventricular nucleus: their possible involvement in neural control of the cardiovascular system. *Brain Res* 1985;329:205–212.

174. Caverson MM, Ciriello J, Calaresu FR. Paraventricular nucleus of the hypothalamus: an electrophysiological investigation of neurons projecting directly to intermediolateral nucleus in the cat. *Brain Res* 1984;305:380–383.

175. Yamashita H, Inenaga K, Koizumi K. Possible projections from regions of paraventricular and supraoptic nuclei to the spinal cord: electrophysiological studies. *Brain Res* 1984;296:373–378.

176. Calaresu FR, Ciriello J. Projections to the hypothalamus from buffer nerves and nucleus tractus solitarius in the cat. *Am J Physiol* 1980;239:R130–R136.

177. Holets V, Elde R. The differential distribution and relationship of serotoninergic and peptidergic fibers to sympathoadrenal neurons in the intermediolateral cell column of the rat: a combined retrograde axonal transport and immunofluorescence study. *Neuroscience* 1982;7:1155–1174.

178. Krukoff TL, Ciriello J, Calaresu FR. Segmental distribution of peptide- and 5-HT-like immunoreactivity in nerve terminals and fibers of the thoracolumbar sympathetic nuclei of the cat. *J Comp Neurol* 1985;240:103–116.

179. Gilbey MP, Coote JH, Fleetwood-Walker S, Peterson DF. The influence of the paraventriculo-spinal pathway, and oxytocin and vasopressin on sympathetic preganglionic neurons. *Brain Res* 1982;251:283–290.

180. Ciriello J, Calaresu FR. Role of paraventricular and supraoptic nuclei in central cardiovascular regulation in the cat. *Am J Physiol* 1980;239:R137–R142.

181. Backman SB, Henry JL. Effects of oxytocin and vasopressin on thoracic sympathetic preganglionic neurons in the cat. *Brain Res Bull* 1984;13:679–684.

182. Ma RC, Dun NJ. Vasopressin depolarizes lateral horn cells of the neonatal rat spinal cord in vitro. *Brain Res* 1985;348:36–43.

183. Porter JP, Brody MJ. The paraventricular nucleus and cardiovascular regulation: role of spinal vasopressinergic mechanisms. *J Hypertens* 1986;4 (suppl 3):S181–S184.

184. Sleight P. *Arterial baroreceptors and hypertension*. Oxford: Oxford University Press, 1980.

185. Talman WT, Perrone MH, Reis DJ. Evidence for L-glutamate as the neurotransmitter of baroreceptor afferent nerve fibers. *Science* 1980;209:813–815.

186. Talman WT, Perrone MH, Scher P, Kwo S, Reis DJ. Antagonism of the baroreceptor reflex by glutamate diethyl ester, an antagonist to L-glutamate. *Brain Res* 1981;217:186–191.

187. Humphrey SJ, McCall RB. Evidence that L-glutamic acid mediates baroreceptor function in the cat. *Clin Exp Hypertens* 1984;6:1311–1329.

188. Talman WT, Granata AR, Reis DJ. Glutamatergic mechanisms in the nucleus tractus solitarius in blood pressure control. *Fed Proc* 1984;43:39–44.

189. Simon JR, DiMicco SK, DiMicco JA, Aprison MH. Choline acetyltransferase and glutamate uptake in the nucleus tractus solitarius and dorsal motor nucleus of the vagus: effect of nodose ganglionectomy. *Brain Res* 1985;344:405–408.

190. Granata AR, Reis DJ. Release of [³H]L-glutamine acid (L-Glu) and [³H]D-aspartic acid (D-Asp) in the area of nucleus tractus solitarius in vivo produced by stimulation of the vagus nerve. *Brain Res* 1983;259:77–93.

191. Gillis RA, Helke CJ, Hamilton BL, Norman WP, Jacobowitz DW. Evidence that substance P is a neurotransmitter of baro- and chemoreceptor afferents in nucleus tractus solitarius. *Brain Res* 1980;181:476–481.

192. Helke CJ, O'Donohue TL, Jacobowitz DM. Substance P as a baro- and chemoreceptor afferent neurotransmitter: immunocytochemical and neurochemical evidence in the rat. *Peptides* 1980;1:1–9.

193. Jacobowitz DM, Helke CJ. Localization of substance P immunoreactive nerves in the carotid body. *Brain Res Bull* 1980;5:195–197.

194. Helke CJ, Jacobowitz DM, Thoa NB. Capsaicin and potassium evoked substance P release from the nucleus tractus solitarius and spinal trigeminal nucleus in vitro. *Life Sci* 1981;29:1779–1785.

195. Helke CJ. Neuroanatomical localization of substance P: implications for central cardiovascular control. *Peptides* 1982;3:479–483.

196. Haeusler G, Osterwalder R. Evidence suggesting a transmitter or neuromodulatory role for substance P at the first synapse of the baroreceptor reflex. *Naunyn Schmiedebergs Arch Pharmacol* 1980;314:111–121.

197. Talman WT, Reis DJ. Baroreflex actions of substance P microinjected into the nucleus tractus solitarii in rat: a consequence of local distortion. *Brain Res* 1981;220:402–407.

198. Kubo T, Kihara M. Blood pressure modulation by substance P in the rat nucleus tractus solitarius. *Brain Res* 1987;413:379–383.

199. Morin-Surun MP, Jordan D, Champagnat J, Spyer KM, Denavit-Saudie M. Excitatory effects of iontophoretically applied substance P on neurons in the nucleus tractus solitarius of the cat: lack of interaction with opiates and opioids. *Brain Res* 1984;307:388–392.

200. Feldman PD, Moises HC. Adrenergic responses of baroreceptive cells in the nucleus tractus solitarii of the rat: a microiontophoretic study. *Brain Res* 1987;420:351–361.

201. Feldman PD, Moises HC. Electrophysiological evidence for alpha 1- and alpha 2-adrenoceptors in solitary tract nucleus. *Am J Physiol* 1988;254:H756–H762.

202. Reis DJ, Joh TH, Nathan MA, Renaud B, Snyder DW, Talman WT. Nucleus tractus solitarii: catecholaminergic innervation in normal and abnormal control of arterial pressure. In: Myer P, Schmitt H, eds. *Nervous system and hypertension.* Toronto: Wiley-Flammarion, 1979; 147–164.

203. Wolf WA, Kuhn DM, Lovenberg W. Blood pressure responses to local application of serotonergic agents in the nucleus tractus solitarii. *Eur J Pharmacol* 1981;69:291–299.

204. Carter DA, Lightman SL. Cardio-respiratory actions of substance P, TRH and 5-HT in the nucleus tractus solitarius of rats: evidence for functional interactions of neuropeptides and amine neurotransmitters. *Neuropeptides* 1985; 6:425–436.

205. Laguzzi R, Reis DJ, Talman WT. Modulation of cardiovascular and electrocortical activity through serotonergic mechanisms in the nucleus tractus solitarius of the rat. *Brain Res* 1984;304:321–328.

206. Shvaloff A, Laguzzi R. Serotonin receptors in the rat nucleus tractus solitarii and cardiovascular regulation. *Eur J Pharmacol* 1986;132: 283–288.

207. Catelli JM, Gikas WJ, Sved AF. GABAergic mechanisms in nucleus tractus solitarius alter blood pressure and vasopressin release. *Brain Res* 1987;403:279–289.

208. Kubo T, Kihara M. Evidence for gamma-aminobutyric acid receptor-mediated modulation of the aortic baroreceptor reflex in the nucleus tractus solitarii of the rat. *Neurosci Lett* 1988;89:156–160.

209. Kubo T, Kihara M. Evidence for the presence of GABAergic and glycine-like systems responsible for cardiovascular control in the nucleus tractus solitarii of the rat. *Neurosci Lett* 1987;74:331–336.

210. Matsuguchi H, Sharabi FM, Gordon FJ, Johnson AK, Schmid PG. Blood pressure and heart rate responses to microinjection of vasopressin into the nucleus tractus solitarius region of the rat. *Neuropharmacology* 1982;21:687–693.

211. King KA, Pang CC. Cardiovascular effects of injections of vasopressin into the nucleus tractus solitarius in conscious rats. *Br J Pharmacol* 1987;90:531–536.

212. Pittman QJ, Franklin LG. Vasopressin antagonist in nucleus tractus solitarius/vagal area reduces pressor and tachycardia responses to paraventricular nucleus stimulation in rats. *Neurosci Lett* 1985;56:155–160.

213. Averill DB, Diz DI, Barnes KL, Ferrario CM. Pressor responses of angiotensin II microinjected into the dorsomedial medulla of the dog. *Brain Res* 1987;414:294–300.

214. Casto R, Phillips MI. Neuropeptide action in nucleus tractus solitarius: angiotensin specificity and hypertensive rats. *Am J Physiol* 1985; 249:R341–R347.

215. Rettig R, Healy DP, Printz MP. Cardiovascular effects of microinjections of angiotensin II into the nucleus tractus solitarii. *Brain Res* 1986; 364:233–240.

216. Campagnole-Santos MJ, Diz DI, Ferrario CM. Baroreceptor reflex modulation by angiotensin II at the nucleus tractus solitarii. *Hypertension* 1988;11:167–171.

217. Petty MA, de-Jong W. Enkephalins induce a centrally mediated rise in blood pressure in rats. *Brain Res* 1983;260:322–325.

218. Petty MA, de-Jong W. Cardiovascular effects of β-endorphin after microinjection into the nucleus tractus solitarii of the anesthetized rat. *Eur J Pharmacol* 1982;81:449–457.

219. Koda LY, Ling N, Benoit R, Madamba SG, Bakhit C. Blood pressure following microinjection of somatostatin related peptides into the rat nucleus tractus solitarii. *Eur J Pharmacol* 1985;113:425–430.

220. Willette RN, Barcas PP, Krieger AJ, Sapru HN. Endogenous GABAergic mechanisms in the medulla and the regulation of blood pressure. *J Pharmacol Exp Ther* 1984;230:34–39.

221. Yamada KA, McAllen RM, Loewy AD. GABA antagonists applied to the ventral surface of the medulla oblongata block the baroreceptor reflex. *Brain Res* 1984;297:175–180.

222. Humphrey SJ, McCall RB. Evidence for γ-aminobutyric acid mediation of the sympathetic nerve inhibitory response to vagal afferent stimulation. *J Pharmacol Exp Ther* 1985;234: 288–297.

223. Sun M-K, Guyenet PG. Arterial baroreceptor and vagal inputs to sympathoexcitatory neurons in rat medulla. *Am J Physiol* 1987;252: R699–R709.

224. Jhamandas JH, Renaud LP. Bicuculline blocks an inhibitory baroreflex input to supraoptic vasopressin neurons. *Am J Physiol* 1987;252: R947–R952.

225. Kasai M, Osaka T, Inenaga K, Kannan H, Yamashita H. Gamma-aminobutyric acid antagonist blocks baroreceptor-activated inhibition of neurosecretory cells in the hypothalamic paraventricular nucleus of rats. *Neurosci Lett* 1987;81:319–324.

226. Barnes KL, Ferrario CM. Differential effects of angiotensin II mediated by the area postrema and the anteroventral third ventricle. In: Buckley JP, Ferrario CM, eds. *Brain peptides and catecholamines in cardiovascular regulation.* New York: Raven Press, 1987;289–300.

227. Faber JE, Brody MJ. Central nervous system action of angiotensin during onset of renal hypertension in awake rats. *Am J Physiol* 1984;247:H349–H360.

228. Johnson AK. The periventricular anteroventral third ventricle (AV3V): its relationship with the subfornical organ and neuronal systems involved in maintaining body fluid homeostasis. *Brain Res Bull* 1985;15:595–601.

229. Bishop VS, Hasser EM, Undesser KP. Vasopressin and sympathetic nerve activity: involvement of the area postrema. In: Buckley JP, Ferrario CM, eds. *Brain peptides and catecholamines in cardiovascular regulation.* New York: Raven Press, 1987;373–382.

230. Hasser EM, DiCarlo SE, Applegate RJ, Bishop VS. Osmotically released vasopressin augments cardiopulmonary reflex inhibition of the circulation. *Am J Physiol* 1988;254:R815–R820.

231. Korner PI, Angus JA. Central nervous control of blood pressure in relation to antihypertensive drug treatment. In: Austin DE, ed. *Antihypertensive drugs.* New York: Pergamon Press, 1982;61–96.

232. Haeusler G. Clonidine-induced inhibition of sympathetic nerve activity: no indication of a central presynaptic or an indirect sympathomimetic mode of action. *Naunyn Schmiedebergs Arch Pharmacol* 1974;286:97–111.

233. Bousquet P, Feldman J, Schwartz J. The medullary cardiovascular effects of imidazolines and some GABA analogues: a review. *J Auton Nerv Syst* 1985;14:263–270.

234. Granata AR, Numao Y, Kumada M, Reis DJ. A1 noradrenergic neurons tonically inhibit sympathoexcitatory neurons of C1 area in rat brain stem. *Brain Res* 1986;377:127–146.

235. Gatti PJ, Hill KJ, Da Silva AMT, Norman WP, Gillis RA. Central nervous system site of action for the hypotensive effect of clonidine in the cat. *J Pharmacol Exp Ther* 1988;245:373–380.

236. Franz DN, Madsen PW, Peterson RG, Sangdee C. Functional roles of monoaminergic pathways to sympathetic preganglionic neurons. *Clin Exp Hypertens* 1982;A4:543–562.

237. McCall RB, Schuette MR, Humphrey SJ, Lahti RA, Barsuhn C. Evidence for a central sympathoexcitatory action of alpha-2 adrenergic antagonists. *J Pharmacol Exp Ther* 1983;224: 501–507.

238. McCall RB, Patel BN, Harris LT. Effects of serotonin₁ and serotonin₂ receptor agonists and antagonists on blood pressure, heart rate and sympathetic nerve activity. *J Pharmacol Exp Ther* 1987;242:1152–1159.

239. Fozard JR, Mir AK, Middlemiss DN. Cardiovascular response to 8-hydroxy-2-(di-N-propylamino) tetralin (8-OH DPAT) in the rat: site of action and pharmacological analysis. *J Cardiovasc Pharmacol* 1987;9:328–347.

240. Ramage AG, Fozard JR. Evidence that the putative 5-HT₁ₐ receptor agonists 8-OH DPAT and ipsapirone have a central hypotensive action that differs from that of clonidine in anesthetized cats. *Eur J Pharmacol* 1987;138:179–191.

241. Verge D, Daval G, Patey A, Gozlan H, El Mestikawy S, Hamon M. Presynaptic 5-HT autoreceptors on serotonergic cell bodies and/or dendrites but not terminals are of the 5-HT₁ₐ subtype. *Eur J Pharmacol* 1985;113:463–464.

242. Dashwood MR, Gilbey MP, Jordan D, Ramage AG. Autoradiographic localization of 5-HT₁ₐ binding sites in the brainstem of the cat. *Br J Pharmacol* 1988;94:386P.

243. McCall RB, Clement ME, Harris LT. Studies on the mechanism of the sympatholytic effect of 8-OH DPAT: lack of correlation between inhibition of serotonin neuronal firing and sympathetic activity. *Brain Res* (in press).

244. Gillis RA, Hill K, Kirby JS, et al. Effect of activation of CNS serotonin 1A receptors on cardiorespiratory function. *J Pharmacol Exp Ther* (in press).

245. Sprouse JS, Aghajanian GK. Electrophysiological responses of serotoninergic dorsal raphe neurons to 5-HT₁ₐ and 5-HT1ᵦ agonists. *Synapse* 1987;1:3–9.

246. Fornal CA, Jacobs BL. Physiological and behavioral correlates of serontonergic single-unit activity. In: Osborne NN, Hamon M, eds. *Neuronal serotonin.* Chichester, England: John Wiley, 1988.

247. Punnen S, Sapru HN. Blockade of cholinergic receptors in the C1 area abolishes hypertensive response to opiates in the A1 area of the ventrolateral medulla. *Brain Res* 1985;336:180–186.

248. Willette RN, Punnen S, Krieger AJ, Sapru HN. Cardiovascular control by cholinergic mechanisms in the rostral ventrolateral medulla. *J Pharmacol Exp Ther* 1984;231:457–463.

249. Punnen S, Willette RN, Krieger AJ, Sapru HN. Medullary pressor area: site of action of intra-venous physostigmine. *Brain Res* 1986;382: 178–184.

250. Reis DJ, Morrison S, Ruggiero DA. The C1 area of the brainstem in tonic and reflex control of blood pressure. State of the art lecture. *Hypertension* 1988;11:8–13.

Cardiovascular Pharmacology, Third Edition,
edited by Michael Antonaccio.
Raven Press, Ltd., New York © 1990.

Renin-Angiotensin System, Converting Enzyme, and Renin Inhibitors

Michael J. Antonaccio and John J. Wright

*Cardiovascular Research and Development, Bristol-Myers Squibb Company,
Wallingford, Connecticut 06492*

The renin-angiotensin system (RAS) has a long history in the regulation of blood pressure and the etiology of hypertension. Almost 100 years ago, Tigerstedt and Bergman (1) coined the word "renin" as a substance derived from kidneys that could raise blood pressure and have potential importance in circulatory control. This discovery remained fallow until 1934 when Goldblatt et al. (2) reported that constriction of a renal artery with contralateral nephrectomy resulted in persistent systemic hypertension. This hypertension, they suggested, could be caused by a circulating pressor agent having its origin in the ischemic kidney. Subsequently, it was found that renin was an enzyme that required a "cofactor" to produce vasoconstriction (3). This pressor substance in the ischemic blood from ischemic kidneys was found to be a peptide called "angiotonin" by Page and Helmer (3) and "hypertensin" by Braun-Menendez et al. (4) until 1958 when it was agreed to combine the names into the compromise term "angiotensin."

RAS

As shown in Fig. 1, the RAS is a closed-loop negative feedback system that responds to a variety of factors that reduce renal perfusion or result in excessive so-dium loss, including hemorrhage, heart failure, hypotension, and sodium depletion (5). Release of renin from specialized cells in the kidney initiates the sequence of events illustrated in Fig. 1. Renin substrate, angiotensinogen, is circulating in the blood and is acted on by renin to produce the biologically inactive decapeptide angiotensin I (AI). AI, in turn, is converted to the octapeptide angiotensin II (AII), mainly in the blood, by angiotensin-converting enzyme (ACE) localized on the endothelium and smooth muscle of blood vessels of lung, kidney, and many other organs. The AII now circulating in the blood has three primary actions that counteract the initial stimulus that led to renin release: it causes powerful arterial vasoconstriction, stimulates the synthesis and release of the sodium-retaining steroid aldosterone from adrenal glands, and acts directly on the kidney to inhibit sodium excretion. By restoration of pressure, renal blood flow, and/or excessive sodium loss by the actions of AII, the initial stimulus for renin secretion is turned off, aided also by the direct inhibitory effect of AII on renin release. The system is then returned to its original status. Inhibition of ACE prevents the conversion of AI to AII (Fig. 1). In addition, because ACE is the same enzyme as kininase II (6), breakdown of kinins is also inhibited to the extent that they are normally degraded by the enzyme.

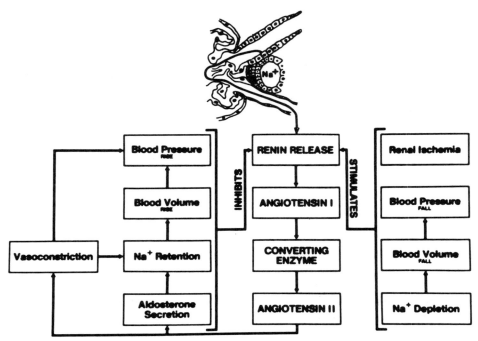

FIG. 1. Diagrammatic representation of the JG apparatus and the factors controlling renin release and AII formation.

The RAS contributes importantly to normal blood pressure regulation and seems to be critically involved in hypertension development and maintenance as well as congestive heart failure (CHF) in which inappropriate control of the RAS is manifest. Specific inhibition of either of the enzymes renin or ACE appears to have excellent beneficial effects in both hypertensive and CHF patients.

RENIN: PURIFICATION, SPECIES DIFFERENCES, AND PROPERTIES

Renin catalyzes the rate-limiting step of the RAS. It is an aspartyl protease, a classification based on the presence of two essential aspartic acid residues at the active site and its susceptibility to inhibition by pepstatin. Human kidney renin was first purified by Yokosowa et al. (7) by conventional chromatographic methods and re-cently by the use of a synthetic renin-inhibiting peptide as an affinity ligand (8).

Renin from a particular organ or species consists of multiple isoenzymes. Renal renins appear to be glycoproteins with quite variable optimal pHs (9). Although renin is an acid protease resembling pepsin, cathepsin D, gastricin, and the fungal protease penicillopepsin, endothiapepsin, and rhizopuspepsin, it is unique in its stringent substrate specificity, which, in turn, depends on the species from which it was derived. Human renin is capable of cleaving human, porcine, canine, bovine, and goat angiotensinogens, whereas human angiotensinogen is a poor substrate for animal renins (9). This has obvious significant implications in the development and testing of renin inhibitors for human clinical use. The specificity of various renins might be accounted for by the differences in angiotensinogens of various species. Human angiotensinogen contains Val-Ile-His-Thr-Glu in positions 11–15, whereas the corresponding positions of horse and cat angiotensinogen contain Leu-Val-Tyr-Ser and Leu-Tyr-Tyr-Ser, respectively (10).

RENIN SYNTHESIS

Animal as well as human renin genes have been cloned and sequenced. For an in-depth review of the subject, the reader is referred to an excellent article by Dzau et al. (11).

The human renin gene is approximately 12.5 Kb in size, containing 10 exons and 9 introns. As might be anticipated, there is substantial homology in the gene structure and protein sequence between human pepsin and renin (11). In addition, there are many sequence homologies among human, rat, and mouse renins in the 5′-flanking regions, portions of the gene that are regulatory in nature. As shown in Fig. 2, human and rat genes exhibit a high degree of homology in the 5′-flanking regions, whereas the mouse renin gene contains a large insertion compared with the human gene (11). It should also be noted that the mouse has two renin genes, *Ren-1* and *Ren-2*, the for-

mer coding for renin in the submandibular gland.

It is interesting to note that transcription of the renin gene is different in kidney in comparison with extrarenal tissue (11). For example, unlike renal renin, extrarenal renin transcription may be initiated at several sites. Because these transcriptional differences may result in translational differences, renins may be formed that are membrane bound and nonsecreted. In turn, these membrane-bound forms of renin, especially in vascular smooth muscle, may involve the local formation of angiotensin, the significance of which will be discussed further below.

Regulation of renin gene expression in rodents has been clearly documented. Sodium depletion, ACE inhibition, β-adrenoceptor stimulation, and renal ischemia all increase renal renin mRNA levels (11–15). Unfortunately, such documentation for renin gene expression is not yet available for humans. However, as shown in Fig. 2, the high degree of homology in the 5′-flanking region sequences of human, mouse, and rat genes strongly suggests that a similarity in the regulation of these genes is likely (11).

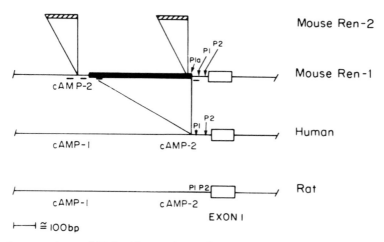

FIG. 2. Overall comparison of 5′-flanking regions of mouse, human, and rat renin genes. Human and rat renin genes exhibit a high degree of homology, whereas the mouse renin gene contains a large insertion compared with the human gene. Position of major promotors (P1a, P1, and P2) are shown as well as two putative cAMP-responsive elements (cAMP-1 and cAMP-2). (From ref. 11.)

MOLECULAR FORMS OF RENIN

Although renal renin is usually present in its active form, there are also precursors of renin that can be activated by limited proteolysis with neutral serine proteases such as trypsin (16). Renin is apparently synthesized by translation of mRNA as an inactive pre-prorenin, which is then processed into a still inactive prorenin, which, in turn, is ultimately converted into active renin either in plasma or its storage granules (10). From work by several groups who have determined the amino acid sequence of renin and its precursors, either directly or through the cloning of its cDNA (17–19), a model for the probable steps in the enzymic processing of renin has been suggested. Pre-prorenin is first converted to prorenin by cleavage between residue Cys-18 and Thr-19; cleavage then takes place at two more sites, Lys-62, Arg-63 and Arg-352, Arg-353. The former removes the "pro" sequence, whereas the latter gives rise to the A and B chains linked by the disulfide bridge (10).

Plasma levels of inactive renin bear a weak direct relationship to active renin levels (16). However, the higher the active renin in the circulation, the lower the proportion of inactive renin, suggesting that higher demands of active renin result in further conversion of inactive to active renin resulting in a lower proportion of the inactive form (16). Factors that acutely alter active renin release seldom cause changes in inactive renin (16). However, in long-term studies, inactive renin usually changes in the same direction as active renin, the exception being during β-adrenoceptor antagonism during which active renin levels fall, whereas inactive renin remains unchanged or decreases (20).

Unlike active plasma renin, which comes essentially from renal sources, inactive renin comes from many extrarenal sources. Also, although active renin is released within minutes of a stimulus, plasma inactive renin release, even if caused by the same stimulus as active renin, appears to require several days (16). It has been suggested that plasma inactive renin levels reflect the level of secretion (16).

RENIN RELEASE

Renal renin release is controlled by the juxtaglomerular (JG) apparatus of the kidney. As shown in Fig. 3, each nephron has a JG apparatus consisting of: (a) granular cells in the media of the renal afferent arteriole that synthesize, store, and release renin; these cells are sympathetically innervated, with renin release being influenced by the activation state of these nerves (vide infra) and (b) macula densa of the distal tubule, the cells of which are in close contact with the JG cells.

PHYSIOLOGICAL CONTROL

There are five fundamental physiological mechanisms for controlling renin release (see [21,22] for excellent in-depth reviews):

1. Intrarenal baroreceptor. Increases in renal perfusion pressure inhibit renin release, whereas decreases in renal pressure stimulate renin release.
2. Catecholamines (sympathetic nervous system/adrenal gland). Stimulation of β-adrenoreceptors on JG cells either by their innervating sympathetic nerves or by circulating epinephrine can increase renin release.
3. Sodium concentration sensed by the macula densa. Renin release is inversely related to the sodium concentration in the macula densa region.
4. Hormones (other than epinephrine). The most important hormones involved in renin release include AII, aldosterone, vasopressin, and prostaglandins. AII inhibits renin release by a direct action of the JG cells by a mechanism independent of aldosterone. AII stimulates aldosterone release that inhibits renin re-

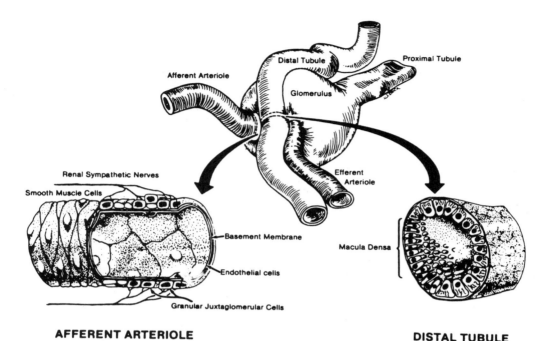

AFFERENT ARTERIOLE   **DISTAL TUBULE**

FIG. 3. Anatomical relationship of the JG cells, which synthesize and release renin, and the afferent arteriole, renal sympathetic nerves, and macula densa cells of the distal tubule. (From ref. 21.)

lease by virtue of its ability to cause sodium retention. Of course, AII also inhibits renin release indirectly by raising blood pressure and decreasing renal blood flow. Vasopressin also inhibits renin release both by a direct action on JG cells as well as increasing blood pressure and depleting sodium. Many prostaglandins have been shown to influence renin release, but prostacyclin (PGI$_2$) formed from arachidonate is probably the most likely endogenous substance responsible for physiological control. PGI$_2$ as well as PGE$_1$, PGE$_2$, PGA$_2$, PGD$_2$, PGG$_2$, and PGH$_2$ all stimulate renin release.

5. Other plasma electrolytes. Potassium suppresses renin release, whereas potassium depletion increases it. Increases in calcium concentration—intracellular as opposed to extracellular—stimulate secretion, whereas calcium depletion increases it. Increases in plasma magnesium concentration stimulate renin release, whereas decreases in magnesium inhibit it.

PHARMACOLOGICALLY INDUCED CHANGES IN RENIN RELEASE

Many drugs are capable of altering renin release, both directly and indirectly. Once again, the reader is referred to the reviews by Keeton and Campbell (21,22) for specific details on the subject. A summary of the pharmacological effects of various agents on renin release is shown in Table 1.

THE RAS AND BLOOD PRESSURE REGULATION

The RAS is a multifaceted system for the maintenance of blood pressure and volume. As mentioned above, AII is the central player in the RAS possessing several prop-

TABLE 1. *Effects of pharmacological agents on renin release* in vivo

Agent	Effect on renin release	Mechanism(s)
α_1-Adrenoceptor agonists	Inhibition	Direct receptor activation on JG cells; increased renal perfusion pressure
α_2-Adrenoceptor agonists	Inhibition	Direct receptor activation on JG cells; reduction in central sympathetic outflow to renal nerves
α_1-Adrenoceptor antagonists	Stimulation	Reflex activation of renal sympathetic nerves; blockade of α_1-presynaptic receptors mediating an increase in renal sympathetic transmitter release
α_2-Adrenoceptor antagonists	Stimulation	Reflex activation of renal sympathetic nerves
β_1-Adrenoceptor agonists	Stimulation (humans)	Direct receptor activation on JG cells
β_2-Adrenoceptor agonists	Stimulation (animals)	Direct receptor activation on JG cells
β_1-Adrenoceptor antagonists	Inhibition	Blockade of β_1-adrenoceptors on JG cells
AII antagonists	Stimulation	Blockade of AII receptor-mediated negative feedback on JG cells
ACE inhibitors	Stimulation	Blockade of AII negative feedback by AII synthesis inhibition
Vasodilators	Stimulation	Reflex activation of renal sympathetic nerves
Diuretics	Stimulation	Decreased Na^+ load to macula densa; activation of renal sympathetic nerves; activation of renal PG formation
Calcium antagonists	Mixed effects	Drug-dependent
Cardiac glycosides	Inhibition	Speculative: inhibition of renal sympathetic nerve activation?
Nonsteroidal antiinflammatories	Inhibition	Inhibition of renal PG formation
Anesthetics	Stimulation	Drug-dependent

erties that allow it to raise blood pressure. The primary hypertensinogenic effects of AII are summarized in Table 2 and the consequences of AII stimulation are schematically shown in Fig. 4. In essence, AII is a direct, powerful vasoconstrictor, more on arteries than veins, and is approximately 40 times as potent as the sympathetic neurotransmitter norepinephrine (NE) (see [23]). AII can also facilitate NE release from sympathetic nerves as well as release both NE and epinephrine by both a direct effect to release neuroeffector stores and an indirect effect by ganglion stimulation. By activation of central receptors, AII can increase sympathetic outflow from the brain to both the vasculature and myocardium. Additionally, AII-mediated NE release can also cause myocardial stimulation, which contributes to blood pressure elevation. Central nervous system activation also results in a dipsogenic effect and release of vasopressin, both of which actions increase plasma volume, further raising blood pressure. Finally, AII can stimulate the adrenal cortex to synthesize and release aldoste-

TABLE 2. *Major actions of AII*

Vasoconstriction
  Direct AII receptor activation
  Sympathetic nerve activation
    Direct transmitter release, both NE and epinephrine, from nerve endings
    Increase in central sympathetic outflow
    Facilitation of NE release
    Ganglionic stimulation
    Postsynaptic adrenergic enhancement
Cardiac stimulation
  Direct AII receptor activation
  Sympathetic nerve activation (as above)
Vasopressin secretion
Dipsogenesis
Aldosterone secretion
Inhibition of Na^+ reabsorption

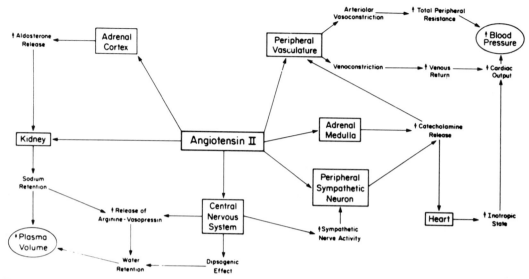

FIG. 4. Role of the renin-angiotensin-aldosterone system in regulation of arterial blood pressure and plasma volume. (From ref. 21.)

rone, a steroid with powerful sodium-retaining properties, also contributing to blood pressure elevation (Fig. 4).

THE VASCULAR WALL RAS

In addition to plasma renin originating from kidneys, there are other sources of renin including brain, heart, adrenals, and blood vessels (see [24,25] for review). With respect to this review, only arterial vascular wall renin will be considered.

The complete RAS can be found in vascular smooth muscle. Vascular renin is synthesized in cultured endothelial and smooth muscle cells, and immunoreactive angiotensinogen as well as AI, AII, and AIII can be measured intracellularly (24). Nonetheless, the source of arterial renin remains controversial. Although many investigators agree that the generation of AII by renin within the vascular wall is probably an important step in the development and maintenance of hypertension, others (26) have argued that the source of renin for this ac-

tivity is probably renal in origin. They have pointed out that renin infusions result in increases in arterial renin and, furthermore, that changes in arterial renin parallel those of plasma renin, results different from those of other investigators (28). Angiotensin release by vascular smooth muscle cells may have important influences on autocrine, paracrine, and perhaps even endocrine function. It has been suggested that peripheral tissues contribute significantly to plasma levels of AI and AII (28). Most evidence suggests that vascular AII may play an important role in the development and maintenance of hypertension. Vascular renin levels are elevated in both renal and spontaneously hypertensive rats, whereas plasma renin activity (PRA) is normal in the chronic stages of the former, and throughout the life span of the latter (see [29–31]). In DOCA-salt hypertension, vascular renin levels are either reduced or normal, but never reach the very low levels of plasma renin in this model (32–34). Furthermore, vascular renin levels are appropriately responsive to various manipulations because they increase with either captopril administration or salt depletion, and decrease with salt loading (30–37). If the vascular RAS were functional, it could contribute to hypertension development and/or maintenance in at least two ways: (a) by a direct vasoconstrictor action of AII on vascular smooth muscle, and (b) facilitation of sympathetic function by increasing the release of NE in the vasculature. Thus, a link is established between the RAS and sympathetic nervous system. PRA is responsible for the increase in blood pressure when it is high (as in the initial phase of renal hypertension) by a direct vasoconstrictor action on vascular smooth muscle as well as by facilitating sympathetic function. However, when PRA is normal, but the vascular RAS is hyperactive, as in both chronic renal and spontaneously hypertensive rats, PRA plays little role in the maintenance of hypertension, whereas the vascular RAS appears to be important in this regard.

It is also clear that the anatomical location of ACE is appropriate for it to have a regulatory role on sympathetic function in the vasculature. The presence of ACE at the adventitiomedial junction of arteries has been demonstrated using a histofluorescent technique (32). Velletri and Bean (38) provided direct biochemical evidence that approximately 58% of total vascular ACE activity was in the adventitia. Finally, Saye et al. (39) demonstrated that conversion of AI to AII was unimpaired in arteries without epithelial cells, only slower. All of the above provided further evidence that vascular ACE is appropriately located (the adventitiomedial border of the arterial wall in close apposition to vascular noradrenergic nerves) to have an important local role in regulating sympathetic function, and it is this ACE, as opposed to plasma ACE, that is important for the antihypertensive action of ACE inhibitors. Hence, drugs interfering with sympathetic function or the synthesis of AII are effective antihypertensives in these models of hypertension.

Furthermore, one might anticipate that, if the vascular RAS affected sympathetic neurotransmission, a drug such as the ACE inhibitor captopril might have an inhibitory effect on responses to sympathetic nerve stimulation and, further, that this inhibition would be preferentially prejunctional and specific for vascular sympathetic responses. Such an inhibitory effect of ACE inhibitors on vascular sympathetic nerve function has been clearly demonstrated by several investigators (40–44). It is important to note that, in those models of hypertension in which the vascular RAS is either normal or reduced such as one kidney renal or one kidney DOCA-salt hypertension, inhibition of ACE by captopril in both these models of hypertension has no significant inhibitory effect on pressor responses to sympathetic nerve stimulation, providing further evidence that an overactive vascular RAS is necessary for a facilitatory role on the sympathetic nervous system. Further support of this concept is provided by the finding that ACE inhibition can also inhibit AII release by vascular tissue (45) and that the antihypertensive effects of ACE inhibitors are much better correlated with inhibition of vascular ACE than plasma ACE (46–51). The potential interactions of the plasma and vascular RAS, sympathetic nerves releasing NE and ACE inhibitors are shown schematically in Fig. 5.

The potential autocrine and paracrine effects of vascular angiotensin have also been proposed (28,52). With respect to blood vessels, the vasoconstricting effects of locally synthesized AII have been discussed. In addition, AII can influence vascular smooth muscle both by a direct growth stimulating effect (53) and an indirect effect by virtue of its ability to facilitate sympathetic activation (54).

Because AII causes an increase in the synthesis of prostaglandins, vascular tone may also be influenced differentially depending on the various contributions of the pressor actions of AII and the dilator ac-

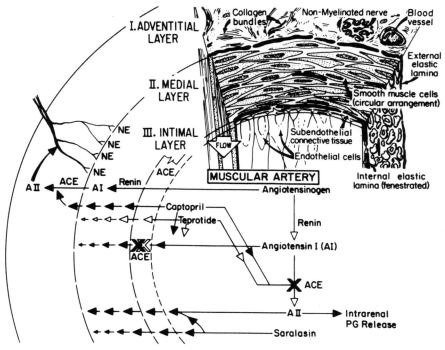

FIG. 5. Schematic representation of an artery showing the proposed interaction of the RAS with the sympathetic noradrenergic system. Renin, either from the plasma or arterial wall, converts angiotensinogen to AI, which is subsequently converted to AII by ACE and facilitates sympathetic function. Blockade of AI formation inhibits sympathetic function by preventing the AII facilitation.

tions of the prostaglandins (25). In fact, the heterogeneity of AII on vascular responsiveness is well documented, having contractile effects on femoral, carotid, and coronary arteries but relaxing canine renal arteries through stimulation of endothelium-mediated prostacyclin synthesis (25,55).

INHIBITORS OF THE RAS

Renin Inhibitors

Agents specifically designed to be renin inhibitors can be classified under the following headings:

1. renin antibodies,
2. renin substrate and pepstatin analogs,
3. renin prosegment analogs.

Renin Antibodies

Studies with antibodies against renin constitute some of the oldest and least satisfying approaches to inhibition of the RAS from the therapeutic standpoint. Although early studies with antisera to kidney extracts were promising in that they inhibited development of hypertension in response to renal ischemia (56), subsequent studies produced variable and conflicting results (57). This was probably mainly due to lack of specificity of the preparations used because the immunogens contained less than 1% of the enzyme (58). Now that renins of various species have been purified to homogeneity, production of specific antibodies has allowed a clearer delineation of the effects of these agents in whole animal preparations.

Goat antibody to purified dog renin was found to be very effective in decreasing blood pressure of normotensive Na^+-depleted dogs as well as one-kidney, one-clip hypertensive dogs but having no effect on sodium-depleted dogs (59). In addition, the reduction in blood pressure was parallel with a reduction in both plasma renin activity and AII levels indicating a specific effect of the antibody on renin. Recently, monoclonal antibodies to specific human renin have been produced (59). These antibodies inhibited human renin but not that of dog, ox, hog, rat, and mouse. Although the use of specific monoclonal antibodies will be useful in understanding substrate interactions, the role of renin in hypertension, etc., the probability of their utility as drugs is small, and no further reference will be made to them in this chapter.

RENIN SUBSTRATE AND PEPSTATIN ANALOGS

Most effort in the design of renin inhibitors for potential therapeutic use has revolved around analogs of the renin substrate angiotensinogen. Determination of the human angiotensinogen amino acid sequence revealed that it differed from the horse, rat, and pig enzyme in that the scissile peptide bond is Leu-Val rather than Leu-Leu (Table 3). In Table 3, the amino acids flanking the scissile peptide bond are described conventionally (60), with P_1-P_n referring to those amino acids on the N-terminal side and P_1-P_n referring to those on the C-terminal side. There are species differences between the sequences on the C-

terminal side, but the sequence on the N-terminal side, corresponding to angiotensin I, is highly conserved. Human renin will cleave human and other mammalian substrates, but only human renin will cleave the human substrate.

Peptide Inhibitors of Renin

Inhibitors specific to renin have been made by preparing peptide fragments of the natural substrate centered on the scissile peptide bond and modifying them in such a way as to render them able to bind to the enzyme but unable to serve as substrates. In this way, renin inhibitory peptide (Table 3) was discovered. This compound was found to exhibit considerable selectivity for the renin of primates (61) ($IC_{50} = 2 \times 10^{-6}$ M vs human renin) and was effective in lowering blood pressure in animal models (61) and in humans (62).

Although the hypotensive effects of renin inhibitory peptide were short-lived, these results prompted a search for more potent, more specific, and more metabolically stable substrate analogs. This search has been heavily influenced by the transition-state analog inhibitor hypothesis (63–65), which states that stable structures resembling transition states for an enzyme reaction will be bound more tightly than the substrate for the enzyme-catalyzed reaction. The transition state for hydrolysis by aspartyl protease is generally assumed to resemble the tetrahedral species generated in this process and much synthetic effort has therefore been directed toward the syntheses of pseudopeptides in which the scissile bond

TABLE 3. *Peptide inhibitors of renin*

					P_6	P_5	P_4	P_3	P_2	P_1	Renin	P_1'	P_2'	P_3'
	1	2	3	4	5	6	7	8	9	10		11	12	13
Human substrate	Asp-	Arg-	Val-	Tyr-	Ile-	His-	Pro-	Phe-	His-	Leu	–	Val-	Ile-	His
Canine substrate	Asp-	Arg-	Val-	Tyr-	Ile-	His-	Pro-	Phe-	His-	Leu	–	Leu-	Val-	Tyr
RIP					Pro-	His-	Pro-	Phe-	His-	Phe	–	Phe-	Val-	Tyr- Lys

RIP, renin inhibitory peptide.

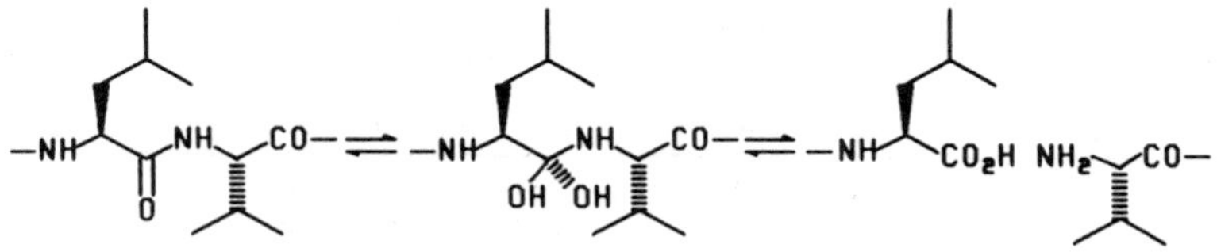

FIG. 6. Renin-catalyzed cleavage of Leu-Val scissile bond of renin substrate.

region of substrate sequences is occupied by a group resembling the tetrahedral species, shown as a partial structure in Fig. 6.

Modified Peptides Containing Statine

Pepstatin (Table 4) is a nonspecific aspartyl protease inhibitor exhibiting exceptionally high potency against members of this family of enzymes, except for renin, against which it is relatively weak. Pepstatin contains the unusual amino acid statine (Fig. 7) that, it has been proposed (66), confers on pepstatin the property of a transition-state analog inhibitor in which statine serves as a transition-state insert. Evidence supporting this hypothesis comes from ^{13}C NMR studies on pepstatin analogs bound to pepsin (67) and by an x-ray study of pepstatin analogs bound to an aspartyl protease from *Rhizopus chinensus* (68). Using an approach based on molecular modeling, Boger et al. proposed (69) that statine may be acting in pepstatin as a dipeptide isostere. In order to exploit this property in the design of renin inhibitors, the Leu-Val dipeptide moiety at the site of bond cleavage was replaced in some human renin substrate sequences

with statine, producing the potent inhibitors *4* and *5* (Table 4).

The modified pseudoheptapeptide statine-containing renin inhibitory peptide (Table 4) is a potent and competitive inhibitor of renin and is selective for renin over other aspartyl proteases (69,70). It is effective in animal models when administered intravenously (71) but has a short duration of action. More recently the highly potent *6* (Table 4) was reported (72).

A requirement for any renin inhibitor that is to be used in the chronic treatment of hypertension is a much longer duration of action than that of either *1* or *4*. Although considerable progress has been made in stabilizing this class of molecules toward proteolysis, it is clear that this is a necessary but not sufficient requirement. An example is provided by the properties of *7* (Table 4), which is short acting although demonstrably stable to proteolysis as a result of the presence in the molecule of two unnatural amino acids, statine and D-proline, and of protecting groups on both terminal amino acids (73). The short duration of action in this case was attributed to biliary excretion. This is not an uncommon excretion pathway for molecules with molecular weights greater than 300 (74).

Similar modifications were, however, successful in producing the prolonged duration of action, relative to unprotected analogs, observed with CGP-29287 (*8*, Table 4) (75). CGP-29287 was also shown to be active when administered by the oral route. However, the magnitude of the hypotensive effect was approximately one thousandth of that observed when it was administered intravenously. Another renin inhibitor that

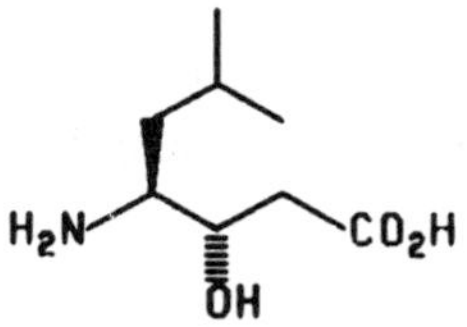

3

FIG. 7. The unusual amino acid statine (Sta).

TABLE 4. *Renin inhibitors containing statine*

		P_6	P_5	P_4	P_3	P_2	P_1P_1'	P_2'	P_3'	IC_{50} (nM) Human renin
2	Pepstatin			Iva -	Val -	Val -	Sta -Ala	-Sta	- OH	22,000
4	SCRIP		Iva - His -	Pro -	Phe -	His -	Sta -Ile	- Phe	- NH$_2$	16
5			Iva - His -	Pro -	Phe -	His -	Sta -Leu	- Phe	- NH$_2$	13
6			Trp(in-Fm) -	Pro -	Phe -	His -	Sta -Val	- Trp(in-Fm)	- NH$_2$	0.38
7			Iva - His - (D)Pro -		Phe -	His -	Sta -Leu	- NH	- Bn	150
8	CGP-29287	Z-Arg - Arg -		Pro -	Phe -	His -	Sta -Ile	- His	- Lys(Boc)OCH$_3$	1.0
9				Iva -	Phe -	Nle -	Sta -Ala	- Sta	- OH	28
10				Boc -	Leu -	His -	Sta -Ile	- NH	- PM	1.7
11	ES-254			Z -	Nal -	His -	Sta -MBA			450
12	ES-305				BNMA -	His -	Sta -MBA			2.4
13				Boc -	Phe -	Phe -	Sta -AHPHA			31
14					Boc -	His -	Sta -Leu	- (ω-lysinol)		2.4

Iva, isovaleryl; Ile, isoleucine; BN, $-CH_2$-Ph; Z, benzyloxycarbonyl; Boc, t-butoxycarbonyl; Nle, norleucine; Nal, naphthylalanine; MBA, 2S-methylbutylamide; BNMA, *bis*(1-naphthyl)methylacetyl; iBu, isobutyl; PM, 2-pyridylmethyl; Sta, statine; SCRIP, statine-containing renin inhibitory peptide.

appears to have an unusually long duration is SR 42128 (*9,* Table 4). SR 42128 is a pepstatin analog in which selectivity for renin has been achieved in large part through replacement, by phenylalanine, of the valine moiety in pepstatin thought to be recognized by the S_3 subsite. The presence of two statine units and a protecting group on the N-terminal amino acid apparently imparts metabolic stability to SR 42128, and significant blood pressure lowering in sodium-depleted conscious monkeys is evident 3 hr after an intravenous dose of 10 mg/kg (76).

An important stimulus to the development of therapeutically useful, low molecular weight inhibitors of renin was the discovery of potent activity associated with the tripeptide aldehyde (77) in which the amino acids of the substrate sequence on the C-terminal side of the scissile bond have been deleted. This finding, together with the activity of some related compounds (78), showed that interaction with S_2 and S_3 subsites was not a requirement for potent inhibition. In contrast, it was found in this compound series that recognition of the S_3 subsite with an aromatic amino acid at the P_3 position was required for potent inhibitory activity to be expressed. The naphthyl group at the P_3 position was found to be superior to the phenyl group in that respect. Replacement, by the same work-

ers, of the leucinal moiety at the C-terminal of ES 188 (*30*) with statine methylbutylamide resulted in a less potent compound, ES-254 (*11,* Table 4) (79). More recently, they have replaced the protected naphthylalanine residue with the highly lipophilic acyl group BNMA (*bis*(1-naphthyl) methylacetyl) to provide a modified dipeptide, ES-305 (*12,* Table 4), a renin inhibitor with an IC_{50} in the nanomolar range (80). Neither ES-254 nor ES-305 has significant activity by the oral route of administration.

A related compound ES-1005 (*14*) is more potent than ES-254 and ES-305 against non-primate renins while retaining its good potency against the human enzyme (81).

In an attempt to produce an inhibitor resistant to proteolysis, two statine-like dipeptide isosteres have been incorporated into the same molecule, *13* (Table 4) (82). The potency of this compound suggests that replacement of the Leu-Phe dipeptide residue by the isostere 2-benzylstatine (AHPHA, notes to Table 4) is acceptable and possibly beneficial in imparting metabolic stability to the molecule.

Renin Inhibitors Containing Modified Statine Moieties

The aldehyde *30* is believed to derive its inhibitory properties from the transformation by enzyme-catalyzed hydration, at the active site of the enzyme, into a tetrahedral species resembling the transition state for the proteolytic step. It has also been found that an analog of pepstatin in which the internal statine moiety was replaced by the corresponding ketone (statone) can function similarly (83,84). In a recent report (85), it was shown that when the statone moiety was incorporated into a renin substrate sequence, the product 15 (Fig. 8) was a weaker inhibitor than the corresponding statine-containing compound 10. However, it was found that incorporation into the same peptide of the fluorinated analog of statone resulted in a considerable enhancement of potency for the resulting modified pseudotetrapeptide 16 (Fig. 8). This result is consistent with the expected stabilization of the tetrahedral species resulting from fluorine substitution (86).

A series of alkyl-substituted statines was

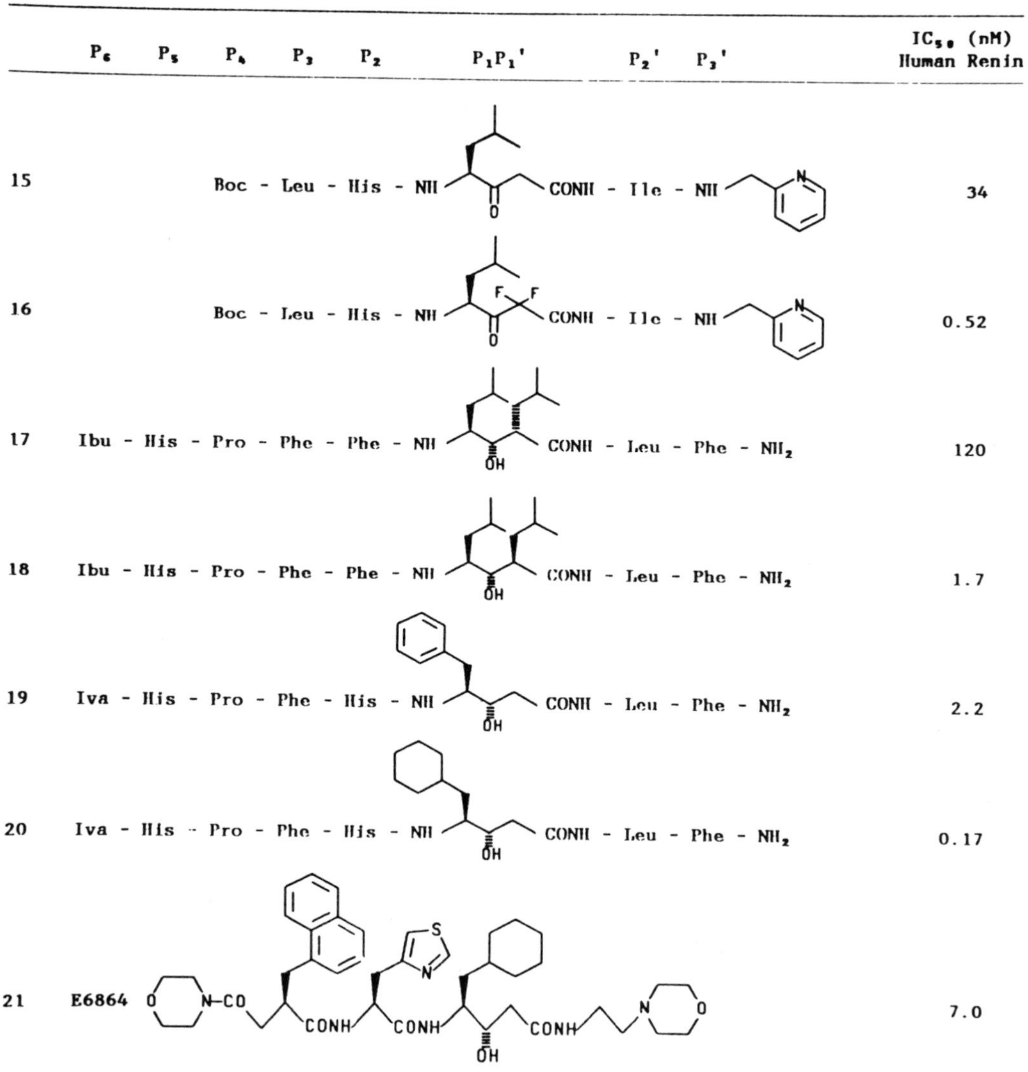

FIG. 8. Renin inhibitors containing modified statine moieties.

incorporated into the pseudoheptapeptides *17* and *18* (Fig. 8) in order to exploit the postulated role of statine as a dipeptide isostere by increasing the degree of hydrophobic interaction at the S_1 subsite (87). Modeling predicted successfully that the 2(R)-alkylstatine analog *18* (Fig. 8) would be more potent than the 2(S)-alkyl analog *17*, but although a more potent compound, it was only slightly more potent than the analog in which the statine was unsubstituted. Further modeling studies by the same group based on the x-ray structure of the rhizopuspepsin-pepstatin complex led to the design of a novel cyclohexylalanine analog of statine (3S,4S-4-amino-3-hydroxy-5-cyclohexylpentanoic acid [ACHPA]) (88), which would, it was predicted, upon incorporation into known inhibitor sequences at the scissile bond region, fit more closely than statine into the hydrophobic pocket that recognizes the statine side-chain methyl groups. This was found to be the case with *20* (Fig. 8), being much more potent than the statine-containing counterpart *5* (Fig. 8) and the phenyl analog *19*.

This incremental increase in *in vitro* potency extends into the *in vivo* situation, with compound *20* being 19 times as potent as *5* in lowering the blood pressure of sodium-deficient dogs when administered by infusion. This result correlates well with the 17-fold greater potency of *20* against dog renin.

One of the most promising renin inhibitors prepared to date, ES-6864 (*21*, Fig. 8), also contains the ACHPA (cyclostatin) moiety. ES-6864 is highly potent, renin specific, and long-acting *in vivo*. Plasma concentrations of ES-6864 in conscious marmosets administered 30 mg/kg reached 1.2 μg/ml at 1 hr, although it was not detected when administered orally at 3 mg/kg. The same dose in sodium-depleted marmosets produced significant blood pressure reduction and almost complete inhibition of PRA. There was no significant increase in heart rate (89).

Transition-State or Intermediate Analogs

In early successful attempts to design transition-state analog or intermediate analog inhibitors of renin (90,91), Szelke et al. incorporated into renin substrate sequences the "reduced peptide" and "hydroxyethylene" dipeptide isosteres to produce potent inhibitors. In the inhibitors *22* and *23* (Fig. 9), the Leu-Val dipeptide flanking the scissile bond of a renin substrate sequence is, in concept, replaced by the transition-state insert Leu (CHNH Val) and in *24* (Fig. 9), the insert is Leu (CHOHCH$_2$)Val. These inhibitors are effective in animal models of hypertension when given intravenously. H-142 (*23*) has been tested in humans (92) and was shown to cause a modest drop in blood pressure of 10 mm Hg with an infusion rate of 17 μg/kg/min.

A cyclohexyl variant of the "reduced peptide" dipeptide isostere was recently reported by Plattner (93) and co-workers who found *26* (Fig. 9) to be approximately 10-fold more potent than the corresponding compound *25* containing the original parent isostere. A further enhancement of potency was associated with the 2-methylbutylamide modification at the C-terminal amino acid in *27* (Fig. 9). A series of cyclohexyl variants of the "hydroxyethylene" transition-state insert has been reported (94), of which *28* (Fig. 9) was one of the most potent inhibitors.

Compound *29* (Fig. 9) appears to represent a significant advance in the search for an orally effective renin inhibitor. By modifying the proteolytically most susceptible peptide linkage (Phe-His) in an inhibitory pseudopentapeptide by N-methylation so as to render the linkage metabolically stable, and by employing the Leu (CHOHCH$_2$)Val dipeptide isostere as the transition-state insert, Thaisrivongs and co-workers (95) succeeded in the synthesis of the long-acting, highly potent, and selective renin inhibitor U-71,039. A comparison of the results obtained after the intravenous administration of U-71,039 with the results obtained after

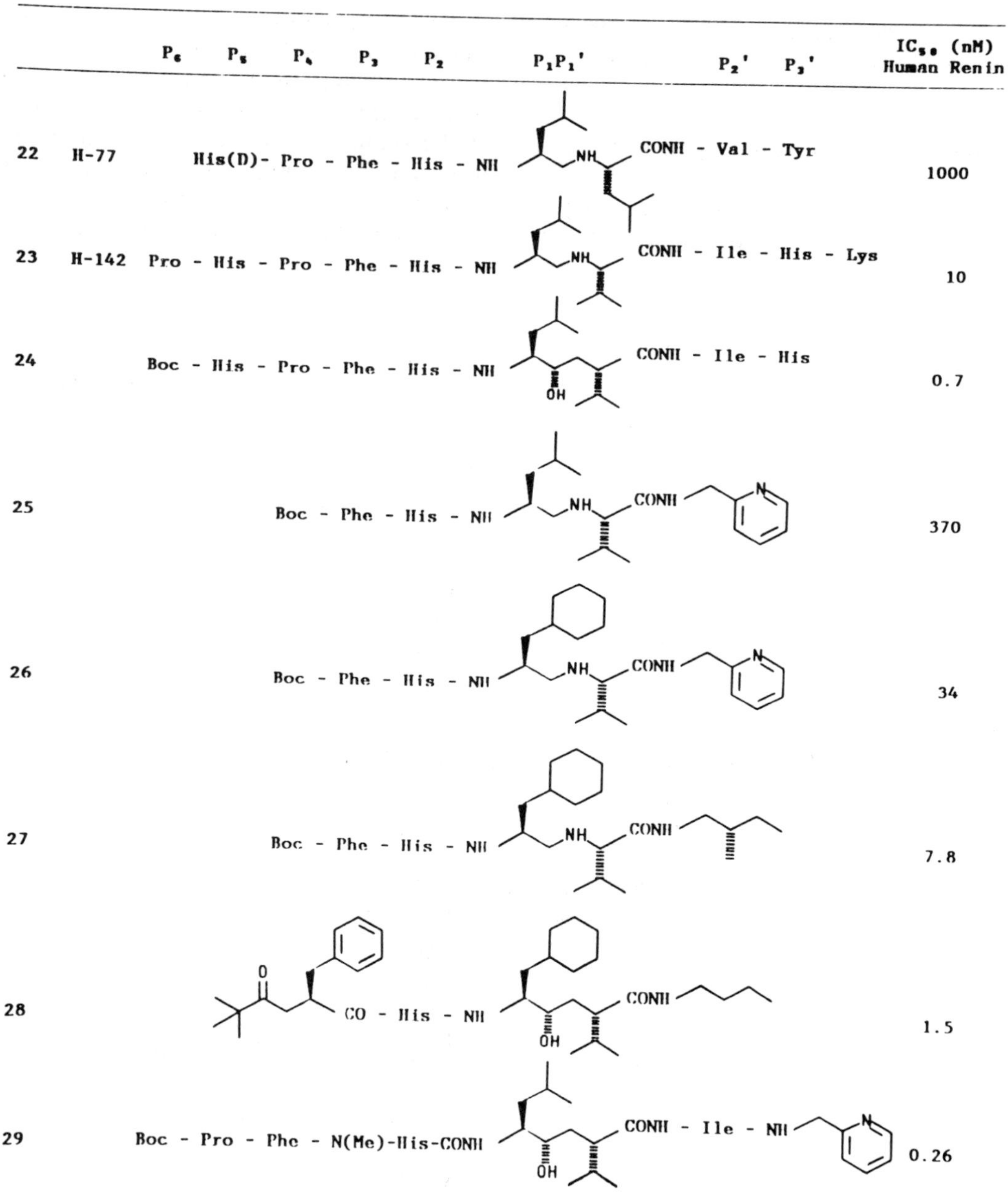

FIG. 9. Transition-state or intermediate analog renin inhibitors.

the oral administration of U-71,039 to hog renin-infused rats and sodium-depleted monkeys implied that at least 10% of the orally administered compound had been absorbed (96). Oral administration of U-71,039 at 50 mg/kg to conscious sodium-depleted monkeys elicited a pronounced hypotensive effect and a decrease in PRA that persisted for 5 hr. It will be interesting to learn if the insertion of a cyclohexyl variant of the "hydroxyethylene" dipeptide isostere present in *29* provides any advantage over *29* in potency or in efficiency of absorption from the gastrointestinal tract.

Renin Inhibitors Containing Novel Moieties

The aldehyde *30* (Fig. 10) is not very effective *in vivo* due presumably to metabolic reduction to the much less potent alcohol. The diol *31* (Fig. 10) was prepared (97) as a potential mimic of the tetrahedral hydrate of an aldehyde group having increased metabolic stability. Although a weak inhibitor, it does possess a high selectivity for human renin versus rat renin or pepsin.

The potent renin inhibitor KRI-1230 (*32*,

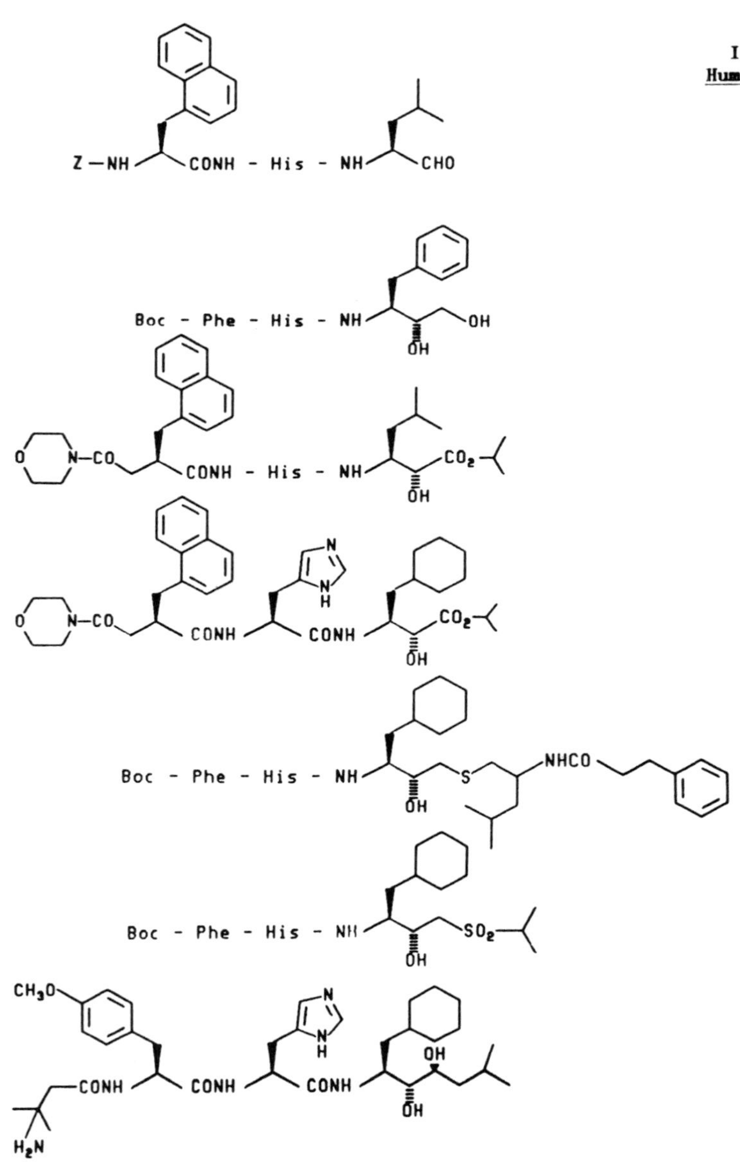

		IC_{50} (nM) Human Renin
30		80
31		2600
32	KRI-1230	7.8
33	KRI-1314	
34		7.0
35		2.0
36	A64662	14

FIG. 10. Renin inhibitors containing novel moieties corresponding to the scissile peptide bond.

Fig. 10) possesses some very interesting features (98,99). It has no peptide bonds and contains the ester of a lower homolog of statine. The corresponding statine-containing analog is considerably less potent ($IC_{50} = 66$ nM). KRI-1230 is stable to liver homogenate and is moderately active upon oral administration.

In common marmosets, the blood pressure drop after a 5-mg/kg injection was comparable with that of an oral dose of 30 mg/kg. In the latter case, the effect was long-lasting. A structurally related compound, KRI-1314 (33, Fig. 11), dose-dependently lowered mean blood pressure in Goldblatt hypertensive marmosets for 5 hr at oral doses of 3 and 10 mg/kg (100).

A series of novel inhibitors were reported recently of which 34 (Fig. 10) is one of the more potent examples (101). A novel feature is that comparison with renin substrate suggests that the isobutyl side-chain may interact with the S_2 subsite. Related compounds including 35 (Fig. 10) have been re-

ported by the same group (102). In both series, compounds containing transition-state inserts having a cyclohexylmethyl side-chain are considerably more potent than those containing an isobutyl side-chain at the same P_1 position. Both series exhibit excellent selectivity for human renin. In a salt-depleted monkey model, an intravenous bolus dose of 1 mg/kg of 34 produced a blood pressure drop comparable in magnitude, but not in duration, with that produced by 0.1 mg/kg of captopril (103). Mean arterial pressure returned to baseline within 30 min after administration of 34. The short half-life is probably the result of instability toward proteases.

The Abbott group also developed compound A-64662 (36, Fig. 10) (104) in which a dihydroxy species serves as the dipeptide isostere. This compound was evaluated initially in normotensive patients, and it was reported that intravenous infusion of A-64662 at 10 to 100 µg/kg reduced PRA and AII levels with concomitant increases

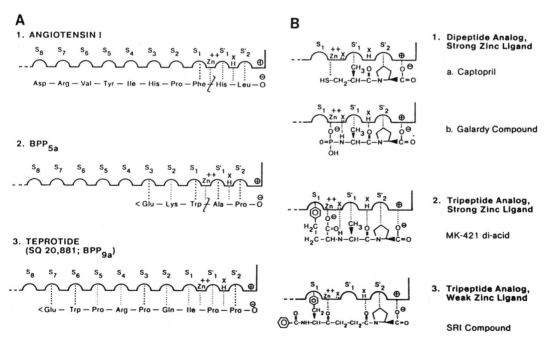

FIG. 11. Hypothetical model of ACE and suggested binding of substrates and inhibitors **(A)** and peptide analog inhibitors **(B)** of the enzyme. S′, obligatory binding site; S, additional binding site.

in active renin and total renin levels (T. Perun, *personal communication*).

Compounds have been placed in Table 4 and Figs. 8 through 10 for convenience, although mechanistically they are probably very closely related. It has been proposed (105) that inhibitors containing statine or the "hydroxyethylene" dipeptide isostere act similarly, functioning more as collected substrate rather than transition-state analog inhibitors, and, on structural grounds, it is likely that most compounds in Table 4 and Figs. 8 through 10 are acting in the same way.

Cyclic Analogs of Renin Substrate

Conformational studies on renin substrate in which a β-turn involving residues 6–9 was proposed (106) led to the design of conformationally restricted analogs having K_i values comparable with the K_m in value for hydrolysis of the natural substrate (107). Related compounds were shown to have a duration of action no longer than the noncyclic analogs (108).

The rapid progress being made in the synthesis of selective, low molecular weight substrate analogs having nanomolar or even subnanomolar inhibitory potencies against renin, together with advances in our capability to protect these molecules from proteolysis augers well for the discovery in the near future of agents that will be effective upon oral administration and suitable for chronic use in humans.

RENIN PROSEGMENT ANALOGS

The primary structure of human pre-prorenin includes a 46 amino acid prosegment shown below. This compound has an IC_{50} value of 3×10^{-4} M (109). A series of small peptides based on the prosegment N-terminal have been shown to inhibit human plasma renin.

Boc-Leu-Lys-Arg-Met-Pro-OCH$_3$

Similar results were found with mouse submaxillary renin (107).

Other reviews of progress in the development of renin inhibitors have been published recently (110–113).

ACE

ACE is a membrane-bound metalloexopeptidase, a peptidyldipeptide carboxyhydrolase (EC 3.4.15.1) that splits off dipeptides from the C-terminal end of peptide substrates (for reviews, see [114–117]). In addition to AI and bradykinin, many other peptides such as leu- and met-enkephalin with widely varying terminal amino acid sequences may serve as substrates for, or inhibitors of, ACE. However, its primary physiological function appears to be connected to its cleavage of the C-terminal dipeptide His-Leu from AI to give AII, and its inactivation of hypotensive kinins by cleavage of the C-terminal dipeptide Phe-Arg.

ACE inhibitors are very effective agents for reducing blood pressure. Their antihypertensive action apparently is derived from their ability to prevent the conversion of AI to AII in the circulation. However, evidence supports the concept that excessive local vascular formation of AII is important in the maintenance of hypertension (see above) and that inhibition of vascular AII formation by ACE inhibitors is important in reducing this hypertension. Several investigators have demonstrated that the antihypertensive effects of ACE inhibitors are much better correlated with inhibition of vascular ACE than plasma ACE (118–121). In these studies, blood pressure and vascular ACE activity remained depressed after immediate cessation of ACE inhibitor therapy, whereas plasma ACE returned quickly to control levels.

As described above, it is also clear that the anatomical location of ACE is appropriate for it to have a regulatory role on sympathetic function in the vasculature. This important local role of ACE in regulating blood pressure, as opposed to plasma ACE, may be critically important for the prolonged antihypertensive action of ACE inhibitors. This proposal has been supported by several reports that indicate that ACE inhibition results in reductions of pressor responses to sympathetic nerve stimulation and NE (122–124).

ACE INHIBITORS

The search for an orally active inhibitor of converting enzyme intensified when the clinical efficacy of a known ACE inhibitor, the nonapeptide teprotide, was demonstrated. The amino acid sequence of ACE is not yet known, and the initial design of synthetic inhibitors of the enzyme was

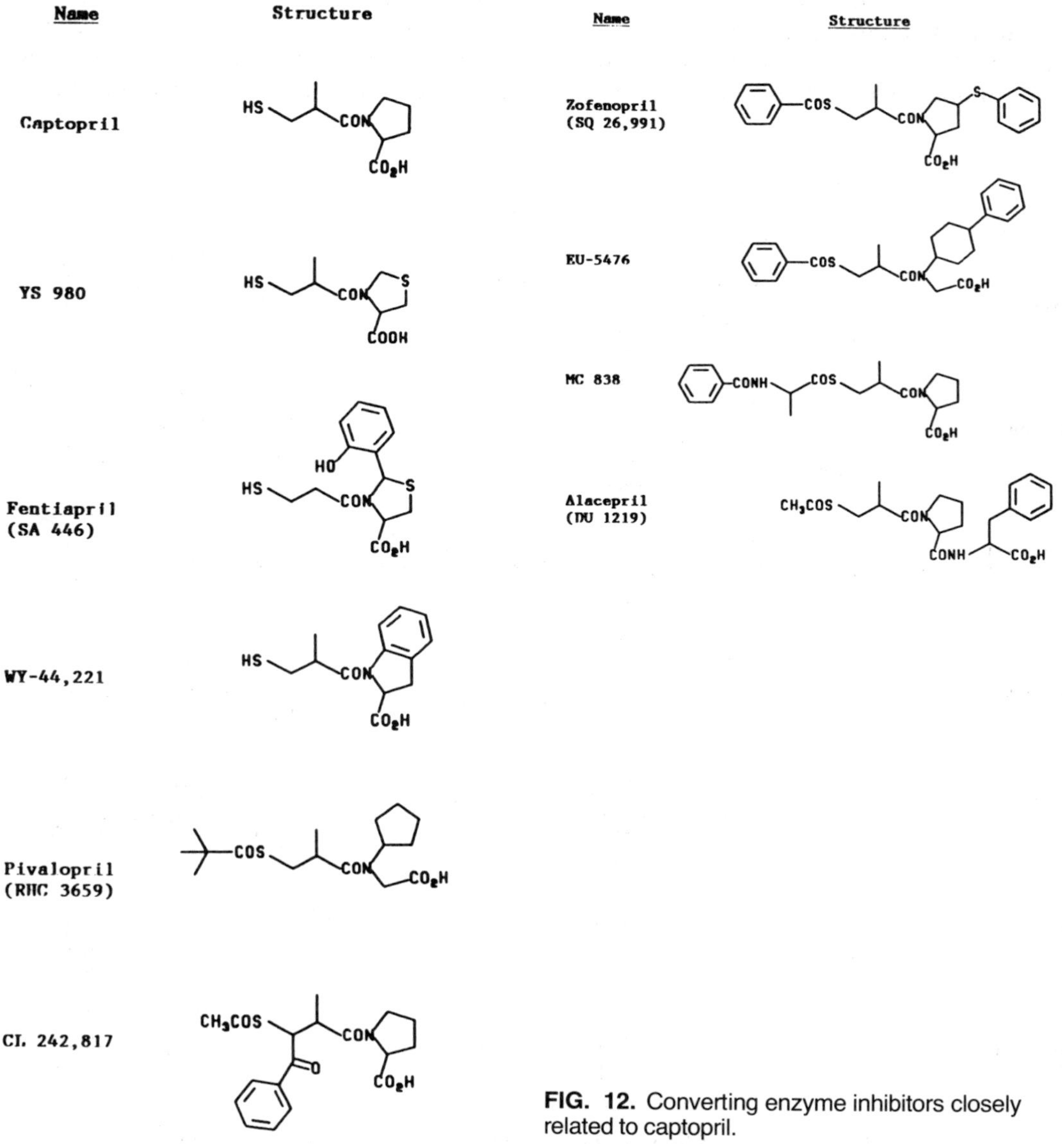

FIG. 12. Converting enzyme inhibitors closely related to captopril.

based on presumed similarities between ACE and the better understood metalloprotease carboxypeptidase A. It was hypothesized that ACE also had Zn^{2+} positioned at the active site to assist in cleavage of the scissile peptide bond. Initial studies were based on the discovery by Byers and Wolfendon (125) that R-2-benzylsuccinic acid was a potent competitive inhibitor of carboxypeptidase A, and the suggestion that the compound was acting as a collected product inhibitor. Modifications of this structure to adjust to the substrate specificity of ACE led eventually to the discovery of captopril (126). The history of its discovery, and subsequently that of enalapril, has been described in numerous reviews (114–117).

The salient features of captopril with respect to binding to ACE are (a) binding of the sulfhydryl to zinc, (b) binding of the proline carboxylic acid to a cationic site on the enzyme, and (c) incorporation of the amino acid proline and a methyl side-chain adjacent to proline. The suggested binding of captopril and other inhibitors to ACE is shown in Fig. 11. Other inhibitors of ACE very similar to captopril, which contain sulfhydryl moieties, and to enalapril, which does not, are shown in Figs. 12 and 13.

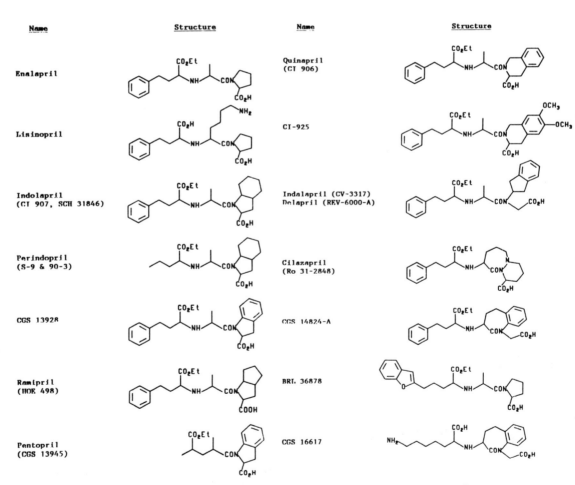

FIG. 13. Converting enzyme inhibitors closely related to enalapril.

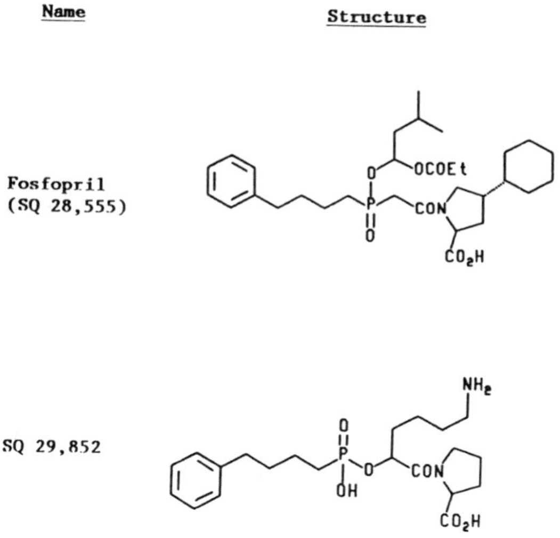

Name   Structure

Fosfopril
(SQ 28,555)

SQ 29,852

FIG. 14. Converting enzyme inhibitors containing phosphorus.

Structures of ACE inhibitors containing phosphorus are shown in Fig. 14. Detailed reviews on the design and proposed binding of newer ACE inhibitors can be found in several reviews (127–129).

HEMODYNAMIC EFFECTS OF ACE INHIBITORS

In every species tested, ACE inhibitors reduced blood pressure in both normotensives and hypertensives, although some differences in efficacy are apparent. As shown in Table 5, ACE inhibitors are very effective in animal models of hypertension. Similarly, ACE inhibitors are effective antihypertensive agents in human mild, moderate, severe, and severe treatment-refractory essential, malignant, and renal vascular hypertension, as well as hypertension caused by chronic renal failure, renal parenchymal disease, and renin-secreting tumors. They are least effective in primary aldosteronism in which PRA is very low. Their efficacy has been demonstrated in many open trials as well as in placebo controlled, double-blind studies. In virtually every study, the antihypertensive effect was enhanced by a

diuretic or a sodium-restricted diet. Although reductions in blood pressure are generally directly related to plasma renin levels, this is not always the case.

In animal and both human essential and renovascular hypertension, acute or chronic administration of ACE inhibitors consistently reduces blood pressure by reducing total peripheral resistance, while cardiac output remains either unchanged or increased (5). Similarly, pulmonary vascular resistance decreases after chronic but not acute ACE inhibitor therapy, suggesting both arterial and venous dilatation. Heart rate was unchanged in these patients.

The hemodynamic effects were significantly correlated to predrug PRA values or plasma AII levels in most studies but not all. Tarazi et al. (130) found that this correlation became much weaker after chronic therapy.

In most studies in animals and human essential hypertensive patients on an unrestricted-sodium diet, ACE inhibitors increased renal blood flow, while decreasing blood pressure, and had no effect on glomerular filtration rate (131,132). As a consequence, filtration fraction decreased. Urinary sodium excretion was unchanged, whereas potassium excretion was decreased.

In studies in hypertensive patients, ACE inhibitors had little or no effect on sodium or potassium excretion or on serum sodium or potassium levels (133,134). Some studies have reported a small but significant increase in serum potassium concentration due to decreases in aldosterone synthesis (135).

Although many ACE inhibitors are in clinical trials, only three are currently approved, namely, captopril, enalapril, and lisinopril. Despite the large number of ACE inhibitors now being tested, there seem to be no important distinguishing characteristic(s) from captopril or enalapril thus far in any of these compounds with respect to efficacy or side effects in the treatment of hypertension or CHF. This is not surprising given the specificity of these drugs for ACE

TABLE 5. *Effects of ACE inhibitors on blood pressure in various animal models of hypertension*

Model	Comments
A. Renal hypertension	
1. Two kidney, one clip	Effective in acute and chronic phase; prevents development
2. Two kidney, two clip	Effective in acute phase; prevents development
3. One kidney, one clip	Effective only after several days of dosing; does not prevent development
4. Two kidney, one wrap	Effective in acute phase
5. Two kidney, two wrap	Effective in acute phase
6. One kidney, one wrap	Effective in acute phase
7. One kidney, Grollman	Effective in acute phase
8. Aortic coarctation	Effective in acute phase
B. Genetic (SHR)	
1. Okamoto-Aoki strain	Modest effect acutely; normalization of blood pressure with chronic dosage; prevents development
2. New Zealand strain	Effective acute
3. Stroke-prone SHR	Greater reductions in blood pressure than in SHR; decreased incidence of stroke; prevents development
C. Steroid hypertension	
1. DOCA-salt	
a. Two kidney	Modest effect acutely
b. One kidney	Inactive
c. Heyman nephritis	Effective acutely
2. Methylprednisolone, two kidney, salt-depleted	Effective acutely
3. Aldosterone, one kidney	Effective after chronic treatment
D. All-salt hypertension	Effective after chronic treatment
E. Unilateral nephrectomy, salt depletion hypertension	Effective acutely; prevents development
F. Psychosocial hypertension	Not effective acutely but normalized blood pressure after 1–7 months

SHR, spontaneously hypertensive rats.

based on their design as described above. Most differences are based on such parameters as selective inhibition of ACE in various target organs (136), penetration in CSF/CNS areas (137), inhibition of sympathetic nerve function either in whole or nephrectomized animals, and in pharmacokinetic differences (138). Perhaps one exception to the pharmacological uniformity of ACE inhibitors has appeared recently. This is BW A575C, which is claimed, not surprisingly based on its structure, to have both ACE inhibitory and β-adrenoceptor antagonist properties (139). The IC_{50} for ACE was 10.7 ± 2.1 nM *cf.* 4.4 ± 0.8 nM for enaliprilat; the pKb against isoproterenol was 7.18 ± 0.05 *cf.* 8.9 ± 0.7 for pindolol. In rats, A575C inhibited AI-induced pressor responses as well isoproterenol-induced tachycardia; in dogs, the drug reduced

blood pressure and heart rate simultaneously, indicating good *in vivo* activity.

There are major differences in potency and pharmacokinetics within these series of ACE inhibitors, but they seem to be of little clinical importance. However, a curious twist to this subject was pointed out by Packer et al. (140) who concluded that large doses of long-acting ACE inhibitors in the treatment of CHF may produce prolonged hypotensive effects that may compromise cerebral and renal function and, therefore, may have disadvantages compared with short-acting agents.

AII ANTAGONISTS

The search for receptor antagonists of angiotensin has largely centered on peptide analogs of angiotensin itself. This has had

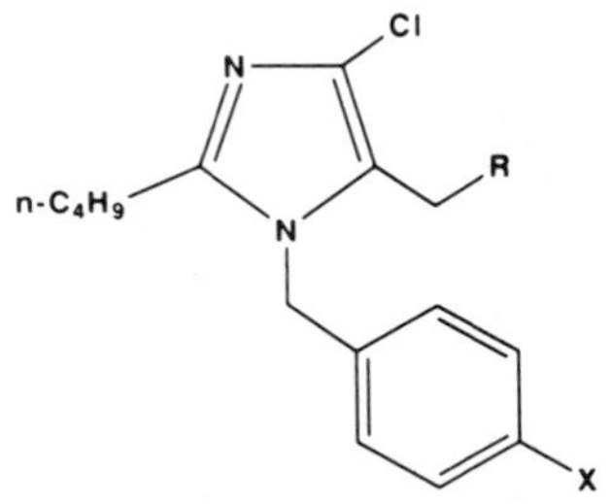

Compound	R	X
EXP6803	COOCH₃	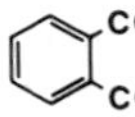 CONH– / COONa
EXP6155	COONa	COONa

FIG. 15. Chemical structures of EXP6155 and EXP6803. (From ref. 143.)

several drawbacks, the primary ones being partial agonist activity and lack of oral efficacy. Recently, however, several nonpeptidic-selective antagonists of angiotensin have been described. Originally, S-8307 and S-8308 were reported to be specific but weak angiotensin antagonists (141,142). Two newer agents, EXP6155 and EXP6803, have demonstrated reasonable potency and selectivity (143) (Fig. 15). These agents selectively blocked responses to AI and AII, but not to KCl, NE, bradykinin, or acetylcholine. In renal artery-ligated rats with elevated renin levels, both agents decreased blood pressure when administered intravenously (but not orally), with no discernible partial agonist activity. Whether clinically useful agents evolve from these prototypes remains to be seen.

ACKNOWLEDGMENT

The authors would like to acknowledge the efforts of Judi Frick who not only typed the manuscript but aided significantly in the editing of the text and references. Her stoicism and good humor during these trying times are gratefully appreciated.

REFERENCES

1. Tigerstedt R, Bergman PG. Niere und Kreislauf. *Scand Arch Physiol* 1898;8:223–271.
2. Goldblatt H, Lynch J, Hanzal R, Ranar F, Sumerville W. Studies on experimental hypertension. I. The production of persistent elevation of systolic blood pressure by means of renal ischemia. *J Exp Med* 1934;59:347–379.
3. Page F, Helmer O. A crystalline pressor substance resulting from the reaction between renin and renin activator. *J Exp Med* 1940;71:29–42.
4. Braun-Menendez E, Fasciolo J, LeLoir C, Mumoz J. La substancia hypertensora de la sangre del rinon isquiniado. *Rev Soc Argent Biol* 1939;15:420–425.
5. Antonaccio MJ. Angiotensin converting enzyme (ACE) inhibitors. *Annu Rev Pharmacol Toxicol* 1982;22:57–87.
6. Yang HYT, Erdos EG, Levin Y. A dipeptidyl carboxypeptidase that converts angiotensin I and inactivates bradykinin. *Biochim Biophys Acta* 1970;214:374–376.
7. Yokosowa H, Inagami T, Hass E. Purification of human renin. *Biochem Biophys Res Commun* 1978;83:306–312.
8. McIntire GD, Lecki B, Hallet A, Szelke M. Purification of human renin by affinity chromatography using a new peptide inhibitor of renin,

H.77 (D-His-Pro-Phe-His-Leu-Val-Tyr). *Biochem J* 1983;211:519–522.

9. Inagami T, Misono K, Chang JJ, Takii Y, Dykes C. Renin and general aspartyl proteases: differences and similarities in structure and function. In: Kostka V, ed. *Aspartic proteinases and their inhibitors.* Berlin: Walter de Gruyter, 1985;319–337.

10. Mathias CJ, May CN, Taylor GM. The renin-angiotensin system and hypertension—basic and clinical aspects. In: Malcolm ADB, ed. *Molecular medicine.* Oxford: IRL Press, 1984;177–208.

11. Dzau VJ, Burt DW, Pratt RE. Molecular biology of the renin-angiotensin system. *Am J Physiol* 1988;255:F563–F573.

12. Dzau VJ, Carlton JE, Brody T. Sequential changes in renin secretion-synthesis coupling in response to acute beta adrenergic stimulation (Abstract). *Clin Res* 1987;35:604A.

13. Ingelfinger JR, Pratt RE, Ellison KE, Dzau VJ. Sodium regulation of angiotensinogen mRNA expression in rat kidney cortex and medulla. *J Clin Invest* 1986;78:1311–1315.

14. Moffatt RB, McGowan RA, Gross KW. Modulation of kidney renin messenger RNA levels during experimentally induced hypertension. *Hypertension* 1986;8:874–882.

15. Nakamara N, Soubrier F, Menard J, Panthier JJ, Rougeon F, Corvol P. Nonproportional changes in plasma renin concentration, renal renin content, and rat renin messenger RNA. *Hypertension* 1985;7:855–859.

16. Sealey JE, Atlas SA. Inactive renin: speculations concerning its secretion and activation. *J Hypertens* 1984;2(Suppl 1):115–123.

17. Rougeon F, Chambrand B, Foote S, Panthier J-J, Nageotte R, Corvol P. Molecular cloning of a mouse submaxillary gland renin cDNA fragment. *Proc Natl Acad Sci USA* 1981;78:6367–6375.

18. Panthier J-J, Foote S, Chambraud D, Strosberg AD, Corvol P, Rougeon F. Complete amino acid sequence and maturation of the mouse submaxillary gland renin precursor. *Nature* 1982;298:90–92.

19. Misono KS, Chang JJ, Inagami T. Amino acid sequence of mouse submaxillary gland renin. *Proc Natl Acad Sci USA* 1982;79:4858–4862.

20. Atlas SA, Sealey JE, Laragh JH, Moon C. Plasma renin and "prorenin" in essential hypertension during sodium depletion, beta-blockade, and reduced arterial pressure. *Lancet* 1977;2:785–788.

21. Keeton TK, Campbell WB. Control of renin release and its alteration by drugs. In: Antonaccio MJ, ed. *Cardiovascular pharmacology.* New York: Raven Press, 1984;65–118.

22. Keeton TK, Campbell WB. The pharmacologic alteration of renin release. *Pharmacol Rev* 1980;32:81–227.

23. Kostis JB, DeFelice EA, Pianko LJ. The renin-angiotensin system. In: Kostis JB, DeFelice EA, eds. *Angiotensin converting enzyme inhibitors.* New York: Alan R Liss, 1987;1–18.

24. Dzau VJ. Significance of the vascular renin-angiotensin pathway. *Hypertension* 1986;8:553–559.

25. Dzau VJ. Vascular renin—angiotensin system in hypertension. New insights into the mechanism of action of angiotensin converting enzyme inhibitors. *Am J Med* 1988;84(Suppl 4A):4–8.

26. Swales JD, Heagerty AM. Vascular renin-angiotensin system: the unanswered questions. *J Hypertens* 1987;5:S1–S5.

27. Antonaccio MJ. The role of the vascular renin-angiotensin system on sympathetic function and vascular responsiveness. In: Bevan JA, Godfraind T, Maxwell RA, Stoclet JC, Worcel M, eds. *Vascular neuroeffector mechanisms.* Amsterdam: Elsevier, 1985;361–365.

28. Campbell DJ. The site of angiotensin production. *J Hypertens* 1985;3:199–207.

29. Antonaccio MJ, Wright JJ. Enzyme inhibitors of the renin-angiotensin system. In: Jucker D, ed. *Progress in drug research,* vol 31. Basel: Birkhauser Verlag, 1987;161–191.

30. Okamura T, Miyazaki M, Inagami T, Toda N. Vascular renin-angiotensin system in two-kidney, one clip hypertensive rats. *Hypertension* 1986;8:560–565.

31. Miyazaki M, Okunishi H, Okamura T, Toda N. Elevated vascular angiotensin converting enzyme in chronic two-kidney, one clip hypertension in the dog. *J Hypertens* 1987;5:155–160.

32. Swales JD, Abramovici A, Beck F, Bing RF, Loudon M, Thurston H. Arterial wall renin. *J Hypertens* 1983;1(Suppl 1):17–22.

33. Antonaccio MJ, Asaad M, Rubin B, Horowitz ZP. Captopril: factors involved in the mechanism of action. In: Horowitz ZP, ed. *Angiotensin converting enzyme inhibitors.* Baltimore: Urban and Schwarzenberg, 1981;161–180.

34. Grinspon DO, Basso N, Ruiz P, Mangiarua E, Taquini AC. Renin-like activity in vascular tissue of DOC-salt hypertensive rats. *Clin Exper Theory Practice* 1985;A7:1269–1282.

35. Thurston H, Swales JD, Bing RF, Hurst BC, Biol M, Marks ES. Vascular renin-like activity and blood pressure maintenance in the rat: studies of the effect of changes in sodium balance, hypertension and nephrectomy. *Hypertension* 1979;1:643–649.

36. Assad MM, Antonaccio MJ. Vascular wall renin in spontaneously hypertensive rats. Potential relevance to hypertension maintenance and antihypertensive effect of captopril. *Hypertension* 1982;4:487–493.

37. Barrett JD, Eggena P, Sambhi MP. Partial characterization of aortic renin in the spontaneously hypertensive rat and its interrelationship with plasma renin, blood pressure and sodium balance. *Clin Sci Mol Med* 1978;55:261–270.

38. Velletri P, Bean BL. Comparison of the time course of action of captopril on angiotensin-converting enzyme with the time course of its antihypertensive effect. *J Cardiovasc Pharmacol* 1981;3:1068–1081.

39. Saye J, Single HA, Peach MJ. Role of endothe-

lium in conversion of angiotensin I to angiotensin II in rabbit aorta. *Hypertension* 1984;6:216–221.

40. Antonaccio MJ, Kerwin L. Pre- and post-junctional inhibition of vascular sympathetic function by captopril in SHR. *Hypertension* 1981;3(Suppl 1):54–62.

41. Sybertz EJ, Sabin CS, Moran R. Influence of angiotensin converting enzyme inhibition with captopril on blood pressure and adrenergic function in normal and sodium restricted rats. *Clin Exp Hypertens* [A] 1981;3:1053–1073.

42. Hatton R, Clough DP. Captopril interferes with neurogenic vasoconstriction in the pithed rat by angiotensin-dependent mechanisms. *J Cardiovasc Pharmacol* 1982;4:116–123.

43. DeJong A, Knape J, VanMeel JCA, et al. Effect of captopril on sympathetic neurotransmission in pithed normotensive rats. *Eur J Pharmacol* 1983;88:231–240.

44. Atkinson J, Sonnay M, Sautel M, Fouda A-K. Chronic treatment of the spontaneously hypertensive rat with captopril attenuates responses to noradrenaline in vivo but not in vitro. *Naunyn Schmiedebergs Arch Pharmacol* 1987;335:624–628.

45. Mizuno K, Nakamaru M, Higashimori K, Inagami T. Local generation and release of angiotensin II in peripheral vascular tissue. *Hypertension* 1988;11:223–229.

46. Sweet CS, Arbegast PT, Gaul SL, Blaine HE, Gross DM. Relationship between angiotensin I blockade and antihypertensive properties of single doses of MK-421 and captopril in spontaneous and renal hypertensive rats. *Eur J Pharmacol* 1981;76:167–176.

47. Cohen ML, Kurz KD. Angiotensin converting enzyme inhibition in tissues from spontaneously hypertensive rats after treatment with captopril or MK-421. *J Pharmacol Exp Ther* 1982;220:63–69.

48. Unger R, Ganten D, Lang RE. Converting enzyme inhibitors: antihypertensive drugs with unexpected mechanisms. *Trends Pharmacol Sci* 1983;4:514–519.

49. Sakaguchi K, Jackson B, Chai SY, Mendelsohn FAO, Johnston CI. Effects of perindopril on tissue angiotensin-converting enzyme activity demonstrated by quantitative in vitro autoradiography. *J Cardiovasc Pharmacol* 1988;12:710–717.

50. Saki K, Shiraki Y, Akima M, et al. Tissue angiotensin-converting enzyme blockade by MC-838 (altiopril calcium) infused intravenously to miniature pigs: comparison with captopril. *Arch Int Pharmacodyn* 1988;294:228–240.

51. Nakamura Y, Nakamura K, Matsukura T, Nakamura K. Vascular angiotensin converting enzyme activity in spontaneously hypertensive rats and its inhibition with cilazapril. *J Hypertens* 1988;6:105–110.

52. Dzau VJ, Safar ME. Large conduit arteries in hypertension: role of the vascular renin-angiotensin system. *Circulation* 1988;77:947–954.

53. Campbell-Boswell M, Robertson AL. Effects of angiotensin II and vasopressin on human smooth cells in vitro. *Exp Mol Pathol* 1981;35:265–276.

54. Dzau VJ, Gibbons GH. Autocrine-paracrine mechanisms of vascular myocytes in hypertension. *Am J Cardiol* 1987;60:99I–103I.

55. Toda N. Endothelium-dependent relation induced by angiotensin II and histamine in isolated arteries of dog. *Br J Pharmacol* 1984;81:301–307.

56. Johnson CA, Wakerlin GE. Antiserum for renin. *Proc Soc Exp Biol Med* 1940;44:277–281.

57. Antonaccio MJ. Inhibitors of the renin-angiotensin system as new antihypertensive agents. *Clin Exp Hypertens* [A] 1982;4:27–46.

58. Haber E. Control of renin action: inhibitors and antibodies. In: Doyle AE, Bearn AG, eds. *Hypertension and the angiotensin system therapeutic approaches*. New York: Raven Press, 1984;133–154.

59. Dzau VJ, Kapelman RI, Barger AC, Slater AC, Haber E. Renin specific antibody for study of cardiovascular homeostasis. *Science* 1980;207:1091–1093.

60. Schechter I, Berger A. On the size of the active site in proteases. I. Papain. *Biochem Biophys Res Commun* 1967;27:157–162.

61. Burton J, Cody RJ Jr, Herd JA, Haber E. Specific inhibition of renin by an angiotensinogen analog: studies in sodium depletion and renin-dependent hypertension. *Proc Natl Acad Sci USA* 1980;77:5476–5479.

62. Zusman RM, Burton J, Christensen D, Nussberger J, Dodds A, Haber E. Hemodynamic effects of a competitive renin inhibitor peptide in humans: evidence for multiple mechanisms of action. *Trans Assoc Am Physicians* 1983;96:365–374.

63. Wolfenden R. Analog approaches to the structure of the transition state in enzyme reactions. *Acc Chem Res* 1972;5:10–18.

64. Wolfenden R. Transition-state affinity as a basis for the design of enzyme inhibitors. In: Gandour RD, Schowen RL, eds. *Transition states of biochemical processes*. New York: Plenum Press, 1978;555–578.

65. Lienhard GE. Enzymatic catalysis and transition-state theory. *Science* 1973;180:149–154.

66. Marciniszyn J Jr, Hartsuck JA, Tang J. Mode of inhibition of acid proteases by pepstatin. *J Biol Chem* 1976;251:7088–7094.

67. Schmidt PG, Bernatowicz MS, Rich DH. Pepstatin binding to pepsin. Enzyme conformation changes monitored by nuclear magnetic resonance. *Biochemistry* 1982;21:6710–6716.

68. Bott R, Subramanian E, Davies DR. Three-dimensional structure of the complex of the *rhizopus chinensis* carboxyl proteinase and pepstatin at 2.5 A resolution. *Biochemistry* 1982;21:6956–6962.

69. Boger J, Lohr NS, Ulm EH, et al. Novel renin inhibitors containing the amino acid statine. *Nature* 1983;303:81–84.

70. Boger J. Renin inhibitors. Design of angioten-

sinogen transition-state analogs containing statine. In: Hurby VK, Rich DJ, eds. *Peptides: structure and function. Proceedings of the Eighth American Peptide Symposium.* Rockford, IL: Pierce Chemical Co, 1983;569–578.

71. Blaine EH, Schorn TW, Boger J. Statine-containing renin inhibitor. Dissociation of blood pressure lowering and renin inhibition in sodium deficient dogs. *Hypertension* 1984; 6(Suppl I):I111–I118.

72. Sawyer TK, Pals DT, Smith CW, et al. "Transition state" substituted renin inhibitor peptides: structure-conformation-activity studies on NIN-formyl-TRP and TRP modified congeners. In: Deber CM, Hurby VJ, Kopple KD, eds. *Peptides—structure and function. Proceedings of the Ninth American Peptide Symposium.* Rockford, IL: Pierce Chemical Co., 1985;729–738.

73. Boger J, Bennett CD, Payne LS, et al. Design of proteolytically-stable, peptidal renin inhibitors and determination of their fate in vivo. *Regul Pept [Suppl]* 1985;4:8–13.

74. Klaassen CD, Watkins JB III. Mechanisms of bile formation, hepatic uptake and biliary excretion. *Pharmacol Rev* 1984;36:1–67.

75. Wood JM, Gulati N, Forgiarini P, Fuhrer W, Hofbauer KG. Effects of a specific and long-acting renin inhibitor in the marmoset. *Hypertension* 1985;7:797–803.

76. DeClaviere M, Cazaubon C, Lacour C, et al. In vitro and in vivo inhibition of human and primate renin by a new potent renin inhibitor: SR 42128. *J Cardiovasc Pharmacol* 1985;7(Suppl 4):858–861.

77. Kokubu T, Hiwada K, Sato Y, et al. Highly potent and specific inhibitors of human renin. *Biochem Biophys Res Commun* 1984;118:929–933.

78. Fehrentz JA, Heitz A, Castro B, Cazaubon C, Nisato D. Aldehydic peptides inhibiting renin. *FEBS Lett* 1984;167:273–276.

79. Kokubu T, Hiwada K, Murakami E, et al. Highly potent and specific inhibitors of human renin. *Hypertension* 1985;7(3 Pt 2):I8–I11.

80. Kokubu T, Hiwada K, Nagae A, et al. Statine-containing dipeptide and tripeptide inhibitors of human renin. *Hypertension* 1986;8(6 Pt 2):II1–II5.

81. Kokubu T, Hiwada, K, Murakami E, et al. In vitro inhibition of human renin by statine-containing tripeptide renin inhibitor (ES-1005). *J Cardiovasc Pharmacol* 1987;10(Suppl 7):S88–S90.

82. Bock MG, DiPardo RM, Evans BE, et al. Dipeptide analogues. Synthesis of a potent renin inhibitor. *J Chem Soc Chem Commun* 1985;3:109–110.

83. Rich DH, Bernatowicz MS, Schmidt PG. Direct ^{13}C NMR evidence for a tetrahedral intermediate in the binding of a pepstatin analogue to porcine pepsin. *J Am Chem Soc* 1982;104:3535–3536.

84. Rich DH, Salituro FG, Holladay MW, Schmidt PG. Design and discovery of aspartyl protease inhibitors. Mechanistic and clinical implications. In: Vida JA, Gordon M, eds. *Conformationally directed drug design.* Washington, DC, American Chemical Society, 1984;211–237.

85. Thaisrivongs S, Pales DT, Kati WM, Turner SR, Thomasco LM, Watt W. Design and synthesis of potent and specific renin inhibitors containing difluorostatine, difluorostatone and related analogues. *J Med Chem* 1986;29:2080–2087.

86. Gelb MH, Svaren JP, Abeles RH. Fluoro ketone inhibitors of hydrolytic enzymes. *Biochemistry* 1985;24:1813–1817.

87. Veber DF, Bock MG, Brady SF, et al. Renin inhibitors containing 2-substituted statine. *Biochem Soc Trans* 1984;12:956–959.

88. Boger J, Payne LS, Perlow DS, et al. Renin inhibitors. Syntheses of subnanomolar, competitive, transition-state analogue inhibitors containing a novel analogue of statine. *J Med Chem* 1985;28:1779–1790.

89. Hiwada K, Kokubu T, Murakami E, et al. A highly potent and long-acting oral inhibitor of human renin. *Hypertension* 1988;11:708–712.

90. Szelke M, Leckie B, Hallett A, et al. Potent new inhibitors of human renin. *Nature* 1982; 229:555–557.

91. Szelke M, Jones DM, Atrash B, Hallett A, Leckie BJ. In: Hruby VJ, Rich DH, eds. *Peptides: structure and function. Proceedings of the Eighth Peptide Symposium.* Rockford, IL: Pierce Chemical Co., 1983;579.

92. Webb DJ, Cumming AM, Leckie BJ, et al. Reduction of blood pressure in man with H-142, a potent new renin inhibitor. *Lancet* 1983;2: 1486–1487.

93. Plattner JJ, Greer J, Fung AKL, et al. Peptide analogues of angiotensinogen effect of peptide chain length on renin inhibition. *Biochem Biophys Res Commun* 1986;139:982–990.

94. Kempf DJ, DeLara E, Plattner JJ, Stein H, Cohen J, Perun TJ. Design and synthesis of renin inhibitors containing novel dipeptide analogues. 191st American Chemical Society Meeting, New York, New York, April 1986; Abstract Medi 10.

95. Thaisrivongs S, Pals DT, Harris DW, Kati WM, Turner SR. Design and synthesis of a potent and specific renin inhibitor with a prolonged duration of action in vivo. *J Med Chem* 1986;29:2088–2093.

96. Pals DT, Thaisrivongs S, Lawson JA, et al. An orally active inhibitor of renin. *Hypertension* 1986;8:1105–1112.

97. Hanson GJ, Baran JS, Lindberg T, et al. Dipeptide glycols: a new class of renin inhibitors. *Biochem Biophys Res Commun* 1985;132:155–161.

98. Miyazaki M, Toda N, Etoh Y, Kubota T, Iizuka K. Newly synthesized, potent human renin inhibitor. *Jpn J Pharmacol* 1986;40(Suppl II):70.

99. Izuka K, Kamijo T, Kubota T, Akahane K, Umeyama H, Kiso Y. New human renin inhibitors containing an unnatural amino acid, norstatine. *J Med Chem* 1988;31:701–704.

100. KRI-1314. *Drugs of the Future* 1988;13:1042–1049.
101. Luly JR, Plattner JJ, Stein H, et al. Renin inhibitors. Peptide analogs of angiotensinogen which display potent and specific inhibition of human renin. *Pharmacologist* 1985;27:260.
102. Luly JR, Soderquist JL, Yi N, et al. Low molecular weight, nanomolar renin inhibitors. 191st American Chemical Society Meeting, New York, New York, April 1986; Abstract Medi 9.
103. Luly JR, Plattner JJ, Stein H, et al. Modified peptides which display potent and specific inhibition of human renin. *Biochem Biophys Res Commun* 1987;143:44–51.
104. Kleinert HD, Martin D, Chekal MA, et al. Effects of the renin inhibitor A-64662 in monkeys and rats with varying baseline plasma renin activity. *Hypertension* 1988;11:613–619.
105. Rich DH. Pepstatin-derived inhibitors of aspartic proteinases. A close look at an apparent transition-state analogue inhibitor. *J Med Chem* 1985;28:263–273.
106. Oliveira MCF, Juliano L, Paiva ACM. Conformations of synthetic tetradecapeptide renin substrate and of angiotensin I in aqueous solution. *Biochemistry* 1977;16:2606–2611.
107. Nakaie CR, Oliveira MCF, Juliano L, Paiva ACM. Inhibition of renin by conformationally restricted analogues of angiotensinogen. *Biochem J* 1982;205:43–47.
108. Boger J, Lohr NS, Ulm EH, et al. Novel renin inhibitors containing the amino acid statine. *Nature* 1983;303:81–84.
109. Cumin F, Evin G, Fehrentz J-A, et al. Inhibition of human renin by synthetic peptides derived from its prosegment. *J Biol Chem* 1985;260:9154–9157.
110. Boger J. Renin inhibition. In: Bailey DM, ed. *Annual reports in medicinal chemistry.* New York: Academic Press, 1985;20:257–266.
111. Antonaccio MJ, Wright JJK. Enzyme inhibitors of the renin-angiotensin system. *Prog Drug Res* 1987;31:161–191.
112. Greenlee WJ. Renin inhibitors. *Pharm Res* 1987;4:364–374.
113. Wood JM, Stanton JL, Hofbauer KG. Inhibitors of renin as potential therapeutic agents. *J Enzyme Inhib (UK)* 1987;1/3:169–185.
114. Cushman DW, Cheung HS, Sabo EF, Ondetti MA. Design of potent competitive inhibitors of angiotensin-converting enzyme. Carboxyalkanoyl and mercaptoalkanoyl amino acid. *Biochemistry* 1977;16:5484-5491.
115. Cushman DW, Cheung HS, Sabo EF, Ondetti MA. Design of new antihypertension drugs. Potent and specific inhibitors of angiotensin-converting enzymes. In: Case DB, Sonnenblick EH, Laragh JH, eds. *Captopril and hypertension.* New York: Plenum Press, 1980;103–113.
116. Petrillo EW Jr, Ondetti MA. Angiotensin-converting enzyme inhibitors: medicinal chemistry and biological actions. *Med Res Rev* 1982;2:1–41.
117. Ondetti MA, Cushman DW. Enzymes of the renin-angiotensin system and their inhibitors. *Annu Rev Biochem* 1982;51:283–308.
118. Sweet CS, Arbegast PT, Gaul SL, Blaine EH, Gross DM. Relationship between angiotensin I blockade and antihypertensive properties of single doses of MK-421 and captopril in spontaneous and renal hypertensive rats. *Eur J Pharmacol* 1981;76:167–176.
119. Velletri P, Bean BL. Comparison of the time course of action of captopril on angiotensin-converting enzyme with the time course of its antihypertensive effect. *J Cardiovasc Pharmacol* 1981;3:1068–1081.
120. Cohen ML, Kurz KD. Angiotensin converting enzyme inhibition in tissues from spontaneously hypertensive rats after treatment with captopril or MK-421. *J Pharmacol Exp Ther* 1982;220:63–69.
121. Unger T, Ganten D, Lang RE. Converting enzyme inhibitors: antihypertensive drugs with unexpected mechanisms. *Trends Pharmacol Sci* 1983;4:514–519.
122. Antonaccio MJ, Kerwin L. Pre- and postjunctional inhibition of vascular sympathetic function by captopril in SHR. Implication of vascular angiotensin II in hypertension and antihypertensive actions of captopril. *Hypertension* 1981;3(3 Pt 2):154–162.
123. Hatton R, Clough. Captopril interferes with neurogenic vasoconstriction in the pithed rat by angiotensin-dependent mechanisms. *J Cardiovasc Pharmacol* 1982;4:116–123.
124. DeJonge A, Knape JT, VanMeel JCA, et al. Effect of captopril on sympathetic neurotransmission in pithed normotensive rats. *Eur J Pharmacol* 1983;88:231–240.
125. Byers LD, Wolfenden R. A potent reversible inhibitor of carboxypeptidase A. *J Biol Chem* 1972;247:606–608.
126. Ondetti MA, Rubin B, Cushman DW. Design of specific inhibitors of angiotensin-converting enzyme: new class of orally active antihypertensive agents. *Science* 1977;196:441–444.
127. Ondetti MA, Cushman DW. Angiotensin-converting enzyme inhibitors: biochemical properties and biological actions. *CRC Crit Rev Biochem* 1984;16:381–411.
128. Cohen ML. Synthetic and fermentation-derived angiotensin-converting enzyme inhibitors. *Annu Rev Pharmacol Toxicol* 1985;25:307–323.
129. Patchett AA, Cordes EH. The design and properties of N-carboxyalkyladipeptide inhibitors of angiotensin-converting enzyme. In: Meister A, eds. *Advances in enzymology.* New York: John Wiley, 1985;1–84.
130. Tarazi RC, Bravo EL, Foread FM, Omvick P, Cody RJ. Hemodynamic and volume changes associated with captopril. *Hypertension* 1980; 2:576–585.
131. Meggs LG, Hollenberg NK. Converting enzyme inhibition and the kidney. *Hypertension* 1980;2:551–557.
132. Mimran A, Brunner HR, Turini GA, Waeber B, Brunner D. Effect of captopril on renal vascu-

lar tone in patients with essential hypertension. *Clin Sci* 1979;57:421S–423S.

133. Brunner HR, Gavras H, Waeber B, et al. Oral angiotensin-converting enzyme inhibitor in long-term treatment of hypertensive patients. *Ann Intern Med* 1979;90:19–23.

134. Morganti A, Pickering TG, Lopey-Ovejero JA, Laragh JH. Endocrine and cardiovascular influences of converting enzyme inhibition with SW 14,225 in hypertensive patients with the supine position and during head up tilt before and after sodium depletion. *J Clin Endocrinol Metab* 1980;50:748–754.

135. MacGregor GA, Markandu ND, Roulston JE, Jones JC. Essential hypertension: effect of an oral inhibitor of angiotensin-converting enzyme. *Br Med J* 1979;2:1106–1109.

136. Cushman DW, Wang FL, Fung WC, Harvey CM, DeForrest JM. Differentiation of angiotensin-converting enzyme (ACE) inhibitors by their selective inhibition of ACE in physiologically important organs. *Am J Hypertens* 1989;2:294–306.

137. Unger T, Badoer E, Ganten D, Lang RE, Rettig R. Brain angiotensin: pathways and pharmacology. *Circulation* 1988;77(Suppl I):I40–I54.

138. Kostis JB. Angiotensin-converting enzyme inhibitors. Emerging differences and new compounds. *Am J Hypertens* 1989;2:57–64.

139. Allan G, Cambridge D, Follenfant MJ, Hardy GW. BW A575C, a novel antihypertensive agent with angiotensin converting enzyme inhibition and β-blocking properties. *Cardiovasc Drug Rev* 1986;315:487P.

140. Packer M, Lee WH, Yushak M, Medina N. Comparison of captopril and enalapril in patients with severe chronic heart failure. *N Engl J Med* 1986;315:847–853.

141. Wong PC, Chiu AT, Price WA, et al. Nonpeptide angiotensin II receptor antagonists. I. Pharmacological characterization of 2-n-butyl-c-chloro-1-(2-chlorobenzyl) imidazole-5-acetic acid sodium salt (S-8307). *J Pharmacol Exp Ther* 1988;247:1–7.

142. Chiu AT, Carini DJ, Johnson AL, et al. Nonpeptide angiotensin II receptor antagonists. II. Pharmacology of S-8308. *Eur J Pharmacol* 1988;157:13–21.

143. Wong PC, Price WA Jr, Chiu AT, et al. Nonpeptide angiotensin II receptor antagonists. IV. EXP 6155 and EXP 6803. *Hypertension* 1989;13:489–497.

Cardiovascular Pharmacology, Third Edition,
edited by Michael Antonaccio.
Raven Press, Ltd., New York © 1990.

Modulation of Neuroeffector Transmission

Michael J. Rand, Henryk Majewski, and David F. Story

Department of Pharmacology, University of Melbourne, Victoria 3052, Australia

LOCAL MODULATION OF TRANSMISSION IN RELATION TO OTHER NEUROEFFECTOR CONTROL MECHANISMS

Control of the cardiovascular system and other autonomically innervated effector systems in the execution of their functions and the maintenance of homeostasis is ultimately exerted by the central nervous system. In addition to neuronal connections to autonomic effector tissues, there are indirect neuroendocrine control mechanisms that operate more diffusely and generally have a slower time course. The output from the autonomic control centers in the central nervous system is regulated by sensory inputs from interoceptors and integrated with higher nervous function.

A schematic diagram of the control of neuroeffector function is given in Fig. 1. After autonomic neurons emerge from the central nervous system, the traffic of nerve impulses is first modulated during ganglionic synaptic transmission. Then, the nerve impulses are conducted to the terminal ramifications at neuroeffector junctions. Local modulatory control of autonomic transmission occurs at both sides of the neuroeffector junctions: at the neuronal terminals, the amounts of the transmitter substances released can be increased or decreased; at the effector cells, the responses can be increased or decreased.

This chapter is mainly concerned with the local modulation of transmitter release at neuroeffector junctions, but references are made to modulation of effector responses and ganglionic transmission when such phenomena are particularly relevant. No attempt is made to deal with the role of the central nervous system in cardiovascular control. However, it should be noted that many of the general principles that emerge from studies of the modulation of neuroeffector transmission are applicable to synaptic transmission in the central nervous system (1,2).

The process of transmitter release has been a target for pharmacological manipulation for many years. The outcome has been a better understanding of the actions of existing drugs together with new understanding of the underlying mechanisms through which they act, and this in turn has led to the development of new drugs. Drugs that affect noradrenergic transmission have not only been used as investigative tools, but are also important therapeutic agents, particularly in the treatment of hypertension (Table 1).

Since the early 1970s, it has been recognized that autonomic transmission can be modulated by a number of endogenously occurring substances acting on receptors associated with the terminal axons (Table 2). Many of these substances are regarded as physiologically significant for the control of neuroeffector function. Several reviews have touched on aspects of the multiplicity

TABLE 1. *Effects on noradrenergic transmission of some drugs with antihypertensive activity*

Effect on transmitter	Examples
Depletion of stores	Reserpine
Inhibition of synthesis	α-Methyl-*p*-tyrosine
Inhibition of metabolism	Pargyline
Change in nature	Methyldopa
Inhibition of release	Guanethidine
	Clonidine
Blockade of action	
At α-adrenoceptors	Prazosin
At β-adrenoceptors	Propranolol

of prejunctional receptors for endogenous substances on sympathetic nerve terminals (3–13).

The apparent complexity of local modulation of transmitter release at noradrenergic neuroeffector junctions was reduced to a systemic order by Westfall in 1977 (4,13), who perceived that there were four general types of modulation, which he designated automodulation, transneuronal modulation, transjunctional modulation, and hormonal modulation. A schematic diagram emphasizing local modulation of neuroeffector transmission in relation to the totality of control mechanisms is given in Fig. 1.

Local modulation of neuroeffector transmission will be discussed under each of the four general types in order to focus on their possible physiological relevance. However, it will be noted that many of the substances involved may engage in more than one type of local modulatory control (Table 2).

The recent growth of knowledge about cotransmission in peripheral neuroeffector systems (14–17) will be given some emphasis; however, research into cotransmitters and their functions is progressing rapidly and it is only possible to provide a glimpse of the present ephemeral scene. The role of cotransmitters in modulation of neuroeffector transmission has been reviewed (13,18). Before dealing with modulation of neuroeffector transmission, it is expedient to review briefly the phenomenon of cotransmission at cardiovascular neuroeffector junctions.

COTRANSMISSION

Historical Introduction

The prevailing concept for many years was that autonomic nerves were either cholinergic or noradrenergic, but Burn and Rand (19,20) in 1959 suggested that noradrenergic nerves also contained a cholinergic mechanism. The hypothesis that acetylcholine is involved in the release of norepinephrine has not been substantiated; how-

TABLE 2. *Endogenously occurring substances having modulatory actions on release of autonomic neurotransmitters and the type of modulation in which they may engage*

Substance	Auto	TNeur	TJunc	Horm
Acetylcholine	+	+		
Adenyl compounds	+	+	+	+
Angiotensin II				+
Corticotrophin				+
Dopamine	+	+		
Epinephrine	+			+
GABA		+		
Histamine				+
NPY	+	+		
Norepinephrine	+	+		
Opioid peptides		+		+
PGs			+	
Serotonin	+			+
VIP	+			

Auto, automodulation; TNeur, transneuronal; TJunc, transjunctional; Horm, hormonal.

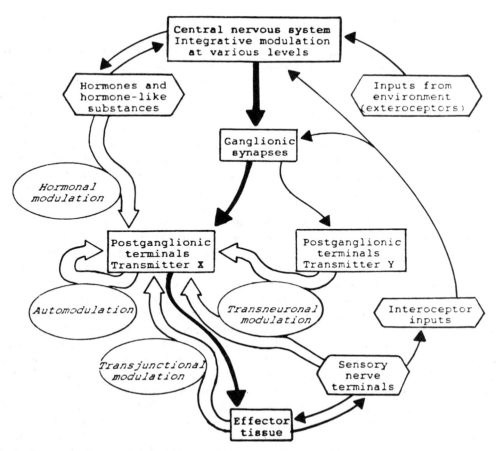

FIG. 1. General scheme of control of autonomic neuroeffector function with emphasis on local modulation. The main control pathway from the central nervous system to the effectors via ganglionic synapses and transmitter release from postganglionic terminals is indicated by thick arrows linking rectangles. The types of modulation of terminal neuroeffector transmission are shown in ellipses and the paths of modulation are indicated by open arrows. Some other modulatory factors are shown in hexagons and the pathways are indicated by thin arrows.

ever, norepinephrine and acetylcholine are both released by many sympathetic nerves (21). The dogma of the invariant nature of autonomic transmitters was further weakened by the concept that substances closely related to the normal transmitter could be utilized as false transmitters, which was first proposed for cholinergic neurons (22) but received a major impetus when it was suggested that α-methylnorepinephrine derived from methyldopa served as a false transmitter in noradrenergic nerves (23). Later, as mentioned below, it was shown

that other substances related to norepinephrine such as dopamine and epinephrine could serve as cotransmitters.

The concept of non-(nor)adrenergic, noncholinergic (NANC) autonomic transmission was first suggested by Burnstock (24) in 1972 who, after reviewing the then available evidence, suggested that the transmitter of many NANC neurons was a purine (probably adenosine triphosphate [ATP]) and proposed the term "purinergic." Subsequently, ATP has become generally accepted as the mediator not only of purinergic transmission but also as a cotransmitter in other neurons (25–27).

An early and striking example of cotransmission came in 1974 from the laboratory of Axelrod et al. (28) where acetylcholine, serotonin, histamine, and octopamine were detected in specifically identified single neurons of the marine invertebrate *Aplysia*. The first coherent general statement about cotransmission came from Burnstock (29) in 1976. Some of the background to Burnstock's preeminence in this field has been reviewed recently (30).

In the late 1970s, the development of immunohistochemical techniques led to the discovery of the widespread presence of peptides with powerful pharmacological activity in neurons. For example, Hökfelt and colleagues (31) detected somatostatin in 60% to 70% of the noradrenergic ganglion cells in prevertebral ganglia of the guinea pig. The discovery of a multitude of other peptides coexisting with classical transmitters in central and peripheral neurons has continued unceasingly (for reviews, see [15,18,32,33]). Neuropeptides have important regulatory roles in cardiovascular function in the central nervous system and at peripheral neuroeffector junctions (34). Peptides that have been detected in perivascular nerve fibers are listed in Table 3; note that some of these fibers are sensory in function, but there is a growing awareness that

they also serve a peripheral control function (see below).

The blood vessels that are predominantly involved in the regulation of systemic peripheral resistance and hence of arterial blood pressure appear to be controlled largely by noradrenergic mechanisms. However, in some vascular beds (e.g., cerebral, intestinal, and genital), the control mechanisms are more complex in that responses to perivascular nerve stimulation are not mimicked precisely by the classical transmitters and perivascular NANC axons are abundant. Cerebral blood vessels have, in addition to sympathetic noradrenergic and cholinergic parasympathetic axons (35), a particularly rich perivascular plexus of nerve fibers containing vasoactive intestinal polypeptide (VIP), peptide histidine isoleucine amide (PHI), substance P, calcitonin gene-related peptide (CGRP), neuropeptide Y (NPY), dynorphin, and serotonin (36–42). Neuropeptides that have been identified in perivascular nerves fibers of erectile tissue of the genitalia include VIP, somatostatin, NPY, and substance P (43–46). There are nonnoradrenergic perivascular fibers containing NPY, VIP, and dynorphin around the guinea pig uterine artery (47).

Another departure from the early dogma about the invariant nature of transmission is the recognition of plasticity in the transmitter system (48). Changes in transmission may occur not only during neuronal development but also in mature neurons; for example, after decentralization, sympathetic postganglionic neurons switch from predominantly noradrenergic to predominantly cholinergic modes of transmission (49) and substance P appears in them (50).

TABLE 3. *Some neuropeptides found in perivascular nerve fibers[a]*

CGRP
Dynorphins
Enkephalins
Galanin
Gastrin releasing peptide
Neurokinin A[b]
NPY
Neurotensin
PHI[b]
Somatostatin
Substance P[c]
VIP[b]

[a]See text for references.
[b]Both produced from preproVIP.
[c]Both produced from β-protachykinin A.

Properties of Cotransmitter Systems

Neurotransmitters can be divided into two broad groups: (a) the so-called classical transmitters, norepinephrine and acetylcholine, and other relatively simple molecules (amines, amino acids, and ATP), and (b) peptides or, more specifically, neuropeptides.

Biosynthesis

A major difference between the two groups is in their intraneuronal biosynthesis. The synthetic enzymes for the classical transmitters are assembled in the cell body and transported to the axon termi-

nals, where the bulk of the transmitter is synthesized to replenish the local stores; however, neuropeptides are synthesized only in the cell body (Fig. 2). One consequence of this is that the rate of replenishment of stores of a peptide cotransmitter in the axon terminals is a function of the rate of axonal transport as well as the rate of synthesis. Axonal transport of neuropeptide cotransmitters appears to be the rate-limiting step in both noradrenergic and cholinergic neurons (51).

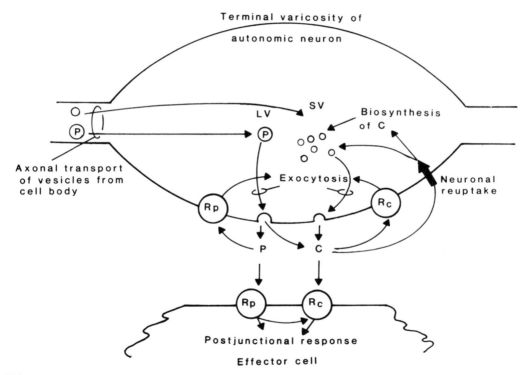

FIG. 2. Features of an autonomic cotransmitter system consisting of a classical transmitter (C, norepinephrine or acetylcholine) and a peptide (P). The transmitter storage vesicles and the enzymes for the biosynthesis of the classical transmitter are formed in the cell body of the neuron and transported along the axon to the terminal varicosities. Large vesicles (LV) contain the peptide cotransmitter that has been synthesized and packaged in the cell body. Both large and small vesicles (SV) contain the classical transmitter (and also contain ATP and may contain other cotransmitters such as epinephrine, dopamine, and serotonin in the case of noradrenergic neurons). The contents of both large and small vesicles are released by exocytosis. Both the peptide and the classical transmitter mediate pre- and postjunctional actions by acting on specific receptors (R_p, R_c): prejunctionally, they modulate subsequent transmitter release; postjunctionally, they mediate effector responses, and the peptide may modulate the response to the classical transmitter. The stores of the classical transmitter are replenished by neuronal reuptake and *de novo* biosynthesis in the terminals (in the case of acetylcholine, the choline moiety is taken up).

Intraneuronal Location

The storage of classical transmitters depends on the location of synthetic enzymes (the final enzyme for biosynthesis of norepinephrine, dopamine-β-hydroxylase, is intravesicular) and the ability of vesicles to take up potential transmitters from the cytoplasm. However, neuropeptides are packaged in vesicles in the cell body, and the intact package is transported to the terminals (Fig. 2). In noradrenergic neurons, peptides are preferentially stored in large (75–110 nm diameter) rather than small (45–55 nm diameter), dense-cored vesicles (52–54). In cholinergic neurons, the main peptide cotransmitter, VIP, is present in large, dense-cored vesicles, whereas the bulk of the acetylcholine is in small, clear vesicles (51,55). In both noradrenergic and cholinergic neurons, the large vesicles may also contain the classical transmitter.

Release

The contents of both the large and small vesicles are released by exocytosis (56,57). However, the conditions for exocytosis differ between large and small vesicles because the large vesicles are mobilized preferentially by higher frequencies of stimulation (58). It is not clear whether this reflects a difference in the mechanism of excitation-secretion coupling between the two types of vesicles or whether it merely reflects the fact that small vesicles greatly outnumber large vesicles so that the probability of their utilization is higher.

Cotransmitters in Noradrenergic Neurons

Amine Cotransmitters

Dopamine

Dopamine comprises between 1% and 5% of the store of catecholamines in noradrenergic nerve terminals (59,60). The rate-limiting enzyme in the neuronal biosynthesis of norepinephrine is generally recognized to be tyrosine hydroxylase, but under certain conditions dopamine-β-hydroxylase may become rate limiting, for example, when the rate of utilization of transmitter is high (60) or when dopamine-β-hydroxylase is inhibited (61), and substantial amounts of dopamine are released by nerve stimulation. In addition, there is evidence that some sympathetic nerves, particularly in the kidney, lack dopamine-β-hydroxylase and are dopaminergic (59).

Dopamine released from noradrenergic or dopaminergic terminals is unlikely to activate postjunctional α- or β-adrenoceptors because dopamine is less potent than norepinephrine as an agonist on them by a factor of 20–100 (62). However, specific dopamine receptors are present in a wide range of tissues (63,64). In the splanchnic and renal vascular beds, activation of dopamine receptors results in vasodilation, and there is evidence that these receptors in the kidney are activated by dopamine from dopaminergic nerves (59). Dopamine of renal origin also produces diuresis and natriuresis and consequently affects cardiovascular control (65). Differences between post- and prejunctional dopamine receptors, established largely on the basis of experiments with a range of agonist and antagonists in anesthetized dogs, led to the postulate that there were two subtypes of dopamine receptors that were designated D_1 and D_2, respectively (66). The action of dopamine on prejunctional receptors is discussed below.

Epinephrine

Epinephrine is found in small amounts in sympathetically innervated tissues (67–69). Some of this epinephrine may be associated with chromaffin cells (70). However, the major location is in sympathetic nerve endings, which take up epinephrine from the circulation (71,72). Removal of the adrenal medullae in rats results in a marked decrease in tissue levels of epinephrine (73,74). Increases in the epinephrine content of sympathetically innervated tissues occur when epinephrine is released from the adrenal medullae by splanchnic nerve stimulation (75–77).

Epinephrine that has been taken up into sympathetic nerve terminals can subsequently be released as a cotransmitter (78–81). The importance of epinephrine as a cotransmitter probably depends on the degree to which it has previously been released from the adrenal medullae, which suggests that after periods of stress it may have a crucial role (82,83). The action of epinephrine on prejunctional α- and β-adrenoceptors is discussed below.

Serotonin

The presence of serotonin in noradrenergic nerve terminals was first demonstrated in the sympathetic nerves to the pineal gland (84). Serotonin can be taken up by noradrenergic nerve terminals and incorporated into the transmitter storage vesicles from which it can be released as a cotransmitter (84–89). The released serotonin can act postjunctionally as a vasoconstrictor (90) and can also act on prejunctional receptors (see below).

Serotonin is present in perivascular nerve terminals of the cerebral vasculature (91, 92), some of which are noradrenergic (41,93), and it may function as a neurovascular transmitter (94). It is not clear whether the serotonin is formed in the axons or taken up from an extraneuronal source (41).

Modulation of neuroeffector transmission by serotonin can arise from its roles as a cotransmitter or as a local hormone (Table 2). Therefore, it is appropriate at this juncture to give a brief account of the complex cardiovascular actions of serotonin and the receptors on which it acts. Serotonin contracts most but relaxes some smooth muscle, it amplifies the contractile response of vascular smooth muscle to other vasoconstrictor agents, it liberates vasoactive substances from endothelial cells, it acts on autonomic neurons to release or inhibit the release of transmitters, and it can also activate α-adrenoceptors (95–98). The actions of serotonin on autonomic neurons have been reviewed by Humphrey and colleagues (99,100) and Fozard (101). The development of selective agonists and antagonists for the various actions of serotonin led to the coining of a nomenclature for the subtypes of receptors on which it acts (Table 4); however, the classification is still in a state of flux and the 5-HT$_1$ subtype has

TABLE 4. *Subtypes of serotonin (5-HT, 5-hydroxytryptamine) receptors*

Subtype	5-HT$_1$-like[a]	5-HT$_2$	5-HT$_3$
Selective agonists	5-Carboxyamido-tryptamine, 8-OH-DPAT, GR-43175	α-Methylserotonin	2-Methylserotonin
Selective antagonists		Ketanserin, ritanserin, cyproheptadine	Cocaine, MDL-7222, ICS 205-930
Peripheral neurons	Inhibition of transmitter release		Transmitter release (depolarization)
Smooth muscle	Contraction or relaxation	Contraction, platelet aggregation	

GR-43175, 3-[2-(dimethylamino)ethyl]-N-methyl-1H-indole-5-methane; ICS 205-930, (3α-tropanyl)-1H-indole-3-carboxylic acid ester; MDL-72222, 1αH,3α,(5αH-tropan-3-yl)3,5-dichlorobenzoate.
[a]The 5-HT$_1$-like subtype is further divided into four subtypes (see ref. 103).
Adapted from refs. 102–104.

been divided into further subtypes: 5-HT$_{1A}$; 5-HT$_{1B}$, and 5-HT$_{1C}$ (102–104).

Serotonin receptors of the 5-HT$_1$ subtype are associated with the terminals of some but not all noradrenergic neurons (99, 105–114). They also occur on the terminals of some autonomic cholinergic nerves (115). A selective ligand for 5-HT$_{1A}$ sites, 8-hy-droxy-2-(di-*n*-propylamino)-tetralin (8-OH-DPAT), lowers blood pressure and heart rate by inhibiting central sympathetic tone and increasing vagal activity (116).

The 5-HT$_2$ receptor subtype subserves contraction of gastrointestinal and vascular smooth muscle, as well as platelet aggregation and depolarization of neurons in the central nervous system.

Serotonin receptors of the 5-HT$_3$ subtype were originally found on cholinergic neurons of the gastrointestinal tract from which their activation results in release of acetylcholine (117–119). They are also present on other types of neurons in the enteric nervous plexuses where activation results in the release of NANC transmitters including substance P (119–121). They have been demonstrated on noradrenergic terminals in the rabbit heart (122) and cat nictitating membrane (114). Activation of 5-HT$_3$ receptors on sensory nerve terminals in intact animals elicits the Bezold-Jarisch reflex (101) and activation of 5-HT$_3$ receptors on cutaneous sensory nerves produces pain and a flare reaction (123). Fozard and colleagues (122,124) showed that 5-HT$_3$ receptors were specifically blocked by metoclopramide and cocaine, which led to the development of more potent selective antagonists (Table 4).

The roles of serotonin in automodulation and as a hormonal modulator of neuroeffector transmission are discussed below.

ATP

The association of ATP with norepinephrine in transmitter storage vesicles has been known for many years (125). It was originally assumed that the ATP formed part of a storage complex that retained the norepinephrine within the vesicles, and it was accepted that ATP would be released along with norepinephrine in exocytosis, but until recently no attention was paid to the possibility that the ATP as well as the norepinephrine played a functional role as a cotransmitter. The role of ATP as a cotransmitter at many sympathetic neuroeffector junctions is now well established (24–27,126–130).

The cardiovascular effects of purines (adenosine and adenosine nucleotides) and their roles in transmission and modulation of transmission have been reviewed (27, 126,131). The receptor subtypes on which purines act (132) are shown in Table 5.

ATP injected intravenously is a vasodilator and was much studied during World War II as a mediator of traumatic shock (133). It is now known that the vasodilation is due to the release of endothelium-derived relaxing factor (EDRF) from endothelial cells (134). However, the ATP released from perivascular sympathetic nerves acts directly on P$_2$-purinoceptors of the smooth muscle to produce a contractile response (135,136). The indirect vasodilation is exerted through endothelial P$_2$-purinoceptors

TABLE 5. *Purinoceptor subtypes*

	Subtype	
	P$_1$	P$_2$
Agonists	Adenosine≥AMP>ADP≥ATP	ATP≥ADP>AMP≥Adenosine
Antagonists	Theophylline	Arylazido amino-propionyl-ATP
	8-Phenyltheophylline	α,β-Methylene-ATP

Adapted from ref. 132.

in the rat femoral artery (135), but in the rabbit ear artery it involves endothelial P_1-purinoceptors (136) and probably requires the breakdown of ATP to adenosine monophosphate (AMP) or adenosine. In pial arteries, activation of P_1- and P_2-purinoceptors on the smooth muscle produces vasodilation and vasoconstriction, respectively, and activation of endothelial P_2-purinoceptors produces vasodilation (137).

In blood vessels, the excitatory junction potentials (EJPs) elicited by sympathetic nerve stimulation are mediated by ATP, and in some blood vessels ATP also contributes to the contractile response (128, 138–144). The EJPs are blocked by guanethidine and abolished after 6-hydroxydopamine-induced sympathectomy (145), indicating that the ATP comes from sympathetic nerves. ATP and norepinephrine released as cotransmitters may act cooperatively to enhance the response in some effectors, for example, the vas deferens (146) and portal vein (147).

In some blood vessels the contractile response to sympathetic nerve stimulation is predominantly mediated by ATP, for example, in the rabbit saphenous (148) and mesenteric artery (141,149) and the dog basilar (150,151) and mesenteric artery (143). In other blood vessels ATP participates to a relatively minor extent, for example, in the rat tail artery (128,152) and rabbit ear artery (127,139). ATP contributes to the pressor responses evoked by stimulating spinal sympathetic nerves in the pithed rat (153) and to the response to hypothalamic stimulation in the rabbit (154). ATP may mediate the residual contractile response of the cat nictitating membrane to sympathetic nerve stimulation after reserpine-induced depletion of norepinephrine stores (155). In the rabbit portal vein neurogenically released ATP acts directly to relax the longitudinal smooth muscle (156,157).

It has been suggested that the purinergic component of responses to sympathetic nerve stimulation is favored by short bursts of stimulation because ATP acts rapidly by opening voltage-operated Ca^{2+} channels, whereas the noradrenergic component is favored by longer trains of stimulation because norepinephrine acts more slowly by opening receptor-operated Ca^{2+} channels (158).

In addition to its role as a cotransmitter, which includes automodulation, ATP (and other adenyl compounds) are involved in other types of modulation of neuroeffector transmission (Table 2): a discussion of these modulatory actions follows.

Peptide Cotransmitters

Peptides that are present in some noradrenergic neurons include somatostatin, enkephalins, NPY (31,159–161), and vasopressin (162). There is compelling evidence that NPY functions as a cotransmitter (see below), but whether the others have a functional role in cardiovascular neuroeffector transmission has yet to be elucidated.

Somatostatin

The somatostatin-containing sympathetic noradrenergic neurons arising in prevertebral ganglia (31,160) innervate the intestinal tract (163,164). There is no evidence for a role of somatostatin in sympathetic cardiovascular control apart from that arising from its effects in the gastrointestinal tract. It has been reported to reduce splanchnic and hepatic blood flow in dogs (165) and humans (166). Intravenous injection of somatostatin in the dog produces a small transient rise in blood pressure (167).

Opioid Peptides

Enkephalins are present in sympathetic ganglia and some autonomically innervated effector tissues, such as the heart (168,169), and the location of enkephalins in some noradrenergic sympathetic terminal axons has been reported (54,170–172).

NPY

Many sympathetic noradrenergic ganglion cells and axons contain NPY (52, 53,161,173–181), and sympathetic cardiovascular terminals are particularly rich in NPY (161,173,175,177,178,180,182–191). NPY-containing fibers are more plentiful around arteries than veins and are more abundant around coronary arteries and arteries in the respiratory, gastrointestinal, and genitourinary tracts than in the liver or kidney. However, not all sympathetic neurons contain NPY; furthermore, not all peripheral NPY-containing neurons are noradrenergic (192).

Tissue levels of NPY are depleted by chemical or surgical sympathectomy (161, 174,178,187,193). Agents that deplete norepinephrine stores such as reserpine or 6-hydroxydopamine also deplete stores of NPY (161,178,182,194,195), but small doses of reserpine reduce the level of norepinephrine to a greater extent than that of NPY (196), presumably because NPY and norepinephrine are not uniformly stored and released.

Both NPY and norepinephrine are released by sympathetic nerve stimulation (197–200). NPY is preferentially released by short bursts of high-frequency stimulation (199,200), which may reflect the differential storage of norepinephrine and NPY. The release of NPY, like the release of norepinephrine, is blocked by guanethidine (197,201,202).

NPY has direct vasoconstrictor activity (186,189,203–206) that is particularly pronounced in cerebral blood vessels (37,204); in most of the commonly studied peripheral vessels of laboratory animals, it is a relatively weak vasoconstrictor (186,207). However, it is a more potent vasoconstrictor than norepinephrine in some human blood vessels (208). The vasoconstrictor effects of NPY are not altered by α- or β-adrenoceptor blockade (204,205,209), but they are inhibited by calcium channel blocking drugs (108) and are absent in a Ca^{2+}-free medium (37,204).

NPY mimics, and may mediate, the slow vasoconstrictor response to sympathetic nerve stimulation remaining after blockade of α-adrenoceptors in the cat submandibular gland (205), dog oral mucosa and dental pulp (210), intestinal blood vessels (174, 211), and human mesenteric vein and renal artery (183). In the cat spleen, after selective depletion of norepinephrine with a low dose of reserpine, vasoconstrictor and splenic capsule contraction responses to sympathetic nerve stimulation are mimicked by NPY (197,212).

High concentrations of NPY are present in the sympathetic axons associated with blood vessels in the carotid body (213). NPY constricts these blood vessels and this results in excitation of the chemoreceptive sensory terminals (214). A component of the vasoconstrictor response to sympathetic nerve stimulation in the carotid body is not blocked by α-adrenoceptor antagonists (215) and may be mediated by NPY (214).

NPY produces coronary vasoconstriction and decreased contractility in the isolated perfused heart of the rabbit (203) and guinea pig (216) but has positive inotropic and chronotropic effects on guinea pig isolated atria (217). In the pig, the positive inotropic response to sympathetic nerve stimulation is abolished by α- and β-adrenoceptor blockade, but the chronotropic response is only partially reduced and may be mediated by NPY (202).

The vasoconstrictor response to NPY in rat tail artery is increased by chronic denervation (218). The mechanism responsible has not been elucidated, but if it is an example of denervation supersensitivity due to up-regulation of receptors, it would indicate that NPY is normally involved in neurovascular function.

NPY has a marked effect in enhancing vasoconstrictor responses to norepinephrine (186,204,207,219,220) and perivascular nerve stimulation (13,37,186,191,207,218–225). The enhancing effects have been observed with concentrations of NPY lower than those producing direct vasoconstriction. In rat mesenteric blood vessels, low concentrations of NPY decrease and higher concentrations increase vasoconstrictor responses to sympathetic nerve stimulation (209). NPY does not potentiate the vasoconstrictor action of norepinephrine in cerebral vessels to the same extent as in peripheral vessels, but the combination of NPY and norepinephrine gives a more prolonged vasoconstriction (186). Vasoconstrictor responses to other agents are also potentiated by NPY (218). The potentiating effect of NPY is abolished by nifedipine (219). It has been reported that the potentiation of the vasoconstrictor action of norepinephrine by NPY is endothelium dependent (226), but this has been contradicted (227).

The prejunctional actions of NPY as a mediator of automodulation and transneuronal modulation are discussed below.

Cotransmitters in Cholinergic Neurons

ATP

In cholinergic neurons, as in noradrenergic neurons, ATP is present in the transmitter storage vesicles from which it is released at cholinergic neuroeffector junctions where it acts as a cotransmitter (26,228).

VIP

VIP is present in many parasympathetic ganglion cells (160,229–235) and in a few sympathetic nonnoradrenergic ganglion cells (160,230,233,236). VIP-containing parasympathetic and sympathetic cholinergic axons are widely distributed in peripheral tissues, particularly in blood vessels, nonvascular smooth muscle, and exocrine glands (236, 237); however, VIP is not detectable in parasympathetic cholinergic axons from the ciliary ganglion or ganglion cells in the bladder (236).

VIP-containing axons are ubiquitous in arterial perivascular plexuses but are more sparse in veins (229,235). They are particularly abundant around blood vessels in exocrine glands (233,234,238) and in skeletal muscle (230). The VIP-containing axons of blood vessels are not affected by sympathectomy or capsaicin-induced degeneration of substance P-containing sensory axons (229,235).

VIP is released by stimulation of the vagus nerve (239) and nerves to salivary glands, particularly by higher frequencies of stimulation (232,240–245). Its effects as a cotransmitter have been most thoroughly studied in the cat submandibular gland, in which parasympathetic nerve stimulation produces salivary secretion and vasodilation. Both effects are mediated by acetylcholine when evoked by low-frequency stimulation, but the vasodilator response elicited with high-frequency stimulation (>2 Hz) is not blocked by atropine (231, 244,246) but can be blocked with an antibody against VIP (242). The atropine-resistant vasodilator response is slowly developing and mimicked by VIP.

Although VIP does not elicit salivary secretion, it potentiates the secretory response to acetylcholine (231,241): the explanation for this effect is that it increases the affinity of the muscarinic receptors for acetylcholine by several orders of magnitude (247). The vasodilator actions of VIP and acetylcholine are merely additive (243). VIP does not affect the bradycardia response to vagal stimulation (167).

VIP is a potent vasodilator and a depressor when injected intravenously (167,248). The mechanism of its vasodilator action differs from that of acetylcholine (249). The presence of VIP as a cotransmitter in cholinergic nerves accounts for the otherwise puzzling phenomenon of atropine-resistant vasodilator responses to nerve stimulation (233,242,246,250,251). In earlier years, many tortuous explanations were devised to account for the atropine resistance of responses elicited by stimulation of nerves that appeared to be cholinergic. VIP is a mediator of neurogenic vasodilator responses in cerebral blood vessels (251–253) and in erectile tissue of the genitalia (46).

The prejunctional actions of VIP in automodulation and transneuronal modulation are discussed below.

Somatostatin

This peptide is present in some vagal fibers (160), including those in the human atrium (254), and particularly concentrated in the right atrium and atrioventricular node (255). It functions as a cotransmitter in the toad heart (256), but little is known about its functional role in mammalian cardiac neurotransmission. It has negative inotropic (257) and chronotropic actions in guinea pig isolated atria (258) but not in rat or rabbit atria (257). It has a negative inotropic action on isolated strips of human right atrium when contractility has been increased by norepinephrine (259).

Opioid Peptides

Enkephalins are colocalized with acetylcholine in some cholinergic neurons (32). In sympathetic ganglia, they are in axon terminals (260) of preganglionic origin (261). They are thought to function as neurotransmitters mediating presynaptic inhibition of acetylcholine release from preganglionic sympathetic terminals (262) and also inhibition of substance-P release from branches of sensory axons in ganglia (263). The roles of enkephalins and substance P in modulating ganglionic transmission are discussed below.

AUTOMODULATION

Automodulation can be defined as the process by which a transmitter substance, once released, can modulate subsequent transmitter release by activating receptors associated with the terminal axons of the neuron, thereby constituting a feedback control loop. The term "autoreceptor" was coined to designate the receptor involved in feedback modulation of transmission. The corresponding term "heteroreceptor" has been used to describe receptors associated with nerve terminals on which endogenous substances other than a transmitter released from those terminals can act to modulate transmission.

The seminal observation that eventually led to the exposition of the concept of automodulation of transmitter release came from studies on sympathetic neuroeffector transmission, in which it was found that blockade of α-adrenoceptors resulted in a large increase in the stimulation-induced release of norepinephrine (264), but the pathway from this observation to the elucidation of the mechanism responsible for the phenomenon was not straightforward (9,11). What finally emerged was that norepinephrine not only mediated the response of the effector cells by acting on the postjunctional receptors but also mediated inhibition of transmitter release by acting on prejunctional α-adrenoceptors, that is, α-adrenoceptors on the noradrenergic nerve terminals. Thus, the release of norepinephrine resulted in the setting up of a negative feedback loop that restrained further release. Blockade of the prejunctional α-adrenoceptors disrupted the feedback inhibition and thereby increased transmitter release.

Feedback inhibition of transmitter release was subsequently recognized to occur at cholinergic neuroeffector junctions and at noradrenergic, cholinergic, dopaminergic, serotonergic, GABAergic, glutaminergic, and glycinergic synaptic junctions in the central nervous system (1,2). Because it is such a widespread phenomenon, the possibility that it is a general property of neurotransmitter release must be entertained.

The conditions under which autoinhibition of noradrenergic transmission comes into operation and the effects of agonist and antagonists of prejunctional receptors on transmitter release have been reviewed recently by Rand and Story (265). The principles that emerge are probably generally applicable to autoinhibition in other transmitter systems. The main ones are as follows.

First, activation of prejunctional receptors by the endogenous mediator of autoinhibition before the first action potential arrives at the axon terminals is unlikely unless there is a high rate of spontaneous release and/or the rate of removal of the spontaneously released mediator is impeded.

Second, autoinhibition does not operate when the frequency of arrival of nerve impulses is very low or when brief (<1 sec) trains of high-frequency impulses are delivered (266).

Third, exogenous agonists acting on prejunctional autoreceptors have their greatest effect in reducing transmitter release at low frequencies of stimulation; in fact, exogenous norepinephrine has its most pronounced effect in inhibiting transmitter release evoked by a single pulse (11).

Fourth, antagonists of prejunctional inhibitory autoreceptors manifest their action in enhancing transmitter release to the greatest extent at an optimal frequency of stimulation after autoinhibition is fully developed. With further increases in frequency, when transmitter release becomes maximally facilitated, blockade of prejunctional receptors produces no further enhancement of release.

A Postulated Physiological Role of Autoinhibition

The role of autoinhibition in neuronal function appears to be in relation to frequency-dependent facilitation of transmitter release. When a train of impulses arrives at axon terminals, the amount of transmitter released per pulse increases with successive pulses until it reaches a plateau level, and the rate of the increase and the plateau level are greater as the fre-

quency increases (265,267). There are limits to the occurrence of frequency-dependent facilitation: at a sufficiently low frequency, the amount of transmitter released per pulse remains constant; beyond an upper limiting frequency, a further increase does not result in faster or greater facilitation. The explanation for frequency-dependent facilitation is related to the role of Ca^{2+} in transmitter release. It is generally accepted that depolarization of the axonal membrane during passage of an action potential opens voltage-dependent Ca^{2+} channels, and the transient increase in the cytoplasmic concentration of free Ca^{2+} triggers mechanisms that culminate in exocytotic release of the transmitter (268). Arrival of a second action potential before the effects produced by the first have dissipated results in release of a greater amount of transmitter. The upper limit to frequency-dependent facilitation occurs when the accumulation of free cytoplasmic Ca^{2+} is maximal, or when the mechanisms involved in exocytosis are fully activated. Autoinhibition provides a braking influence on frequency-dependent facilitation; therefore, when autoinhibition is blocked, frequency-dependent facilitation is enhanced (Fig. 3).

Automodulation of Noradrenergic Neuroeffector Transmission

Automodulation of transmitter release from sympathetic noradrenergic nerve terminals calls for consideration not only of norepinephrine but also of other substances released as cotransmitters, including dopamine, epinephrine, serotonin, ATP, and NPY. The sympathetic nerve terminals are endowed with specific receptors for each of these substances that may mediate automodulation not only of their own release but also of norepinephrine and the other cotransmitters. With the notable exception of epinephrine acting on prejunctional β-adrenoceptors, cotransmitters are inhibitory modulators.

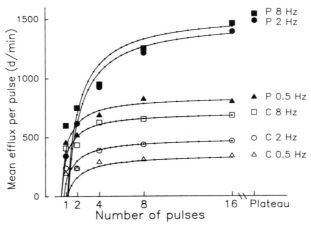

FIG. 3. Data illustrating the relationship between frequency-dependent facilitation of transmitter norepinephrine release and autoinhibition. The efflux of radioactivity from [³H]norepinephrine-labeled rat atria evoked by field stimulation of the intramural sympathetic nerves was used as an index of transmitter norepinephrine release. The amount of radioactivity released per pulse of stimulation increased and approached a plateau level with increasing number of pulses in the train of stimulation (1, 2, 4, 8, and 16 pulses). Increases in the frequency of stimulation (0.5, 2, and 8 Hz) resulted in faster rates of rise in the amount released per pulse with increasing number of pulses, and higher plateau levels. When autoinhibition was removed by blocking prejunctional α-adrenoceptors with phentolamine (3 μM), the rates of rise in the amounts of norepinephrine released and the plateau levels were increased, reflecting unopposed frequency-dependent facilitation of transmitter release. Symbols above the labels 1–16 are data from groups of experiments ($n = 5$) with stimulation at 0.5 Hz (△,▲) 2 Hz (○,●), or 8 Hz (□,■) in the absence (C,△,○,□) or presence (P,▲,●,■) of phentolamine. The hyperboli were derived from lines of best fit to the data, and the symbols above the label Plateau are calculated equilibrium plateau values. (From Standford-Starr, Story, and Rand, *unpublished observations.*)

Prejunctional α-Adrenoceptors

The reviews by Langer (6–8,269), Rand and colleagues (11,12), Vizi (5), Gillespie (9), Westfall (4), and particularly those by Starke (3,270) provide comprehensive accounts of the development of the concept and the relevant literature. Other reviews cover the subject from various perspectives (10,271–275). Some reviews take the line that the concept of autoinhibition through prejunctional α-adrenoceptors is unwarranted (276,277): the opposing views have been debated (278,279).

As mentioned earlier, the existence of prejunctional α-adrenoceptors subserving automodulation came to light during the investigation of the increase in stimulation-induced release of norepinephrine produced by α-adrenoceptor antagonists; it be-

came clear that they did so by blocking the prejunctional α-adrenoceptors involved in the inhibitory feedback loop mediated by norepinephrine of neurogenic origin. In the course of these investigations, it was observed that exogenous norepinephrine and a number of other α-adrenoceptor agonists inhibited stimulation-induced norepinephrine release. During the study of the effects of various agonists and antagonists on the prejunctional receptors of noradrenergic terminals, it became apparent that they differed in a number of respects from the α-adrenoceptors of effector tissues (280). It was suggested that α-adrenoceptors comprised two subtypes designated as α_1- and α_2-adrenoceptors, corresponding respectively to their post- and prejunctional locations (8). Subsequently, agonists and antagonists with relative specificity for

TABLE 6. *Agonists and antagonists with relative selectivity for the α_1- and α_2-subtypes of adrenoceptor in descending order of selectivity for α_1-adrenoceptors*

Agonists	Ratio (α_1/α_2)	Antagonists
	>100	Prazosin
Methoxamine	100–10	Corynanthine
Phenylephrine		Clozapine
		Azapetine
Norepinephrine	1–10	Phentolamine
Epinephrine	0.1–1	Piperoxan
Naphazoline		Tolazoline
Oxymetazoline		Dihydroergotamine
Clonidine		
α-Methylnorepinephrine		
Tramazoline	0.01–0.1	Yohimbine
BHT 920		
UK14304	<0.01	Rauwolscine
		Idazoxan

each subtype were identified and others were developed. Further studies with these drugs showed that α_2-adrenoceptors were more widely distributed, being present in platelets, adipocytes, Langerhans cells, and some smooth muscle cells (281). Furthermore, there is evidence for the association of α_1-adrenoceptor with some noradrenergic terminals where they participate along with α_2-adrenoceptors in automodulation (280,282,283). The α_1- and α_2-subtypes of adrenoceptors are now defined in terms of the relative potencies of agonists that activate them and antagonists that block them (Table 6).

Are Prejunctional α-Adrenoceptors Functional In Vivo?

Experiments with isolated tissues have established firmly that activation of α_2-adrenoceptors on sympathetic nerve terminals decreases the stimulation-induced release of norepinephrine, and this system subserves automodulation. However, if prejunctional α_2-adrenoceptors and automodulation of noradrenergic transmission are physiologically operational, their function must be demonstrated *in vivo*. The evidence is reviewed in the following paragraphs.

The α_2-adrenoceptor agonist clonidine inhibits the rate of norepinephrine release in the pentobarbitone-anesthetized rabbit largely by acting within the central nervous system to decrease sympathetic activity (72). However, in pithed rabbits in which the spinal sympathetic outflow is electrically stimulated, clonidine still inhibits the rate of norepinephrine release, although to a much lesser extent (284). The inhibitory effect of clonidine on stimulation-induced norepinephrine release in pithed rabbits is blocked by yohimbine but not by corynanthine, indicating that it is due to α_2-adrenoceptor activation (284). The finding in pithed rabbits suggests that a peripheral action may contribute to the effect of clonidine in the anesthetized rabbit. Moreover, the α_2-adrenoceptor agonist α-methylnorepinephrine, which does not readily penetrate the blood-brain barrier, significantly decreases the norepinephrine release rate in conscious rabbits, suggesting that activation of peripheral α_2-adrenoceptors inhibits norepinephrine release under physiological conditions (285). In pithed rabbits, α-methylnorepinephrine decreases the rate of norepinephrine release during electrical stimulation of the spinal sympathetic outflow to the same extent as in conscious rabbits (284), confirming a peripheral site of action.

If negative feedback modulation of norepinephrine release operates *in vivo,* blockade of α_2-adrenoceptors should enhance norepinephrine release. In conscious rabbits, the α_2-adrenoceptor antagonists yohimbine and rauwolscine increase the norepinephrine release rate whereas the selective α_1-adrenoceptor antagonist corynanthine does not (285). Yohimbine and rauwolscine can increase sympathetic activity by an action in the central nervous system (286); however, when this effect is dampened by pentobarbitone anesthesia, yohimbine and rauwolscine still enhance the norepinephrine release rate (287) and are probably acting peripherally because in the pithed rabbit with stimulated spinal sympathetic outflow, these two drugs enhance norepinephrine release to about the same extent as in the anesthetized rabbit (284).

In the conscious rat, yohimbine increases markedly the plasma norepinephrine level (288). Furthermore, the increase in plasma norepinephrine level produced by the nonselective α-adrenoceptor blocking drug phentolamine is greater than that produced by equihypotensive doses of the α_1-adrenoceptor blocking drug prazosin or the directly acting vasodilator hydralazine (288). In the pithed rat with stimulated sympathetic outflow, yohimbine also enhances significantly the plasma norepinephrine level (289). On the other hand, it has been reported that phentolamine and hydralazine increase plasma norepinephrine levels in the conscious rabbit to the same extent in equihypotensive doses (290), but this is at variance with other reports from whole animal experiments that are consistent with the physiological operation of a negative feedback loop resulting from activation of prejunctional α-adrenoceptors (291–293).

Studies in human subjects have not clearly substantiated a role for prejunctional α_2-adrenoceptors in automodulation, despite evidence for their presence in human isolated tissues. Clonidine reduces the norepinephrine release rate into plasma in humans (294), but this is mainly due to an effect in the central nervous system. Local infusion of clonidine into the human forearm does not inhibit norepinephrine release as measured by the arteriovenous difference in plasma norepinephrine (295). Furthermore, it has been reported that the intravenous infusion of α-methylnorepinephrine does not decrease the plasma norepinephrine level (296); however, the dose of α-methylnorepinephrine used may have been too low to activate prejunctional α_2-adrenoceptors (285).

In contrast to these studies, the α_2-adrenoceptor agonist guanfacine decreases plasma norepinephrine levels after the central effects on α_2-adrenoceptors have been blocked by idazoxan (297). Idazoxan increases plasma norepinephrine levels in human subjects (298), but a central action cannot be excluded. Local administration of yohimbine into the circulation of the human forearm enhances significantly plasma norepinephrine levels, but only after norepinephrine has been released by tyramine (299).

Taken together, studies in whole animals substantially support the view that prejunctional α-adrenoceptors at sympathetic nerve endings are operationally engaged in inhibitory automodulation of noradrenergic transmission. However, further work is required to demonstrate convincingly the physiological operation of prejunctional α_2-adrenoceptors in humans.

Role of α_2-Adrenoceptors in Postjunctional Modulation of Neuroeffector Transmission

There are postjunctional as well as prejunctional α_2-adrenoceptors (281). Activation of α_2-adrenoceptors at neuroeffector junctions may modulate the effector response as well as the amount of transmitter released from sympathetic nerve terminals. In the rat tail artery, activation of the postjunctional α_2-adrenoceptors enhances vasoconstrictor responses to sympathetic nerve stimulation, norepinephrine, phenylephrine, ATP, and vasopressin (300,301). Similarly, pressor responses to sympathetic nerve stimulation, norepinephrine and phenylephrine in the pithed rat are enhanced by α_2-adrenoceptor agonists (302). These enhancing effects are produced by amounts of α_2-adrenoceptor agonists that are much lower than those necessary to act prejunctionally to inhibit norepinephrine release or postjunctionally to produce vasoconstriction directly.

Modulation of Release of Cotransmitters by Activation of Prejunctional α_2-Adrenoceptors

ATP

Because ATP and norepinephrine are present in the same transmitter storage vesicles and both are released by exocytosis, all of the considerations applying to automodulation of norepinephrine release apply to noradrenergic modulation of ATP release.

Epinephrine

The release of epinephrine as a cotransmitter in sympathetic nerves appears to be regulated by the same prejunctional receptor mechanisms as norepinephrine (78).

NPY

Activation of prejunctional α_2-adrenoceptors with clonidine inhibits the release of NPY (201). In animals treated with clonidine, the NPY levels are increased in the heart (303) and spleen (304), presumably because the rate of replenishment by axonal transport exceeds the rate of release by the depressed tonic sympathetic drive. There is a feedback inhibitory effect of norepinephrine on NPY release because blockade of prejunctional α-adrenoceptors with the selective antagonist yohimbine or the nonselective antagonists phentolamine (172,199,201,305) and phenoxybenzamine (199,202) enhances NPY release.

Opioid Peptides

The release of the leu-enkephalin precursor α-neoendorphin from cardiac sympathetic nerves of the guinea pig heart is increased by blockade and decreased by activation of prejunctional α_2-adrenoceptors (172).

Automodulation by Cotransmitters in Noradrenergic Neurons

Feedback modulatory loops mediated by cotransmitters of noradrenergic neurons are shown in Fig. 4.

Prejunctional Purinoceptors

As well as mediating some components of neuroeffector responses to sympathetic nerve stimulation as described above, ATP released as a cotransmitter may also be involved in automodulation. The prejunctional receptors for adenyl compounds are P_1-purinoceptors and their activation results in inhibition of norepinephrine release (126,306). Adenosine and AMP are relatively selective for the P_1-subtype, whereas ATP is relatively selective for P_2-purinoceptors (Table 5); however, ATP is rapidly broken down to AMP and adenosine. Blockade of prejunctional P_1-purinoceptors with theophylline results in increased stimulation-induced release of both ATP and norepinephrine (307). This effect has been attributed to ATP-mediated autoinhibition; however, it is difficult to exclude the pos-

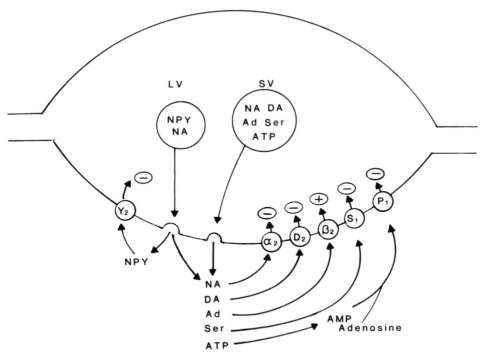

FIG. 4. Automodulatory feedback loops that may be mediated by cotransmitters of noradrenergic neurons and the main subtype of prejunctional receptor on which each cotransmitter acts. NA, norepinephrine (α_2-adrenoceptor); NPY, neuropeptide Y (Y_2); DA, dopamine (D_2); Ad, epinephrine (β_2-adrenoceptor); Ser, serotonin (S_1, referred to as the 5-HT$_1$-like subtype of serotonin receptor in the text); ATP, or its breakdown products (P_1-purinoceptor). Note that ATP may be a cotransmitter in all noradrenergic neurons, and NPY is a cotransmitter in many (but probably in the majority of those concerned with cardiovascular control). However, DA, Ad, and Ser only serve functionally as cotransmitters under certain circumstances; furthermore, with all of the cotransmitters, feedback modulation only occurs under certain conditions (see text). The feedback loops are all inhibitory on transmitter release, with the exception of that mediated by Ad acting on β_2-adrenoceptors.

sibility that it is mediated by adenosine released from non-neuronal tissue, and is thus an example of transjunctional modulation (see below).

Activation of prejunctional P_1-purinoceptors inhibits release of ATP and norepinephrine in various vascular preparations (308–311). It has been reported that the prejunctional inhibition resulting from P_1-purinoceptor activation is less in spontaneously hypertensive (SHR) than in normotensive Wistar-Kyoto (WKY) rats (312), but the postjunctional vasoconstrictor role of ATP is greater in SHR than in WKY (144). It was suggested that the lesser prejunctional inhibition of transmitter release together with

the greater postjunctional vasoconstrictor action of ATP may contribute to the greater sympathetic tone in hypertension. However, no evidence for the involvement of ATP in the hypertensive state was found in a recent study (313).

Prejunctional NPY Receptors

In contrast to its postjunctional actions in producing vasoconstriction and potentiating other vasoconstrictors, NPY acts prejunctionally to inhibit stimulation-induced transmitter release. The prejunctional inhibition of transmitter release has been stud-

ied most intensively in isolated vasa deferentia of the rat, mouse, and guinea pig, in
which NPY reduces contractile responses to
field stimulation of the intramural nerves without affecting responses to norepinephrine and
inhibits the stimulation-induced release of norepinephrine (162,217,222,314–318).

In isolated preparations of blood vessels,
despite the enhancement of vasoconstrictor
responses to perivascular nerve stimulation, NPY decreases the release of norepinephrine in rat femoral artery (222), portal
vein (319), mesenteric blood vessels (209),
and in rabbit ear artery (225), as shown in
Fig. 5. However, it has been reported that
NPY does not inhibit stimulation-induced
norepinephrine release from cerebral arteries (320). Inhibition of stimulation-induced
norepinephrine release has also been observed in guinea pig atria (217).

It is presumed that NPY released as a
cotransmitter from noradrenergic neurons
mediates an inhibitory feedback effect. The
simplest way to demonstrate the operation
of an inhibitory feedback loop is to block
the prejunctional receptors on which the
mediator acts. However, at the present time
no antagonist for NPY has been developed;
therefore, the case for the participation of
NPY in automodulation rests on the cir-
cumstantial evidence presented.

As far as its effects on vascular neuroeffector transmission are concerned, it has
been suggested that NPY may function to
conserve transmitter by inhibiting release
by activating prejunctional NPY receptors
while reinforcing the response by activating
postjunctional NPY receptors during periods of prolonged, intense sympathetic
drive (225,321).

Comparisons of the spectrum of effects
of NPY with some of its C-terminal fragments suggest there are subtypes of NPY
receptors. The postjunctional receptors,
designated Y_1, are activated only by intact
NPY, but the prejunctional Y_2 receptors
can also be activated by the 13–36 C-terminal fragment (322).

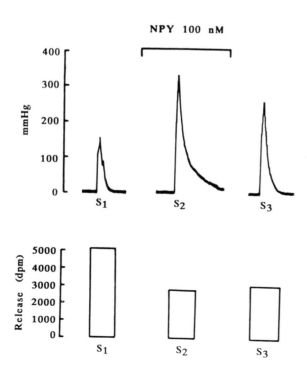

FIG. 5. Effects of NPY in enhancing the
vasoconstriction and inhibiting the norepinephrine release evoked by sympathetic
nerve stimulation. Data from an experiment with an isolated perfused segment of
rabbit ear artery previously incubated with
[³H]norepinephrine to label transmitter
stores. The perivascular sympathetic
nerves were stimulated at 1 Hz for 30 sec
at S_1, S_2, and S_3, 25 min apart. Upper
tracings are increases in perfusion pressure indicating vasoconstrictor responses.
Lower columns are stimulation-induced ef-
fluxes of radioactivity indicating norepinephrine release. NPY (100 nM) was present during S_2. (From ref. 225.)

Prejunctional Serotonin Receptors

Serotonin that has been taken up into noradrenergic neurons is released by nerve impulses and can mediate an inhibitory feedback effect on noradrenergic transmission by acting on prejunctional serotonin receptors (89,111,323). These receptors are of the 5-HT$_1$-like subtype (Table 4).

Prejunctional Dopamine Receptors

Dopamine has prejunctional actions and is as potent as norepinephrine in inhibiting stimulation-induced release of norepinephrine in the rabbit ear artery (324–326), cat spleen, and nictitating membrane (327). Noradrenergic terminals in some sympathetically innervated tissues are endowed

with specific dopamine receptors because the prejunctional inhibitory action of dopamine is blocked by dopamine receptor antagonists but not by α-adrenoceptor antagonists (6,11,326,328–331). When dopamine levels in noradrenergic terminals are raised by inhibition of dopamine-β-hydroxylase and loading with dopamine (326,329) or dopa (332), the amount of dopamine released as a cotransmitter is sufficient to mediate an inhibitory feedback loop.

During prolonged periods of intense sympathetic nerve activity, transmitter stores of norepinephrine become depleted and the proportion of dopamine increases (333). The postulated physiological role of prejunctional dopamine receptors on noradrenergic nerves is to provide a restraint on release when transmitter stores are running low (329). This would not necessarily

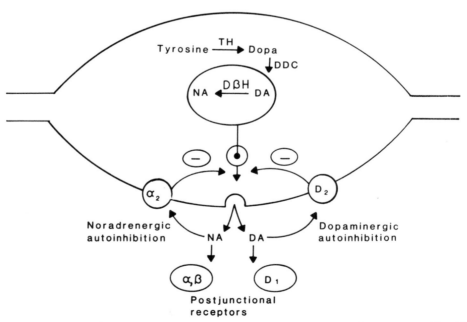

FIG. 6. Automodulation by norepinephrine and dopamine in a cotransmitter system. The biosynthesis of epinephrine (NA) is shown within a terminal noradrenergic varicosity. Tyrosine hydroxylase (TH) converts tyrosine to dopa and then dopa decarboxylase (DDC) converts dopa to dopamine (DA), which is taken up into vesicles where dopamine-β-hydroxylase (DβH) converts it to norepinephrine. If dopamine-β-hydroxylase becomes rate limiting, dopamine accumulates and is released together with norepinephrine and may mediate an additional feedback inhibitory loop by acting on prejunctional dopamine receptors (D$_2$).

compromise the postjunctional response because vasoconstrictor responses to sympathetic nerve stimulation are at first decreased by dopamine but then gradually recover in the continued presence of dopamine despite the decreased release of norepinephrine (326). Prolonged stimulation of sympathetic nerve terminals of the dog mesenteric artery with a high K^+ medium leads to a decrease in the norepinephrine/dopamine ratio and to a relative increase in the release of dopamine that mediates feedback inhibition through prejunctional dopamine receptors (334). A schema of dopamine-mediated autoinhibition is shown in Fig. 6.

Prejunctional Opioid Receptors

Opioids, particularly δ-receptor agonists such as the enkephalins, inhibit the nerve stimulation-induced release of norepinephrine from some autonomic nerve terminals (see below). If opioids were released as cotransmitters and the nerve terminals were endowed with opioid δ-receptors, it would be expected that they would mediate an autoinhibitory feedback loop. However, blockade of opioid receptors with naloxone does not result in an increase in stimulation-induced release of autonomic transmitters or an increased effector response except in two tissues, the rabbit pulmonary and ear arteries. In these tissues, the vasoconstrictor responses to norepinephrine as well as to sympathetic nerve stimulation are increased (335), indicating a postjunctional site of action. Thus, there is no evidence that endogenous opioids engage in automodulation of noradrenergic transmission.

Prejunctional β-Adrenoceptors

The first evidence for the existence of prejunctional β-adrenoceptors subserving facilitation of norepinephrine release came from Adler-Graschinsky and Langer in 1975 (336), who found that isoproterenol increased the stimulation-induced release of norepinephrine from guinea pig atria. This effect has been observed in many other sympathetically innervated tissues from a number of species using several β-adrenoceptor agonists (for reviews, see [82, 337]). It was further suggested that norepinephrine released from sympathetic nerves could activate prejunctional β-adrenoceptors and enhance norepinephrine release (336), thereby forming a positive feedback loop. However, later observations showed that norepinephrine is almost ineffective in enhancing norepinephrine release and only does so if its inhibitory effect on prejunctional α-adrenoceptors is blocked (82). If prejunctional β-adrenoceptors were activated by neuronally released norepinephrine, β-adrenoceptor blocking drugs should inhibit norepinephrine release, but this has only rarely been observed (82,337). Prejunctional β-adrenoceptors are of the $β_2$-subtype (82,337), on which epinephrine is considerably more potent than norepinephrine as an agonist. Thus, epinephrine is a possible physiological activator of prejunctional β-adrenoceptors and has been shown to facilitate norepinephrine release from many isolated tissues (including human tissues) in concentrations that are within the range occurring physiologically in plasma of 0.5 to 10 nm (83).

Epinephrine may alter norepinephrine release through activation of either inhibitory prejunctional α-adrenoceptors or facilitatory prejunctional β-adrenoceptors at sympathetic nerve endings. In animal and human isolated tissues, low concentrations of epinephrine (0.5–10 nm) enhance norepinephrine release by activating prejunctional β-adrenoceptors, whereas higher concentrations (30–1,000 nm) inhibit norepinephrine release by activating prejunctional α-adrenoceptors (82,83). Similar effects of epinephrine have been found *in vivo* (338). It is likely that the only physiological effect of epinephrine at sympathetic nerve terminals in humans is on prejunctional β-adrenoceptors, since the plasma epinephrine level only rises to approximately 6 nM even in stressful situations (339,340).

The release of epinephrine from sympathetic nerve terminals as a cotransmitter with norepinephrine can result in the activation of prejunctional β-adrenoceptors to enhance subsequent norepinephrine release as has been observed *in vitro* (78,80) and *in vivo* (77). The participation of epinephrine as a cotransmitter may have several important consequences. First, by accumulating epinephrine, noradrenergic nerves can concentrate the relatively low levels of epinephrine found in plasma. Second, the epinephrine taken up into nerve endings has a half-life of several hours (82), and this marked persistence allows for occasional bursts of epinephrine secretion from the adrenal medulla to be accumulated in nerves and then to have a prolonged effect on sympathetic neurotransmission. The incorporation of epinephrine into noradrenergic terminals and subsequently its release

and action are shown diagrammatically in Fig. 7.

There has been substantial verification in humans for the facilitatory effect of epinephrine on norepinephrine release from sympathetic nerves. Epinephrine and other β-adrenoceptor agonists enhance norepinephrine release in a variety of human tissues (83). Furthermore, infusions of epinephrine increase plasma norepinephrine levels (341,342). It also has been reported that epinephrine infusion produces a rise in plasma norepinephrine levels and blood pressure after the epinephrine infusion has ceased (343,344). This effect is blocked by propranolol (343). Similarly, epinephrine released from the adrenal medulla by glucagon produces a prolonged rise in plasma norepinephrine levels that persists after return of the plasma epinephrine to basal levels (343). The most likely interpretation of these findings is that epinephrine is taken up into sympathetic nerve terminals and

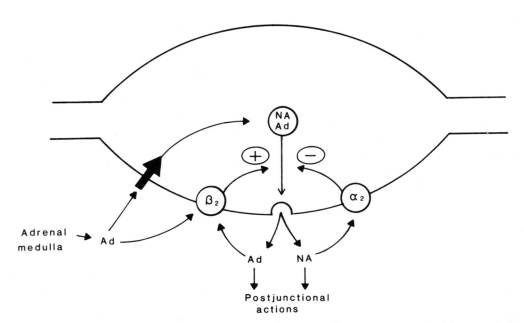

FIG. 7. Epinephrine (Ad) secreted from the adrenal medulla can activate prejunctional β₂-adrenoceptors on noradrenergic nerve terminals. The epinephrine is also taken up into the terminals and then incorporated into the transmitter storage vesicles, from which it can be subsequently released as a cotransmitter. The released epinephrine can mediate facilitatory automodulation by acting on the prejunctional β₂-adrenoceptors.

subsequently released as a cotransmitter that mediates a persistent facilitation of norepinephrine release.

Considerable evidence has now accumulated that the effect of epinephrine in enhancing norepinephrine release may be implicated in the development of hypertension in animals and humans, and there are several reviews on the subject (82,83,345).

Automodulation of Cholinergic Neuroeffector Transmission

Acetylcholine, like norepinephrine, not only mediates neuroeffector transmission but also exerts a feedback inhibitory effect by activating muscarinic autoreceptors. Agonists acting on the prejunctional cholinoceptors of postganglionic autonomic cholinergic nerves inhibit transmitter release and antagonists increase release by disrupting autoinhibition. There are several reviews on the subject (5,346–348). Autoinhibition of cholinergic transmission has been much studied in parasympathetically innervated tissues, including the heart (349), but there have been only a few studies on blood vessels.

It has been known for more than 50 years that blood vessels in skeletal muscle in the cat and dog are innervated by cholinergic sympathetic postganglionic fibers because vasodilator responses can be elicited by sympathetic nerve stimulation and these are enhanced by physostigmine and reduced by atropine (350). Blood vessels in the cephalic (233,351–353), coronary (354), and uterine (355) vascular beds are also innervated by cholinergic fibers, stimulation of which elicits vasodilator responses. Acetylcholine generally acts indirectly as a vasodilator by releasing EDRF, although a direct relaxant action on smooth muscle has been demonstrated at some cholinergic vascular neuroeffector junctions (see below). Another mechanism by which cholinergic nerves could produce vasodilation is by an action of the released acetylcholine on prejunctional muscarinic cholinoceptors of noradrenergic vasoconstrictor nerves to inhibit norepinephrine release (see the section on transneuronal modulation).

At the skeletal muscle neuroeffector junction, acetylcholine mediates a facilitatory feedback loop by acting on prejunctional nicotinic cholinoceptors that differ from the postjunctional ones (356,357). This type of cholinergic automodulation has not so far been described in autonomic cardiovascular control systems.

Cholinergic-Purinergic Cotransmission

The prejunctional inhibitory actions of ATP (or its breakdown products AMP and adenosine) on cholinergic transmission have been reviewed (26,228). There is little information about this in relation to cardiovascular control.

Cholinergic-VIPergic Cotransmission

The pre- and postjunctional effects of acetylcholine and VIP as cotransmitters and the interactions between them are summarized in Fig. 8.

VIP inhibits the stimulation-induced release of acetylcholine, and acetylcholine inhibits the release of VIP (18,231). Blockade of prejunctional cholinoceptors with atropine increases not only the stimulation-induced release of acetylcholine by disrupting autoinhibition but also increases the release of VIP from the salivary gland (232,242,244). The increased loss of VIP from the axon terminals in the presence of atropine results in a substantial depletion of VIP stores and the decreased activation of the VIP receptors results in their upregulation (358).

TRANSNEURONAL MODULATION

Transneuronal modulation is the modulation of transmitter release from one type

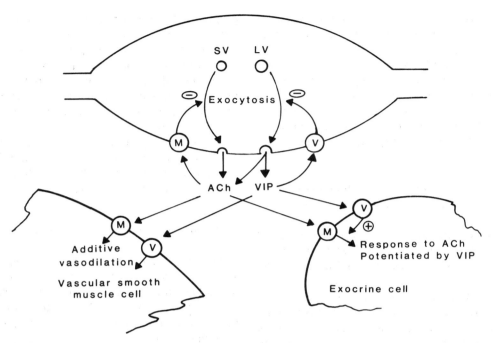

FIG. 8. Pre- and postjunctional interactions between VIP and acetylcholine (ACh) in the cotransmitter system of the parasympathetic nerve supply to the salivary gland. Acetylcholine is stored in small vesicles (SV), whereas VIP is in large vesicles (L) together with acetylcholine. When released exocytotically in response to nerve stimulation, acetylcholine acts on muscarinic cholinoceptors (M) prejunctionally to inhibit transmitter release and postjunctionally to produce vasodilation and salivary secretion, and VIP acts on its receptors (V) prejunctionally to inhibit transmitter release and postjunctionally to produce vasodilation, which is additive to that produced by acetylcholine and to potentiate the secretory response to acetylcholine.

of neuron by a transmitter released from terminals of another type of neuron. For transneuronal modulation to operate, the terminals of the two different kinds of neurons must be located in reasonable proximity, at least within the range of influence of the released transmitter mediating the effect. At peripheral neuroeffector junctions, most attention has been paid to transneuronal modulation between noradrenergic and cholinergic terminals in those tissues receiving a dual innervation. More recently, transneuronal modulation arising from the juxtaposition of nerve terminals containing NANC transmitters (including sensory nerve terminals) to noradrenergic and cholinergic terminals has been considered.

Cholinergic Modulation of Noradrenergic Transmission

The modulation of norepinephrine release from sympathetic nerves by acetylcholine and other cholinomimetic drugs has been dealt with in a number of reviews (359–362). There are two main ways in which acetylcholine and other cholinoceptor agonists interact with noradrenergic neuroeffector transmission. First, cholinoceptor agonists with activity at nicotinic cholinoceptors, such as nicotine, acetylcholine, and DMPP (*N,N*-dimethyl-*N*-phenylpiperazinium) evoke release of norepinephrine from sympathetic nerve terminals by a mechanism that is calcium dependent and involves exocytosis of the transmitter storage vesicles. Second, cholinoceptor agonists such as acetylcholine, methacholine, and pilocarpine act at prejunctional muscarinic cholinoceptors to inhibit stimulation-induced norepinephrine release. This section will deal with the inhibitory effect of acetylcholine and other muscarinic cholinoceptor agonists on noradrenergic transmitter release in cardiovascular tissues. The phenomenon of nicotinic stimulation of noradrenergic nerve terminals will not be considered, but the reader is referred to a recent review that dealt, among others, with this topic (362).

The existence of muscarinic cholinoceptors at noradrenergic nerve terminals was first proposed to explain the effect of muscarinic cholinoceptor agonists in inhibiting the efflux of norepinephrine evoked by nicotinic agonists in perfused rabbit hearts (363,364). Subsequently it was found that responses to sympathetic nerve stimulation and the associated stimulation-induced efflux of norepinephrine from perfused hearts was also subject to inhibition by muscarinic agonists (365). Inhibition of stimulation-induced norepinephrine release from sympathetic nerves by activation of prejunctional muscarinic cholinoceptors has been demonstrated in numerous isolated tissue preparations including many vascular preparations (362).

Norepinephrine release induced by nicotinic agonists and electrical stimulation of nerve axons or terminals is inhibited by muscarinic agonists, as is release evoked by depolarizing concentrations of K^+ (366–368). However, the release of norepinephrine by mechanisms not involving exocytosis, such as that induced by indirectly acting sympathomimetic amines, is not inhibited by muscarinic agonists (365,369,370).

It is generally accepted that muscarinic cholinoceptors comprise M_1 and M_2 subclasses (371). It appears that the muscarinic cholinoceptors located postjunctionally on most peripheral effector cells are of the M_2 type. In general, it has not been possible to

differentiate between postjunctional and prejunctional muscarinic cholinoceptors on sympathetic nerve terminals by the use of selective agonists and antagonists of the subtypes (372–375). However, there is evidence to suggest that muscarinic cholinoceptors on sympathetic nerve terminals may differ between tissues. For example, the selective M_1-cholinoceptor agonist McN-A-343 inhibits noradrenergic transmission in the rabbit ear artery (376) but not in the rabbit heart (377) or pulmonary artery (378,379). Moreover, the relative antagonistic potencies of gallamine, stercuronium, and pancuronium in blocking the effect of carbachol at prejunctional muscarinic cholinoceptors differ between rabbit ear artery and other tissues (380).

In tissues that receive both a noradrenergic and a cholinergic innervation, it is possible that acetylcholine released from cholinergic nerves may activate prejunctional muscarinic cholinoceptors on noradrenergic nerves to decrease norepinephrine release (Fig. 9). Where there is such a dual innervation, effector cells generally respond to the two transmitters in the opposite sense; therefore, the inhibitory effect of transmitter acetylcholine on noradrenergic transmission would serve to reinforce its postjunctional action. Electromicrographic studies reveal close apposition of cholinergic and noradrenergic terminal networks in several tissues, including the heart (381,382) and some blood vessels (383–386).

In the case of the heart there is considerable evidence that transmitter acetylcholine can modulate norepinephrine release from sympathetic nerves. Thus, in the rabbit isolated heart, vagal stimulation reduces norepinephrine release and responses to sympathetic nerve stimulation (387,388). Evidence for the activation of inhibitory prejunctional muscarinic cholinoceptors of sympathetic nerves by transmitter acetylcholine has been obtained from experiments with isolated rabbit atria subjected to field stimulation of intrinsic sympathetic and parasympathetic nerves (389,390); how-

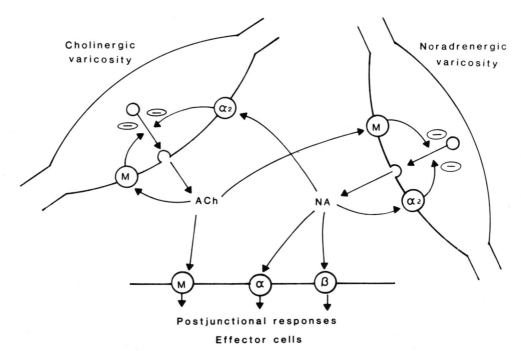

FIG. 9. Transneuronal modulation between cholinergic and noradrenergic neuroeffector transmission and cholinergic and noradrenergic automodulation. The subtypes of adrenoceptors and muscarinic cholinoceptors involved in postjunctional responses depend on the particular effector tissue. The subtypes of muscarinic cholinoceptors involved in automodulation and transneuronal modulation have not yet been determined definitively and may differ between neuroeffector junctions in different tissues. The adrenoceptors of cholinergic terminals involved in inhibitory transneuronal modulation also depend on their location: they are generally α_2-adrenoceptors (see text), but in some tissues they are α_1-adrenoceptors (415), and it has been suggested that they are β-adrenoceptors in the respiratory tract (418). Note that additional automodulation and transneuronal modulation may be mediated by VIP and NPY released as cotransmitters from cholinergic and noradrenergic terminals, respectively.

ever, no such interaction was found with guinea pig isolated atria (389,391). Acetylcholine released by stimulation of cardiac parasympathetic nerves in the dog *in vivo* inhibits norepinephrine release and the responses to cardiac sympathetic nerve stimulation (392,393).

Experiments with rabbit isolated atria have revealed that two populations of muscarinic cholinoceptors are involved in the inhibitory modulation of noradrenergic transmission by neuronally released acetylcholine (394). Stimulation of both the extrinsic vagus and sympathetic nerves for 3-min periods at 3 Hz in such a way that the

pulses applied to the vagus precede those applied to the sympathetic nerve inhibits norepinephrine release when the interval between the pulses is 3 to 10 msec or 200 to 283 msec, but there is no significant inhibition when the delay is 30 to 167 msec. Both the early and late inhibitions are blocked by atropine. However, stimulation with a delay of 100 msec between pulses does inhibit norepinephrine release when M_1-cholinoceptors are selectively blocked with pirenzepine (395). It was first suggested that the early inhibition may involve modulation of the conductance of an ion channel and the late inhibition effect may be mediated by a prostanoid (394). Subsequently it was suggested that neuronally released acetylcholine acts prejunctionally on M_2-cholinoceptors to inhibit, and on M_1-cholinoceptors to enhance norepinephrine release (395).

Some blood vessels receive a cholinergic innervation, either in the form of sympathetic cholinergic postganglionic fibers or postganglionic parasympathetic fibers. Such blood vessels are known to be present in the skin on the face and neck, skeletal muscle, and penile erectile tissue. Cholinergic vasodilation has also been observed in blood vessels of the cat salivary gland (233), nasal mucosa (396), tongue (250,351), and brain (351), in dog coronary (95) and gastric (397) arteries, in guinea pig uterine artery (355), and in rabbit lingual artery (353). The dilator action of acetylcholine in many blood vessels is mediated by EDRF (134,398). In the rabbit pulmonary artery, removal of the endothelium reverses the dilator response to acetylcholine to a constriction, but the inhibitory effect of acetylcholine on noradrenergic transmission is unaltered (399). Moreover, in the cholinergically innervated lingual artery of the rabbit, the vasodilator action of transmitter acetylcholine does not involve EDRF (353).

The vasodilator responses to cholinergic nerve stimulation in blood vessels receiving a dual cholinergic-noradrenergic innervation could be due to inhibition of noradrenergically maintained vasoconstrictor tone (370), but the extent to which this occurs is not known. However, blood vessels with a cholinergic innervation in which endogenously released acetylcholine has been shown to inhibit norepinephrine release include the dog coronary (400) and gastric arteries (397). There is an interaction between noradrenergic and cholinergic perivascular axon terminals of cerebral blood vessels (386). Interactions between noradrenergic and cholinergic terminals are illustrated in Fig. 9. However, most blood vessels do not receive a cholinergic innervation; therefore, the role of muscarinic cholinoceptors subserving inhibition of noradrenergic transmission on sympathetic nerve terminals in the vast majority of blood vessels is unknown.

Noradrenergic Modulation of Cholinergic Transmission

Evidence that α-adrenoceptors might serve a modulatory role in cholinergic neuroeffector transmission was first obtained in the myenteric plexus of the gastrointestinal tract (401). There have been many reports that α-adrenoceptor agonists decrease the efflux of acetylcholine from isolated intestinal preparations both under resting conditions and during periods of field stimulation of the intramural nerves (402–406). The prejunctional α-adrenoceptors of cholinergic nerve terminals in the myenteric plexus are of the α_2-subtype (407–410). They appear to be involved in transjunctional modulation of cholinergic transmission in that they are activated by norepinephrine released from adjacent noradrenergic terminals (405,411,412).

There have been relatively few studies concerned with the possibility of noradrenergic modulation of cholinergic transmission in cardiovascular tissues. Not surprisingly, virtually all of the information available relates to cholinergic transmission in the heart, where the juxtaposition of noradrenergic and cholinergic nerve terminals would seem to provide the opportunity for reciprocal interaction between the two transmitter systems (see previous section; 11,391). In addition to transmitter interactions at the neuroeffector level, there is also the possibility of noradrenergically mediated modulation of cholinergic transmission at cardiac intramural ganglionic synapses.

In isolated perfused rabbit hearts, the responses to stimulation of the extrinsic vagus nerve are reduced by the selective α_2-adrenoceptor agonists oxymetazoline and naphthazoline (413). In guinea-pig atria, α-adrenoceptor agonists reduce the field stimulation-induced release of radioactivity that had been incorporated into the cholinergic transmitter stores as [^{3}H]acetylcholine, but the negative chronotropic response is unaltered (414). In rat isolated atria, acetylcholine release from intramural cholinergic nerves is inhibited by norepinephrine acting on prejunctional α-adrenoceptors that appear to be of the α_1-subtype (415). In guinea pig atria, α-adrenoceptor agonists also inhibit the stimulation-induced efflux of acetylcholine, but prejunctional α_2-adrenoceptors are involved (414).

In contrast to the gastrointestinal tract, the evidence for a modulatory role of neuronally released norepinephrine on cholinergic transmission in the heart is sparse. In guinea pig atria neither phentolamine, idazoxan, nor prazosin have any effect on the release of [^{3}H]acetylcholine, which has been incorporated into cholinergic transmitter stores (414). Moreover, depletion of the noradrenergic transmitter pool by reserpine pretreatment does not alter stimulation-induced acetylcholine release in guinea pig atria (416).

Transneuronal Modulation Involving NANC Mediators

There are many examples of nerve stimulation-induced responses of effector tissue that cannot be ascribed to noradrenergic or cholinergic mechanisms (417), and as mentioned previously NANC transmission appears to be of functional significance for neuroeffector transmission in some vascular beds. The increasing awareness of the significance of NANC transmission for the control of lung function, particularly that mediated by neuropeptides, has been emphasized by Barnes (418). The possibility of interactions between NANC transmitters and classical transmitters through actions on prejunctional receptors has been recognized but has yet to be thoroughly explored.

NPYergic Modulation of Cholinergic Transmission

There is evidence that NPY released as a cotransmitter from noradrenergic terminals can modulate cholinergic transmission. NPY inhibits the bradycardia produced by vagal stimulation in guinea pig isolated atria (217) and in the intact guinea pig, rabbit (203), and dog (419). The evidence indicates that this is due to inhibition of acetylcholine release from the postganglionic terminals, but an additional inhibition of ganglionic transmission has not been excluded (420). NPY inhibits the cholinergic contractile response of the rat uterus to field stimulation of the intramural nerves (421,422).

Stimulation of cardiac sympathetic nerves produces a long-lasting inhibition of the bradycardia response to vagal stimulation that is not mimicked by norepinephrine and not affected by adrenoceptor blockade (419). This effect is mimicked by NPY (419,423). Pretreatment with guanethidine, which blocks release of both NPY and norepinephrine, abolishes the inhibitory effect of sympathetic stimulation on responses to vagal stimulation (424). The inhibitory effect of sympathetic stimulation on vagal bradycardia is greater when the sympathetic nerves are stimulated at a high (20 Hz) rather than a low (5 Hz) frequency with the same number of pulses (425), which is consistent with the effect being mediated by NPY.

Sympathetic Modulation of VIPergic Transmission

VIPergic transmission is not only subject to automodulation but also to transneuronal modulation, because the release of VIP evoked by parasympathetic nerve stimulation in the cat intestine and the vasodilator response produced by it are inhibited by sympathetic nerve stimulation (426). Conversely, VIP reduces the vasoconstrictor response to sympathetic nerve stimulation (427), but the mechanism of this effect has not been elucidated.

Cholinergic Modulation of Purinergic Transmission

It would be expected that activation of prejunctional muscarinic cholinoceptors would inhibit transmission at those sympathetic neuroeffector junctions where ATP mediates postjunctional responses. In fact, acetylcholine reduces the amplitude of ATP-mediated EJPs elicited by stimulation of perivascular sympathetic axons in the rabbit saphenous artery by an action that does not depend on the endothelium (428). The possibility exists, therefore, for the transneuronal modulation of purinergic transmission, but this does not appear to have been demonstrated.

Modulation of Autonomic Transmission by γ-Aminobutyric Acid

The evidence for a functional role of γ-aminobutyric acid- (GABA) containing peripheral neurons has been reviewed (429). Some effector tissues contain GABA in amounts equivalent to those in the central nervous system (430). Both $GABA_A$ and $GABA_B$ receptor subtypes are fairly widely distributed at prejunctional as well as postjunctional locations. Activation of GABA receptors, probably of the $GABA_A$ subtype, stimulates cholinergic neurons in the intestine (431) and gallbladder (432). Activation of prejunctional receptors, probably of the $GABA_B$ subtype, inhibits transmitter release from cholinergic neurons in the gut (431) and from noradrenergic neurons in the rabbit pulmonary artery (433), mouse and guinea pig atria, and the rat vas deferens (434) and anococcygeus muscle (435). Thus, the possibility exists for transneuronal modulation of noradrenergic and

cholinergic transmission by GABAergic neurons but has yet to be demonstrated.

Other Examples of Modulation of NANC Transmission

There have been few studies on the modulation of NANC transmission in cardiovascular effectors with the exception of those on the well-recognized cotransmitters mentioned earlier. However, there are data on the modulation of NANC transmitter release in other tissues. In the anococcygeus muscle, stimulation-induced norepinephrine and NANC inhibitory transmission are both inhibited by somatostatin (436) and muscarinic agonists (437). In intestinal preparations, NANC inhibitory transmission is inhibited by α_2-adrenoceptor agonists (438,439). NPY decreases the response to stimulation of intrinsic NANC nerves in the guinea pig urinary bladder (217). These examples point to the possibility of transneuronal modulation of NANC transmission by noradrenergic and cholinergic mechanisms.

Transmitters of Sensory Neurons and Their Roles in Modulation of Autonomic Neuroeffector Transmission

The relevance of sensory neurons to the functioning and modulation of neuroeffector transmission is that they send peripheral axons to blood vessels and sympathetic ganglia and contain substances with potent pharmacological activity that are released and produce local actions when the sensory terminal axons are activated. These substances include ATP and a number of neuropeptides. In addition to their actions on effector tissues, many of these substances may also act on autonomic nerve terminals and thereby engage in transneuronal modulation. The full physiological significance of the local reactions to activation of sensory nerve terminals remains to be elucidated: most attention has been paid to the role they play in reactions to noxious stimuli (440). In experimental studies in which stimulation is applied to efferent nerve terminals within a tissue, the sensory nerve terminals will also be activated, and even stimulation of extrinsic nerve trunks does not avoid the possibility of activation of sensory nerve terminals because peripheral nerve trunks contain both efferent and afferent axons. For these reasons, effects of the pharmacologically active substances released from sensory nerve terminals of autonomic neuroeffector transmission demand attention.

ATP is released from sensory nerve terminals by antidromic stimulation (441). Its role in mediating the vasodilation produced by antidromic sensory nerve stimulation is not clear: ATP acts directly on P_2-purinoceptors of most vascular smooth muscle to produce vasoconstriction, but it can also act on endothelial cells to release EDRF and thereby indirectly cause vasodilation. Antidromic vasodilation occurs in small blood vessels with only few smooth muscle cells between the adventitial nerve terminals and the endothelial cells, so it is possible that ATP traverses the media and the predominant effect is due to EDRF release from the endothelial cells. A further possibility for the vasodilation produced by antidromic stimulation of sensory nerves is inhibition of sympathetic vasoconstrictor tone by activation of prejunctional P_1-purinoceptors.

The ways in which sensory neurokinins may affect vascular function have been summarized by Regoli and D'Orleans-Juste (442) as (a) blood-borne or local hormones mediating vasodilation by releasing EDRF, (b) neurotransmitters mediating vasoconstriction in some blood vessels and possibly some vascular beds, (c) modulators of sympathetic transmission, and (d) mediators of sensory nerve influences on local blood flow.

In perivascular nerve fibers, substance P and the related neurokinins coexist with CGRP in axons that are distinct from noradrenergic axons and are presumed to be afferents (41,191,443–446). Both substance P and CGRP are vasodilators (see below).

Substance P and Other Neurokinins

In the early days of research on substance P, it was identified by bioassay, but its precise localization has only been possible since the development of highly sensitive immunochemical methods; however, unless special safeguards are taken these do not discriminate between substance P and other closely related neurokinins (440). In the following account, the term substance P may also include other neurokinins. This group of biologically active peptides, including many of nonmammalian origin, are collectively termed tachykinins.

Substance P is synthesized in the cell bodies of primary afferent neurons and transported to the central and peripheral terminals. The importance of the peripheral distribution of substance P is emphasized by the finding that approximately 80% of that formed in the cell bodies is transported along the peripheral axon branches (447,448). Substance P-containing axons that are presumably peripheral axons of primary sensory neurons are present in many effector tissues (440). In the cardiovascular system, they are in the heart (449) and blood vessels where they form perivascular networks (443).

Substance P mimics the vasodilation, extravasation of plasma, contraction of nonvascular smooth muscle, and increased mucociliary activity produced by antidromic stimulation of sensory nerves and probably mediates these effects (450,451). Some of the effects of substance P appear to involve interactions with sympathetic neuroeffector control because the vasodilation and extravasation of plasma produced by injection of substance P into the rat femoral artery are only fully revealed after chemical sympathectomy or guanethidine to remove sympathetic vasoconstrictor tone (451). Somatostatin and an enkephalin analog inhibit responses to antidromic nerve stimulation but not to substance P, suggesting that they inhibit release of substance P (452).

Substance P is present in cerebral perivascular axons and is a potent cerebral vasodilator *in vitro* and *in situ* (445). Axon terminals containing substance P are in close proximity to those containing norepinephrine in cerebral blood vessels (453). In addition to mediating vasodilation, substance P released from perivascular sensory axons may impose a restraint on vasoconstriction because transection of the trigeminal nerve in the cat results in prolongation of the vasoconstrictor action of norepinephrine on cerebral blood vessels (39).

Substance P-containing sensory terminals in sympathetic ganglia form synapses with autonomic ganglion cells (454). It has been known for some years that substance P enhances ganglionic transmission (455), and more recently the basis for this has been shown to be that substance P pro-

duces a slow excitatory postsynaptic potential that lowers the threshold for excitation and can even initiate action potentials (456). Stimulation of the sensory collateral axons to sympathetic ganglia produces a similar slow excitatory postsynaptic potential to that produced by substance P (263). The use of substance P antagonists has shown that this is mediated by substance P (456). It has been suggested that substance P-containing sensory axon collaterals and sympathetic postganglionic neurons could constitute a peripheral reflex mechanism (456) as shown in Fig. 10.

A major advance in tachykinin research arising from the development of synthetic analogs with agonistic and/or antagonistic activity has been the identification of neurokinin receptor subtypes (457), which, with their implications for cardiovascular neuroeffectors, are shown in Table 7. Their distribution and contributions to the overall response vary considerably between tissues. In the dog carotid artery, only NK_1 receptors are present; in rabbit pulmonary artery and mesenteric vein there are both

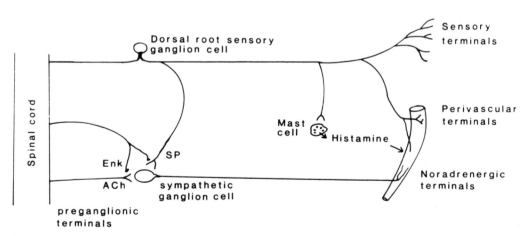

FIG. 10. Peptidergic modulatory influences on synaptic transmission in sympathetic ganglia. Branches of substance P-containing sensory axons (SPergic) impinge on ganglion cells and substance P released as a transmitter elicits slow excitatory postsynaptic potentials, thereby facilitating transmission initiated by fast excitatory postsynaptic potentials mediated by acetylcholine released from sympathetic preganglionic terminals (AChergic). Enkephalin-containing terminals (Enkergic) impinge on the AChergic and SPergic terminals where enkephalins inhibit transmitter release. See text for details.

TABLE 7. *Neurokinin receptor subtypes and cardiovascular consequences for their activation*

Subtype	Neurokinin	Response to activation
NK_1	SP≥NKA≥NKB	Release of EDRF (vasodilation)
NK_2	NKA>NKB≫SP	Contraction of smooth muscle; facilitation of transmitter release
NK_3	NKB>NKA≥SP	Contraction of longitudinal smooth muscle of rat portal vein; activation of cholinergic neurons; extravasation of plasma

SP, substance P; NKA, neurokinin A; NKB, neurokinin B.

NK_1 and NK_2 receptors; in rat portal vein there are only NK_3 receptors.

The complexity of the interactions between the cardiovascular responses to neurokinins is dramatically highlighted when the responses to selective agonists for the receptor subtypes are injected intravenously in rats (457). Agonists for the NK_1 receptor have a depressor action due to vasodilation that is accompanied by reflex tachycardia. Activation of NK_2 receptors produces a small transient fall in blood pressure and a pronounced tachycardia due to facilitation of norepinephrine release from cardiac sympathetic nerves (458). NK_3 receptor agonists produce bradycardia due to release of acetylcholine from vagal cholinergic neurons and a fall in blood pressure due to vasodilation accentuated by extravasation of plasma.

CGRP

There is CGRP-like immunoreactivity in the cardiovascular system of several species in blood vessels (459,460) and heart (461,462). CGRP coexists with substance P in cerebral perivascular axons (463) and is also a potent cerebral vasodilator (459). The amount of CGRP associated with cerebral blood vessels increases after sympathectomy (464).

CGRP, like substance P, is a depressor when injected intravenously and a potent vasodilator (445,465,466), but the two peptides act by different mechanisms: the vasodilator action of substance P is endothelium dependent, but that of CGRP is not (467). CGRP potentiates the action of substance P in producing extravasation of plasma protein (468). This effect is apparently due to inhibition by CGRP of the breakdown of substance P (469).

CGRP has positive chronotropic and inotropic actions (193,259,467,469–471). It differs in this respect from other sensory neuropeptides (substance P, neurokinins A and B) and from VIP, which do not have cardiac stimulant activity (446,467). The cardiac actions of CGRP are not exerted through a noradrenergic mechanism but, like β-adrenoceptor agonists, CGRP activates adenylate cyclase (472).

There are CGRP-containing nerves in the vas deferens (473). CGRP inhibits the twitch response to field stimulation (474,475) and reduces contractile responses to norepinephrine and ATP (473). CGRP hyperpolarizes the smooth muscle membrane but does not alter the amplitude of EJPs, therefore its effect is postjunctional (473). CGRP relaxes rat splenic strips precontracted with norepinephrine (470).

TRANSJUNCTIONAL MODULATION

Transjunctional modulation involves the action on transmitter release of substances released from effector cells. This type of modulation has been particularly studied by Hedqvist (476,477). The main mediators are adenosine and prostaglandin (PG) E_2: both are liberated when effector cells are activated and both inhibit stimulation-induced

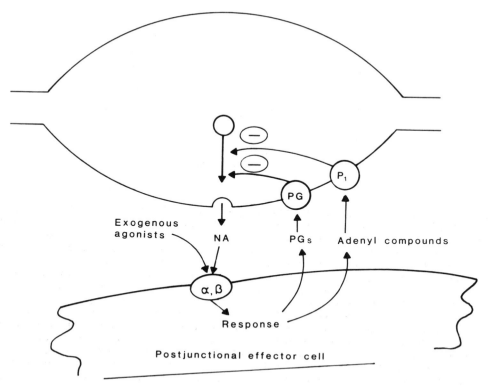

FIG. 11. Transjunctional modulation of transmitter release resulting from activation of prejunctional receptor by substances released from effector cells that have been stimulated by the transmitter (for example, norepinephrine, NA) or by an exogenous agonist. PGs (generally PGEs, acting on PG receptors) and adenyl compounds (adenosine or AMP, acting on P_1-purinoceptors) are common examples of such substances.

release of norepinephrine (Fig. 11). When both are eliminated (PG synthesis blocked by indomethacin and the prejunctional action of adenosine blocked by theophylline), the increase in the stimulation-induced release of norepinephrine from the kidney is as great as that produced by blocking prejunctional α-adrenoceptors (477). It appears, therefore, that the magnitude of transjunctional modulation is as great as that of automodulation in limiting noradrenergic transmission, at least in the kidney. From a teleological point of view, the functional significance of transjunctional modulation is to impose a restraint on excessive activation of effector cells.

Adenyl Compounds

Adenyl compounds are released when effector tissues are activated: whichever adenyl compound is released, it would be rapidly broken down to adenosine, so this is the main one to be considered as a mediator of transjunctional modulation of noradrenergic transmission. In the kidney, adenosine is released from effector cells by sympathetic nerve stimulation, and its release is blocked by α-adrenoceptor antagonists (478). Adenosine has vasoconstrictor activity in the kidney (479) and potentiates the vasoconstrictor action of norepinephrine (306); however, as described above, it also

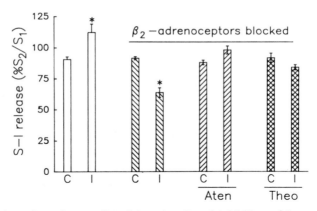

FIG. 12. Evidence for adenosine-mediated transjunctional inhibition of transmitter release in rat isolated atria. The atria were labeled with [^{3}H]norepinephrine and the stimulation-induced (**S**-I) efflux of radioactivity was used as an index of transmitter norepinephrine release. In each experiment, two periods of field stimulation (2 Hz for 60 sec) were given 30 min apart, and the efflux in the second (S_2) was expressed as a percentage of that in the first (S_1). In the hatched columns, isoproterenol (0.1 μM) was present during the second period of stimulation, and the open columns are corresponding control experiments. Values are the means of four to eight experiments and the vertical bars represent the S.E.M. Significant differences ($P<0.05$, Student's t-test) from the corresponding control are indicated by *. All experiments were carried out in the presence of atropine (1 μM) and phentolamine (1 μM). The first pair of columns shows that isoproterenol facilitates norepinephrine release by acting on prejunctional β_2-adrenoceptors. In the experiments marked β_2-adrenoceptors blocked, the selective antagonist ICI 118,551 (0.1 μM) was present to block the prejunctional β_2-adrenoceptors: this revealed an inhibitory effect of isoproterenol on norepinephrine release. The inhibitory effect was abolished by blockade of postjunctional β_1-adrenoceptors with atenolol (3 μM, Aten), or of prejunctional P_1-purinoceptors with theophylline (100 μM, Theo), indicating that it arose from isoproterenol-stimulated atrial tissue and was due to an adenyl compound. (From Mian, Majewski, and Rand, *unpublished observations.*)

inhibits stimulation-induced release of norepinephrine. The adenosine released from effector cells in the kidney appears to contribute to the vasoconstrictor response to sympathetic nerve stimulation because the response is reduced by theophylline (478). However, theophylline also blocks the prejunctional inhibitory action of adenosine, so that sympathetic nerve stimulation releases a greater amount of norepinephrine (477).

Evidence for transjunctional inhibition of noradrenergic transmission in rat isolated atria is presented in Fig. 12.

PGs

In the early days of research on PGs it was noticed that particularly those of the E series decreased the rise in blood pressure (480) and the tachycardia (481) produced by catecholamines. However, in some autonomic effector tissues they either do not affect the responses to catecholamines or they enhance them.

The more marked effect of PGs on autonomic effectors is modulation of neurotransmission (for reviews, see [3,4,476, 482]). PGEs decrease responses to sympathetic nerve stimulation by decreasing norepinephrine release in the cat spleen, rabbit heart and kidney, guinea pig vas deferens, and in blood vessels (476). However, enhancement of vasoconstrictor responses to sympathetic nerve stimulation by PGE$_2$, despite inhibition of norepinephrine release, has been observed in the rat isolated perfused kidney (483).

Activation of tissues by norepinephrine or sympathetic nerve stimulation releases PGs (predominantly PGE with smaller amounts of PGA and PGF) from spleen, kidney (476), and heart (476,484). In addition, some of the PGs released by sympathetic stimulation may be of neuronal origin (485). Inhibition of PG synthesis results in larger responses to sympathetic nerve stimulation in spleen, heart, and vas deferens, and greater release of norepinephrine (476), and larger vasoconstrictor responses to norepinephrine (486).

In contrast to PGs of the E series, those of the F series, particularly $F_{2\alpha}$, enhance stimulation-induced release of norepinephrine in some tissues (487). $PGF_{2\alpha}$ enhances vasoconstrictor responses to perivascular nerve stimulation and reflex stimulation without affecting responses to norepinephrine, but in veins it enhances responses to both (488). The venoconstrictor and vasoconstrictor actions of $PGF_{2\alpha}$ depend on the integrity of the sympathetic innervation (488), which probably reflects facilitation of transmitter release by the sympathetic tone *in vivo*.

The inhibition of transmitter release by PGE_1 appears to extend to cholinergic terminals because it inhibits the bradycardia response to vagal stimulation in the rabbit without affecting the response to acetylcholine (489).

HORMONAL MODULATION

Hormonal modulation in this context is the alteration by hormones of transmitter release by activation of specific receptors associated with the nerve terminals. The term hormone is used in the broad sense to include not only endocrine hormones but also so-called local hormones and autacoids. Epinephrine, which acts on prejunctional β-adrenoceptors to facilitate noradrenergic transmission, has been dealt with previously as a cotransmitter that engages in automodulation, because this is the more

important aspect of its action in modulating neuroeffector transmission.

Angiotensin II

Angiotensin II has long been considered a major hormonal factor for the regulation of cardiovascular function. The classical renin-angiotensin system comprises three components: (a) the enzyme renin, synthesized and released by the juxtaglomerular cells of the kidney; (b) the α_2-globulin precursor, angiotensinogen, present in plasma; and (c) angiotensin-converting enzyme, associated primarily with pulmonary vascular endothelial cells. In addition, it is now recognized that many tissues, including the heart and blood vessels, have the capacity to synthesize angiotensin II. It seems likely that angiotensin II produced locally in cardiovascular tissues also subserves a regulatory role in cardiovascular function. Locally produced angiotensin II would be more appropriately considered a local hormone or autacoid than a circulating hormone.

The effects of angiotensin II on cardiovascular function depend not only on its direct vasoconstrictor and cardiac stimulant actions and ability to enhance the synthesis and release of aldosterone but also on several specific interactions with the sympathetic nervous system. The interactions between angiotensin II and the sympathetic nervous system are of particular interest because they may provide for close integration of the neural and hormonal cardiovascular control systems.

Angiotensin II enhances the activity of the sympathetic nervous system at several levels: it promotes increased efferent sympathetic tone by acting on neurons in the central nervous system (490,491), it activates sympathetic ganglion cells (492–494), it stimulates adrenal chromaffin cells to release catecholamines (495), and it facilitates noradrenergic neuroeffector transmission by actions at both pre- and postjunctional sites. The major prejunctional action of angiotensin II on noradrenergic nerve terminals is to enhance stimulation-induced transmitter release (3,4): it has also been reported to increase the rate of synthesis of norepinephrine (496) and inhibit neuronal reuptake of the transmitter (497). The major postjunctional interaction between angiotensin II and noradrenergic neuroeffector function is to increase the responsiveness of effector cells to the transmitter and also to other vasoconstrictor agents (498). The prejunctional action of angiotensin II in enhancing transmitter release appears to be quantitatively more important than its postjunctional sensitizing action (499–501).

Angiotensin II facilitates stimulation-induced norepinephrine release by activating specific prejunctional receptors, and the effect is blocked by angiotensin-II receptor antagonists (502–504). The threshold concentration of angiotensin II for enhancement of norepinephrine release in guinea pig isolated atria is less than 100 pM (504) and in rat caudal arteries enhancement of vasoconstrictor responses to stimulation is produced by angiotensin II in concentrations approximately one-tenth of those required to produce vasoconstriction (503).

There are numerous reports of enhancement by angiotensin II of vasoconstrictor responses to sympathetic nerve stimulation *in situ,* for example, in the vasculatures of rat mesentery (505) and the dog hind paw (502). Similarly, many studies have demonstrated that pressor responses to stimulation of the spinal sympathetic outflow in pithed rats are enhanced by angiotensin II (499).

Evidence for facilitation of noradrenergic transmission by endogenous angiotensin II has been obtained in various species by using inhibitors of the renin-angiotensin system. Thus, in anesthetized cats, inhibition of converting enzyme or blockade of angiotensin II receptors with saralasin enhances the fall in blood pressure produced by activation of sympathetic reflexes by negative pressure applied to the lower body (506). Similarly converting-enzyme inhibitors and saralasin attenuate stimulation-

induced pressor responses in pithed rats (507–509). Such findings indicate that there is ongoing facilitation of vascular and/or cardiac noradrenergic transmission by endogenous angiotensin II (507,510). More direct evidence that the facilitatory influence of endogenous angiotensin II on noradrenergic transmission *in vivo* involves enhancement of transmitter release has been obtained in pithed rabbits in which the spinal sympathetic outflow was stimulated (511) and in which the converting-enzyme inhibitor captopril and saralasin reduce the release rate of norepinephrine.

In addition to the interactions of angiotensin II with noradrenergic neuroeffector transmission cited above, angiotensin II releases PGs from effector cells in many tissues (512,513). The PGs so produced generally act to oppose the pre- and postjunctional effects of angiotensin II, as has been observed in the rat isolated perfused heart (514). After inhibition of cyclooxygenase by indomethacin or meclofenemate, the facilitatory effect of angiotensin II on noradrenergic transmission in anesthetized dogs is enhanced (515).

The enzymatic production of angiotensin II from peptide precursors has been demonstrated in many tissues, including the heart and blood vessels. The presence of renin-like activity in nonrenal tissues was first deduced from the ability of the tissues to form angiotensin I and angiotensin II from peptide precursors. More recently, immunofluorescent techniques have revealed the presence of renin in a wide variety of tissues and cell types, including vascular endothelial cells (516) and vascular smooth muscle (517). Synthesis of renin has been demonstrated in cultured aortic smooth muscle, in endothelial cells (517,518), and the heart (519). However, much of the renin present in blood vessel walls may not be synthesized locally but derive from circulating renin of renal origin (519–522). Vascular wall renin has a much longer half-life than plasma renin (519) and has been shown to be released by physiological stimuli such as hemorrhage (523). In addition to renin itself, other less specific enzymes such as acid proteases may be involved in angiotensin-II formation in cardiovascular tissues.

Angiotensin-converting enzyme is also present in the heart and vasculature. It is generally accepted that angiotensin-converting enzyme is synthesized and stored in vascular endothelial cells (524,525). However, in an isolated preparation of the rat caudal artery, the ability of angiotensin I to enhance vasoconstrictor responses to sympathetic stimulation, presumably as a consequence of lcoal production of angiotensin II, does not depend on the presence of a functional endothelium (526). In rats the highest cardiac levels of angiotensin-converting enzyme activity are in the atria (519). In addition, an isoangiotensin-converting enzyme is present in bovine atria (527).

Although there is still uncertainty about the physiological role of local renin-angiotensin systems in cardiovascular tissues, it is an attractive possibility that locally produced angiotensin II may function as a modulator of sympathetic neuroeffector transmission, as shown in Fig. 13. In the isolated mesenteric vasculature of SHR,

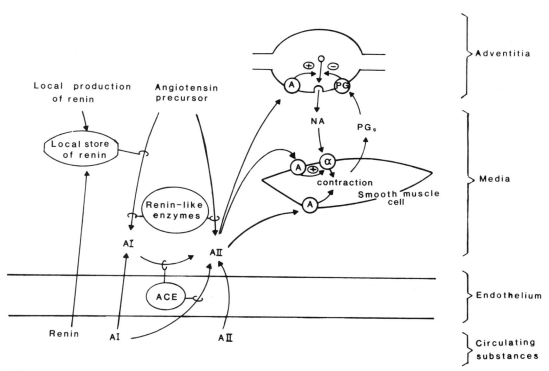

FIG. 13. Schema for the local generation of angiotensin II (AII) and its interaction with noradrenergic transmission in the blood vessel wall. An angiotensin precursor in the vessel wall may be converted to angiotensin I (AI) by either renin sequestered from plasma or synthesized locally, or by renin-like enzymes. Proteases in the vessel wall may also convert an angiotensin precursor directly to AII. Angiotensin-converting enzyme, which is associated mainly with endothelial cells, converts AI from plasma, or locally generated AI to AII. AII may also enter the vascular wall from plasma. AII acts at receptor sites on vascular smooth muscle cells to sensitize them to the action of transmitter norepinephrine, to produce vasoconstriction and stimulate PG production (PGs). AII also acts on prejunctional receptors of sympathetic nerve terminals to enhance transmitter release. The enhancing effect of AII on transmitter release may be opposed by a prejunctional inhibitory action of the PGs released from the vascular smooth muscle cells.

constrictor responses to sympathetic stimulation are enhanced by tetradecapeptide renin substrate and also by hog renin substrate, and in each case the enhancement is blocked by angiotensin-converting-enzyme inhibitors and saralasin (500). In isolated caudal arteries from normotensive Wistar rats, tetradecapeptide renin substrate and angiotensin I enhance stimulation-induced vasoconstriction and norepinephrine release. However, whereas the facilitatory effects of both tetradecapeptide and angiotensin I on responses and transmitter efflux are blocked by saralasin, only the effects of angiotensin I are blocked by converting-enzyme inhibitors (528). Converting-enzyme inhibitors also fail to prevent the facilitatory effect of tetradecapeptide renin substrate on noradrenergic transmission guinea pig isolated atria (503) and rat isolated kidneys (530). Such findings would suggest that tetradecapeptide renin substrate may itself have agonist activity at prejunctional angiotensin-II receptors or alternatively, that some cardiovascular tissues have the capacity to convert the tetradecapeptide to angiotensin II by a pathway that is independent of angiotensin-converting enzyme. In fact, tetradecapeptide renin substrate may be converted directly to angiotensin II by peptidases such as tonin (531) and cathepsin D (532).

In pithed rats (533) and pithed rabbits (511), saralasin and captopril decrease the norepinephrine release rate during stimulation of the sympathetic outflow, suggesting that there is tonic modulation of norepinephrine release by endogenous angiotensin II. However, no such sympathoinhibitory effect of saralasin or captopril is observed in acutely nephrectomized animals (511,533). This does not necessarily rule out the possibility of local angiotensin-II production being important in the modulation of norepinephrine release, but it does suggest that renin of renal origin is the critical determinant of endogenous angiotensin-II effects in the whole animal.

Activation of β-adrenoceptors releases renin from the juxtaglomerular cells of the kidney and thereby increases plasma renin activity (534). The possibility of the existence of a counterpart of this mechanism for local angiotensin-II production in blood vessels has been raised because the effect of isoproterenol in enhancing vasoconstrictor responses to sympathetic stimulation in rat isolated mesenteric vascular beds is reduced, not only by β-adrenoceptor antagonists but by captopril and saralasin (535). Direct evidence that β-adrenoceptor activation enhances angiotensin-II production has been obtained in rat isolated mesenteric vasculature (536). In rat isolated vena cava, a major part of the β-adrenoceptor enhancement of transmitter norepinephrine release is mediated by locally produced angiotensin II (537). The β-adrenoceptors involved in the stimulation of angiotensin-II production in the vena cava are probably located on the smooth muscle cells because isoproterenol is more effective in enhancing transmitter release when applied to the intimal rather than the adventitial surface. Moreover, the effect is unchanged after removing the endothelium (537).

The findings of a functional link between β-adrenoceptors and local angiotensin-II production in blood vessels does not negate the existence of facilitatory prejunctional β-adrenoceptors. Indeed, in mesenteric vascular preparations, blockade of the renin-angiotensin system does not abolish the facilitatory effect of isoproterenol on noradrenergic transmission (535,537). Moreover, in other tissues the facilitatory effect of β-adrenoceptor agonists is independent of angiotensin-II production. This has been shown to be the case in guinea pig atria (529) and in rat kidney (538) and anococcygeus muscle (539). Furthermore, in mouse atria and rat tail artery (540), the β-adrenoceptor agonist isoproterenol still enhances norepinephrine release in the presence of maximal facilitatory concentrations of angiotensin II. Isoproterenol also enhances norepinephrine release when the angiotensin-II mechanism has been desensitized by a high concentration of angiotensin II.

Corticotrophin (Adrenocorticotrophic Hormone)

In isolated preparations of rabbit pulmonary artery and aorta, corticotrophin$_{1-24}$ enhances stimulation-induced norepinephrine release (541–543) but not the release of norepinephrine induced by tyramine (542). Peptides related to corticotrophin (corticotrophin$_{1-24}$, α-melanocyte stimulating hormone, and the full amino-acid sequence of porcine corticotrophin) increase norepinephrine release, whereas corticotrophin$_{4-10}$ has no effect. The rank order of potency of these peptides on noradrenergic transmission is the same as that for increasing glucocorticoid production in isolated adrenal cortex cells (542). Corticotrophin$_{7-38}$, which is a weak antagonist of corticotrophic activity, antagonizes the facilitatory effect of corticotrophin$_{1-24}$ on norepinephrine release in rabbit pulmonary artery (542).

Norepinephrine release evoked by stimulation of the sympathetic outflow in the pithed rabbit is facilitated by corticotrophin at plasma levels close to the physiological range (544). Furthermore, in the rabbit isolated heart the concentration of corticotrophin$_{1-24}$ (0.1 nM) that is effective in enhancing norepinephrine release in response to stimulation of the extrinsic sympathetic nerves is within the physiological range (545).

Although prejunctional facilitatory corticotrophin receptors are associated with the terminals of both cardiac and vascular sympathetic nerves in the rabbit (541–543, 545), they are not demonstrable in rat or guinea pig pulmonary artery or rat atria (543). However, the facilitatory effect of corticotrophin$_{1-24}$ on norepinephrine release in the rabbit pulmonary artery is revealed by blockade of prejunctional α-adrenoceptors, suggesting that activation of prejunctional α-adrenoceptors buffers the response to activation of prejunctional corticotrophin receptors (543).

Opioids

Endogenous opioids can be regarded as humoral modulators of neuroeffector transmission because their main sources are the adrenal medulla (440) and the anterior lobe of the pituitary (546). They are released into the circulation in various forms of shock (547,548).

Noradrenergic Transmission

The effects of opioids on noradrenergic neuroeffector transmission have been comprehensively reviewed (335,549,550,551). Morphine has an inhibitory action at only a few sites, notably the cat nictitating membrane and the mouse vas deferens. However, at several neuroeffector sites, opioid peptides are inhibitory whereas morphine is not, for example, in the cat spleen, in vasa deferentia of the rat and rabbit, in rabbit ear, pulmonary and mesenteric arteries, portal vein, heart and atria, and in guinea pig atria. At those neuroeffector sites where morphine has an inhibitory action, the endogenous opioids met- and leu-enkephalin are considerably more potent. The differences between morphine and opioid peptides are explained by the distribution of opioid receptor subtypes (Table 8) and the relative activity of agonists on the receptor subtypes: morphine acts predominantly on μ-receptors whereas the enkephalins act predominantly on δ- and κ-receptors. The differences between species, tissues, and agonists explain reports of lack of an effect under particular circumstances (553). The situation is further complicated by the fact that a particular receptor may be present, but the manifestation of its activation is only revealed under certain circumstances. Thus, in the rabbit jejunal artery,

TABLE 8. *Types of prejunctional opioid receptors identified at various neuroeffector sites*

Cat	
Nictitating membrane	μ
Spleen	δ,?κ
Rabbit	
Ear artery	δ,κ
Mesenteric artery	δ,κ
Pulmonary artery	κ
Portal vein	δ,κ
Vas deferens	κ
Atria	
Noradrenergic	κ
Cholinergic	μ,δ
Rat	
Tail artery	ε
Vas deferens	κ
Atria	
Noradrenergic	?δ
Cholinergic	δ
Mouse	
Vas deferens	μ,δ,κ
Guinea pig	
Atria	
Noradrenergic	κ,?δ
Cholinergic	None

See refs. 13, 335, 549, 540.

the inhibitory effect of κ-receptor agonists can be observed only after blockade of prejunctional α_2-adrenoceptors (335,552).

Intravenous injections of enkephalins decrease the blood pressure and heart rate in anesthetized rats (547) but raise the blood pressure in conscious rats (554). Opioid peptides lower the blood pressure in pithed rabbits in which the pressure is elevated by electrical stimulation of the sympathetic outflow by acting on prejunctional receptors of the noradrenergic nerve terminals to decrease the release of norepinephrine (335,555–557). A stable analog of met-enkephalin (DAMA) decreases pressor responses in pithed rats to stimulation of the spinal sympathetic outflow or sympathetic ganglia (558).

The endogenous opioids released in shock apparently play a part in mediating the hypotensive state by inhibiting sympathetic vasomotor tone because the opioid receptor antagonist naloxone raises the blood pressure (559–561) and increases the plasma level of norepinephrine (562).

Cholinergic Transmission

Morphine inhibits responses to cholinergic nerve stimulation in the intestine and heart of various species by depressing the release of acetylcholine (563). The slowing of the rate of beating of isolated atria of the rat and rabbit produced by field stimulation of intramural cholinergic nerves is inhibited by stable analogs of opioid peptides without the response to acetylcholine being affected, but these opioids have no effect on cholinergic transmission in guinea pig isolated atria (553,564). Opioid peptides inhibit stimulation-induced release of acetylcholine from the rabbit perfused heart (565) and isolated atria (553). Although it is likely that the inhibitory effects of opioids on responses to vagal stimulation are due to depression of acetylcholine release from postganglionic rather than preganglionic terminals, this has not been conclusively demonstrated.

Histamine

Histamine has profound effects on cardiovascular tissues by acting on H_1 and H_2 receptors of vascular smooth muscle and it has cardiac stimulant activity that is exerted on H_2 receptors (566–568).

Histamine is present in appreciable quantities in the heart and blood vessels. Although it is mostly stored in mast cells (569), there is some evidence for its presence in sympathetic nerves (568,570–572). In tissues labeled with [^{3}H]histamine, radioactivity is released by sympathetic nerve stimulation (573,574), and there is evidence suggesting that it mediates vasodilation (575,576).

Histamine, in amounts that have no other actions, decreases responses to sympathetic nerve stimulation in dog blood vessels (577,578) and heart (579). In guinea pig isolated atria, histamine increases the rate and force of beating, but inhibits these responses to sympathetic nerve stimulation and inhibits norepinephrine release by acting on prejunctional receptors that do not conform to either the H_1- or H_2-subtypes although they more closely resemble the H_2-subtype (580).

There is no evidence that endogenous histamine modulates cardiac sympathetic function under normal conditions (580). However, in anaphylactic reactions in guinea pigs, histamine is released in sufficient quantities to produce marked changes in cardiac activity (568). The stimulation-induced release of norepinephrine is decreased in anaphylaxis, but histamine does not mediate this effect (581).

Bradykinin

Bradykinin stimulates sympathetic ganglion cells (492,493) and releases catecholamines from the adrenal medulla (582). However, bradykinin decreases the stimulation-induced release of norepinephrine in the rabbit isolated heart and pulmonary artery, but this is due to bradykinin-induced production of PGs (583). In the rat isolated vas deferens, bradykinin increases contractile responses to field stimulation of the intramural nerves (584), presumably by facilitating transmitter release.

Adenyl Compounds

Adenyl compounds are released from myocardial cells in hypoxia and when myocardial activity is increased and are thought to be mediators of coronary vasodilation (585). The relative contributions of prejunctional inhibition of release of vasoconstrictor transmitters and postjunctional direct and indirect vasodilation have not been elucidated.

Mediators from Platelets

Platelets contain a number of potent pharmacologically active substances that subserve physiological roles that come into play when the mediators are released by damage to or aggregation of platelets. These substances may be engaged in complex interactions with other factors having modulatory effects on vascular smooth muscle and neurovascular transmission (Fig. 14).

Serotonin

In peripheral tissues the main source of serotonin is the enterochromaffin cells. Serotonin released from enterochromaffin cells can exert a local effect consisting of activation of reflex vasodilation resulting from release of VIP (586), but the main thing to be considered here is that the serotonin released from enterochromaffin cells is taken up by platelets.

A striking example of the modulation of neurovascular transmission by serotonin released from aggregating platelets is provided by observations on dog isolated coronary artery segments by Cohen (586a, 586b). In this tissue, norepinephrine released by stimulating the perivascular axons acts on postjunctional β-adrenoceptors to produce vasodilation. Serotonin (and adenyl compounds) released from platelets in contact with the intimal surface can diffuse through the medial layer in a sufficient amount to inhibit stimulation-induced norepinephrine release from the axons at the adventitial-medial border and thereby reduce the vasodilator response to noradrenergic nerve stimulation.

Adenyl Compounds

Adenyl compounds as well as serotonin liberated during aggregation of platelets can exert direct vascular effects as well as an

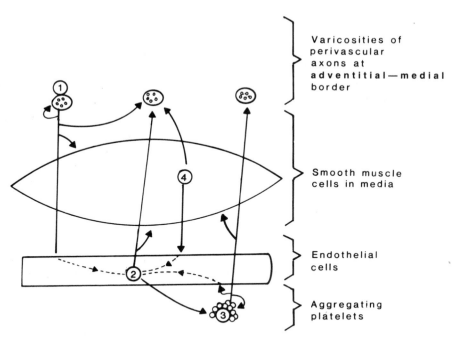

FIG. 14. Diagrammatic representation of possible interactions of modulatory influences on vascular smooth muscle. 1: Transmitters released by nerve impulses may act directly on the smooth muscle or indirectly by releasing active substances from the endothelial cells; they may also mediate automodulation and transneuronal modulation of transmitter release. 2: Stimuli acting on endothelial cells release active substances that act on the smooth muscle, may affect platelet aggregation, and may modulate neurotransmission. 3: Substances released from platelets can affect platelet aggregation, stimulate the release of active substances from endothelial cells, act on the smooth muscle, and modulate neurotransmission. 4: Activation of the smooth muscle may release substances that can mediate transjunctional modulation of neurotransmission and may release active substances from endothelial cells.

inhibitory effect on noradrenergic transmission (586b).

Thromboxane

An analog of thromboxane A$_2$ decreases norepinephrine release in the guinea pig isolated mesenteric artery (587) and the thromboxane-mimetic U46619 reduces the vasoconstrictor response to sympathetic nerve stimulation without affecting that to norepinephrine in the rat autoperfused mesenteric vasculature (588), suggesting a prejunctional inhibitory action. However, in the rat anococcygeus muscle U44619 enhances contractile responses to sympathetic nerve stimulation and norepinephrine (589),

and in the perfused rat kidney U46619 enhances vasoconstrictor responses to sympathetic nerve stimulation but does not affect norepinephrine release (483). In the rabbit vas deferens, U46619 enhances norepinephrine release and the contractile response to norepinephrine (590). Further studies are necessary to clarify the effects of thromboxane on norepinephrine release and to determine whether it functions as a modulator of autonomic neuroeffector transmission.

Mediators from Vascular Endothelial Cells

Endothelial cells are the source of substances with marked pharmacological activity, and these substances, like the substances released from platelets, could have influences on vascular neuroeffector function.

Much attention was focused on endothelial cells after the discovery by Furchgott and Zawadzki in 1980 (591) that acetylcholine relaxed vascular smooth muscle indirectly by releasing a mediator termed EDRF. Subsequently it was found that several other vasodilator substances acted in the same way (for reviews, see [134,398, 592,593]). EDRF has recently been identified as nitric oxide or a closely related substance (594). Apart from EDRF, endothelial cells are the source of other vasodilator substances including prostacyclin and possibly acetylcholine since they contain choline acetyltransferase (595).

There is also evidence that endothelial cells are the source of one or more substances mediating vasoconstriction in response to stretch, anoxia, and other stimuli (354,596). Recently a potent vasoconstrictor peptide, endothelin, has been isolated from endothelial cells (597). Endothelial cells are also a potential source of angiotensin II because they contain converting enzyme (524,525).

The possible effects of neurotransmitters from perivascular axon terminals in releasing endothelium-derived substances has been discussed by Vanhoutte (354): he considered it unlikely that norepinephrine, acetylcholine, serotonin, or ATP of neurogenic origin acted indirectly on endothelial cells in controlling the function of vascular smooth muscle, but it was possible that substance P might do so. If vasodilator responses to cholinergic nerve stimulation entailed the release of EDRF, it would imply that acetylcholine released from the axon terminals in the adventitia would have to traverse the media to reach the endothelial cells before it could act. In fact, in the cholinergically innervated cat auricular and rabbit lingual arteries, vasodilator responses to acetylcholine and perivascular nerve stimulation occur in the absence of endothelium (353).

The matter to be discussed here is whether endothelium-derived substances modulate vascular neuroeffector transmission. The influences of EDRF and prostacyclin on neuroeffector transmission have received surprisingly little attention. Somewhat more is known about the effects of the much more recently discovered mediator endothelin (see below). The possible interactions between endothelium-derived substances, platelet-derived substances, and neurovascular transmission are shown in Fig. 14.

Prostacyclin

Vasoconstrictor responses to both norepinephrine and sympathetic nerve stimulation are reduced by prostacyclin in isolated blood vessels (598) and in the autoperfused mesenteric vascular bed of the cat (599) but to unequal extents in the rat (588), suggesting a prejunctional action. However, prostacyclin does not affect stimulation-induced norepinephrine release in the rat isolated kidney (483).

Endothelin

Endothelin has been reported to have a powerful and long-lasting vasoconstrictor action on isolated arteries from various regions of several species and a long-lasting pressor effect in the anesthetized rat (597). Vasoconstrictor responses were readily blocked by dihydropyridine calcium antagonists, so it was suggested that endothelin may be an endogenous agonist for voltage-dependent calcium channels. It was more potent on isolated ring segments of rat renal artery from SHR than from WKY, suggesting a possible role in hypertension (600).

Endothelin acts not only on vascular smooth muscle and endothelial cells, but has pre- and postjunctional effects on neuroeffector mechanisms. It was reported to reduce vasoconstrictor responses and release of norepinephrine elicited by perivascular nerve stimulation in the guinea pig

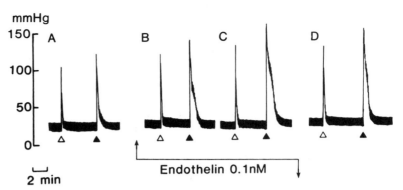

FIG. 15. Effects of endothelin (0.1 nм) on vasoconstrictor responses to norepinephrine (△, 25 ng) and perivascular nerve stimulation (▲, 2 Hz, 10 sec) in an isolated segment of endothelium-denuded rat tail artery perfused at 4 ml/min. **A:** Control responses. **B** and **C:** Responses during infusion of endothelin after 10 (**B**) and 55 min (**C**): note the slow development of the enhancements of vasoconstrictor responses and the prolongation of a second phase in the response to norepinephrine. **D:** 60 min after cessation of exposure to endothelin: note the persistence of the enhancements. (From Wong-Dusting, La, and Rand, *unpublished observations.*)

isolated femoral artery (601). However, in the rabbit ear artery, 10 nM endothelin increases the stimulation-induced release of norepinephrine but, paradoxically, it decreases vasoconstrictor responses to nerve stimulation and norepinephrine (602). In a concentration below that having vasoconstrictor activity, endothelin (100 pM) produces a slowly developing but pronounced enhancement of vasoconstrictor responses to norepinephrine and sympathetic nerve stimulation in isolated perfused rabbit ear and rat tail artery segments (Fig. 15).

On rat isolated atria, endothelin was reported to have a potent positive inotropic action but no chronotropic activity (603). However, we found that it increased both the rate and force of beating in rat (602) and guinea pig isolated atria (602a). It inhibited responses to isoproterenol (602) and norepinephrine (Reid et al., *unpublished observations*).

The cardiovascular effects of endothelin in whole animals are complex. The original report showed that 1 nmol/kg injected intravenously in the anesthetized rat produced a transient fall in blood pressure before the onset of the pronounced pressor effect (597). In the pithed rat, intravenous injec-

tions of endothelin in doses of 0.1 to 1 nmol/kg produce falls in blood pressure with only slight secondary rises, but injections into the aortic arch produce only rises in blood pressure (Xiao et al., *unpublished observations*). Endothelin releases eicosanoids from rat and guinea pig lung (604), which might explain the depressor effects.

ACKNOWLEDGMENTS

This work was supported by a program grant from the National Health and Medical Research Council of Australia. Dr. H. Majewski is a Wellcome Australian Senior Research Fellow.

REFERENCES

1. Starke K. Presynaptic receptors. *Annu Rev Pharmacol Toxicol* 1981;21:7–30.
2. Chesselet M-F. Presynaptic regulation of neurotransmitter release in the brain. *Neuroscience* 1984;12:347–376.
3. Starke K. Regulation of noradrenaline release by presynaptic receptor systems. *Rev Physiol Biochem Pharmacol* 1977;77:1–124.
4. Westfall TC. Local regulation of adrenergic neurotransmission. *Physiol Rev* 1977;57:659–728.

5. Vizi ES. Presynaptic modulation of neurochemical transmission. *Prog Neurobiol* 1979;12:181–290.

6. Langer SZ. Presynaptic regulation of catecholamine release. *Biochem Pharmacol* 1974;23:1793–1800.

7. Langer SZ. Presynaptic receptors and their role in the regulation of transmitter release. *Br J Pharmacol* 1977;60:481–497.

8. Langer SZ. Presynaptic regulation of the release of catecholamines. *Pharmacol Rev* 1981;32:337–362.

9. Gillespie JS. Presynaptic receptors in the autonomic nervous system. In: Szekeres L, ed. *Adrenergic activators and inhibitors, vol 54/1: Handbook of experimental pharmacology.* Berlin: Springer, 1980;353–425.

10. Vanhoutte PM, Verbeuren TJ, Webb RC. Local modulation of adrenergic neuroeffector interaction in the blood vessel wall. *Physiol Rev* 1981;61:151–247.

11. Rand MJ, McCulloch MW, Story DF. Prejunctional modulation of noradrenergic transmission by noradrenaline, dopamine and acetylcholine. In: Davies DS, JL Reid, eds. *Central action of drugs in blood pressure regulation.* London: Pitman Medical, 1975;94–132.

12. Rand MJ, McCulloch MW, Story DF. Catecholamine receptors on nerve terminals. In: Szekeres L, ed. *Adrenergic activators and inhibitors, vol 54/1: Handbook of experimental pharmacology.* Berlin: Springer, 1980;223–266.

13. Rand MJ, Majewski H, Wong-Dusting H, Story DF, Loiacono RE, Ziogas J. Modulation of neuroeffector transmission. *J Cardiovasc Pharmacol* 1987;10(Suppl 12):S33–S44.

14. Hökfelt T, Johansson O, Ljungdahl A, Lundberg JM, Schultzberg M. Peptidergic neurones. *Nature* 1980;284:515–521.

15. Cuello AC. *Cotransmission.* London: Macmillan, 1982.

16. Burnstock G. Autonomic neuromuscular junctions: current developments and future directions. *J Anat* 1986;146:1–30.

17. Burnstock G. The changing face of autonomic neurotransmission. *Acta Physiol Scand* 1986;126:67–91.

18. Bartfai T, Iverfeldt K, Fisone G, Serfözö P. Regulation of the release of coexisting neurotransmitters. *Annu Rev Pharmacol Toxicol* 1988;28:285–310.

19. Burn JH, Rand MJ. Sympathetic postganglionic mechanism. *Nature* 1959;184:163–165.

20. Burn JH, Rand MJ. Acetylcholine in adrenergic transmission. *Annu Rev Pharmacol* 1965;5:163–182.

21. Burnstock G. Do some sympathetic neurones release both noradrenaline and acetylcholine? *Prog Neurobiol* 1978;11:205–222.

22. Bowman WC, Rand MJ. Actions of triethylcholine on neuromuscular transmission. *Br J Pharmacol* 1961;17:176–195.

23. Day MD, Rand MJ. Some observations on the pharmacology of α-methyldopa. *Br J Pharmacol* 1964;22:84–96.

24. Burnstock G. Purinergic nerves. *Pharmacol Rev* 1972;24:509–581.

25. Burnstock G. Present status of purinergic neurotransmission—implications for vascular control. In: Nobin A, Owman C, Aneklo-Nobin B, eds. *Neuronal messengers in vascular function.* Amsterdam: Elsevier, 1987;327–340.

26. Burnstock G. The co-transmitter hypothesis, with special reference to the storage and release of ATP with noradrenaline and acetylcholine. In: Cuello AC, ed. *Cotransmission.* London: Macmillan, 1982;151–163.

27. Su C. Purinergic neurotransmission and neuromodulation. *Annu Rev Pharmacol Toxicol* 1983;23:397–411.

28. Brownstein MJ, Saavedra JM, Axelrod J, Zeman GH, Carpenter DO. Coexistence of several putative neurotransmitters in single identified neurons of *Aplysia. Proc Natl Acad Sci USA* 1974;71:4662–4665.

29. Burnstock G. Do some nerve cells release more than one transmitter? *Neuroscience* 1976;1:239–248.

30. Rand MJ, Mitchelson F. The guts of the matter: contribution of studies on smooth muscle to discoveries in pharmacology. In: Parnham MJ, Bruinvels J, eds. *Discoveries in pharmacology, vol 3.* Amsterdam: Elsevier, 1986;19–61.

31. Hökfelt T. Elfvin L-G, Elde R, Schultzberg M, Goldstein M, Luft R. Occurrence of somatostatin-like immunoreactivity in some peripheral sympathetic noradrenergic neurons. *Proc Natl Acad Sci USA* 1977;74:3587–3591.

32. Lundberg JM, Hökfelt T. Coexistence of peptides and classical neurotransmitters. *Trends Neurosci* 1983;6:325–333.

33. Iversen LL. Amino acids and peptides: fast and slow chemical signals in the nervous system? *Proc R Soc Lond [Biol]* 1984;221:245–260.

34. Said SI. Neuropeptides in cardiovascular regulation. In: Buckley JP, Ferrario CM, eds. *Brain peptides and catecholamines in cardiovascular regulation.* New York: Raven Press, 1987;93–107.

35. Edvinsson L, MacKenzie ET. Amine mechanisms in cerebral circulation. *Pharmacol Rev* 1976;28:275–348.

36. Edvinsson L, McCulloch J. Distribution and vasomotor effects of peptide HI (PHI) in feline cerebral blood vessels in vitro and in situ. *Regul Pept* 1985;10:345–356.

37. Edvinsson L. Characterization of the contractile effect of neuropeptide Y in feline cerebral arteries. *Acta Physiol Scand* 1985;125:33–41.

38. Itakura T, Okuno T, Nakakita K, et al. A light and electron microscopic immunohistochemical study of vasoactive intestinal polypeptide- and substance P-containing fibers along the cerebral blood vessels: comparison with aminergic and cholinergic nerve fibers. *J Cereb Blood Flow Metab* 1984;4:407–414.

39. McCulloch J, Uddmann R, Kingman TA, Edvinsson L. Calcitonin gene-related peptide: functional role in cerebrovascular regulation. *Proc Natl Acad Sci USA* 1986;83:5731–5735.

40. Moskowitz MA, Brezina LR, Kuo C. Dynorphin B-containing perivascular axons and sensory neurotransmitter mechanisms in brain blood vessels. *Cephalalgia* 1986;6:81–86.
41. Owman C, Chang J-Y, Ekblad E, Steinbusch HWM. Immunohistochemical investigation of the relationship between different neuropeptides and amine transmitters in monkey and guinea-pig cerebral arteries. In: Nobin A, Owman C, Aneklo-Nobin B, eds. *Neuronal messengers in vascular function.* Amsterdam: Elsevier, 1987;355–370.
42. Owman C, Hardebo JE, eds. *Neural regulation of brain circulation.* Amsterdam: Elsevier, 1986.
43. Steers WD, McConnell J, Benson GS. Anatomical localization and some pharmacological effects of vasoactive intestinal polypeptide in human and monkey corpus cavernosum. *J Urol* 1984;132:1048–1053.
44. Gu J, Polak JM, Probert L, et al. Peptidergic innervation of human male genital tract. *J Urol* 1983;130:386–391.
45. Adrian TE, Gu J, Allen JM, Tatemoto K, Polak JM, Bloom SR. Neuropeptide Y in the human male genital tract. *Life Sci* 1984;35:2643–2648.
46. Andersson KE, Hedlund H, Fovaeus M. Interactions between classical neurotransmitter and some neuropeptides in human penile erectile tissues. In: Nobin A, Owman C, Aneklo-Nobin B, eds. *Neuronal messengers in vascular function.* Amsterdam: Elsevier, 1987;505–524.
47. Morris JL, Gibbins IL, Furness JB, Costa M, Murphy R. Colocalization of neuropeptide Y, vasoactive intestinal polypeptide and dynorphin in non-noradrenergic axons of the guinea pig uterine artery. *Neurosci Lett* 1985;62:31–37.
48. Hendry IA. Phenotypic plasticity of sympathetic adrenergic and cholinergic neurones. *Trends Pharmacol Sci* 1985;6:126–129.
49. Holton P, Rand MJ. Sympathetic vasodilatation in the rabbit ear. *Br J Pharmacol* 1962;19:513–526.
50. Black IB, Kessler JA, Adler JE, Bohn MC. Regulation of substance P expression and metabolism in vivo and in vitro. *Ciba Found Symp* 1982;91:107–122.
51. Lundberg JM, Fried G, Fahrenkrug J, et al. Subcellular fractionation of cat submandibular gland: comparative studies on the distribution of acetylcholine and vasoactive intestinal polypeptide (VIP). *Neuroscience* 1981;6:1001–1010.
52. Fried G, Terenius L, Hökfelt T, Goldstein M. Evidence for differential localization of noradrenaline and neuropeptide Y (NPY) in neuronal storage vesicles isolated from rat vas deferens. *J Neurosci* 1985;5:450–458.
53. Fried G, Terenius L, Brodin E, et al. Neuropeptide Y, enkephalin and noradrenaline coexist in sympathetic neurons innervating the bovine spleen. Biochemical and immunohistological evidence. *Cell Tissue Res* 1986;243:495–508.
54. Douglas RH, Duff RB, Thureson-Klein Å, Klein RL. Enkephalin contents reflect noradrenergic large dense cored vesicle populations in vasa deferentia. *Regul Pept* 1986;14:193–210.
55. Johansson O, Lundberg JM. Ultrastructural localization of VIP-like immunoreactivity in large dense-core vesicles of 'cholinergic-type' nerve terminals in cat exocrine glands. *Neuroscience* 1981;6:847–862.
56. Fillenz M, Howe PRC. Depletion of noradrenaline stores in sympathetic nerve terminals. *J Neurochem* 1975;24:683–688.
57. Thureson-Klein Å. Exocytosis from large and small dense cored vesicles in noradrenergic nerve terminals. *Neuroscience* 1983;10:245–252.
58. Fried G, Lundberg JM, Theodorsson-Norheim E. Subcellular storage and axonal transport of neuropeptide Y (NPY) in relation to catecholamines in the cat. *Acta Physiol Scand* 1985;125:145–154.
59. Bell C. Dopamine release from sympathetic nerve terminals. *Prog Neurobiol* 1988;30:193–208.
60. Bell C. Dopamine: precursor or neurotransmitter in sympathetically innervated tissues? *Blood Vessels* 1987;24:234–239.
61. Hope W, Majewski H, McCulloch MW, Rand MJ, Story DF. Modulation of sympathetic transmission by neuronally-released dopamine. *Br J Pharmacol* 1979;67:185–192.
62. Goldberg LI. Cardiovascular and renal actions of dopamine: potential clinical applications. *Pharmacol Rev* 1972;24:1–30.
63. Lokhandwala MF, Barrett RJ. Cardiovascular dopamine receptors: physiological, pharmacological and therapeutic implications. *J Auton Pharmacol* 1982;3:189–215.
64. Willems JL, Buylaert WA, Lefevre RA, Bogaert MG. Neuronal dopamine receptors on autonomic ganglia and sympathetic nerves and dopamine receptors in the gastrointestinal system. *Pharmacol Rev* 1985;37:165–216.
65. Bell C. Endogenous renal dopamine and control of blood pressure. *Clin Exp Hypertens* 1987;A9:955–975.
66. Goldberg LI, Kohli JD. Peripheral dopamine receptors: a classification based on potency series and specific antagonism. *Trends Pharmacol Sci* 1983;4:64–66.
67. Dahlöf C, Abrahamsson T, Eriksson BM, Ablad B. Is prejunctional β-adrenoceptor mediated facilitation of neuronal noradrenaline release controlled by neuronal or adrenal medullary adrenaline? In: Vizi ES, ed. *Advances in pharmacological research and practice. Vol II: Modulation of neurochemical transmission.* New York: Pergamon, 1979;157–167.
68. Goodall McC. Studies of adrenaline and noradrenaline in mammalian hearts and suprarenals. *Acta Physiol Scand* 1951;24:1–51.
69. Rehn NO. Effect of decentralization on the content of catecholamines in the spleen and kidney of the cat. *Acta Physiol Scand* 1958;42:309–312.

70. von Euler US. Adrenergic neuro-hormones. *Comp Endocrinol* 1963;1:209–238.
71. Anden NE. Uptake and release of dextro and laevo-adrenaline in noradrenaline stores. *Acta Pharmacol Toxicol* 1964;21:59–75.
72. Majewski H, Hedler L, Starke K. The noradrenaline release rate in the anaesthetized rabbit: facilitation by adrenaline. *Naunyn Schmiedebergs Arch Pharmacol* 1982;321:337–362.
73. Dahlöf C. Studies on β-adrenoceptor mediated facilitation of sympathetic neurotransmission. *Acta Physiol Scand* 1981;500:1–147.
74. Majewski H, Alade PI, Rand MJ. Adrenaline and stress-induced increases in blood pressure in rats. *Clin Exp Pharmacol Physiol* 1986;13:283–288.
75. Raab W, Giggee W. Die Katecholamine des Herzens. *Arch Exp Pathol Pharmacol* 1953;219:248–262.
76. Langer SZ, Vogt M. Noradrenaline release from isolated muscles of the nictitating membrane of the cat. *J Physiol* 1971;214:159–171.
77. Schmidt HHHW, Schurr C, Hedler L, Majewski H. Local modulation of noradrenaline release in vivo: presynaptic β₂-adrenoceptors and adrenaline. *J Cardiovasc Pharmacol* 1984;6:641–649.
78. Guimaraes S, Brandao F, Paiva MQ. A study of the adrenoceptor-mediated feedback mechanisms by using adrenaline as a false transmitter. *Naunyn Schmiedebergs Arch Pharmacol* 1978;305:185–188.
79. Majewski H, McCulloch MW, Rand MJ, Story DF. Adrenaline activation of prejunctional β-adrenoceptors in guinea-pig atria. *Br J Pharmacol* 1980;71:435–444.
80. Majewski H, Rand MJ, Tung LH. Activation of prejunctional β-adrenoceptors in rat atria by adrenaline applied exogenously or released as a cotransmitter. *Br J Pharmacol* 1981;73:669–679.
81. Berecek KH, Brody MJ. Evidence for a neurotransmitter role for epinephrine derived from the adrenal medulla. *Am J Physiol* 1982;242:H593–H601.
82. Majewski H. Modulation of noradrenaline release through activation of presynaptic β-adrenoceptors. *J Auton Pharmacol* 1983;3:47–60 [Corrigenda 155].
83. Majewski H, Rand MJ. A possible role of epinephrine in the development of hypertension. *Med Res Rev* 1986;6:197–225.
84. Jain-Etcheverry G, Zieher LM. Coexistence of monoamines in peripheral adrenergic neurones. In: Cuello AC, ed. *Cotransmission*. London: Macmillan, 1982;189–206.
85. Thoa NB, Eccleston D, Axelrod J. The accumulation of ¹⁴C-serotonin in the guinea-pig vas deferens. *J Pharmacol Exp Ther* 1969;169:68–73.
86. Verbeuren TJ, Jordaens F, Herman AG. Accumulation and release of [³H]5-hydroxytryptamine in saphenous veins and cerebral arteries of the dog. *J Pharmacol Exp Ther* 1983;226:579–588.
87. Edvinsson L, Birath E, Uddmann R, et al. Indoleamine mechanisms in brain vessels; locali-

zation, concentration, uptake and in vitro responses of 5-hydroxytryptamine. *Acta Physiol Scand* 1984;121:291–299.
88. Cohen RA. Platelet-induced neurogenic coronary arterial contractions due to accumulation of the false neurotransmitter, 5-hydroxytryptamine. *J Clin Invest* 1985;75:286–292.
89. Cohen RA. Inhibition of adrenergic neurotransmission in canine tibial artery after exposure to 5-hydroxytryptamine in vitro. *J Pharmacol Exp Ther* 1987;242:493–499.
90. Cohen RA, Zitnay KM, Weisbrod RM. Accumulation of 5-hydroxytryptamine leads to dysfunction of adrenergic nerves in canine coronary artery following intimal damage in vivo. *Circ Res* 1987;61:829–833.
91. Griffith SG, Lincoln J, Burnstock G. Serotonin as a neurotransmitter in cerebral arteries. *Brain Res* 1982;247:388–392.
92. Scatton B, Duverger D, l'Heureux R, et al. Neurochemical studies on the existence, origin and characteristics of the serotonergic innervation of small pial vessels. *Brain Res* 1985;345:219–229.
93. Chang JY, Owman C. Immunohistochemical and pharmacological studies on serotonergic nerves and receptors in brain vessels. *Acta Physiol Scand* 1986;127(Suppl 552):49–53.
94. Saito A, Lee TJ-F. Serotonin as an alternative transmitter in sympathetic nerves of large cerebral arteries of the rabbit. *Circ Res* 1987; 60:220–228.
95. Cohen RA, Shepherd JT, Vanhoutte PM. Neurogenic cholinergic prejunctional inhibition of sympathetic beta adrenergic relaxation in the canine coronary artery. *J Pharmacol Exp Ther* 1984;229:417–421.
96. Van Neuten JM, Janssens WJ, Vanhoutte PM. Serotonin and vascular reactivity. *Pharmacol Res Commun* 1985;17:585–608.
97. Vanhoutte PM. *Serotonin and the cardiovascular system*. New York: Raven Press, 1985.
98. Houston DS, Vanhoutte PM. Serotonin and the vascular system: role in health and disease and implications for therapy. *Drugs* 1986;31:149–163.
99. Humphrey PPA, Feniuk W, Watts AD. Prejunctional effects of 5-hydroxytryptamine on noradrenergic nerves in the cardiovascular system. *Fed Proc* 1983;42:218–222.
100. Humphrey PPA, Feniuk W. Pharmacological characterization of functional neuronal receptors for 5-hydroxytryptamine. In: Nobin A, Owman C, Aneklo-Nobin B, eds. *Neuronal messengers in vascular function*. Amsterdam: Elsevier 1987;3–19.
101. Fozard JR. Neuronal 5-HT receptors in the periphery. *Neuropharmacol* 1984;23:1473–1486.
102. Bradley PB, Engel G, Feniuk W, et al. Proposals for the classification and nomenclature of functional receptors for 5-hydroxytryptamine. *Neuropharmacology* 1986;25:563–575.
103. Van Heuven-Nolsen D. 5-HT receptor subtype-specific drugs and the cardiovascular system. *Trends Pharmacol Sci* 1987;9:423–433.

104. Humphrey PPA, Richardson BP. Classification of 5-HT receptors and binding sites: an overview. In: Mylecharane EJ, Angus JA, de la Lande IS, Humphrey PPA, eds. *Serotonin: actions, receptors, pathophysiology.* London: Macmillan, 1989;204–221.

105. McGrath MA. 5-Hydroxytryptamine and neurotransmitter release in canine blood vessels. *Circ Res* 1977;41:428–435.

106. Feniuk W, Humphrey PPA, Watts AD. Presynaptic inhibitory action of 5-hydroxytryptamine in dog isolated saphenous vein. *Br J Pharmacol* 1979;67:247–254.

107. Feniuk W, Humphrey PPA, Watts AD. Modification of the vasomotor actions of methysergide in the femoral arterial bed of the anaesthetised dog by changes in sympathetic nerve activity. *J Auton Pharmacol* 1981;1:127–132.

108. Watts AD, Feniuk W, Humphrey PPA. A prejunctional action of 5-hydroxytryptamine and methysergide on noradrenergic nerves in dog isolated saphenous vein. *J Pharm Pharmacol* 1981;33:515–520.

109. Engel G, Göthert M, Müller-Schweinitzer E, Schlicker E, Sistonen L, Stadler PA. Evidence for common pharmacological properties of [³H]5-hydroxytryptamine binding sites, presynaptic 5-hydroxytryptamine autoreceptors in CNS and inhibitory presynaptic 5-hydroxytryptamine receptors on sympathetic nerves. *Naunyn Schmiedebergs Arch Pharmacol* 1983;324:116–124.

110. Su C, Urano T. Excitatory and inhibitory effects of 5-hydroxytryptamine in mesenteric arteries of spontaneously hypertensive rats. *Eur J Pharmacol* 1985;106:283–290.

111. Cohen RA. Serotonergic prejunctional inhibition of canine coronary adrenergic nerves. *J Pharmacol Exp Ther* 1985;235:76–80.

112. Charlton KG, Bond RA, Clarke DE. An inhibitory prejunctional 5-HT₁-like receptor in the isolated perfused rat kidney. *Naunyn Schmiedebergs Arch Pharmacol* 1986;332:8–15.

113. Göthert M, Schlicker E, Kollecher P. Receptor-mediated effects of serotonin and 5-methoxytryptamine on noradrenaline release in the rat vena cava and in the heart of the pithed rat. *Naunyn Schmiedebergs Arch Pharmacol* 1986;332:124–130.

114. Adler-Graschinsky E, Elgoyhen AB, Butta NV. Different receptor subtypes mediate the dual presynaptic effects of 5-hydroxytryptamine on peripheral sympathetic neurones. *J Auton Pharmacol* 1989;9:3–13.

115. North RA, Henderson G, Katayama Y, Johnson SM. Electrophysiological evidence for presynaptic inhibition of acetylcholine release by 5-hydroxytryptamine in the enteric nervous system. *Neuroscience* 1980;5:581–586.

116. Fozard JR, Mir AK, Middlemiss DN. The cardiovascular responses to 8-hydroxy-2(di-n-propylamino) tetralin (8-OH-DPAT) in the rat: site of action and pharmacological analysis. *J Cardiovasc Pharmacol* 1987;9:328–347.

117. Gaddum JH, Picarelli ZP. Two kinds of trypt-amine receptor. *Br J Pharmacol* 1957;12:323–328.

118. Hendrix TR, Atkinson M, Clifton JA, Inglefinger J. The effect of 5-hydroxytryptamine on intestinal motor function in man. *Am J Med* 1957;23:886–893.

119. Costa M, Furness JB. The sites of action of 5-hydroxytryptamine in nerve muscle preparations from the guinea-pig small intestine and colon. *Br J Pharmacol* 1979;65:237–248.

120. Drakontides AB, Gershon MD. 5-Hydroxytryptamine receptors in the mouse duodenum. *Br J Pharmacol* 1968;33:480–492.

121. Buccheit KH, Engel G, Mutschler E, Richardson BP. Studies of the contractile effect of 5-hydroxytryptamine (5-HT) in the isolated longitudinal muscle strip from guinea-pig ileum. *Naunyn Schmiedebergs Arch Pharmacol* 1985;329:36–41.

122. Fozard JR, Mobarok Ali ATM, Newgrosh G. Blockade of serotonin receptors on autonomic neurones by (–)-cocaine and some related compounds. *Eur J Pharmacol* 1979;59:195–210.

123. Richardson BP, Engel G, Donatsch P, Stadler PA. Identification of serotonin M-receptor subtypes and their specific blockade by a new class of drugs. *Nature* 1985;316:126–131.

124. Fozard JR, Mobarok Ali ATM. Blockade of neuronal tryptamine receptors by metoclopramide. *Eur J Pharmacol* 1978;49:109–112.

125. Geffen LB, Livett BG. Synaptic vesicles in sympathetic neurons. *Physiol Rev* 1971;51:98–157.

126. Burnstock G, Kennedy C. A dual function for adenosine 5'-triphosphate in the regulation of vascular tone. Excitatory cotransmitter with noradrenaline from perivascular nerves and locally released inhibitory intravascular agent. *Circ Res* 1986;58:319–330.

127. Head J, Stitzel RE, de la Lande IS, Johnson SM. Effect of chronic denervation on activities of monoamine oxidase and catechol-O-methyl transferase and on contents of noradrenaline and adenosine-triphosphate in rabbit ear artery. *Blood Vessels* 1977;14:229–239.

128. Sneddon P, Burnstock G. ATP as a cotransmitter in rat tail artery. *Eur J Pharmacol* 1985;106:149–152.

129. Sneddon P, Burnstock G. Pharmacological evidence that adenosine triphosphate and noradrenaline are cotransmitters in the guinea-pig vas deferens. *J Physiol* 1984;347:561–580.

130. Sneddon P, Westfall DP. Pharmacological evidence that adenosine triphosphate and noradrenaline are cotransmitters in the guinea-pig vas deferens. *J Physiol* 1984;347:561–580.

131. Fredholm BB, Hedqvist P. Modulation of neurotransmission by purine nucleotides and nucleosides. *Biochem Pharmacol* 1980;29:1635–1643.

132. Burnstock G. A basis for distinguishing two types of purinergic receptor. In: Bolis L, Straub RW, eds. *Cell membrane receptors for drugs and hormones.* New York: Raven Press, 1978;107–118.

133. Green HN, Stoner HB. *Biological actions of the adenosine nucleotides.* London: Lewis, 1950.

134. Furchgott RF. Role of endothelium in responses of vascular smooth muscle. *Circ Res* 1983;53:557–573.

135. Kennedy C, Delbro D, Burnstock G. P_2-purinoceptors mediate both vasodilation (via the endothelium) and vasoconstriction of the isolated rat femoral artery. *Eur J Pharmacol* 1985;107:161–168.

136. Kennedy C, Burnstock G. ATP produces vasodilation via P_1 purinoceptors and vasoconstriction via P_2 purinoceptors in the isolated rabbit central ear artery. *Blood Vessels* 1985;22:145–155.

137. Hardebo JE, Kåhrström J, Owman C. P_1- and P_2-purine receptors in brain circulation. *Eur J Pharmacol* 1987;144:323–352.

138. Ishikawa S. Actions of ATP and α,β-methylene ATP on neuromuscular transmission and smooth muscle membrane of the rabbit and guinea-pig mesenteric arteries. *Br J Pharmacol* 1985;86:777–787.

139. Suzuki H. Electrical responses of smooth muscle cells of the rabbit ear artery to adenosine triphosphate. *J Physiol* 1985;359:401–415.

140. Cheung DW, Fujioka M. Inhibition of the excitatory junction potential in the guinea-pig saphenous artery by ANAPP. *Br J Pharmacol* 1986;89:3–5.

141. von Kügelgen I, Starke K. Noradrenaline and adenosine triphosphate as co-transmitters of neurogenic vasoconstriction in rabbit mesenteric artery. *J Physiol* 1985;367:435–455.

142. Flavahan NA, Vanhoutte PM. Sympathetic purinergic vasoconstriction and thermosensitivity in a canine cutaneous vein. *J Pharmacol Exp Ther* 1986;239:784–789.

143. Muramatsu I. Evidence for sympathetic, purinergic transmission in the mesenteric artery of the dog. *Br J Pharmacol* 1986;87:478–480.

144. Vidal M, Hicks PE, Langer SZ. Differential effects of α,β-methylene ATP on responses to nerve stimulation in SHR and WKY tail arteries. *Naunyn Schmiedebergs Arch Pharmacol* 1986;332:384–390.

145. Miyahara H, Suzuki H. Effects of tyramine on noradrenaline outflow and electrical responses induced by field stimulation in the perfused rabbit ear artery. *Br J Pharmacol* 1985;86:405–416.

146. Holck MI, Marks BH. Purine nucleoside and nucleotide interactions on normal and subsensitive α-adrenoceptor responsiveness in guinea-pig vas deferens. *J Pharmacol Exp Ther* 1978;205:104–117.

147. Kennedy C, Burnstock G. ATP causes postjunctional potentiation of noradrenergic contractions in the portal vein of guinea-pig and rat. *J Pharm Pharmacol* 1986;38:307–309.

148. Burnstock G, Warland JJI. A pharmacological study of the rabbit saphenous artery in vivo: a vessel with a large purinergic contractile response to sympathetic nerve stimulation. *Br J Pharmacol* 1987;90:319–330.

149. Ramme D, Regenold JT, Starke K, Busse R, Illes P. Identification of the neurotransmitter in jejunal branches of the rabbit mesenteric artery. *Naunyn Schmiedebergs Arch Pharmacol* 1987;336:267–273.

150. Muramatsu I, Fujiwara J, Miura A, Sakakibara Y. Possible involvement of adenine nucleotides in sympathetic neuroeffector mechanisms of dog basilar artery. *J Pharmacol Exp Ther* 1981;216:401–409.

151. Muramatsu I, Kigoshi S. Purinergic and non-purinergic innervation in the cerebral arteries of the dog. *Br J Pharmacol* 1987;92:901–908.

152. Cheung DW. Two components in the cellular response of rat tail arteries to nerve stimulation. *J Physiol* 1982;328:461–468.

153. Flavahan NA, Grant TL, Grieg J, McGrath JC. Analysis of the α-adrenoceptor-mediated, and other, components in the sympathetic vasopressor responses of the pithed rat. *Br J Pharmacol* 1985;86:265–274.

154. Shimada SG, Stitt JT. An analysis of the purinergic component of active muscle vasodilatation obtained by electrical stimulation of the hypothalamus in rabbits. *Br J Pharmacol* 1984;83:577–589.

155. Langer SZ, Pinto JEB. Possible involvement of a transmitter different from norepinephrine in residual responses to nerve stimulation of cat nictitating membrane after pretreatment with reserpine. *J Pharmacol Exp Ther* 1976;196:697–713.

156. Burnstock G, Crowe R, Wong HK. Comparative pharmacological and histochemical evidence for purinergic inhibitory innervation of the portal vein of the rabbit, but not guinea-pig. *Br J Pharmacol* 1979;65:377–388.

157. Reilly WM, Saville VL, Burnstock G. An assessment of the antagonistic activity of reactive blue at P_1- and P_2-purinoceptors: supporting evidence for purinergic transmission in the rabbit portal vein. *Eur J Pharmacol* 1987;140:47–53.

158. Kennedy C, Saville VL, Burnstock G. The contributions of noradrenaline and ATP to the response of the rabbit central ear artery to sympathetic nerve stimulation depend on the parameters of stimulation. *Eur J Pharmacol* 1986;122:291–300.

159. Schulzberg M, Hökfelt T, Terenius L, et al. Enkephalin immunoreactive nerve fibers and cell bodies in sympathetic ganglia of the guinea-pig and rat. *Neuroscience* 1979;4:249–270.

160. Lundberg JM, Hökfelt T, Änggård A, et al. Organization principles in the peripheral sympathetic nervous system: subdivision by coexisting peptides (somatostatin-, avian pancreatic polypeptide- and vasoactive intestinal polypeptide-like immunoreactive materials). *Proc Natl Acad Sci USA* 1982;79:1301–1307.

161. Lundberg JM, Terenius L, Hökfelt T, et al. Neuropeptide Y (NPY)-like immunoreactivity in peripheral noradrenergic neurons and effects of NPY on sympathetic function. *Acta Physiol Scand* 1982;116:477–480.

162. Hanley MR, Benton HP, Lightman SL, et al.

A vasopressin-like peptide in the mammalian sympathetic nervous system. *Nature* 1984; 309:258–261.

163. Costa M, Furness JB. Somatostatin is present in a subpopulation of noradrenergic nerve fibres supplying the intestine. *Neuroscience* 1984;13:911–919.

164. Macrae IM, Furness JB, Costa M. Distribution of subgroups of noradrenaline neurons in the coeliac ganglion of the guinea-pig. *Cell Tissue Res* 1986;244:173–180.

165. Samnegård H, Thulin L, Andreen M, Tydén G, Hallberg D, Efendic S. Circulatory effects of somatostatin in anesthetized dogs. *Acta Chir Scand* 1979;145:209–212.

166. Tydén G, Samnegård H, Thulin L, Muhrbeck O, Efendic S. Circulatory effects of somatostatin in anesthetized man. *Acta Chir Scand* 1979;145:443–446.

167. Kilborn MJ, Potter EK, McCloskey DI. Effects of periods of conditioning stimulation and of neuropeptides on vagal action at the heart. *J Auton Nerv Syst* 1986;17:131–142.

168. Hughes J, Kosterlitz HW, Smith TW. The distribution of methionine-enkephalin and leucine-enkephalin in the brain and peripheral tissues. *Br J Pharmacol* 1977;61:639–647.

169. Lang RE, Hermann K, Dietz R, et al. Evidence for the presence of enkephalins in the heart. *Life Sci* 1983;32:399–406.

170. Wilson SP, Klein RL, Chang K-J, Gasparis MS, Viveros OH, Yang W-H. Are opioid peptides co-transmitters in noradrenergic vesicles of sympathetic nerves? *Nature* 1980;288:707–709.

171. Weihe E, McKnight AT, Corbett AD, Kosterlitz HW. Proenkephalin- and prodynorphin-derived opioid peptides in guinea-pig heart. *Neuropeptides* 1985;5:453–456.

172. Archelos J, Xiang JZ, Reinecke M, Lang RE. Regulation of release and function of neuropeptides in the heart. *J Cardiovasc Pharmacol* 1987;10(Suppl 12):S45–S50.

173. Lundberg JM, Terenius L, Hökfelt T, Goldstein M. High levels of neuropeptide Y (NPY) in peripheral noradrenergic neurons in various mammals including man. *Neurosci Lett* 1983; 42:167–172.

174. Sundler F, Moghimzadeh E, Håkanson R, Ekelund M, Emson P. Nerve fibers in the gut and pancreas of the rat displaying neuropeptide Y immunoreactivity. Intrinsic and extrinsic origin. *Cell Tissue Res* 1983;230:487–493.

175. Furness JB, Costa M, Papka RE, Della NG, Murphy R. Neuropeptides contained in peripheral cardiovascular nerves. *Clin Exp Hypertens* 1984;A6:91–106.

176. Furness JB, Costa M, Emson PC, et al. Distribution, pathways and reactions to drug treatment of nerves with neuropeptide Y and pancreatic polypeptide-like immunoreactivity in the guinea pig digestive tract. *Cell Tissue Res* 1983;234:71–92.

177. Allen JM, Gjörstrup P, Björkman J-A, Ek L, Abrahamsson T, Bloom SR. Studies on cardiac distribution and function of neuropeptide Y. *Acta Physiol Scand* 1986;126:405–411.

178. Allen JM, Polak JM, Rodrigo J, Darcey K, Bloom SR. Localisation of neuropeptide Y in nerves of the rat cardiovascular system and the effect of 6-hydroxydopamine. *Cardiovasc Res* 1985;19:570–577.

179. Allen JM, Schon F, Todd N, Yeats JC, Crockard HA, Bloom SR. Presence of neuropeptide Y in human circle of Willis and its possible role in cerebral vasospasm. *Lancet* 1984;2:550–552.

180. Uddmann R, Ekblad E, Edvinsson L, Håkanson R, Sundler F. Neuropeptide Y-like immunoreactivity in perivascular nerve fibres of the guinea-pig. *Regul Pept* 1985;10:243–257.

181. Uddmann R, Sundler F, Emson P. Occurrence and distribution of neuropeptide-Y-like immunoreactive nerves in the respiratory tract and middle ear. *Cell Tissue Res* 1984;237:321–327.

182. Lundberg JM, Saria A, Änggård A, Hökfelt T, Terenius L. Neuropeptide Y and noradrenaline interaction in peripheral cardiovascular control. *Clin Exp Hypertens* 1984;A6:1961–1972.

183. Lundberg JM, Torssel L, Sollevi A, et al. Neuropeptide Y and sympathetic vascular control in man. *Regul Pept* 1985;13:41–52.

184. Gu J, Adrian TE, Tatemoto K, Polak JM, Allen JM, Bloom SR. Neuropeptide tyrosine (NPY)—a major cardiac neuropeptide. *Lancet* 1983;1:1008–1010.

185. Gu J, Polak JM, Allen JM, et al. High concentrations of a novel peptide, neuropeptide Y, in the innervation of mouse and rat heart. *J Histochem Cytochem* 1984;32:467–472.

186. Ekblad E, Edvinsson L, Wahlestedt C, Uddmann R, Håkanson R, Sundler F. Neuropeptide Y coexists and co-operates with noradrenaline in perivascular nerve fibres. *Regul Pept* 1984;8:225–235.

187. Ganten D, Lang RE, Archelos J, Unger T. Peptidergic systems: effects on blood vessels. *J Cardiovasc Pharmacol* 1984;6(Suppl 4):S589–S607.

188. Sternini C, Brecha N. Distribution and colocalization of neuropeptide Y- and tyrosine hydroxylase-like immunoreactivity in the guinea pig heart. *Cell Tissue Res* 1985;241:93–102.

189. Edvinsson L, Emson P, McCulloch J, Tatemoto K, Uddmann R. Neuropeptide Y: immunocytochemical localization to and effect upon feline pial arteries and veins in vitro and in situ. *Acta Physiol Scand* 1984;122:155–163.

190. Edvinsson L, Håkanson R, Wahlestedt C, Uddmann R. Effects of neuropeptide Y on the cardiovascular system. *Trends Pharmacol Sci* 1987;8:231–235.

191. Jansen I, Uddmann R, Hocherman M, et al. Localization and effects of neuropeptide Y, vasoactive intestinal polypeptide, substance P, and calcitonin gene-related peptide in human temporal arteries. *Ann Neurol* 1986;20:496–501.

192. Potter EK. Neuropeptide Y as an autonomic neurotransmitter. *Pharmacol Ther* 1988;37:251–273.

193. Dalsgaard C-J, Franco-Cereceda A, Saria A, Lundberg JM, Theodorsson-Norheim E, Hökfelt T. Distribution and origin of substance P

and neuropeptide Y immunoreactive nerves in the guinea-pig heart. *Cell Tissue Res* 1986; 243:477–485.

194. Lundberg JM, Al-Saffar A, Saria A, Theodorsson-Norheim E. Reserpine-induced depletion of neuropeptide Y from cardiovascular nerves and adrenal gland due to enhanced activation. *Naunyn Schmiedebergs Arch Pharmacol* 1986;332:163–168.

195. Morris JL, Murphy R, Furness JB, Costa M. Partial depletion of neuropeptide Y from noradrenergic perivascular and cardiac axons by 6-hydroxydopamine and reserpine. *Regul Pept* 1986;13:147–162.

196. Lundberg JM, Saria A, Franco-Cereceda A, Hökfelt T, Terenius L, Goldstein M. Differential effects of reserpine and 6-hydroxydopamine on neuropeptide Y (NPY) and noradenaline in peripheral nerves. *Naunyn Schmiedebergs Arch Pharmacol* 1985;328:331–340.

197. Lundberg JM, Änggård A, Theodorsson-Norheim E, Pernow J. Guanethidine-sensitive release of NPY-like immunoreactivity in the cat spleen by sympathetic nerve stimulation. *Neurosci Lett* 1984;52:175–180.

198. Lundberg JM, Martinsson A, Hemsén A, et al. Co-release of neuropeptide-Y and catecholamines during physical exercises in man. *Biochem Biophy Res Commun* 1985;133:30–36.

199. Lundberg JM, Rudehill A, Sollevi A, Theodorsson-Norheim E, Hamberger B. Frequency- and reserpine-dependent chemical coding of sympathetic transmission: differential release of noradrenaline and neuropeptide Y from pig spleen. *Neurosci Lett* 1986;63:96–100.

200. Allen JM, Bircham PMM, Bloom SR, Edwards AV. Release of neuropeptide Y in response to splanchnic nerve stimulation in the conscious calf. *J Physiol* 1984;357:401–408.

201. Dahlöf C, Dahlöf P, Lundberg JM. α_2-Adrenoceptor-mediated inhibition of nerve stimulation-evoked release of neuropeptide Y (NPY)-like immunoreactivity in the pithed guinea-pig. *Eur J Pharmacol* 1986;131:279–283.

202. Rudehill A, Sollevi A, Franco-Cereceda A, Lundberg JM. Neuropeptide Y (NPY) and the pig heart: release and coronary vasoconstrictor effects. *Peptides* 1986;7:821–826.

203. Allen JM, Bircham PMM, Edwards AV, Tatemoto K, Bloom SR. Neuropeptide Y (NPY) reduces myocardial perfusion and inhibits the force of contraction of the isolated perfused rabbit heart. *Regul Pept* 1983;6:247–253.

204. Edvinsson L, Emson P, McCulloch J, Tatemoto K, Uddmann R. Neuropeptide Y: cerebrovascular innervation and vasomotor effects in the cat. *Neurosci Lett* 1983;43:79–84.

205. Lundberg JM, Tatemoto K. Pancreatic polypeptide family (APP, BPP, NPY and PYY) in relation to alpha-adrenoceptor sympathetic vasoconstriction resistant to adrenoceptor blockade. *Acta Physiol Scand* 1982;116:393–402.

206. Rioux F, Bachelard H, Martel JC, St-Pierre S. The vasoconstrictor effects of neuropeptide Y and related peptides on the guinea-pig isolated heart. *Peptides* 1986;7:27–31.

207. Edvinsson L, Ekblad E, Håkanson R, Wahlestedt C. Neuropeptide Y potentiates the effect of various vasoconstrictor agents on rabbit blood vessels. *Br J Pharmacol* 1984;83:519–525.

208. Pernow J, Lundberg JM, Kaijser L. Vasoconstrictor effects in vivo and plasma disappearance rate of neuropeptide Y in man. *Life Sci* 1987;40:47–54.

209. Westfall TC, Carpentier S, Chen X, Beinfeld MC, Naes L, Meldrum MJ. Prejunctional and postjunctional effects of neuropeptide Y at the noradrenergic neuroeffector junction of the perfused mesenteric arterial bed of the rat. *J Cardiovasc Pharmacol* 1987;10:716–722.

210. Edwall B, Gazelius B, Fazekas A, Theodorsson-Norheim E, Lundberg JM. Neuropeptide Y (NPY) and sympathetic control of blood in oral mucosa and dental pulp in the cat. *Acta Physiol Scand* 1985;125:253–264.

211. Hellström PM, Olerup O, Tatemoto K. Neuropeptide Y may mediate effects of sympathetic nerve stimulation on colonic motility and blood flow in the cat. *Acta Physiol Scand* 1985;124:613–624.

212. Lundberg JM, Fried G, Pernow J, Theodorsson-Norheim E, Änggård A. NPY—a mediator of reserpine-resistant, nonadrenergic vasoconstriction in cat spleen after preganglionic denervation? *Acta Physiol Scand* 1986;126:151–152.

213. Kondo H, Kuramoto H, Fujita T. Neuropeptide tyrosine-like immunoreactive nerve fibres in the carotid body chemoreceptors of rats. *Brain Res* 1986;372:353–356.

214. Potter EK, McCloskey DI. Excitation of carotid body chemoreceptors by neuropeptide-Y. *Resp Physiol* 1987;67:357–365.

215. O'Regan RG. Response of carotid body chemosensory activity and blood flow to stimulation of sympathetic nerves in the cat. *J Physiol* 1981;315:81–98.

216. Franco-Cereceda A, Lundberg JM, Dahlhöf C. Neuropeptide Y and sympathetic control of heart contractility and coronary vascular tone. *Acta Physiol Scand* 1985;124:361–369.

217. Lundberg JM, Hua X-Y, Franco-Cereceda A. Effects of neuropeptide Y (NPY) on mechanical activity and neurotransmission in the heart, vas deferens and urinary bladder of the guinea-pig. *Acta Physiol Scand* 1984;121:325–332.

218. Neild TO. Actions of neuropeptide Y on innervated and denervated rat tail arteries. *J Physiol* 1987;386:19–30.

219. Pernow J, Saria A, Lundberg JM. Mechanisms underlying pre- and postjunctional effects of neuropeptide Y in sympathetic vascular control. *Acta Physiol Scand* 1986;126:239–249.

220. Wahlestedt C, Edvinsson L, Ekblad E, Håkanson R. Neuropeptide Y potentiates noradrenaline-evoked vasoconstriction: mode of action. *J Pharmacol Exp Ther* 1985;234:735–741.

221. Dahlöf C, Dahlöf P, Lundberg JM. Neuropeptide Y (NPY): enhancement of blood pressure increase upon α-adrenoceptor activation and direct pressor effects in pithed rats. *Eur J Pharmacol* 1985;109:289–291.

222. Lundberg JM, Pernow J, Dahlöf C, Tatemoto K. Pre- and postjunctional effects of NPY on sympathetic control of rat femoral artery. *Acta Physiol Scand* 1985;123:511–513.
223. Glover WE. Increased sensitivity of the rabbit ear artery to noradrenaline following perivascular nerve stimulation may be a response to neuropeptide Y released as a cotransmitter. *Clin Exp Pharmacol Physiol* 1985;12:227–230.
224. Hanko J, Törnebrandt K, Hardebo JE, Kåhrström J, Nobin A, Owman C. Neuropeptide Y induces and modulates vasoconstriction in intracranial and peripheral vessels of animals and man. *J Auton Pharmacol* 1986;6:117–124.
225. Wong-Dusting H, Rand MJ. Pre- and postjunctional effects of neuropeptide Y on the rabbit isolated ear artery. *Clin Exp Pharmacol Physiol* 1988;15:411–418.
226. Daly RN, Hieble JP. Neuropeptide Y modulates adrenergic neurotransmission by an endothelium dependent mechanism. *Eur J Pharmacol* 1987;138:445–446.
227. Buchanan F, Neild TO, Parkington HC. Potentiating action of neuropeptide Y is not endothelium-dependent. *Proc Austral Physiol Pharmacol Soc* 1989;20:19P.
228. Burnstock G. Purinergic modulation of cholinergic transmission. *Gen Pharmacol* 1980;11:15–18.
229. Larsson L-I, Fahrenkrug J, Schaffalitzky de Muckadell OB, Sundler F, Håkanson R, Rehfelt JF. Localization of vasoactive intestinal polypeptide (VIP) to central and peripheral neurons. *Proc Natl Acad Sci USA* 1976;73:3197–3200.
230. Lundberg JM, Hökfelt T, Schultzberg M, Uvnas-Wallensten K, Kohler C, Said SI. Occurrence of vasoactive intestinal polypeptide (VIP)-like immunoreactivity in certain cholinergic neurons of the cat: evidence from combined immunohistochemistry and acetylcholinesterase staining. *Neuroscience* 1979;4:1539–1559.
231. Lundberg JM, Änggård A, Fahrenkrug J, Hökfelt T, Mutt V. Vasoactive intestinal polypeptide in cholinergic neurons of exocrine glands: functional significance of coexisting transmitters for vasodilation and secretion. *Proc Natl Acad Sci USA* 1980;77:1651–1655.
232. Lundberg JM, Änggård A, Emson P, Fahrenkrug J, Hökfelt T. Vasoactive intestinal polypeptide and cholinergic mechanisms in cat nasal mucosa. Studies on choline acetyltransferase and release of vasoactive intestinal polypeptides. *Proc Natl Acad Sci USA* 1981;78:5255–5259.
233. Lundberg JM. Evidence for the existence of vasoactive intestinal polypeptide (VIP) and acetylcholine in neurons of cat exocrine glands. Morphological, anatomical and functional studies. *Acta Physiol Scand* 1981(Suppl 496):1–57.
234. Lundberg JM, Änggård A, Fahrenkrug J, Johansson O, Hökfelt T. Vasoactive intestinal polypeptide in cholinergic neurons of exocrine glands. In: Said SI, ed. *Vasoactive intestinal peptide*. New York: Raven Press, 1982;373–389.
235. Della NG, Papka RE, Furness JB, Costa M. Vasoactive intestinal peptide-like immunoreactivity in nerves associated with the cardiovascular system of guinea-pigs. *Neuroscience* 1983;9:605–619.
236. Hökfelt T, Schultzberg M, Lundberg JM, et al. Distribution of vasoactive intestinal polypeptide in the central and peripheral nervous system as revealed by immunocytochemistry. In: Said SI, ed. *Vasoactive intestinal peptide*. New York: Raven Press, 1982;65–90.
237. Håkanson R, Sundler F, Uddmann R. Distribution and topography of peripheral VIP nerve fibres: functional implications. In: Said SI, ed. *Vasoactive intestinal peptide*. New York: Raven Press, 1982;121–144.
238. Sundler F, Alumets J, Håkanson R, Fahrenkrug J, Schaffalitzky de Muckadell OB. Peptidergic (VIP) nerves in the pancreas. *Histochemistry* 1978;55:173–176.
239. Bloom SR, Edwards AV. Effects of autonomic stimulation on the release of vasoactive intestinal peptide from the gastrointestinal tract in the calf. *J Physiol* 1980;299:437–452.
240. Uddmann R, Fahrenkrug J, Malm L, Alumets J, Håkanson R, Sundler F. Neuronal VIP in salivary glands: distribution and release. *Acta Physiol Scand* 1980;110:31–38.
241. Lundberg JM, Änggård A, Fahrenkrug J. Complementary role of vasoactive intestinal polypeptide (VIP) and acetylcholine for cat submandibular gland blood flow and secretion. I. VIP release. *Acta Physiol Scand* 1981;113:317–327.
242. Lundberg JM, Änggård A, Fahrenkrug J. Complementary role of vasoactive intestinal polypeptide (VIP) and acetylcholine for cat submandibular gland blood flow and secretion. II. Effects of cholinergic antagonists and VIP antiserum. *Acta Physiol Scand* 1981;113:329–336.
243. Lundberg JM, Anggård A, Fahrenkrug J. Complementary role of vasoactive intestinal polypeptide (VIP) and acetylcholine for cat submandibular gland blood flow and secretion. III. Effects of local infusions. *Acta Physiol Scand* 1982;114:329–337.
244. Lundberg JM, Änggård A, Fahrenkrug J, Lundgren G, Holmstedt B. Corelease of VIP and acetylcholine in relation to blood flow and salivary secretion in cat submandibular salivary gland. *Acta Physiol Scand* 1982;115:525–528.
245. Andersson KE, Bloom SR, Edwards AV, Jarhult J. Effects of stimulation of the chorda tympani in bursts on submaxillary responses in the cat. *J Physiol* 1982;322:469–483.
246. Bloom SR, Edwards AV. Vasoactive intestinal polypeptide in relation to atropine resistant vasodilatation in the submaxillary gland of the cat. *J Physiol* 1980;300:41–53.
247. Lundberg JM, Hedlund B, Bartfai T. Vasoactive intestinal polypeptide enhances muscarinic ligand binding in cat submandibular salivary gland. *Nature* 1982;295:147–149.
248. Said SI, Mutt V. Polypeptide with broad biolog-

ical activity: isolation from small intestine. *Science* 1970;169:1217–1218.

249. Itoh T, Sasaguri T, Makita Y, Kanmura Y, Kuriyama H. Mechanisms of vasodilation induced by vasoactive intestinal polypeptide in rabbit mesenteric artery. *Am J Physiol* 1985; 249:H231–H240.

250. Lundberg JM, Änggård A, Fahrenkrug J, VIP as a mediator of hexamethonium-sensitive, atropine-resistant vasodilatation in the cat tongue. *Acta Physiol Scand* 1982;116:387–392.

251. Bevan JA, Brayden JE. Non-adrenergic neural vasodilator mechanisms. *Circ Res* 1987;60: 309–320.

252. Lee TJ-F, Saito A, Berezin I. Vasoactive intestinal polypeptide-like substance: the potential transmitter for cerebral vasodilation. *Science* 1984;224:898–901.

253. Edvinsson L, Håkanson R, Sundler F, Jansen I, Uddmann R. Peptide-containing nerve fibres in human arteries and veins: vasomotor responses to the neuropeptides. In: Nobin A, Owman C, Aneklo-Nobin B, eds. *Neuronal messengers in vascular function.* Amsterdam: Elsevier, 1987;199–209.

254. Franco-Cereceda A, Lundberg JM, Hökfelt T. Somatostatin: an inhibitory parasympathetic transmitter in the human heart. *Eur J Pharmacol* 1986;132:101–102.

255. Day S, Gu J, Polak J, Bloom S. Somatostatin in the human heart and comparison with guinea-pig and rat heart. *Br Heart J* 1985;53:153–157.

256. Campbell G, Gibbins IL, Morris JB, et al. Somatostatin is contained in and released from cholinergic nerves in the heart of the toad *Bufo marinus. Neuroscience* 1982;7:2012–2023.

257. Quirion R, Regoli D, Rioux F, St-Pierre S. An analysis of the negative inotropic action of somatostatin. *Br J Pharmacol* 1979;66:251–257.

258. Diez J, Tamargo J. Effect of somatostatin on ^{45}Ca fluxes in guinea-pig isolated atria. *Br J Pharmacol* 1987;90:309–314.

259. Franco-Cereceda A, Bengtsson L, Lundberg JM. Inotropic effects of calcitonin gene-related peptide, vasoactive intestinal polypeptide and somatostatin on the human right atrium in vitro. *Eur J Pharmacol* 1987;134:69–76.

260. Hervonen A, Linnoila I, Pickel VM, et al. Localization of [met^5]- and [leu^5]-enkephalin-like immunoreactivity in nerve terminals in human paravertebral sympathetic ganglia. *Neuroscience* 1981;6:323–330.

261. Dalsgaard C-J, Hökfelt T, Schultzberg M, et al. Origin of peptide-containing fibers in the inferior mesenteric ganglion of the guinea pig: immunohistochemical studies with antisera to substance P, enkephalin, vasoactive intestinal polypeptide, cholecystokinin and bombesin. *Neuroscience* 1983;9:191–211.

262. Konishi S, Tsunoo A, Otsuka M. Enkephalins presynaptically inhibit cholinergic transmission in sympathetic ganglia. *Nature* 1979;282:515–516.

263. Jiang Z-G, Dun NJ, Karczmar AG. Substance P: a putative sensory transmitter in mammalian autonomic ganglia. *Science* 1982;217:739–741.

264. Brown GL, Gillespie JS. The output of sympathetic transmitter from the spleen of the cat. *J Physiol* 1957;138:81–102.

265. Rand MJ, Story DF. Conditions required for the inhibitory feedback loop in noradrenergic transmission. In: Feigenbaum JJ, Hanani M, eds. *The presynaptic regulation of neurotransmitter release.* London and Tel Aviv: Freund (in press).

266. Story DF, McCulloch MW, Rand MJ, Standford-Starr. Conditions required for the inhibitory feedback loop in noradrenergic transmission. *Nature* 1981;293:62–65.

267. Stjärne L. Basic mechanisms and local feedback control of secretion of adrenergic and cholinergic neurotransmitters. In: Iversen LL, Iversen SD, Snyder SH, eds. *Handbook of psychopharmacology, vol 6.* New York: Plenum Press, 1975;179–233.

268. Augustine GJ, Charlton MP, Smith SJ. Calcium action in synaptic transmitter release. *Annu Rev Neurosci* 1987;10:633–693.

269. Langer SZ, Armstrong JM. Prejunctional receptors and the cardiovascular system: pharmacological and therapeutic relevance. In: Antonaccio MJ, ed. *Cardiovascular Pharmacology,* 2nd ed. New York: Raven Press, 1984;197–213.

270. Starke K. Presynaptic α-autoreceptors. *Rev Physiol Biochem Pharmacol* 1987;107:73–146.

271. Bacq ZM. Les contrôles de la libération des médiateurs aux terminations des nerfs andrénergiques. *J Physiol* 1976;72:371–473.

272. Doxey JC, Roach AG. Presynaptic α-adrenoceptor; in vitro methods and preparations utilized in the evaluation of agonists and antagonists. *J Auton Pharmacol* 1980;1:73–99.

273. Kirkepar SM. Factors influencing transmission at adrenergic synapses. *Prog Neurobiol* 1975;4:165–210.

274. Lokhandwala MF. Presynaptic receptor systems on cardiac sympathetic nerves. *Life Sci* 1979;245:1823–1832.

275. Wikberg J. The pharmacological classification of α_1 and α_2 receptors and their mechanism of action. *Acta Physiol Scand* 1979(Suppl 468):1–99.

276. Kalsner S. Feedback regulation of neurotransmitter release through adrenergic presynaptic receptors: time for a reassessment. In: Kalsner S, ed. *Trends in autonomic pharmacology, vol 2.* Baltimore-Munich: Urban & Schwartzenberg, 1982;385–425.

277. Kalsner S. Is there feedback regulation of neurotransmitter release by autoreceptors? *Biochem Pharmacol* 1985;34:4085–4097.

278. Kalsner S. The presynaptic receptor controversy. *Trends Pharmacol Sci* 1982;3:11–16,18–21.

279. Rand MJ, McCulloch MW, Story DF. Feedback modulation of noradrenergic transmission. *Trends Pharmacol Sci* 1982;3:8–11,16–18.

280. Starke K. α-Adrenoceptor subclassification. *Rev Physiol Biochem Pharmacol* 1981;88:199–236.

281. Ruffolo RR, Nichols AJ, Hieble JP. Functions

mediated by alpha-2 adrenergic receptors. In: Limbird LE, ed. *The alpha-2 adrenergic receptors.* Clifton, NJ: Humana Press, 1988;187–280.

282. Story DF, Standford-Starr CA, Rand MJ. Evidence for the involvement of α_1-adrenoceptors in negative feedback regulation of noradrenergic transmitter release in rat atria. *Clin Sci* 1985;68(Suppl 10):111s–115s.

283. Rump LC, Majewski H. Modulation of norepinephrine release through α_1- and α_2-adrenoceptors in rat isolated kidney. *J Cardiovasc Pharmacol* 1987;9:500–507.

284. Majewski H, Hedler L, Starke K. Evidence for a physiological role of presynaptic α-adrenoceptors: modulation of noradrenaline release in pithed rabbit. *J Cardiovasc Pharmacol* 1983;324:256–263.

285. Majewski H, Hedler L, Starke K. Modulation of noradrenaline release in the conscious rabbit through α-adrenoceptors. *Eur J Pharmacol* 1983;93:255–264.

286. McCall RB, Schmitts MR, Humphrey SJ, Lahti RA, Barsuhn C. Evidence for a central sympathetic excitatory action of alpha-2 adrenergic antagonists. *J Pharmacol Exp Ther* 1983; 224:501–507.

287. Majewski H, Rump LC, Hedler L, Starke K. Effects of α_1- and α_2-blocking drugs on the noradrenaline release rate in the anaesthetized rabbit. *J Cardiovasc Pharmacol* 1983;5:703–711.

288. Graham RM, Stephenson WH, Pettinger WA. Pharmacological evidence for a functional role of the prejunctional alpha-adrenoceptor in noradrenergic transmission in the conscious rat. *Naunyn Schmiedebergs Arch Pharmacol* 1980; 311:129–138.

289. Zukowska-Grojec Z, Bayorh MA, Kopin IJ. Effect of desepramine on the effects of α-adrenoceptor inhibitors on pressor responses and release of norepinephrine into plasma of pithed rats. *J Cardiovasc Pharmacol* 1983; 5:297–301.

290. Hamilton CA, Reid JL, Zamboulis C. The role of presynaptic α-adrenoceptors in the regulation of blood pressure in the conscious rabbit. *Br J Pharmacol* 1982;75:417–424.

291. Yamaguchi N, De Champlain J, Nadeau RA. Regulation of norepinephrine release from cardiac sympathetic fibres in the dog by presynaptic α- and β-adrenoceptors. *Circ Res* 1977;41:108–117.

292. Heyndrickx GR, Vilaine JP, Moerman EJ, Leusen I. Role of prejunctional α_2-adrenergic receptors in the regulation of myocardial performance during exercise in conscious dogs. *Circ Res* 1984;54:683–693.

293. Saeed M, Sommer O, Holtz J, Bassenge E. α-Adrenoceptor blockade by phentolamine causes β-adrenergic vasodilation by increased catecholamine release due to presynaptic α-blockade. *J Cardiovasc Pharmacol* 1982;4:44–52.

294. Esler M, Jennings G, Korner P, Blomberry P, Sacharias N, Leonard P. Measurement of total

and organ specific norepinephrine kinetics in humans. *Am J Physiol* 1984;247:E21–E28.

295. Kiowski W, Hulthen VL, Ritz R, Bühler FR. Prejunctional α_2-adrenoceptors and norepinephrine release in the forearm of normal humans. *J Cardiovasc Pharmacol* 1985;7(Suppl 6):S144–S148.

296. Fitzgerald GA, Watkins T, Dollery CT. Regulation of norepinephrine release by peripheral alpha receptor stimulation. *Clin Pharmacol Ther* 1981;29:160–167.

297. Brown MJ, Struthers AD, Burrin JM, Di Silvio L, Brown DC. The physiological and pharmacological role of presynaptic α- and β-adrenoceptors in man. *Br J Clin Pharmacol* 1985;20:649–658.

298. Elliot HL, Jones CR, Vincent J, Lawrie CB, Reid JL. The alpha adrenoceptor antagonist properties of idazoxan in normal subjects. *Clin Pharmacol Ther* 1985;36:190–196.

299. Jie K, Van Brummeln P, Vermey P, Timmermans PBMWM, Van Zwieten PA. Modulation of noradrenaline release by peripheral presynaptic α_2-adrenoceptors in humans. *J Cardiovasc Pharmacol* 1987;9:407–413.

300. Xiao X-H, Medgett IC, Rand MJ. The α_2-adrenoceptor agonists clonidine, TL99 and DPI enhance vasoconstrictor responses to sympathetic nerve stimulation in the rat tail artery preparation. *Clin Exp Pharmacol Physiol* 1987; 14:903–906.

301. Xiao X-H, Rand MJ. α_2-Adrenoceptor agonists enhance responses to certain other vasoconstrictor agonists in the rat tail artery. *Br J Pharmacol* 1989;96:539–546.

302. Xiao X-H, Rand MJ. Effects of the α_2-adrenoceptor agonist UK14304 on pressor responses in pithed rats. *Proc Austral Physiol Pharmacol Soc* 1989;20:4P.

303. Nagata A, Franco-Cereceda A, Svensson TH, Lundberg L. Clonidine treatment elevates the content of neuropeptide Y in cardiac nerves. *Acta Physiol Scand* 1986;128:321–322.

304. Franco-Cereceda A, Nagata M, Svensson TH, Lundberg JM. Differential effects of clonidine and reserpine treatment on neuropeptide Y content in some sympathetically innervated tissues of the guinea-pig. *Eur J Pharmacol* 1987;142:267–273.

305. Lundberg JM, Pernow J, Franco-Cereceda A, Rudehill A. Effects of antihypertensive drugs on sympathetic vascular control in relation to neuropeptide Y. *J Cardiovasc Pharmacol* 1987;10(Suppl 12):S51–S68.

306. Hedqvist P, Fredholm BB. Effects of adenosine on adrenergic neurotransmission: prejunctional inhibition and postjunctional enhancement. *Naunyn Schmiedebergs Arch Pharmacol* 1976;293:217–223.

307. Katsuragi T, Su C. Augmentation by theophylline of [^{3}H]purine release from vascular adrenergic nerves: evidence for presynaptic autoinhibition. *J Pharmacol Exp Ther* 1982;220:152–156.

308. Su C. Purinergic inhibition of adrenergic trans-

mission in rabbit blood vessels. *J Pharmacol Exp Ther* 1978;204:351–361.

309. De Mey JG, Burnstock G, Vanhoutte PM. Modulation of the evoked release of noradrenaline in canine saphenous vein via presynaptic receptors for adenosine but not ATP. *Eur J Pharmacol* 1979;55:401–405.

310. Husted S, Nedergaard OA. Inhibition of adrenergic neuroeffector transmission in rabbit pulmonary artery and aorta by adenosine and adenine nucleotides. *Acta Pharmacol Toxicol* 1981;49:334–353.

311. Burnstock G, Crowe R, Kennedy C, Török J. Indirect evidence that purinergic modulation of perivascular adrenergic neurotransmission in the portal vein is a physiological process. *Br J Pharmacol* 1984;82:359–368.

312. Kamikawa Y, Cline WH, Su C. Diminished purinergic modulation of the vascular adrenergic neurotransmission in spontaneously hypertensive rats. *Eur J Pharmacol* 1980;66:347–353.

313. Muir TC, Wardle KA. Vascular smooth muscle responses in normo- and hypertensive rats to sympathetic nerve stimulation and putative transmitters. *J Auton Pharmacol* 1989;9:23–34.

314. Allen JM, Adrian TE, Tatemoto K, Polak JM, Hughes J, Bloom SR. Two novel related peptides, neuropeptide Y (NPY) and peptide YY (PYY) inhibit the contraction of electrically stimulated mouse vas deferens. *Neuropeptides* 1982;3:71–77.

315. Ohhashi I, Jacobowitz DM. The effects of pancreatic polypeptides and neuropeptide Y on the rat vas deferens. *Peptides* 1983;4:381–386.

316. Lundberg JM, Stjärne L. Neuropeptide Y (NPY) depresses the secretion of ³H-noradrenaline and the contractile response evoked by field stimulation in rat vas deferens. *Acta Physiol Scand* 1984;120:477–479.

317. Huidobro-Toro PJ, Rohde G, Tatemoto K. Neuropeptide Y (NPY): an endogenous modulator of non-adrenergic transmission in rat vas deferens? *Eur J Pharmacol* 1985;109:317–318.

318. Serfözö P, Bartfai T, Vizi ES. Presynaptic effects of neuropeptide Y on [³H]noradrenaline and [³H]acetylcholine release. *Regul Pept* 1986;15:117–123.

319. Dahlöf C, Dahlöf P, Tatemoto K, Lundberg JM. Neuropeptide Y (NPY) reduces field stimulation-evoked release of noradrenaline and enhances force of contraction in the rat portal vein. *Naunyn Schmiedebergs Arch Pharmacol* 1985;328:327–330.

320. Edvinsson L, Skärby T. Interaction of peptides present in perivascular nerves on the smooth muscle of the cat cerebral arteries and on the stimulation-evoked efflux of ³H-noradrenaline. *J Auton Pharmacol* 1984;4:193–198.

321. Wahlestedt C, Edvinsson L, Ekblad E, Håkanson R. Effects of neuropeptide Y at sympathetic neuroeffector junctions: existence of Y₁- and Y₂-receptors. In: Nobin A, Owman C, Aneklo-Nobin B, ed. *Neuronal messengers in vascular function.* Amsterdam: Elsevier, 1987; 231–242.

322. Wahlestedt C, Yanaihara N, Håkanson R. Evidence for different pre- and post-junctional receptors for neuropeptide Y and related peptides. *Regul Pept* 1986;13:307–318.

323. Meehan AG, Story DF. Interaction of the prejunctional inhibitory action of 5-hydroxytryptamine on noradrenergic transmission with neuronal uptake in rabbit isolated ear artery. *J Pharmacol Exp Ther* 1989;248:342–347.

324. McCulloch MW, Rand MJ, Story DF. Evidence for a dopaminergic mechanism for modulation of adrenergic transmission in the ear artery. *Br J Pharmacol* 1973;49:141.

325. Hope W, Law M, McCulloch MW, Rand MJ, Story DF. Effects of some catecholamines on noradrenergic transmission in the rabbit ear artery. *Clin Exp Pharmacol Physiol* 1976;3:15–28.

326. Hope W, McCulloch MW, Rand MJ, Story DF. Modulation of noradrenergic transmission in the rabbit ear artery by dopamine. *Br J Pharmacol* 1978;64:527–537.

327. Enero MA, Langer SZ. Inhibition by dopamine of ³H-noradrenaline release elicited by nerve stimulation in the isolated cat's nictitating membrane. *Naunyn Schmiedebergs Arch Pharmacol* 1975;289:179–203.

328. Hope W, McCulloch MW, Story DF, Rand MJ. Effects of pimozide on noradrenergic transmission in rabbit isolated ear arteries. *Eur J Pharmacol* 1977;46:101–111.

329. Hope W, Majewski H, McCulloch MW, Rand MJ, Story DF. Evidence for a modulatory role of dopamine in sympathetic transmission. *Circ Res* 1980;46(Suppl I):177–179.

330. Langer SZ, Dubocovich ML. Physiological and pharmacological role of the regulation of noradrenaline release by presynaptic dopamine receptors in the peripheral nervous system. In: Imbs J-L, Schwartz J, eds. *Peripheral dopaminergic receptors.* Oxford: Pergamon, 1979; 233–245.

331. Bell C, Lang WJ. Is there a place for dopamine in autonomic neuromuscular transmission? In: Kalsner S, ed. *Trends in autonomic pharmacology, vol 2.* Baltimore, Munich: Urban & Schwarzenberg, 1982;263–284.

332. Lokhandwala MF, Buckley JP. The effect of *l*-dopa on peripheral sympathetic nerve function: role of presynaptic dopamine receptors. *J Pharmacol Exp Ther* 1978;204:362–371.

333. Snider SR, Almgren O, Carlsson A. The occurrence and functional significance of dopamine in some peripheral adrenergic nerves of the rat. *Naunyn Schmiedebergs Arch Pharmacol* 1973;278:1–12.

334. Soares-da-Silva P. Evidence for dopaminergic cotransmission in dog mesenteric arterial vessels. *Br J Pharmacol* 1988;95:218–224.

335. Starke K, Illes P, Ramme D, et al. Peripheral prejunctional opioid receptors in cardiovascular control. In: Nobin A, Owman C, Aneklo-Nobin B, eds. *Neuronal messengers in vascular function.* Amsterdam: Elsevier, 1987;247–269.

336. Adler-Graschinsky E, Langer SZ. Possible role

of a β-adrenoceptor in the regulation of noradrenaline release by nerve stimulation through a positive feedback mechanism. *Br J Pharmacol* 1975;53:43–50.

337. Misu Y, Kubo T. Presynaptic β-adrenoceptors. *Med Res Rev* 1986;6:197–225.

338. Majewski H, Hedler L, Schurr C, Starke K. Dual effect of adrenaline on noradrenaline release in the pithed rabbit. *J Cardiovasc Pharmacol* 1985;7:251–257.

339. Dominiak P, Grobecker H. Elevated plasma catecholamines in young hypertensive and hyperkinetic patients: effect of pindolol. *Br J Clin Pharmacol* 1982;13(Suppl 2):81S–90S.

340. Cryer PE. Physiology and pathophysiology of the human sympathoadrenal neuroendocrine system. *N Engl J Med* 1980;303:436–444.

341. Musgrave IF, Bachman AW, Jackson RV, Gordon RD. Increased plasma noradrenaline during low dose adrenaline infusion in resting man and during sympathetic stimulation. *Clin Exp Pharmacol Physiol* 1985;12:285–289.

342. Vincent HH, Boomsma F, Man in't Veld AJ, Schalekamp MADH. Beta-receptor stimulation by adrenaline elevates plasma noradrenaline and enhances the pressor responses to cold exposure and isometric exercise. *J Hypertens* 1983;1(Suppl 2):74–70.

343. Nezo M, Miura Y, Adachi M, et al. The effects of epinephrine on norepinephrine release in essential hypertension. *Hypertension* 1985;7:187–195.

344. Blankestijn PJ, Man in't Veld AJ, Tulen J, et al. Support for adrenaline-hypertension hypothesis: 18 hour pressor effect after 6 hours adrenaline infusion. *Lancet* 1988;2:1386–1389.

345. Rand MJ, Majewski H. Adrenaline mediates a positive feedback loop in noradrenergic transmission: its possible role in the development of hypertension. *Clin Exp Hypertens* 1984;A6:347–370.

346. Molenaar PC, Polak HL. Inhibition of acetylcholine release by activation of acetylcholine receptors. *Prog Pharmacol* 1980;3:39–41.

347. Kilbinger H. Presynaptic muscarinic receptors modulating acetylcholine release. *Trends Pharmacol Sci* 1984;5:103–105.

348. Szerb JC. Autoregulation of acetylcholine release. In: Langer SZ, Starke K, Dubocovich ML, eds. *Presynaptic receptors*. Oxford: Pergamon, 1979;292–298.

349. Löffelholz K, Brehm R, Lindmar R. Hydrolysis, synthesis and release of acetylcholine in the isolated heart. *Fed Proc* 1984;43:2603–2606.

350. Bülbring E, Burn JH. The sympathetic dilator fibres in the muscles of the cat and dog. *J Physiol* 1935;83:483–501.

351. Bevan JA, Buga GM, Jope RS, Moritoki H. Further evidence for a muscarinic component to the neural vasodilator innervation of cerebral and cranial extracerebral arteries of the cat. *Circ Res* 1982;51:421–429.

352. Eckenstein F, Baughman RW. Two types of cholinergic innervation in cortex, one co-localized with vasoactive intestinal polypeptide. *Nature* 1984;309:153–155.

353. Brayden JE, Large WA. Electrophysiological analysis of neurogenic vasodilatation in the isolated lingual artery of the rabbit. *Br J Pharmacol* 1986;89:163–171.

354. Vanhoutte PM. Interactions between nerves, smooth muscle and endothelium in vascular responses. In: Nobin A, Owman C, Aneklo-Nobin B, eds. *Neuronal messengers in vascular function*. Amsterdam: Elsevier, 1987;295–304.

355. Bell C. Dual vasoconstrictor and vasodilator innervation of the uterine arterial supply in the guinea-pig. *Circ Res* 1968;23:279–289.

356. Bowman WC, Marshall IG, Gibb AJ, Harborne AJ. Feedback control of transmitter release at the neuromuscular junction. *Trends Pharmacol Sci* 1988;9:16–20.

357. Wessler I. Control of transmitter release from the motor nerve by presynaptic nicotinic and muscarinic autoreceptors. *Trends Pharmacol Sci* 1989;10:110–114.

358. Hedlund B, Abens J, Bartfai T. Vasoactive intestinal polypeptide and muscarinic receptors: supersensitivity induced by long-term atropine treatment. *Science* 1983;220:519–521.

359. Vanhoutte PM. Cholinergic inhibition of adrenergic transmission. *Fed Proc* 1977;36:2444–2449.

360. Fozard J. Cholinergic mechanisms in adrenergic function. In: Kalsner S, ed. *Trends in autonomic pharmacology, vol 1*. Baltimore, Munich: Urban & Schwarzenberg, 1979;145–195.

361. Muscholl E. Peripheral muscarinic control of norepinephrine release in the cardiovascular system. *Am J Physiol* 1980;239:H713–H720.

362. Rand MJ, Story DF. Modulation of norepinephrine release from sympathetic nerve terminals by cholinomimetic drugs and cholinergic nerves. In: Feigenbaum JJ, Hanani M, eds. *The presynaptic regulation of neurotransmitter release*. London and Tel Aviv: Freund (*in press*).

363. Löffelholz K. Untersuchunger über die Noradrenalin-Freisetzung durch Acetylcholin an perfundierten Kaninchenherzen. *Arch Pharmak Exp Pathol* 1967;258:108–122.

364. Lindmar R, Löffelholz K, Muscholl E. A muscarinic mechanism inhibiting the release of noradrenaline from peripheral adrenergic nerve fibres by nicotinic agents. *Br J Pharmacol* 1968;32:280–294.

365. Löffelholz K, Muscholl E. A muscarinic inhibition of noradrenaline release evoked by postganglionic sympathetic nerve stimulation. *Arch Exp Pathol Pharmacol* 1969;265:1–15.

366. Haeusler G, Thoenen H, Haefely W, Heuerlimann A. Electrical events in cardiac adrenergic nerves and noradrenaline release from the cat heart induced by acetylcholine and KCl. *Naunyn Schmiedebergs Arch Pharmacol* 1968;261:389–411.

367. Muscholl E. Cholinomimetic drugs and the release of the adrenergic transmitter. In: Schümann HJ, Kroneberg G, eds. *New aspects of*

storage and release mechanisms of catechol-amines. Berlin: Springer, 1970;168–186.

368. Dubey MP, Muscholl E, Pfeiffer A. Muscarinic inhibition of potassium induced noradrenaline release and its dependence on the calcium concentration. Naunyn Schmiedebergs Arch Pharmacol 1975;291:1–15.

369. Vanhoutte PM, Lorenz RR, Tyce GM. Inhibition of norepinephrine-^{3}H release from sympathetic nerve endings in veins by acetylcholine. J Pharmacol Exp Ther 1973;185:386–394.

370. Vanhoutte PM. Inhibition by acetylcholine of adrenergic neurotransmission in vascular smooth muscle. Circ Res 1974;34:317–326.

371. Hammer R, Berrie CP, Birdsall NJM, Burgen ASV, Hulme EC. Pirenzepine distinguishes between different subclasses of muscarinic receptors. Nature 1980;283:90–92.

372. Muscholl E. Presynaptic muscarine receptors and inhibition of release. In: Paton DM, ed. Adrenergic neurones. Oxford: Pergamon, 1979; 87–110.

373. Fuder H, Rink D, Muscholl E. Sympathetic nerve stimulation on the perfused rat heart. Affinities of N-methylatropine and pirenzipine at pre and postsynaptic muscarinic receptors. Naunyn Schmiedebergs Arch Pharmacol 1982; 318:210–219.

374. Fuder H. The affinity of pirenzepine and other antimuscarinic compounds for pre- and postsynaptic muscarinic receptors of the isolated rabbit heart. Scand J Gastroenterol 1982; 17(Suppl 72):79–85.

375. Lauer JA, Steinsland OS. Pirenzepine has similar affinities for pre- and post-junctional muscarinic receptors. Fed Proc 1983;42:1145.

376. Rand MJ, Varma B. The effects of cholinomimetic drugs on responses to sympathetic nerve stimulation and noradrenaline in the rabbit ear artery. Br J Pharmacol 1970;38:758–770.

377. Fozard JR, Muscholl E. Effects of several muscarinic agonists on cardiac performance and the release of noradrenaline from sympathetic nerves of the perfused rabbit heart. Br J Pharmacol 1972;45:616–629.

378. Nedergaard OA. Modulation by the muscarinic agonist McN-A-343 of noradrenaline release from vascular sympathetic neurones. J Cardiovasc Pharmacol 1980;2:629–643.

379. Nedergaard OA. Dual effect of the muscarinic agonist McN-A-343 on vascular neuroeffector transmission. Acta Pharmacol Toxicol 1981; 49:354–365.

380. Li CK, Mitchelson F. The selective antimuscarinic action of stercuronium. Br J Pharmacol 1980;70:313–321.

381. Ehinger B, Falck B, Sporrung B. Possible axo-axonal synapses between peripheral adrenergic and cholinergic nerve terminals. Z Zellforsch 1970;107:508–521.

382. Cooper T. Terminal innervation of the heart. In: Randall WC, ed. Nervous control of the heart. Baltimore: Williams & Wilkins, 1965; 130.

383. Graham JDP, Lever JD, Spriggs TLB. An ex-

amination of adrenergic axons around pancreatic arterioles of the cat for the presence of acetylcholinesterase by high resolution autoradiographic and histochemical methods. Br J Pharmacol 1968;33:15–20.

384. Iwayama T, Furness JB, Burnstock G. Dual adrenergic and cholinergic innervation of the cerebral arteries of the rat, an ultrastructural study. Circ Res 1970;26:635–646.

385. Nielsen KC, Owman Ch, Sporrong B. Ultrastructure of the autonomic innervation apparatus in the main pial arteries of rats and cats. Brain Res 1971;27:25–32.

386. Edvinsson L, Falck B, Owman B. Possibilities for a cholinergic action on smooth musculature and sympathetic axons in brain vessels mediated by muscarinic and nicotinic receptors. J Pharmacol Exp Ther 1977;200:117–126.

387. Löffelholz K, Muscholl E. Inhibition by parasympathetic nerve stimulation of the release of the adrenergic transmitter. Naunyn Schmiedebergs Arch Pharmacol 1970;276:181–184.

388. Langley AE, Gardiner RW. Effect of atropine and acetylcholine on nerve stimulated output of noradrenaline and dopamine-beta-hydroxylase from isolated rabbit and guinea-pig hearts. Naunyn Schmiedebergs Arch Pharmacol 1977; 297:251–256.

389. Hope W, McCulloch MW, Rand MJ, Story DF. Cholinergic effects on adrenergic transmission in rabbit and guinea-pig isolated atria. Proc Austral Physiol Pharmacol Soc 1974;5:213–214.

390. Muscholl E, Muth A. The effects of physostigmine on the vagally induced muscarinic inhibition of noradrenaline release from the isolated perfused rabbit atria. Naunyn Schmiedebergs Arch Pharmacol 1982;320:160–169.

391. Story DF, Allen GS, Glover AB, et al. Modulation of adrenergic transmission by acetylcholine. Clin Exp Pharmacol Physiol 1975(Suppl 2):27–33.

392. Levy MN, Blattberg B. Effect of vagal stimulation on the overflow of norepinephrine into the coronary sinus during cardiac sympathetic nerve stimulation in the dog. Circ Res 1976;38:81–85.

393. Lokhandwala MF, Cavero I, Buckley JP. Influence of pentobarbital anaesthesia on the effects of certain autonomic blocking agents on heart rate. Eur J Pharmacol 1973;24:274–277.

394. Habermeier-Muth A, Muscholl E. Short and long-latency muscarinic inhibition of noradrenaline release from rabbit atria induced by vagal stimulation. J Physiol 1988;401:277–293.

395. Muscholl E, Forsyth KM, Habermeier-Muth A. A presynaptic excitatory M1 muscarine receptor at postganglionic cardiac adrenergic fibres that is activated by endogenous acetylcholine. Naunyn Schmiedebergs Arch Pharmacol 1989;339:R88.

396. Eccles R, Wilson H. The autonomic innervation of the nasal blood vessels of the cat. J Physiol 1974;238:549–560.

397. Van Hee R, Vanhoutte PM. Cholinergic inhibi-

tion of adrenergic neurotransmission in the canine gastric artery. *Gastroenterology* 1978;74:1266–1270.

398. Furchgott RF. The role of endothelium in responses of vascular smooth muscle to drugs. *Annu Rev Pharmacol Toxicol* 1984;24:175–197.

399. Loiacono RE, Story DF. Acetylcholine induced inhibition of responses to field stimulation in rabbit pulmonary artery is unaffected by endothelium removal. *J Pharm Pharmacol* 1984;26:262–264.

400. Cohen RR, Shepherd JT, Vanhoutte PM. Neurogenic cholinergic prejunctional inhibition of sympathetic beta adrenergic relaxation in the canine coronary artery. *J Pharmacol Exp Ther* 1984;229:417–421.

401. McDougal MD, West GB. The inhibition of the peristaltic reflex by sympathomimetic amines. *J Physiol* 1954;120:41–52.

402. Schäumann W. Zusammenhauge zwischender Wirkung der Anagetica und Sympathomimetica auf den Meerschweinen-Dunndarm. *Arch Exp Pathol Pharmacol* 1958;233:112–124.

403. Vizi ES. The inhibitory action of noradrenaline and adrenaline on release of acetylcholine from guinea-pig ileum longitudinal strips. *Naunyn Schmiedebergs Arch Pharmacol* 1968;259:199–200.

404. Beani L, Biachi C, Crema A. The effects of catecholamines and sympathetic stimulation on the release of acetylcholine from guinea-pig colon. *Br J Pharmacol* 1969;36:1–17.

405. Paton WDM, Vizi E. The inhibitory action of noradrenaline and adrenaline on acetylcholine output by guinea-pig ileum longitudinal muscle strips. *Br J Pharmacol* 1969;35:10–28.

406. Kosterlitz HW, Lydon RJ, Watt AJ. The effects of adrenaline, noradrenaline and isoprenaline on inhibitory α- and β-adrenoceptors in the longitudinal muscle of the guinea-pig ileum. *Br J Pharmacol* 1970;39:398–413.

407. Drew GM. Pharmacological characterization of the presynaptic α-adrenoceptors regulating cholinergic activity in the guinea-pig ileum. *Br J Pharmacol* 1978;64:293–300.

408. Wikberg JES. Differentiation between pre- and postjunctional alpha-receptors in guinea-pig ileum and rabbit aorta. *Acta Physiol Scand* 1978;103:225–239.

409. Tanaka T, Starke K. Binding of ^{3}H-clonidine to an alpha-adrenoceptor in membranes of guinea-pig ileum. *Naunyn Schmiedebergs Arch Pharmacol* 1979;309:207–215.

410. Andréjak M, Pommier Y, Mouille P, Schmitt H. Effects of some alpha-adrenoceptor agonists and antagonists on the guinea-pig ileum. *Naunyn Schmiedebergs Arch Pharmacol* 1980;314:83–87.

411. Knoll J, Vizi ES. Effect of frequency of stimulation on the inhibition by noradrenaline of the acetylcholine output from parasympathetic nerve terminals. *Br J Pharmacol* 1971;42:263–272.

412. Kilbinger H, Wessler I. Increase by alpha-adrenolytic drugs of acetylcholine release evoked by field stimulation of the guinea-pig ileum.

Naunyn Schmiedebergs Arch Pharmacol 1979;309:255–257.

413. Starke K. Alpha sympathomimetic inhibition of adrenergic and cholinergic transmission in the rabbit heart. *Naunyn Schmiedebergs Arch Pharmacol* 1972;274:18–45.

414. Loiacono RE, Story DF. Effect of α-adrenoceptor agonists and antagonists on cholinergic transmission in guinea-pig isolated atria. *Naunyn Schmiedebergs Arch Pharmacol* 1987;334:40–47.

415. Wetzel GT, Goldstein D, Brown JM. Acetylcholine release from rat atria can be regulated through an α_1-adrenergic receptor. *Circ Res* 1985;56:763–766.

416. Dieterich HA, Lindmar R, Löffelholtz K. The role of choline in the release of acetylcholine in isolated hearts. *Naunyn Schmiedebergs Arch Pharmacol* 1978;301:207–215.

417. Burnstock G. Neurotransmitters and trophic factors in the autonomic nervous system. *J Physiol* 1981;313:1–35.

418. Barnes PJ. Airway neuropeptides and asthma. *Trends Pharmacol Sci* 1987;8:24–27.

419. Potter EK. Prolonged non-adrenergic inhibition of cardiac vagal action following sympathetic stimulation: neuromodulation by neuropeptide Y? *Neurosci Lett* 1985;54:117–121.

420. Potter EK. Presynaptic inhibition of cardiac vagal postganglionic nerves by neuropeptide Y. *Neurosci Lett* 1987;83:101–106.

421. Stjernqvist M, Emson P, Owman C, Sjöberg N-O, Sundler F, Tatemoto K. Neuropeptide Y in the female reproductive tract of the rat. Distribution of nerve fibers and motor effects. *Neurosci Lett* 1983;39:279–284.

422. Owman C, Stjernqvist M, Helm G, Kannisto P, Sjöberg N-O, Sundler P. Comparative histochemical distribution of nerve fibres storing noradrenaline and neuropeptide Y (NPY) in human ovary, fallopian tube and uterus. *Med Biol* 1986;64:57–65.

423. Kilborn MJ, Potter EK, McCloskey DI. Neuromodulation of the cardiac vagus: comparison of neuropeptide Y and related peptides. *Regul Pept* 1985;12:155–161.

424. Potter EK. Guanethidine blocks neuropeptide-Y-like inhibitory action of sympathetic nerves on cardiac vagus. *J Auton Nerv Syst* 1987;21:87–90.

425. Gardner TD, Potter EK. Dependence of non-adrenergic inhibition of cardiac vagal action on peak frequency of sympathetic stimulation in the dog. *J Physiol* 1988;405:115–122.

426. Sjöqvist A, Fahrenkrug J. Sympathetic nerve activation decreases the release of vasoactive intestinal polypeptide from the feline intestine. *Acta Physiol Scand* 1986;127:419–423.

427. Järhult J, Hellstrand P, Sundler F. Immunohistochemical localization and vascular effects of vasoactive intestinal polypeptide in skeletal muscle of the cat. *Cell Tissue Res* 1980;207:55–64.

428. Komori K, Suzuki H. Heterogeneous distribution of muscarinic receptors in the rabbit saphenous artery. *Br J Pharmacol* 1987;92:657–664.

429. Erdö SL. Peripheral GABAergic mechanisms. *Trends Pharmacol Sci* 1985;6:205–208.

430. Jessen KR, Mirsky ME, Dennison ME, Burnstock G, GABA may be a neurotransmitter in the vertebrate peripheral nervous system. *Nature* 1979;281:71–74.

431. Ong J, Kerr DIB. GABA$_A$- and GABA$_B$-receptor-mediated modification of intestinal motility. *Eur J Pharmacol* 1983;89:9–17.

432. Saito N, Taniyama K, Tanaka C. ^{3}H-Acetylcholine release from guinea-pig gall bladder evoked by GABA through the bicuculline-sensitive GABA receptor. *Naunyn Schmiedebergs Arch Pharmacol* 1984;326:45–48.

433. Starke K, Weitzell R. τ-Aminobutyric acid and postganglionic sympathetic transmission in the pulmonary artery of the rabbit. *J Auton Pharmacol* 1980;1:45–51.

434. Bowery NG, Doble A, Hill DR, et al. Bicuculline-insensitive GABA receptors on peripheral autonomic nerve terminals. *Eur J Pharmacol* 1981;71:53–70.

435. Hughes PR, Morgan PF, Stone TW. Inhibitory action of τ-aminobutyric acid on the excitatory but not inhibitory innervation of the rat anococcygeus muscle. *Br J Pharmacol* 1982;77:691–695.

436. Priestly T, Woodruff GN. The inhibitory effect of somatostatin peptides on the rat anococcygeus muscle in vitro. *Br J Pharmacol* 1988; 94:87–96.

437. Li CG, Rand MJ. Prejunctional inhibition of non-adrenergic non-cholinergic transmission in the rat anococcygeus muscle. *Eur J Pharmacol* 1989;168:107–110.

438. Fontaine J, Grivegnee A, Reuse J. Adrenoceptors and regulation of intestinal tone in the isolated colon of the mouse. *Br J Pharmacol* 1984;81:231–243.

439. Kojima S, Sakato M, Shimo Y. An α_2-adrenoceptor-mediated inhibition of non-adrenergic non-cholinergic inhibitory responses of the isolated proximal colon of the guinea-pig. *Asia Pacific J Pharmacol* 1988;3:69–75.

440. Marley P, Livett BG. Neuropeptides in the autonomic nervous system. *CRC Crit Rev Clin Neurobiol* 1985;1:201–283.

441. Holton P. The liberation of adenosine triphosphate on antidromic stimulation of sensory nerves. *J Physiol* 1959;145:494–504.

442. Regoli D, D'Orléans-Juste P. Substance P and neurokinins in vascular neuroeffector transmission. In: Bevan J, Majewski H, Maxwell RA, Story DF, eds. *Vascular neuroeffector mechanisms*. Oxford: ICSU Press, 1988;131–139.

443. Furness JB, Papka RE, Della NG, Costa M, Eskay RL. Substance P-like immunoreactivity in nerves associated with the vascular system of guinea-pigs. *Neuroscience* 1982;7:447–459.

444. Uddmann R, Edvinsson L, Ekman R, Kingman I, McCulloch J. Innervation of the feline cerebral vasculature by nerve fibers containing calcitonin gene-related peptide: trigeminal origin and co-existence with substance P. *Neurosci Lett* 1985;62:131–136.

445. Edvinsson L, McCulloch J, Uddmann R. Substance P: immunohistochemical localization and effect upon cat pial arteries in vitro and in situ. *J Physiol* 1981;318:251–258.

446. Lundberg JM, Franco-Cereceda A, Hua X, Hökfelt T, Fischer JA. Co-existence of substance P and calcitonin gene-related peptide-like immunoreactivities in sensory nerves in relation to cardiovascular and bronchoconstrictor effects of capsaicin. *Eur J Pharmacol* 1985;108:315–319.

447. Brimijoin S. Lundberg JM, Brodin E, Hökfelt T, Nilsson G. Axonal transport of substance P in the vagus and sciatic nerves of the guinea pig. *Brain Res* 1980;191:443–457.

448. Harmar A, Keen P. Synthesis and central and peripheral axonal transport of substance P in a dorsal root ganglion-nerve preparation in vitro. *Brain Res* 1982;231:379–385.

449. Wharton J, Polak JM, McGregor GP, Bishop AE, Bloom SE. The distribution of substance P-like immunoreactive nerves in the guinea pig heart. *Neuroscience* 1981;6:2193–2204.

450. Pernow B. Substance P—a putative mediator of antidromic vasodilation. *Gen Pharmacol* 1983;14:13–16.

451. Pernow B. Substance P. *Pharmacol Rev* 1983; 35:85–141.

452. Lembeck F, Donnerer J, Barthó L. Inhibition of neurogenic vasodilation and plasma extravasation by substance P antagonists, somatostatin and [D-Met^2,Pro^5]enkephalinamide. *Eur J Pharmacol* 1982;85:171–176.

453. Matsuyama T, Wanaka AS, Yoneda S, et al. Fine structure and interrelationship between peptidergic and catecholaminergic nerve fibers in the cerebral artery. *Acta Physiol Scand* 1986;127(Suppl 552):17–20.

454. Dalsgaard C-J, Hökfelt T, Elfvin L-G, Skirboll L, Emson P. Substance P-containing primary sensory neurones projecting to the inferior mesenteric ganglion: evidence from combined retrograde tracing and immunohistochemistry. *Neuroscience* 1982;7:647–654.

455. Beleslin D, Radnarovic B, Varagic V. The effect of substance P on the superior cervical ganglion of the cat. *Br J Pharmacol* 1960;15:10–13.

456. Konishi S, Otsuka M. Blockade of slow excitatory postsynaptic potential by substance P antagonists in guinea-pig sympathetic ganglia. *J Physiol* 1985;361:115–130.

457. Regoli D, Drapeau G, Dion S, Couture R. New selective agonists for neurokinin receptors: pharmacological tools for receptor characterization. *Trends Pharmacol Sci* 1988;9:290–295.

458. Holzer-Petsche U, Schmimek U, Amann R, Lembech F. In vivo and in vitro actions of mammalian tachykinins. *Naunyn Schmiedebergs Arch Pharmacol* 1985;330:130–135.

459. Edvinsson L. Functional role of perivascular peptides in the control of the cerebral circulation. *Trends Neurosci* 1985;8:126–131.

460. Saito A, Goto K. Depletion of calcitonin gene-related peptide (CGRP) by capsaicin in cerebral arteries. *J Pharmacobiodyn* 1986;9:613–619.

461. Saito A, Ishikawa T, Kimura S, Goto K. Role

of calcitonin gene-related peptide (CGRP) as cardiotonic neurotransmitter in guinea pig left atria. *J Pharmacol Exp Ther* 1987;243:721–736.

462. Miyauchi T, Ishikawa T, Sugishita Y, Saito A, Goto K. Effects of capsaicin on nonadrenergic noncholinergic nerves in the guinea pig atria: role of calcitonin gene-related peptide as cardiac neurotransmitter. *J Cardiovasc Pharmacol* 1987;10:675–682.

463. Gulbenkian S, Merighi A, Wharton J, Varndell IM, Polak JM. Ultrastructural evidence for the coexistence of calcitonin gene-related peptide and substance P in secretory vesicles of peripheral nerves in the guinea pig. *J Neurocytol* 1986;15:535–542.

464. Schon F, Ghatei M, Allen JM, Mulderry PK, Kelly JS, Bloom SR. The effect of sympathectomy on calcitonin gene-related peptide levels in the rat trigeminovascular system. *Brain Res* 1985;348:197–200.

465. Brain SD, Williams TJ, Tippins JR, Morris HR, MacIntyre I. Calcitonin gene-related peptide is a potent vasodilator. *Nature* 1985;313:54–56.

466. Hanko J, Hardebo JE, Kåhrström J, Owman C, Sundler F. Calcitonin gene-related peptide is present in mammalian cerebrovascular nerve fibers and dilates pial and peripheral arteries. *Neurosci Lett* 1985;57:91–95.

467. Edvinsson L, Fredholm BB, Hamel E, Jansen I, Verrecchia C. Perivascular peptides relax cerebral arteries concomitant with stimulation of cyclic adenosine monophosphate accumulation or release of an endothelium-derived relaxing factor in the cat. *Neurosci Lett* 1985;58:213–217.

468. Gamse R, Saria A. Potentiation of tachykinin-induced plasma protein extravasation by calcitonin gene-related peptide. *Eur J Pharmacol* 1985;114:61–66.

469. Le Grevés P, Nyberg F, Terenius L, Hökfelt T. Calcitonin gene-related peptide is a potent inhibitor of substance P degradation. *Eur J Pharmacol* 1985;115:309–311.

470. Sigrist S, Franco-Cereceda A, Mutt L, Henecke H, Lundberg JM, Fischer JA. Specific receptor and cardiovascular effects of calcitonin gene-related peptide. *Endocrinol* 1986;119:381–389.

471. Tippins JR, Morris HR, Panico M, et al. The myotropic and plasma calcium modulating effects of calcitonin gene related peptide (CGRP). *Neuropeptides* 1984;4:425–434.

472. Ishikawa T, Okamura N, Saito A, Goto K. Comparison of the effects of calcitonin gene-related peptide and isoproterenol on the myocardial contractility and adenylate cyclase activity in the rat heart. *J Mol Cell Cardiol* 1987;19:723–728.

473. Goto K, Kimura S, Saito A. Inhibitory effect of calcitonin gene-related peptide on excitation and contraction of smooth muscles of the rat vas deferens. *J Pharmacol Exp Ther* 1987;241:635–641.

474. Ohhashi I, Jacobowitz DM. Effect of calcitonin gene-related peptide on the neuroeffector mechanism of sympathetic nerve terminals in rat vas deferens. *Peptides* 1985;6:987–991.

475. Al-Kazwini SJ, Craig RK, Marshall I. Postjunctional inhibition of contractor responses in the mouse vas deferens by rat and human calcitonin gene-related peptide (CGRP). *Br J Pharmacol* 1986;88:173–180.

476. Hedqvist P. Basic mechanisms of prostaglandin action on autonomic neurotransmission. *Annu Rev Pharmacol Toxicol* 1977;17:259–279.

477. Hedqvist P. Evidence for transsynaptic modulation of adrenergic transmitter secretion. In: Yoshida M, Hagihara Y, Ebashi S, eds. *Neurotransmitters–receptors,* Proc 8th IUPHAR Congress. Oxford: Pergamon, 1982;103–107.

478. Fredholm BB, Hedqvist P. Release of ^{3}H-purines from [^{3}H]-adenosine labelled rabbit kidney following sympathetic nerve stimulation and its inhibition by α-adrenoceptor blockade. *Br J Pharmacol* 1978;64:239–245.

479. Thurau K. Renal hemodynamics. *Am J Med* 1964;36:687–719.

480. Bergstrom S, Carlson LA, Oro L. Effect of prostaglandins on catecholamine induced changes in the free fatty acids of plasma and in blood pressure in the dog. *Acta Physiol Scand* 1964;60:170–180.

481. Carlson LA, Oro L. Effect of prostaglandin E$_1$ on blood pressure and heart rate in the dog. *Acta Physiol Scand* 1966;67:89–99.

482. Horton EW. Prostaglandins at adrenergic nerve-endings. *Br Med Bull* 1973;29:148–151.

483. Rump LC, Schollmeyer P. Effect of endogenous and synthetic prostanoids on ^{3}H-noradrenaline release and vascular tone in rat isolated kidney. *Br J Pharmacol* 1989;97:819–828.

484. Khan MT, Malik KU. Sympathetic nerve stimulation of isolated rat heart: release of a prostaglandin-like substance and the inhibitory effect of prostaglandin on the output of [^{3}H]-norepinephrine. *Adv Prostaglandin Thromboxane Res* 1980;8:1241–1243.

485. Stjärne L. Prostaglandin E restricting noradrenaline secretion—neuronal in origin? *Acta Physiol Scand* 1972;86:574–576.

486. Zimmerman BG, Ryan MJ, Gomer S, Kraft T. Effect of prostaglandin synthesis inhibitors indomethacin and eicosa-5,8,11,14-tetraynoic acid on adrenergic responses in dog's cutaneous vasculature. *J Pharmacol Exp Ther* 1973;187:315–323.

487. Vanhoutte PM, Webb RC, Collins MG. Pre- and postjunctional adrenergic mechanisms and hypertension. *Clin Sci* 1980;59:211s–223s.

488. Powell JR, Brody MJ. Peripheral facilitation of reflex vasoconstriction by prostaglandin F$_{2\alpha}$. *J Pharmacol Exp Ther* 1973;187:495–500.

489. Wennmalm Å, Hedqvist P. Inhibition by prostaglandin E$_1$ of parasympathetic neurotransmission in the rabbit heart. *Life Sci* 1971;10:465–470.

490. Bickerton RK, Buckley JP. Evidence for a central mechanism in angiotensin induced hypertension. *Proc Soc Exp Biol Med* 1961;106:834–836.

491. Scroop GC, Lowe RD. Efferent pathways of the cardiovascular response to vertebral artery

infusions of angiotensin in the dog. *Clin Sci* 1969;37:605–619.

492. Lewis GP, Reit E. The action of angiotensin and bradykinin on the superior cervical ganglion of the cat. *J Physiol* 1965;179:538–553.

493. Trendelenburg U. Observations on the ganglion-stimulating action of angiotensin and bradykinin. *J Pharmacol Exp Ther* 1966;154:418–425.

494. Reit E. Actions of angiotensin on the adrenal medulla and autonomic ganglia. *Fed Proc* 1972;31:1338–1343.

495. Peach MJ. Adrenal medullary stimulation induced by angiotensin I, angiotensin II and analogues. *Circ Res* 1971;29(Suppl II):107–117.

496. Roth RH. Action of angiotensin on adrenergic nerve endings: enhancement of norepinephrine biosynthesis. *Fed Proc* 1972;31:1358–1364.

497. Khairallah PA. Action of angiotensin on adrenergic norepinephrine uptake. *Fed Proc* 1972; 31:1351–1357.

498. Zimmerman BG. Adrenergic facilitation by angiotensin: does it serve a physiological function? *Circ Res* 1983;53:121–130.

499. Day MD, Owen DAA. Potentiation by angiotensin of responses to endogenously released noradrenaline in the pithed rat. *Arch Int Pharmacodyn* 1969;179:469–479.

500. Malik KU, Nasjletti A. Facilitation of adrenergic transmission by locally generated angiotensin II in rat mesenteric arteries. *Circ Res* 1976;38:26–30.

501. Zimmerman BG. Actions of angiotensin on adrenergic nerve endings. *Fed Proc* 1978;37:199–202.

502. Zimmerman BG, Kraft E. Blockade by saralasin of adrenergic potentiation induced by renin-angiotensin system. *J Pharmacol Exp Ther* 1979;210:101–105.

503. Ziogas J, Story DF, Rand MJ. Facilitation of noradrenergic transmission by locally generated angiotensin II of guinea-pig isolated atria and in the perfused caudal artery of the rat. *Clin Exp Pharmacol Physiol* 1984;11:413–418.

504. Ziogas J, Story DF, Rand MJ. Effects of locally generated angiotensin II on noradrenergic transmission in guinea-pig isolated atria. *Eur J Pharmacol* 1985;106:11–18.

505. Cline WH. Enhanced in vivo responsiveness of presynaptic angiotensin II receptor-mediated facilitation of vascular adrenergic neurotransmission of spontaneously hypertensive rats. *J Pharmacol Exp Ther* 1985;232:661–669.

506. Hatton R, Clough DP, Adigun SA, Conway J. Functional interaction between angiotensin and sympathetic reflexes in cats. *Clin Sci* 1982; 62:51–56.

507. Boura ALA, Rechtman MP, Walters WA. Attenuation by captopril of pressor responses to sympathetic stimuli: effects of procedures reducing the activity of the renin-angiotensin system. *J Auton Pharmacol* 1982;3:203–211.

508. De Jonge A, Knape JTA, Van Meel JCA, et al. Effect of converting enzyme inhibition and angiotensin receptor blockade on the vasoconstriction mediated by α_1- and α_2-adrenoceptor stimulation in pithed normotensive rats. *Naunyn Schmiedebergs Arch Pharmacol* 1982; 321:309–313.

509. Satoh S, Yoneyama F, Susuki-Kusaba M. Effects of cilazaprilat and enalaprilat on the sympathetically mediated pressor response in pithed rats. *Asia Pacific J Pharmacol* 1988; 3:231–239.

510. Kaufman LJ, Vollmer RR. Endogenous angiotensin II facilitates sympathetically mediated hemodynamic responses in pithed rats. *J Pharmacol Exp Ther* 1985;235:128–134.

511. Majewski H, Hedler L, Schurr C, Starke K. Modulation of noradrenaline release in the pithed rabbit: a role for angiotensin II. *J Cardiovasc Pharmacol* 1984;6:888–896.

512. Gimbrone MA, Alexander RW. Angiotensin II stimulation of prostaglandin production in cultured human vascular endothelium. *Science* 1975;189:219–220.

513. Blumberg AL, Nichikawa K, Denny SE, Marshall GP, Needlemann P. Angiotensin (AI, AII, AIII) receptor characterization. Correlation of prostaglandin release with peptide degradation. *Circ Res* 1977;41:154–158.

514. Lanier SM, Malik KU. Attenuation by prostaglandins of the facilitatory effect of angiotensin II at adrenergic prejunctional sites in the Krebs-perfused rat heart. *Circ Res* 1982;51:594–601.

515. Lanier SM, Malik KU. Facilitation of adrenergic transmission in the canine heart by intra-coronary infusion of angiotensin II: effect of prostaglandin synthesis inhibition. *J Pharmacol Exp Ther* 1983;227:676–682.

516. Lilly LS, Pratt RE, Alexander RW, Gimbrone MA, Dzau VJ. Cultured vascular endothelial cells contain the complete renin-angiotensin system. *Clin Res* 1983;31:A332.

517. Re RN. Cellular biology of the renin-angiotensin systems. *Arch Intern Med* 1984;144:2037–2041.

518. Dzau VJ. Significance of the vascular renin-angiotensin pathway. *Hypertension* 1986;8:553–559.

518a. Rosenthal J, Von Lutterotti N, Thurnreiter M, et al. Suppression of renin-angiotensin system in the heart of spontaneously hypertensive rats. *J Hypertens* 1987;5(Suppl):S23–S31.

519. Swales JD. Arterial wall or plasma renin in hypertension? *Clin Sci* 1979;56:293–298.

520. Fordis CM, Megorden JS, Ropchak TG, Keiser HR. Absence of renin-like activity in rat aorta and microvessels. *Hypertension* 1983;5:635–641.

521. Ganten D, Schelling P, Vecsei P, Ganten U. Isorenin of extrarenal origin: "the tissue angiotensinogenase systems." *Am J Med* 1976;60:760–772.

522. Loudon M, Thurston H, Swales JD. Arterial wall uptake of renal renin and blood pressure control. *Hypertension* 1983;5:629–634.

523. Ganten D, Hayduk K, Brecht HM, Boucher R, Genest J. Evidence of renin release or production in splanchnic territory. *Nature* 1970;226:551–552.

524. Hail V, Gimbrone MA, Peyton MP, Wilcox GM, Pisano JJ. Angiotensin metabolism by cultured human vascular endothelial and smooth muscle cells. *Microvasc Res* 1979;17:314–329.

525. Takada Y, Hiwada K, Unno M, Kokubo T. Immunocytochemical localization of angiotensin converting enzyme at the ultrastructural level in the human lung and kidney. *Biomed Res* 1982;3:169–174.

526. Story DF, Ziogas J. Role of the endothelium on the facilitatory effects of angiotensin I and angiotensin II on noradrenergic transmission in the caudal artery of the rat. *Br J Pharmacol* 1986;87:249–255.

527. Harris RB, Wilson JB. Atrial tissue contains a metallo dipeptidyl carboxyhydrolase not present in ventricular tissue: partial purification and characterization. *Arch Biochem Biophys* 1984;233:667–675.

528. Ziogas J, Story DF. Effect of locally generated angiotensin II on noradrenergic neuroeffector function in the rat isolated caudal artery. *J Hypertens* 1987;5(Suppl 2):S47–S51.

529. Ziogas J, Story DF. Tissue and species variability in the involvement of angiotensin II in the isoprenaline-induced enhancement of transmitter noradrenaline release. *Proc Tenth Int Congr Pharmacol* 1987;P1395.

530. Böke T, Malik KU. Enhancement by locally generated angiotensin II of release of the adrenergic transmitter in the isolated rat kidney. *J Pharmacol Exp Ther* 1983;226:900–907.

531. Boucher R, Asselin J, Genest J. A new enzyme leading to the direct formation of angiotensin II. *Circ Res* 1974;34(Suppl):203–209.

532. Hackenthal E, Hackenthal R, Hilgenfeldt U. Isorenin pseudorenin, cathepsin D and renin: a comparative enzymatic study of angiotensin-forming enzymes. *Biochim Biophys Acta* 1978; 552:574–588.

533. Majewski H. Angiotensin II and noradrenergic transmission in the pithed rat. *J Cardiovasc Pharmacol* 1989;14:622–630.

534. Keeton TK, Campbell WB. The pharmacologic alteration of renin release. *Pharmacol Rev* 1980; 31:81–227.

535. Kawasaki H, Cline WH, Su C. Involvement of the vascular renin-angiotensin system in beta adrenergic receptor-mediated facilitation of vascular neurotransmission in spontaneously hypertensive rats. *J Pharmacol Exp Ther* 1984;231:23–32.

536. Nakamara M, Jackson EK, Inagami T. β-Adrenoceptor-mediated release of angiotensin II from mesenteric arteries. *Am J Physiol* 1986; 250:H144–H148.

537. Göthert M, Kollecker P. Subendothelial β_2-adrenoceptors in the rat vena cava: facilitation of noradrenaline release via local stimulation of angiotensin II synthesis. *Naunyn Schmiedebergs Arch Pharmacol* 1986;334:156–165.

538. Rump LC, Majewski H. Beta adrenoceptor facilitation of norepinephrine release is not dependent on local angiotensin II formation in the rat isolated kidney. *J Pharmacol Exp Ther* 1987;243:1107–1112.

539. Li CG, Majewski H, Rand MJ. Facilitation of noradrenaline release from sympathetic nerves in rat anococcygeus muscle by activation of prejunctional β-adrenoceptors and angiotensin II receptors. *Br J Pharmacol* 1988;95:385–392.

540. Rajanayagam MAS, Musgrave IF, Rand MJ, Majewski H. Facilitation of noradrenaline release by isoprenaline is not mediated by angiotensin II in mouse atria and rat tail artery. *Arch Int Pharmacodyn* 1989;299:185–189.

541. Göthert M. $ACTH_{1-24}$ increases stimulation-evoked noradrenaline release from sympathetic nerves by acting on presynaptic ACTH receptors. *Eur J Pharmacol* 1981;76:285–296.

542. Göthert M. Facilitatory effects of adrenocorticotropic hormone and related peptides on Ca^{2+}-dependent noradrenaline release from sympathetic nerves. *Neuroscience* 1984;11:1001–1009.

543. Costa M, Majewski H. Facilitation of noradrenaline release from sympathetic nerves through activation of ACTH receptors, β-adrenoceptors and angiotensin II receptors. *Br J Pharmacol* 1988;95:993–1001.

544. Szabo B, Hedler L, Schurr C, Starke K. ACTH increases noradrenaline release in pithed rabbits with electrically stimulated sympathetic outflow. *Eur J Pharmacol* 1987;136:391–399.

545. Szabo B, Hedler L, Schurr C, Starke K. ACTH increases noradrenaline release in the rabbit heart. *Naunyn Schmiedebergs Arch Pharmacol* 1988;338:368–372.

546. Smyth DG. β-Endorphin and related peptides in pituitary, brain, pancreas and antrum. *Br Med Bull* 1983;39:25–30.

547. Lang RE, Buickner UB, Kempel B, et al. Opioid peptides and blood pressure regulation. *Clin Exp Hypertens* 1982;A4:249–269.

548. Elam R, Bergmann F, Feuerstein G. Simultaneous changes of catecholamines and leu-enkephalin-like immuno-reactivity in plasma and cerebrospinal fluid of cats undergoing acute hemorrhage. *Brain Res* 1984;303:313–317.

549. Szabó B, Ramme D, Starke K. Opioid receptors in the sympathetic supply to heart and blood vessels. In: Stumpe KO, Kraft K, Faden AL, eds. *Opioid peptides and blood pressure control*. Berlin: Springer, 1988;129–140.

550. Illes P, Bucher B. Opioid receptor types at noradrenergic neurons and their role in blood pressure regulation. In: Stumpe KO, Kraft K, Faden AL, eds. *Opioid peptides and blood pressure control*. Berlin: Springer, 1988;190–205.

551. Henderson G, Hughes J, Kosterlitz HW. Modification of catecholamine release by narcotic analgesics and opioid peptides. In: Paton DM, ed. *The release of catecholamines from adrenergic neurons*. Oxford: Pergamon, 1979;217–228.

552. Ramme D, Illes P, Späth L, Starke K. Blockade of α_2-adrenoceptors permits the operation of

otherwise silent opioid κ-receptors at the sympathetic axons of rabbit jejunal arteries. *Naunyn Schmiedebergs Arch Pharmacol* 1986; 334:48–55.

553. Wong-Dusting H, Rand MJ. Effect of [D-Ala^2,Met^5]enkephalinamide and [D-Ala^2,D-Leu^5] eukephalin on cholinergic and noradrenergic neurotransmission in isolated atria. *Eur J Pharmacol* 1985;111:65–72.

554. Thornhill JA, Ewen M, Wilfong AA, Gregor L, Saunders WS. Pressor effects of systemic administration of methionine and leucine enkephalin in the conscious rat. *Can J Physiol Pharmacol* 1987;64:1353–1360.

555. Ensinger H, Hedler L, Schurr C, Starke K. Ethylketacyclazocine decreases noradrenaline release and blood pressure in the rabbit at a peripheral opioid receptor. *Naunyn Schmiedebergs Arch Pharmacol* 1984;328:20–23.

556. Ensinger H, Hedler L, Szabo B, Starke K. Bremazocine causes sympatho-inhibition and hypotension in rabbits by activating peripheral K-receptors. *J Cardiovasc Pharmacol* 1986; 8:470–475.

557. Szabo B, Hedler L, Ensinger H, Starke K. Opioid peptides decrease noradrenaline release and blood pressure in the rabbit at peripheral receptors. *Naunyn Schmiedebergs Arch Pharmacol* 1986;332:50–56.

558. Wong-Dusting H, Rand MJ. Inhibition of sympathetic neurotransmission by the opioid δ-receptor agonist DAMA in the pithed rat. *Clin Exp Pharmacol Physiol* (submitted).

559. Faden AI, Holaday JW. Opiate antagonists: a role in the treatment of hypovolemic shock. *Science* 1979;205:317–318.

560. Peters WP, Friedman PA, Johnson MW, Mitch WE. Pressor effect of naloxone in septic shock. *Lancet* 1981;1:529–532.

561. Holaday JW. Cardiovascular effects of endogenous opiate system. *Annu Rev Pharmacol Toxicol* 1983;23:541–594.

562. Schadt JC, Gaddis RR. Endogenous opiate peptides may limit norepinephrine release during hemorrhage. *J Pharmacol Exp Ther* 1985; 232:656–660.

563. Lees GM, Kosterlitz HW, Waterfield AA. Characteristics of morphine-sensitive release of neurotransmitter substances. In: Kosterlitz HW, Collier HOJ, Villareal JE, eds. *Agonist and antagonist actions of narcotic analgesic drugs.* London: Macmillan, 1972;142–152.

564. Wong-Dusting H, Rand MJ. Effects of the opioid peptides [Met^5]enkephalin-Arg^6-Phe^7 and [Met^5]enkephalin-Arg^6-Gly^7-Leu^8 on cholinergic neurotransmission in the rabbit isolated atria. *Clin Exp Pharmacol Physiol* 1987;14:725–730.

565. Weitzell R, Illes P, Starke K. Inhibition via opioid μ- and δ-receptors of vagal transmission in rabbit isolated heart. *Naunyn Schmiedebergs Arch Pharmacol* 1984;328:186–190.

566. Owen DAA. Histamine receptors in the cardiovascular system. *Gen Pharmacol* 1977;8:141–156.

567. Levi R, Owen DAA, Trzeciakowski J. Actions of histamine on the heart and vasculature. In: Ganelin R, Parsons M, eds. *Pharmacology of histamine receptors.* London: Wright, 1982; 236–297.

568. Wolff AW, Levi R. Histamine and cardiac arrhythmias. *Circ Res* 1986;58:1–16.

569. Giotti A, Guidotti A, Mannaioni PF, Zilleti L. The influence of adrenotropic drugs and noradrenaline on the histamine release in cardiac anaphylaxis in vitro. *J Physiol* 1966;184:924–941.

570. Howland RD, Spector D. Disposition of histamine in mammalian blood vessels. *J Pharmacol Exp Ther* 1972;182:239–245.

571. Ryan MJ, Brody MJ. Distribution of histamine in the canine autonomic system. *J Pharmacol Exp Ther* 1970;174:123–132.

572. Ryan MJ, Brody MJ. Neurogenic and vascular stores of histamine in the dog. *J Pharmacol Exp Ther* 1972;181:83–91.

573. Tuttle RS, McClearly M. Effects of sympathetic nerve activity on labelling and release of histamine in the cat. *Am J Physiol* 1970; 218:143–148.

574. Lioy F, White KP. ^{14}C-histamine release during vasodilatation induced by lumbar ventral root stimulation. *Pflugers Arch* 1973;342:319–324.

575. Beck L, Schon D, Pollard AA, Wyse DG. Increased concentration of radiolabelled histamine in the venous effluent of dog gracilis muscle during reflex vasodilation. *Res Commun Chem Pathol Pharmacol* 1971;12:415–428.

576. Heitz DC, Brody MJ. Possible mechanism of histamine release during active vasodilatation. *Am J Physiol* 1975;225:1351–1357.

577. McGrath MA, Shepherd JT. Inhibition of adrenergic neurotransmission in canine vascular smooth muscle by histamine. Mediation by H$_2$-receptors. *Circ Res* 1976;39:566–573.

578. Powell JR. Effects of histamine in vascular sympathetic neuroeffector transmission. *J Pharmacol Exp Ther* 1979;208:360–365.

579. Lokhandwala MF. Inhibition of sympathetic nervous system by histamine: studies with H$_1$ and H$_2$-receptor antagonists. *J Pharmacol Exp Ther* 1978;206:115–122.

580. Rand MJ, Story DF, Wong-Dusting HK. Effects of impromidine, a specific H$_2$-receptor agonist, and 2-(2-pyridyl)-ethylamine, an H$_1$-receptor agonist, on stimulation-induced release of [^{3}H]-noradrenaline in guinea-pig isolated atria. *Br J Pharmacol* 1982;76:305–311.

581. Wong-Dusting H, Story DF, Rand MJ. Are the prejunctional histamine receptors on sympathetic nerve terminals in guinea-pig isolated atria activated during anaphylaxis in vitro? *J Pharm Pharmacol* 1982;34:653–657.

582. Staszewska-Barczak J, Vane JR. The release of catecholamines from adrenal medulla by peptides. *Br J Pharmacol* 1967;30:655–667.

583. Starke K, Peskar BA, Schumacher KA, Taube HD. Bradykinin and postganglionic sympa-

thetic transmission. *Naunyn Schmiedebergs Arch Pharmacol* 1977;299:23–32.

584. Llona I, Vavrek R, Stewart J, Huidobro-Toro JP. Identification of pre- and postsynaptic bradykinin receptor sites in the vas deferens: evidence for different structural prerequisites. *J Pharmacol Exp Ther* 1987;241:608–614.

585. Berne RM, Rubio R, Dobson JG, Curnish RR. Adenosine and adenine nucleotides as possible mediators of cardiac and skeletal muscle blood flow regulation. *Circ Res* 1971;28/29(Suppl 1):115–119.

586. Eklund S, Fahrenkrug J, Jodal M, et al. Vasoactive intestinal polypeptide, 5-hydroxytryptamine and reflex hyperaemia in the small intestine of the cat. *J Physiol* 1980;302:549–557.

586a. Cohen RA, Weisbrod RM. Can vasoactive substances released during intravascular thrombosis influence coronary adrenergic nerves? *Blood Vessels* 1986;23:62.

586b. Cohen RA. Adenine nucleotides and 5-hydroxytryptamine released by aggregating platelets inhibit adrenergic neurotransmission in canine coronary artery. *J Clin Invest* 1986;77:369–375.

587. Makita Y. Effects of prostaglandin I_2 and carbocyclic thromboxane A_2 on smooth muscle cells and neuromuscular transmission in the guinea-pig mesenteric artery. *Br J Pharmacol* 1983;78:517–527.

588. Li DMF, De Garis RM, Dusting GJ. Inhibition of vasoconstrictor mechanisms by dazoxiben in the rat mesenteric vasculature. *Eur J Pharmacol* 1985;110:351–356.

589. Timini KSA, Bedwani JR, Stanton AWB. Effects of prostaglandin E_2 and a prostaglandin endoperoxide analogue on neuroeffector transmission in the rat anococcygeus muscle. *Br J Pharmacol* 1978;63:167–176.

590. Trachte GJ. Thromboxane agonist (U46619) potentiates norepinephrine efflux from adrenergic nerves. *J Pharmacol Exp Ther* 1986;237:473–477.

591. Furchgott RF, Zawadzki JV. The obligatory role of endothelial cells in the relaxation of arterial smooth muscle by acetylcholine. *Nature* 1980;288:373–376.

592. Furchgott RF. The requirement for endothelial cells in the relaxation of arteries by acetylcholine and some other vasodilators. *Trends Pharmacol Sci* 1981;2:173–176.

593. Vanhoutte PM, Rubanyi GM, Miller VM, Houston DS. Modulation of vascular smooth muscle contraction by the endothelium. *Annu Rev Physiol* 1986;48:307–320.

594. Palmer RMJ, Ferrige AG, Moncada S. Nitric oxide release accounts for the biological activity of endothelium-derived relaxing factor. *Nature* 1987;327:524–526.

595. Parnavelas JG, Kelly W, Burnstock G. Ultrastructural localization of choline acetyltransferase in vascular endothelial cells in rat brain. *Nature* 1985;316:408–409.

596. Harder DR. Pressure-induced myogenic activation of cat cerebral arteries is dependent on intact endothelium. *Circ Res* 1987;60:102–107.

597. Yanagisawa M, Kurihara H, Kimura S, et al. A novel potent vasoconstrictor peptide produced by vascular endothelial cells. *Nature* 1988;332:411–415.

598. Armstrong JM, Thirsk G, Salmon JA. Effects of prostacyclin (PGI_2), 9-oxo-$PGF_{1\alpha}$ and PGE_2 on sympathetic nerve function in mesenteric arteries and veins of the rabbit in vitro. *Hypertension* 1979;1:309–315.

599. Lippton H, Chapnick BM, Hyman A, Kadowitz PJ. Inhibition of vasoconstrictor responses by prostacyclin (PGI_2) in the feline vascular bed. *Arch Int Pharmacodyn Ther* 1979;241:214–223.

600. Tomobe Y, Miyauchi T, Saito A, et al. Effects of endothelin on the renal artery from spontaneously hypertensive and Wistar Kyoto rats. *Eur J Pharmacol* 1988;152:373–374.

601. Wiklund NP, Öhlen A, Cederqvist B. Inhibition of adrenergic neuroeffector transmission by endothelin in the guinea-pig femoral artery. *Acta Physiol Scand* 1988;134:311–312.

602. Wong-Dusting H, Reid JJ, Rand MJ. Paradoxical effects of endothelin on cardiovascular neurotransmission. *Clin Exp Pharmacol Physiol* 1989;16:229–233.

602a. Reid JJ, Wong-Dusting HK, Rand MJ. The effect of endothelin on noradrenergic transmission in rat and guinea-pig atria. *Eur J Pharmacol* 1989;168:93–96.

603. Hu JR, von Harsdorf R, Land RE. Endothelin has potent inotropic effects in rat atria. *Eur J Pharmacol* 1988;158:275–278.

604. Antunes E, de Nucci G, Vane JR. Endothelin releases eicosanoids from and is removed by isolated perfused lungs of the guinea-pig. *J Physiol* 1988;407:40P.

Cardiovascular Pharmacology, Third Edition,
edited by Michael Antonaccio.
Raven Press, Ltd., New York © 1990.

Ischemic Heart Disease: Pathophysiology and Pharmacologic Management

Judith K. Mickelson, Paul J. Simpson, and Benedict R. Lucchesi

Department of Pharmacology, The University of Michigan Medical School,
Ann Arbor, Michigan 48109-0626

The spectrum of ischemic heart disease has many presentations, ranging from asymptomatic or "silent" ischemia to sudden death and within this range of presentations are stable exertional angina, variant angina, unstable angina, acute myocardial infarction, and postinfarction angina. Coronary artery disease is the most common single cause of death in the United States today. The annual cost of diagnosing and treating ischemic heart disease is substantial. Most often patients present with some form of chest pain, which may or may not have all the characteristics of typical angina pectoris.

ANGINA PECTORIS

More than 200 years ago, in the first written account of angina pectoris, Heberden (1) described it as a

disorder of the breast marked with strong and peculiar symptoms. . . . Those who are afflicted with it are seized while they are walking (more especially if it be up hill, and soon after eating), with a painful and most disagreeable sensation in the breast, which seems as if it would extinguish life, if it were to increase or to continue; but the moment they stand still, all this uneasiness vanishes. . . . Males are most liable to this

disease, especially such as have passed their fiftieth year. After it has continued a year or more, it will not cease as instantaneously upon standing still, and it will come on not only when persons are walking, but when they are lying down.

By the late 18th century, angina pectoris was thought to indicate cardiac disease, but it was not until 1928 that inadequate myocardial oxygenation was defined as the physiological determinant common to the anginal state, irrespective of the nature of the responsible cardiac disease (2). The coronary circulation is responsible for carrying blood into the myocardium, providing nutrition to cardiac cells, and removing metabolites. The coronary arteries must respond rapidly to meet the demands of the systemic circulation and the myocardium itself. In this section, a review of those factors known to regulate myocardial oxygen supply and demand will be followed by a discussion of the therapeutic options available for the treatment of angina pectoris and ischemic heart disease.

MYOCARDIAL AND CORONARY ANATOMY

Within the myocardium, each muscle fiber originates from the fibrous rings at the base of the heart, those more superficial descend to the apex and form the vortex spirals. These then loop upward as deeper fibers to reinsert into the annulus fibrosis (Fig. 1). There are four major muscle bands that can be dissected free: (a) a superficial sinospiral that originates and inserts at the tricuspid valve ring, (b) the superficial bulbospiral that originates and inserts at the mitral valve ring, (c) deep sinospirals that surround both ventricles, and (d) deep bulbospirals that encircle the left ventricle. Overall the fibers resemble "figure eights" with origins and insertions at the base and a fulcrum at the apex. The ventricle represents a single muscle mass dividing and branching into interconnected fascicles. Approximately 10 times as many fibers are oriented circumferentially as longitudinally, and this ratio increases from apex to base of the left ventricle (3).

The development of coronary arteriography in 1958 (4) and coronary artery bypass surgery in 1968 (5,6) furthered interest in human coronary anatomy greatly. In humans, the two coronary arteries originate from the right and left coronary sinuses, respectively, just above the aortic valve (Fig. 2). The left main coronary artery is relatively and variably short (1.0 mm–3.0 cm), dividing into the left anterior descending and left circumflex arteries. Sometimes there is a third branch at this point, called the ramus intermedius. The anterior descending coronary artery courses anteriorly around the pulmonary artery and lies anteriorly in the interventricular groove, on the interventricular septum, giving off branches that penetrate the septal tissue (septal perforating) or course out over the surface of the left ventricle at acute angles (diagonal branches). This major artery variably wraps around the apex and extends some distance posteriorly along the posterior interventricular groove. The circumflex artery travels posteriorly under the left atrial appendage in the left atrioventricular groove giving off branches that course an-

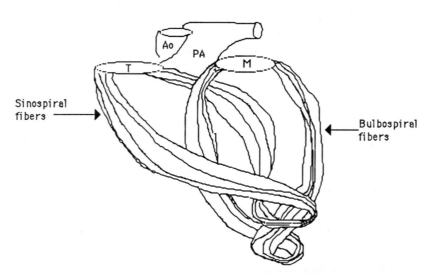

FIG. 1. Myocardial muscle fibers. The superficial muscle fibers originate from the fibrous rings at the base of the heart and descend to the apex to form the vortex spirals. These loop upward and reinsert into the annulus fibrosis. The superficial sinospiral originates and inserts at the tricuspid valve ring (T) and the superficial bulbospiral originates and inserts at the mitral valve ring (M). Ao, aorta; PA, pulmonary artery.

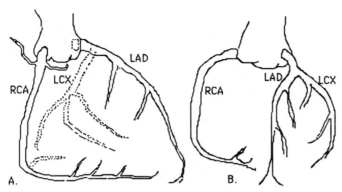

FIG. 2. Anatomy of human epicardial coronary arteries. Two coronary arteries arise from the aorta just above the valve in the right and left coronary sinus, respectively. The left main coronary artery is short and divides into the left anterior descending (LAD) and left circumflex (LCX) arteries. The LAD travels anteriorly in the interventricular groove and the LCX travels posteriorly under the left atrial appendage in the left atrioventricular groove. The right coronary artery (RCA) courses in the right atrioventricular sulcus toward the crux of the heart in the posterior interventricular groove. The arteries are shown in the right anterior oblique (**A**) and left anterior oblique with cranial angulation (**B**) views.

teriorly (obtuse marginals) on the surface of the left ventricle. In approximately 10% of cases the artery reaches the posterior interventricular groove and courses anteriorly in it as the posterior descending branch. In slightly less than half of human hearts, the sinus node branch arises from the circumflex. From the posterior descending branch arises the artery to the atrioventricular node, a small artery that travels superiorly to reach the node. The right coronary artery travels in the right atrioventricular sulcus toward the posterior interventricular groove to the crux of the heart where it bifurcates, with one branch turning anteriorly as the posterior descending artery in most cases (90%) and the other emerging to the left of the interventricular groove and running parallel to the obtuse marginal branches as the posterolateral left ventricular branch(es). The most proximal branch of the right coronary is the conus artery that often arises from a separate ostium (50%) and courses around the conus of the right ventricle near the pulmonary valve. The sinus node artery arises from the proximal right coronary artery a little more than half the

time. Other branches of the right coronary artery are small and supply the right ventricular free wall (acute marginals) and right atria.

The epicardial coronary arteries branch from the right and left coronary artery over the surface of the heart, dividing as described above. When they reach the 1- to 3-mm size, they begin to send tributaries into the myocardium, which quickly subdivide in two manners to supply nutrients. One group branches quickly into a very fine network that distributes itself in the epicardial 75% to 80% of the myocardium. The other group branches less frequently reaching the subendocardium where they subdivide, forming large looping arcades that anastomose freely (7).

The coronary arteries supply the specialized conducting cells of the myocardium. There are four major components: sinoatrial node, internodal pathways in the atria, atrioventricular node, and the His-Purkinje system (Fig. 3). The initiation of electrical activity in the heart lies in the sinoatrial node, a group of fine muscle fibers lying near the junction of the superior vena cava with the right atrium (8). Activity is

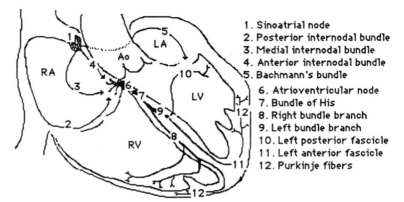

1. Sinoatrial node
2. Posterior internodal bundle
3. Medial internodal bundle
4. Anterior internodal bundle
5. Bachmann's bundle

6. Atrioventricular node
7. Bundle of His
8. Right bundle branch
9. Left bundle branch
10. Left posterior fascicle
11. Left anterior fascicle
12. Purkinje fibers

FIG. 3. Diagram of the system in the heart for generating and conducting impulses. The impulse normally originates in the sinoatrial node (1) and travels along intraatrial pathways (2–5) to the atrioventricular node (6). The impulse is slowed in this node and the bundle of His (7) then rapidly disperses to the ventricles (8–12). RA, right atrium; LA, left atrium; Ao, aorta; RV, right ventricle; LV, left ventricle.

spontaneous, and, although other regions of the heart can also act as pacemakers, normally the rate of activity is highest in this region and thus sets the pace. The electrical activity spreads through the atria via internodal pathways that cross into the ventricle at one point, usually the atrioventricular node. The atrioventricular node is composed of specialized cells that conduct the impulse relatively slowly so that atrial contraction precedes ventricular contraction. The conducting fibers from the atrioventricular node are large and form the bundle of His in the interventricular septum, which subsequently divides into the right and left bundle, the left bundle bifurcating immediately into a left anterior and left posterior fascicle. The terminal portions of these bundles are composed of Purkinje fibers arborizing throughout both ventricles and ensuring rapid and synchronous conduction and subsequent contraction.

The heart is supplied with afferent pain fibers and efferent fibers to the myocytes and coronary vessels. The vagus nerve, which when stimulated is cardio-inhibitory, slows the heart beat, and causes a negative inotropic effect on both the atria and ven-

tricles. The dorsal nucleus of the vagus is located in the brainstem medullary center, in the floor of the fourth ventricle. The cardiac fibers separate from the trunk of the vagus in the neck between the origins of the superior and inferior laryngeal branches. These fibers enter the deep and superficial cardiac plexuses, traveling to the atrial muscle with postganglionic fibers innervating the conduction tissue (Fig. 4). Some vagal fibers distribute to the ventricular muscle and coronary arteries. The cardioaccelerator and positive inotropic innervation originate from cells in the lateral horns of the upper thoracic segments of the spinal cord fibers (intermediolateral cell column) that leave the cord via the anterior nerve roots and enter the sympathetic chain of ganglia to connect with cells in the inferior, middle, and superior cervical ganglia. The first thoracic and inferior cervical ganglia are often fused to form the stellate ganglion. Stimulation of the left stellate ganglion causes greater increase in inotropy than heart rate, whereas right stellate stimulation causes the opposite effect. The postganglionic fibers from these ganglia form the inferior, middle, and superior car-

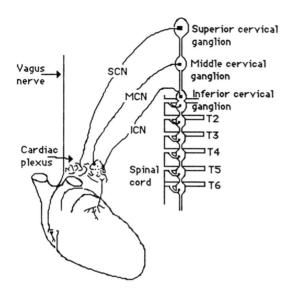

FIG. 4. Cardiac innervation. Cardio-inhibitory input arises from stimulation of the vagus nerve, slowing the heart rate and causing a negative inotropic effect. Cardio-accelerator and positive inotropic input originates in the sympathetic chain of ganglion including the superior, middle, and inferior cervical ganglia and the first six thoracic ganglia (T1–6). SCN, superior cardiac nerve; MCN, middle cardiac nerve; ICN, inferior cardiac nerve.

diac nerves that pass directly to the heart. Those from the right side terminate in the sinoatrial node and atria, whereas those from the left side travel mainly to the atrioventricular node, bundle of His, and ventricle.

MYOCARDIAL METABOLISM

Myocardial energy metabolism can be divided into those events that make energy available for cardiac function and those that relate to energy utilization. Normally the determinants of myocardial oxygen demand are based on oxygen consumption of the heart functioning as an aerobic organ. The substrates and oxygen that are delivered by the coronary circulation pass through the extracellular space and traverse the cell membranes entering the cytosol. There the substrates are modified for entry into mitochondria that produce energy via oxidative phosphorylation. There are many substrates that can be funneled into the mitochondria (Fig. 5). In the heart, oxidation of free fatty acids predominates, providing 60% to 90% of the energy. Free

fatty acid metabolism occurs in cells as acylCoA-fatty acid is processed via the acylCoA-carnitine transferase system. Cytosolic acylCoA-fatty acids may be oxidized in the mitochondria to acetylCoA, the two carbon fragments that can enter the Krebs cycle, and the reduced flavin and nicotinamide dinucleotides are fully oxidized to CO_2 and water with the production of adenosine triphosphate (ATP) by the electron transport chain.

During ischemia, oxidative phosphorylation is reduced and the anaerobic production of ATP proceeds at a slower rate (Fig. 6). Lactate and hydrogen ions increase. High-energy phosphate use exceeds production. Intracellular levels of ATP, adenosine diphosphate (ADP), creatine phosphate (CP), and the adenosine nucleotide pool (ΣAD) decrease. Metabolic products like adenosine monophosphate (AMP), inosine (INO), hypoxanthine (HPX), xanthine (X), and adenosine (ADO) increase. This phase of ischemia may last 15 min. During this time the myocardium is acontractile; however, a sufficient amount of high-energy phosphate is produced to maintain the cells' structural, electrical, and interstitial

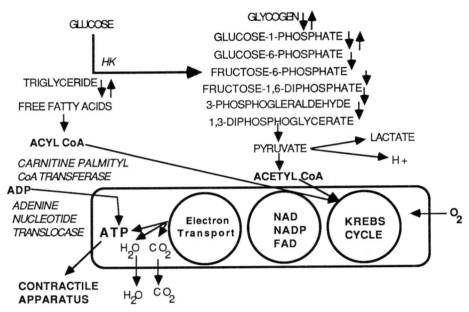

FIG. 5. Energy production in the myocardium. Normally myocardial metabolism is aerobic and the rates of electron transport and oxidative phosphorylation are controlled by available ADP. Oxidation of free fatty acids to two carbon fragments that enter the mitochondria and the Krebs cycle results in reduced flavin and nicotinamide dinucleotides, which are reoxidized via electron transport to yield ATP, water, and carbon dioxide.

integrity. Sometime around 60 min of ischemia, the transformation from reversible to irreversible cell damage occurs (Fig. 7). Anaerobic glycolysis slows and stops; high-energy phosphate stores are exhausted. There are plasmalemmal defects; mitochondria swell and calcium influx forms deposits in the abnormal mitochondria. The increased calcium activates endogenous phospholipases from lysosomes, free radicals appear, and lipid peroxidation occurs.

During later stages of ischemic injury, the membrane defects enlarge, which results in an equilibration between intra- and extracellular fluid components (Fig. 8). There is an efflux of enzymes and cofactors and an even greater influx of calcium from the extracellular fluid (9).

The immediate physiological response to ischemia is akinetic or dyskinetic wall motion in the central ischemic zone. This affects not only contractility or systolic func-

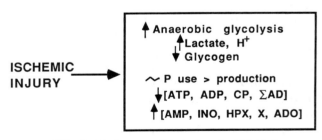

FIG. 6. Early reversible ischemia (15 min).

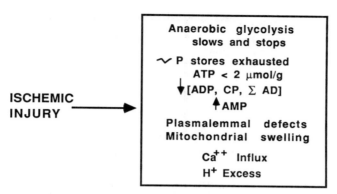

FIG. 7. Early irreversible ischemia (60 min).

tion but also diastolic function because diastolic relaxation is impaired and the left ventricular end-diastolic pressure rises. When end-diastolic pressure rises, the coronary perfusion gradient decreases and myocardial perfusion is jeopardized. The clinical effects of ischemia on myocardial contractility become overt if a significant portion of the left ventricle is involved: signs of heart failure and symptoms like angina or breathlessness may appear.

DETERMINANTS OF MYOCARDIAL OXYGEN CONSUMPTION

The balance between myocardial oxygen supply and demand primarily depends on the factors that control the consumption of oxygen and utilization of energy by the heart (Fig. 9). Oxygen consumption depends on oxygen delivery, which in turn is controlled by arterial oxygen content, oxygen extraction by the myocardium (coronary arteriovenous oxygen difference), and coronary blood flow. Overall myocardial oxygen or energy requirements are determined by the development of wall stress or tension in the heart and the contractility of the myocardium (10). Development of myocardial wall stress is directly related to left ventricular volume (chamber size) and pressure (blood pressure) and is inversely related to wall thickness (11). When the heart dilates, the myocardium hypertrophies, or blood pressure is elevated, total myocardial oxygen requirements increase. Catecholamines or digitalis augment myocardial contractility and increase oxygen consumption; however, β-adrenergic block-

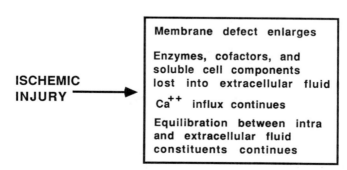

FIG. 8. Late irreversible ischemia (24 hr).

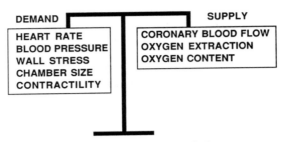

FIG. 9. Myocardial oxygen balance.

ing agents decrease myocardial contractility and decrease oxygen consumption. Because the heart rate determines the fraction of time that myocardial wall stress is exerted, oxygen consumption is directly proportional to the heart rate and can be significantly increased by tachycardia. Estimation of myocardial oxygen consumption (MVO_2) is based on the Fick principle: the product of coronary blood flow per minute and the coronary arteriovenous difference. In normal resting human subjects, values for MVO_2 average approximately 8.5 ml/min of O_2 per 100 g of left ventricle (12).

During periods of increased oxygen demand, three mechanisms are theoretically available for increasing myocardial oxygen delivery: (a) increasing arterial oxygen content, (b) increasing oxygen extraction by the myocardium, and (c) increasing coronary blood flow. The oxygen-carrying capacity of the blood is not a variable that can be increased immediately on demand. In situations in which hypoxemia is present long enough or specialized ventilation equipment is used, then oxygen content of the blood may be increased. The myocardium extracts a high (greater than any other tissue) and relatively fixed amount of oxygen from the blood perfusing the heart and oxygen delivery cannot be increased to any great extent via increased extraction during stress (13). Thus, the factor that usually controls oxygen delivery is coronary blood flow, and blood flow is inversely related to coronary vascular resistance. Compressive forces within the myocardium influence vascular resistance, especially during sys-

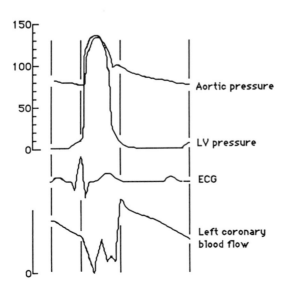

FIG. 10. Cardiac cycle. The aortic and left ventricular pressures are displayed at the top of the figure. The ECG is placed in the center for determining timing intervals. The left coronary blood flow occurs predominantly during early diastole and reaches zero during peak left ventricular systolic contraction.

tole with a significantly greater effect on the subendocardium than on the subepicardium. Intramyocardial pressure affects coronary pressures and the former depends on intraventricular pressure, which is lowest during diastole. Accordingly, a large portion of coronary blood flow to the left ventricle occurs during diastole (Fig. 10). Increases in heart rate diminish the duration of diastole, consequently decreasing subendocardial blood flow.

CORONARY BLOOD FLOW

Coronary blood flow is also influenced by anatomic, hydraulic, mechanical, and metabolic factors. Blood flow in the coronary arteries depends in part on driving pressure and resistance of the coronary vascular bed. Coronary vasomotor tone under normal conditions is relatively high and thus resistance is also relatively high. Changes in tone of the vascular bed are mediated by metabolic, pharmacological, neural, and myogenic factors. During periods of enhanced myocardial oxygen demand, the capacity of the normal coronary circulation to maintain adequate blood flow is great. As demand increases, ADO is released and dilates the arteries appropriately. Adenosine has been identified as a primary mediator of this coronary flow autoregulatory function, although other hormonal factors have been implicated in this control.

Superimposed on some of these autoregulatory factors is the varying tonic influence of the sympathetic nervous system. Both α- and β-adrenergic receptor agonist activity has been demonstrated in the coronary vasculature. Infusion of norepinephrine induces a brief fall, followed by a sustained rise in coronary vascular resistance. The early dilatation can be largely eliminated by β-adrenergic blockade, and the later increase in coronary vascular resistance can be prevented by α-adrenergic receptor blockade. The stimulation of para-

sympathetic receptors leads to reflex vasodilation. Intracoronary Veratrum alkaloids induce reflex bradycardia and hypotension (the Bezold-Jarisch reflex), and the afferent limb of this reflex involves the vagus nerve (14). Despite the demonstration of the activity of β-adrenergic agonists and antagonists *in vitro,* under physiological conditions direct effects of β-adrenergic antagonists on the coronary vascular bed are not prominent.

THE ENDOTHELIUM AND CONTROL OF CORONARY BLOOD FLOW

Endothelium-dependent Relaxation

The endothelium, once considered to be a simple layer of nucleated cells that served as a barrier has now gained significant importance in capillary transport, regulation of plasma lipids, hemostasis, angiogenesis, and the control of vascular tone. The intimate apposition of the endothelium to the vascular smooth muscle permits the endothelium to provide an important influence over the control of smooth muscle tone and the control of vasomotion. Furchgott and Zawadzki (15) observed that acetylcholine-induced relaxation of rabbit isolated aortic strips and a variety of other isolated vessels depended on the presence of an intact endothelium. The removal of the endothelial cells by mechanical or enzymatic procedures abolished the relaxation induced by acetylcholine or other muscarinic agonists and in some instances resulted in contraction of vascular smooth muscle (Fig. 11). It soon became apparent that acetylcholine was acting on endothelial cell muscarinic receptors to induce the formation and release of one or possibly several substances capable of relaxing vascular smooth muscle. Initially it was suggested that the responsible mediator of smooth muscle relaxation was a product derived from the action of lipoxygenase acting on arachidonic acid (15,16), which subsequently enhanced the

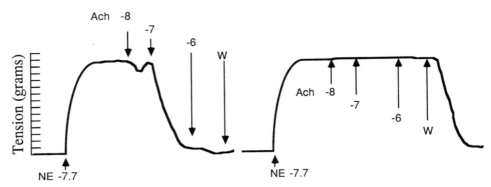

FIG. 11. Schematic representation illustrating the smooth relaxing effect of acetylcholine on a pre-contracted (norepinephrine, NE) vascular strip with an intact endothelium **(left)**. Removal of the endothelium is associated with an inability of acetylcholine to relax the precontracted vessel **(right)**. The observation suggests that the endothelium responds to acetylcholine with the formation of a smooth muscle relaxing mediator referred to as EDRF.

activity of cGMP in vascular smooth muscle. The use of an ingenious "sandwich" preparation consisting of recording the contraction from an endothelium-free strip that was closely approximated to a vascular strip with an intact endothelium allowed the conclusion that a diffusible relaxing substance was released on the addition of acetylcholine (Fig. 12). This substance was referred to as endothelium-dependent relaxing factor or EDRF (16,17).

The release of EDRF is not unique to the action of acetylcholine but can be observed with a wide variety of agonists known to induce vascular smooth muscle relaxation (Table 1). On the other hand, a number of agents known to relax vascular smooth muscle are effective in the absence of an intact endothelium. ADO, AMP, isoproterenol, papaverine, prostacyclin, and, most important, the nitrovasodilators glyceryl trinitrate and nitroprusside do not require the presence of an intact endothelium to initiate vascular smooth muscle relaxation.

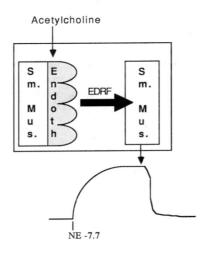

FIG. 12. Schematic representation of an *in vitro* study using the "sandwich" technique in which a vessel stripped with intact endothelium is placed in contact with an endothelium-free vascular strip from which contractile recordings are made. Stimulation of the intact vascular strip with acetylcholine results in the relaxation of the precontracted endothelial-free vascular smooth muscle (Sm. Mus.). The relaxation is due to the formation of EDRF by the endothelium (Endoth.).

TABLE 1. *Agents mediating endotheliuim-dependent relaxation*

Acetylcholine	Histamine
A23187	Serotonin
Arachidonic acid	Thrombin
Arginine-containing peptides	Vasoactive intestinal polypeptide
Bradykinin	Vasopressin

Nitric Oxide and EDRF

Approximately 1 year before the observation of an endothelial-derived relaxing factor, Gruetter et al. (18) reported that nitric oxide (NO) gas added to the buffer medium bathing precontracted arterial vascular strips resulted in a rapid but brief relaxation of the vascular smooth muscle. The response to NO could be prevented by hemoglobin or methylene blue. Furchgott et al. (16) had observed that free radicals, including NO, could activate soluble guanylate cyclase and that nitrovasodilators resulted in smooth muscle relaxation coincident with the generation of NO, as reported by others (19). Based on these observations, Furchgott et al. (15) speculated that the factor responsible for endothelium-dependent relaxation of vascular smooth muscle, EDRF, was acting by increasing the activity of cGMP. Several subsequent studies (20–23) provided confirmation of the hypothesis demonstrating the relationship between EDRF and activation of guanylate cyclase. The measured increase in the cyclic nucleotide occurs in the smooth muscle cell (20,22,24) through the direct activation of soluble guanylate cyclase (25,26). It is postulated that the activation of the cyclic nucleotide results in smooth muscle relaxation as a result of cGMP-dependent phosphorylation and dephosphorylation of the myosin light chain (27).

EDRF is a labile substance with a half-life that varies between 6 and 50 sec. The original concept held that EDRF was derived from the action of lipoxygenase on arachidonic acid. However, this concept has now been determined to be incorrect, as suggested by the observation that methylene blue or hemoglobin inhibited the relaxation of vascular smooth muscle in response to nitrovasodilators and prevented the activation of guanylate cyclase. Both methylene blue and hemoglobin inhibited the endothelium-dependent relaxation of blood vessels and the increase in cGMP. Methylene blue and hemoglobin are believed to inhibit smooth muscle relaxation reacting directly with EDRF (22,28) or more likely due to the competitive binding of NO by the ferrous heme moieties of hemoglobin and soluble guanylate cyclase (28). The limited half-life and the ability of hemoglobin to inactivate EDRF would confine the action of the vasodilator to the smooth muscle in proximity to the site of endothelial-cell production. The hemoglobin bound to haptoglobin in plasma, as well as the heme in the red cells, would prevent vascular activity at a site removed from the point of release. Hemoglobin does not penetrate the intact endothelial cell and thus would not interfere with EDRF acting on the underlying smooth muscle.

Endothelium-dependent relaxation is also prevented by several reducing agents that give rise to the formation of superoxide anion. It is the latter that inactivates EDRF (29). It is worth noting that superoxide dismutase (SOD), through its ability to dismutate the oxygen radical, prolongs the half-life of EDRF that is released from endothelial cells in response to acetylcholine (30). This observation provides additional evidence that the superoxide anion can mediate an inhibition of EDRF and, under some circumstances, superoxide anion may serve as an endothelium-derived contracting factor (31).

Canine coronary arterial rings without endothelium were precontracted by prostaglandin $F_{2\alpha}$ and superfused with perfusate that had passed through an intact segment

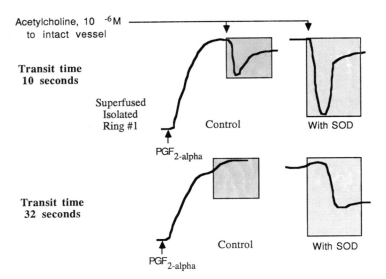

FIG. 13. Schematic representation illustrating the potentiation of EDRF by the antioxidant enzyme SOD. See text for full description. (Adapted from data in ref. 30.)

of canine femoral artery (Fig. 13). Relaxation of the isolated vascular rings becomes less pronounced as the transit time increases from segment 1 to segment 2. Relaxation of the isolated endothelium-free rings was enhanced by the addition of SOD to the perfusate, thereby suggesting that EDRF is subject to degradation by the presence of superoxide anion and that the vasodilator action of EDRF can be preserved by the free radical scavenger (30).

Basal Formation of EDRF and Loss of Endothelial Function

There is a basal rate of formation and release of EDRF from all vascular endothelial cells of all blood vessels studied. There is considerable variability among vessels obtained from different sites with respect to the rate of EDRF formation and the responsiveness of the individual vessels (32). It is of interest to note that EDRF activity is high in coronary arteries (33,34) and is consistent with the observation that its vasodilator effect is greater in vessels in which the activator calcium needed for contrac-

tion stems from extracellular sources as opposed to being mobilized from intracellular storage sites. The basal release of EDRF is related to the rate of blood flow, increasing as a function of flow due to shear stress on the surface of the endothelium (35,36).

The loss of endothelial function and the failure to form EDRF can result in what would ordinarily be a vasodilator response to a response that involves an increase in vascular tone or an unmasking of a constrictor response, which otherwise would have been prevented by the basal release of the endogenous vasodilator. The removal of the endothelium from isolated vessel segments is associated with contraction of vascular smooth muscle, which may be a result of a loss of the basal release of EDRF. The loss of the endothelium and the ability to regulate the movement of plasma or blood into the interstitial space may be an additional mechanism whereby EDRF is inhibited as a result of extravascular accumulation of hemoglobin. Ordinarily, hemes that are restricted to the vascular space would not be expected to inhibit the action of NO, which is released intracellularly—a response that is susceptible to inhibition by methylene blue. The production of EDRF by the endothelium is an energy-dependent process. It is possible, therefore, that ischemia or hypoxia would interrupt the basal production of the vasodilator, leading to alterations in vascular tone (37).

EDRF and Platelet Function

EDRF and the nitrovasodilator, sodium nitroprusside, activate soluble guanylate cyclase in platelets as they are known to do in vascular smooth muscle. As a result of an increase in cGMP activity, platelets are prevented from aggregating (38,39). It is of interest to note that organic nitrovasodilators do not activate guanylate cyclase in platelets. The vasodilator and antiaggregatory actions of EDRF would be additive or synergistic with those related actions of prostacyclin. The action of EDRF depends on activation of guanylate cyclase and an increase in intracellular cGMP, whereas the action of prostacyclin depends on an increase in cAMP via activation of adenylate cyclase. There is evidence that NO (EDRF) synergizes with prostacyclin to inhibit platelet aggregation and that the antiaggregation activity of both compounds when given together is apparent under conditions in which either of them alone is ineffective in preventing platelet aggregation. NO is also active in preventing platelet adhesion to vascular endothelium and may serve an important function in preventing the initiating phases of platelet thrombus formation at the critical interface between the platelet and the endothelial cell.

The formation and release of EDRF serve to amplify and coordinate vascular responses to primary changes in resistance throughout the coronary vascular bed. The flow-related formation of EDRF will influence the reactive hyperemic response of the coronary bed that occurs after a period of flow deprivation. That portion of the increase in coronary blood flow mediated by EDRF may account for the failure to attribute the reactive hyperemic response entirely to the actions of adenosine. This component of the autoregulatory mechanism for the control of coronary blood flow would be impaired under conditions in which the endothelium is removed. Thus, the regional production and release of EDRF may be lacking in the pathophysiological states associated with damage to the endothelium. There is a decrease in EDRF activity in experimental models of atheroma (40,41) and hypertension (42,43), as well as in diabetes (44) and aging (43). Each of these conditions is associated with an increased incidence of vascular thrombosis that may be related in part to the loss of a local physiological mechanism by which platelet adhesion and aggregation are modulated.

The Mechanism of Action of Nitrovasodilators

The organic nitrate and nitrite esters, inorganic nitrite, and nitroso compounds elicit a relaxation of vascular smooth muscle by a mechanism dependent on the conversion of the nitrovasodilator to the active NO, either by spontaneous release in aqueous media or through their ability to react with thiol compounds resulting in unstable S-nitrosothiols (Fig. 14). It was postulated that the lipid soluble vasodilators such as glyceryl trinitrate, isoamyl nitrite, nitroprusside, and other agents in this class had to penetrate the vascular smooth muscle cells and react with free thiols in order to form the unstable S-nitrosothiols. The latter reactant would then bring about an activation of guanylate cyclase, leading to an increase in cGMP that would participate in relaxation of vascular smooth muscle (45). Subsequent studies led to the conclusion that NO is the active species of several vasodilators and that cGMP was the second messenger involved in both the vasodilator response and the inhibition of platelet aggregation (46). A number of studies have

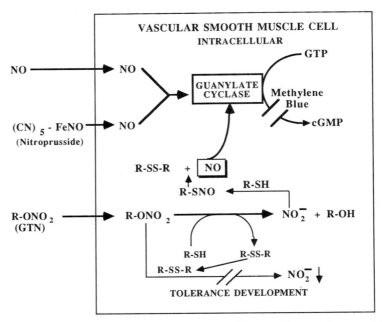

FIG. 14. The proposed mechanism of action of nitrovasodilators. See text for complete description. (Modified from ref. 58.)

now concluded that EDRF and NO are pharmacologically and chemically identical (47–50). The presence of free sulfhydryls or thiols potentiate the nitrite activation of guanylate cyclase as thiols decrease the stability of nitrites and enhance the formation of NO.

The continued administration of glyceryl trinitrate results in a development of tolerance that is not associated with a simultaneous tolerance to nitroprusside. Tolerance to the vasodilator action of glyceryl trinitrate is accompanied by a tolerance to the increase in cGMP. On the other hand, cross-tolerance was not seen in response to nitroprusside, S-nitrosothiols, or NO (51). The tolerance to glyceryl trinitrate could be reversed by exposure of smooth muscle to sulfhydryl-reducing agents. This is in keeping with the concept that organic nitrate esters require the presence of cysteine for the generation of S-nitrosocysteine and NO to bring about relaxation of vascular smooth muscle (51).

A number of possible pathways for the formation of NO have been suggested and include enzymatic and nonenzymatic mechanisms. Recent evidence suggests that L-arginine can serve as the precursor for endothelial cell-derived NO (EDNO). Endothelial cells can synthesize ^{15}NO from labeled L-arginine and the structural analogs of arginine, N^G-monomethyl arginine, as well as L-canavanine, and could prevent endothelial-dependent vascular relaxation (52). High molecular weight polyamino acids, composed of basic amino acids L-arginine, L-lysine, or L-ornithine, cause endothelium-dependent vascular smooth muscle relaxation associated with the formation of EDNO (53). The polyamino acids and A23187 released a similar EDNO from artery and vein that possessed similar half-lives, were inhibited by superoxide anion as well as by oxyhemoglobin, and potentiated by SOD. Tolerance to the smooth muscle relaxant effects and the increase in cGMP were observed to occur if exposure of the vessels to the polyamino acids was prolonged. Cross-tolerance extended to other endothelium-dependent vasodilators but not to that of glyceryl trinitrate or isoproterenol. The poly-amino acid-induced tolerance was accompanied by a reduction in the formation of EDNO. The suggestion was made that the basic polyamino acids serve as partial substrates for the enzyme system that catalyzes the conversion of L-arginine to NO. If arginine is the natural substrate for the enzyme, the enzyme could become desensitized on prolonged contact with the poly-amino acids, thereby giving rise to the phenomenon of tolerance. The basic amino acid may serve as an alternate or partial substrate that would compete with arginine for binding to the enzyme. Recent studies have demonstrated that EDNO is released from vascular segments by endothelium-dependent vasodilators and is associated with endothelium-dependent relaxation of smooth muscle (54). The NO released is present in the effluent of the vessel and is not transformed significantly, thus permitting it to be subject to bioassay as opposed to perfused organs in which NO is converted rapidly to a mixture of NO_2- and other NO-derived, biologically inactive molecules (55).

The receptor for NO is believed to be the heme moiety of soluble guanylate cyclase. The interaction of NO with the cyclase-bound heme forms the nitrosyl-heme adduct, which is the activated form of the enzyme. The interaction of the enzyme with NO and EDNO in preparations of vascular smooth muscle and platelets is identical. The lipophilicity and its small molecular size allow NO to diffuse rapidly from its site of formation in the endothelial cell and to gain access to the vascular smooth muscle or to come in contact with platelets in proximity to the vascular endothelium. EDNO is most likely released luminally as well as abluminally (56). Due to its instability and the fact that it is neutralized by hemoglobin, the most significant action of EDNO would be expressed in cell-cell mediated responses in which the predominant effect would be on the vascular smooth muscle. Based on its biological properties, it seems logical to suggest that NO is the autocoid responsible for the local control of vascular and platelet responses. The biological actions and properties of EDRF and EDNO have been reviewed recently (57,58) and should be consulted by the interested reader.

Endothelium-dependent Contraction

In addition to serving as a barrier to the transport of solutes from the vascular compartment and an "organ" with significant metabolic activity, endothelium possesses autocrine and paracrine functions. The endothelium is situated so as to be able to participate in the moment-to-moment control of vasomotor tone. Most attention has been devoted in the study of the endothelium and its capacity to synthesize vasodilators, such as prostacyclin and EDRF, and its important role in mediating the vascular responses to pharmacological interventions, which are classified as endothelium-dependent vasodilators. Of more recent significance is the recognition that the endothelium may express vasoconstricting substances (59,60) and may facilitate increases in vascular smooth muscle tone in response to anoxia. Subsequent inquiry into this phenomenon led to the description of the synthesis and secretion of a potent polypeptide vasoconstrictor found in endothelial cell culture media (61,62). The polypeptide was noted to produce a calcium-dependent, sustained contraction of vascular smooth muscle. The response could be inhibited by the calcium channel antagonist, verapamil, and was unaffected by other receptor antagonists. The polypeptide vasoconstrictor has been isolated and purified from cultured porcine endothelial cells (63). The peptide contains 21 amino acids (Fig. 15). Molecular weight estimated at 2,492 shows little homology with other known vasoactive peptides and has been termed endothelin-1 (ET-1). The amino-acid sequence of porcine and human

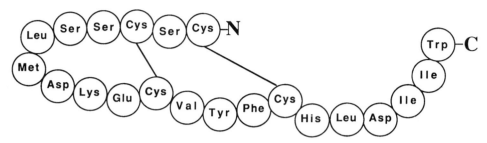

FIG. 15. Structure of ET-1.

ET-1 are identical (64), whereas only small portions of the structure are conserved in ET obtained from the vessels of rats (ET-3) (65). Porcine and human ETs are produced from an approximately 200-residue precursor peptide termed preproendothelin-1 (ppET-1). The mRNA for ppET-1 is expressed in cultured endothelial cells as well as in porcine and aortic intima *in situ*. The expression of ppET-1 mRNA is under the control of humoral and mechanical stimuli, which would suggest that the vasoconstrictor peptide has an important physiological function in modulation of vascular responses.

The pharmacological properties of ET-1 are summarized in Table 2. The pharmacological actions of ET-1 may have a relationship with events that involve coronary spasm or sustained increases in arterial blood pressure in the anesthetized or conscious rat. The rapid response in the blood pressure to the intravenous administration of ET-1 suggests that it is transported across the endothelial cell where it gains access to the smooth muscle of the blood vessel and elicits vasospasm.

In addition to exerting an effect on vascular smooth muscle, ET-1 is an effective positive inotropic agent, as well as being able to influence the rate of depolarization in the sinoatrial node. The major site of action of the peptide, however, is on the vascular bed with the pulmonary and renal arteries being the most responsive. The vasoconstriction is antagonized in a competitive manner by calcium channel antag-

onists. It is postulated that ET-1 acts via the L-type calcium channel in porcine coronary artery, thereby inducing a positive inward movement of calcium ion leading to smooth muscle contraction. The ET-1 receptor is believed to be separate from the calcium channel because the binding sites of ET-1 and nicardipine to porcine endothelium were independent and both have been separated chemically in myocardial tissue (66). ET-1-induced contraction of vascular smooth muscle is associated with an immediate, but brief, increase in intracellular free calcium ion concentration that is followed by a slow decrease to a new sustained concentration. The immediate increase in free calcium occurs even in the absence of extracellular calcium, whereas the sustained increase depends on the inward movement of the ion from the extracellular environment. The sustained in-

TABLE 2. *Pharmacological properties of ET-1*

Slow onset of action in contracting coronary artery smooth muscle
Sustained contracture of isolated coronary artery vessels
More potent than angiotensin: EC_{50} 4.0×10^{-10} M
Action dependent on extracellular calcium ion
Antagonized competitively by calcium channel antagonists
Intravenous administration causes sustained increase in blood pressure
Exhibits a positive inotropic action
Exhibits a positive chronotropic action
Smooth muscle contraction induced by ET-1 is potentiated by hemoglobin
ET-1 acts on receptors or channels that differ from the dihydropyridine-sensitive channels

crease in free calcium ion in response to ET-1 is prevented by calcium channel antagonists, such as nicardipine, thereby suggesting that the secondary increase in free calcium ion is derived from an influx of the ion, whereas the initial and rapid increase is from an intracellular storage site.

ADO AND THE CONTROL OF CORONARY ARTERY BLOOD FLOW

Autoregulatory mechanisms tend to maintain myocardial perfusion to provide the tissue with adequate oxygenation regardless of the moment-to-moment changes in arterial perfusion pressure. Thus, autoregulation of the coronary vascular bed is influenced by myocardial oxygen consumption. A number of mechanisms have been suggested as participating in autoregulation of the coronary vascular bed and include tissue pressure, as well as myogenic and metabolic factors. The effects of ADO on the coronary vasculature have been appreciated for many years (67), and it is considered one of the principal factors that participate in autoregulation in the coronary vascular bed.

It is well established that changes in regional myocardial metabolism influence autoregulation in the coronary vascular bed. A number of potential mediators capable of altering vascular smooth muscle tone have been studied and include oxygen, carbon dioxide, potassium ion, and degradation products derived from increased regional metabolic activity within heart muscle. In the latter category, ADO has received the greatest attention.

Drury and Szent-Gyorgyi (68) first demonstrated the vasoactivity of ADO in the coronary vascular bed. Subsequently, the nucleoside was crystallized from extracts of cardiac muscle, and it was suggested that ADO is the physiological regulator of the coronary circulation (69). During periods of increased metabolic demand or decreases in regional myocardial blood flow, the deg-

radation of ATP exceeds that of synthesis, thereby resulting in cellular loss of purine bases. The latter, which include HPX, INO, and ADO, accumulate in the interstitial fluid and can also be detected in the coronary sinus blood. ADO is known to exert a marked relaxant effect on coronary artery smooth muscle (70,71). The vasodilator action of ADO, when given exogenously, has recently been suggested as being mediated via an endothelium-dependent mechanism (72)—a view that is not in keeping with the observation that vessels deprived of endothelium still relax in response to the nucleoside. Furthermore, ADO released from the cardiac myocyte into the interstitial fluid would approach the vascular smooth muscle from the abluminal side and not come into contact with the vascular endothelium. It is also important to recognize that the vascular endothelium rapidly converts ADO to HPX and INO. A number of excellent reviews provide a summary of the potential role of ADO in the control of the coronary vascular bed (73–75).

ADO is believed to act on the surface of vascular smooth muscle cells via a specific receptor(s) that ultimately leads to an inhibition of Ca^{2+} entry into the cell, thereby resulting in relaxation of vascular smooth muscle and vasodilation (67). Although the nature of the ADO receptor on the coronary vascular smooth muscle has not been established, it is suggested that it is an A_2 receptor. This conclusion is based on the rank order of potency of ADO analogs that reduce coronary vessel smooth muscle tone (76). The rank order of potency of the ADO analogs in relaxing the coronary vascular smooth muscle supports the presence of A_2 receptors as being the predominant type. These studies did not attempt to differentiate between A_2 receptors on the endothelial cell as opposed to those on the vascular smooth muscle. The subclassification of ADO receptors is based on the efficacy of a variety of ADO receptor agonists such as (R)-phenylisopropyladenosine, cyclohexyladenosine, and cyclopentyladenosine, which have a high affinity for A_1 ADO receptors as compared with the 5'-N-ethylcarboxamidoadenosine or 5'-N-cyclopropylcarboxamido-adenosine, which possess a high affinity for A_2 ADO receptors. The A_1 receptors are predominantly in cardiac muscle, whereas the A_2 receptors are in the vascular smooth muscle. The evidence to date suggests that exogenously administered ADO acts via the endothelial cell where it activates A_2 receptors, which in turn are coupled to the vascular smooth muscle and induce relaxation by a yet-to-be described mechanism. On the other hand, the endogenous release of ADO from the cardiac myocyte is more likely to act directly on the A_1 receptor of vascular smooth muscle, possibly leading to an increase in the intracellular concentration of cGMP (77). However, the true mechanism by which ADO elicits relaxation of coronary vascular smooth muscle is not known for certain, although it has been demonstrated that ADO interferes with calcium ion uptake in smooth muscle, which is depolarized by high concentrations of potassium (78).

It is important to note that the vasodilatory effects of exogenously administered ADO may be antagonized competitively by the previous administration of alkylxanthines such as theophylline. On the other hand, dipyridamole, which is capable of preventing the uptake of ADO into cells and thus its degradation, will potentiate the vasodilator action of the nucleoside. Despite the ability of a number of pharmacological interventions to modify the effects of exogenously administered ADO, the same ADO receptor antagonists or uptake blockers fail to influence the actions of endogenously released ADO. The differential action of the ADO antagonists and uptake blockers may be due to the fact that exogenously administered agents are exerting their respective effects via the luminal side of the vessel, whereas endogenously released ADO is approaching the vascular smooth muscle from the interstitial space.

Although ADO is considered as being a major factor in the control of the coronary vascular resistance, it is not the only meta-bolic factor capable of influencing the state of the vascular smooth muscle. Prostaglandins, kinins, potassium, and other cellular metabolites are able to influence smooth muscle tone in the coronary vascular bed.

CORONARY ATHEROSCLEROSIS

The development of atherosclerosis begins in the second decade of life, much sooner than any clinical suspicion exists regarding coronary artery disease. These lesions begin as fatty streaks, lipid accumulations along collagen and elastin fibers, or contained as droplets in lipid-laden foam cells within the intima (Fig. 16). The atherosclerotic lesion appears to affect the intima and smooth muscle cells begin to proliferate covered by a layer(s) of endothelial cells and thickened intima. As the atherosclerotic plaques develop, they accumulate cellular debris and cholesterol crystals, and calcification occurs. The plaques are eccentric and may limit coronary blood flow as they encroach on the luminal dimensions (stenosis) and may become a nidus for thrombosis (Fig. 17A). The plaque may fissure or rupture with exposure of subendothelial thrombogenic materials or internal hemorrhage may occur with expansion to occlude the lumen acutely (Fig. 17B and C).

Normal epicardial coronary arteries dilate and constrict in response to appropriate stimuli; however, atheromatous lesions in diseased vessels cause a hemodynamic stenosis and modify the ability of these arteries to dilate appropriately. The physiological consequences of atherosclerotic coronary artery disease on myocardial perfusion and subsequently on myocardial function are multiple and at present only partially defined (79). Coronary artery stenoses represent a fixed resistance interposed between the aorta and the variable resistance arterioles. This structural change functionally converts the coronary circulation from the normal pressure-independent system into a potentially compromised pressure-

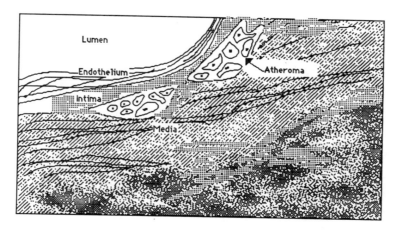

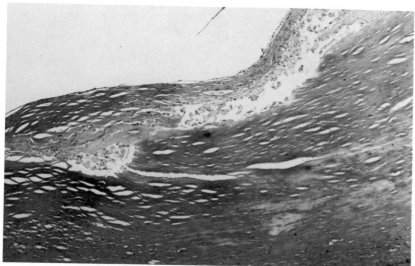

FIG. 16. Early coronary atherosclerosis. This segment of right coronary artery was obtained from a patient dying within 24 hr of an acute myocardial infarction. In this area there was no arterial narrowing but early atheroma appear as foam cells in the intima, covered by a thickened intimal layer and normal endothelium. There is no disruption of the endothelium in this segment.

dependent system. One of the mechanical factors determining coronary blood flow is the pressure gradient that forces blood into the myocardium during diastole. This pressure gradient is related to the difference between diastolic aortic pressure and the filling pressure in the left ventricle. In the normal heart, a coronary perfusion pressure of ≥60 mm Hg is required to maintain adequate flow to meet the oxygen demands of the myocardium. In contrast to normal vessels where perfusion pressure is not as critical, aortic diastolic pressure in the patient with atherosclerotic coronary disease needs to be sufficiently high to maintain an adequate perfusion pressure with elevated left ventricular filling pressures to force blood through the stenotic segments. Thus, in many patients with coronary disease, myocardial blood flow is extremely sensitive to perfusion pressure and hypotension is poorly tolerated. In some patients, ade-

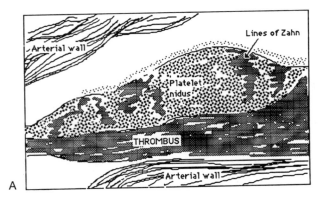

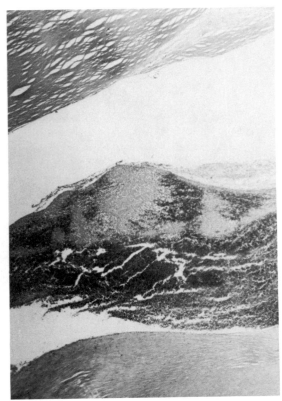

FIG. 17. Coronary thrombus. This segment of the right coronary artery was obtained from the same patient described in Fig. 16. A nonocclusive thrombus is present within the lumen (**A**). The thrombus contains a platelet-rich nidus and red blood cells; lines of Zahn are present in the thrombus placing its formation as an antemortum event. Higher magnifications show an area of thrombus that contains atheromatous plaque. Disruption of the plaque either occurred spontaneously or at the time of PCTA performed as a salvage procedure when tissue plasminogen activator failed to induce thrombolysis (**B,C**).

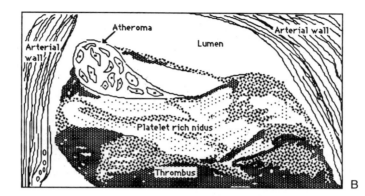

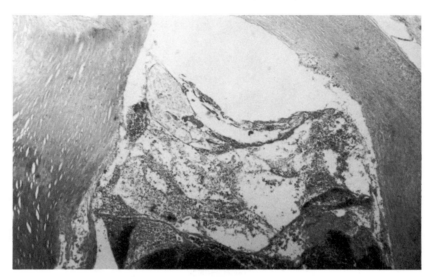

FIG. 17. *Continued.*

quate collateral blood supply has developed in response to chronic ischemia and extremes in blood pressure may be tolerated without symptoms (80).

In coronary artery disease, collateral vessel formation is stimulated and vascular supplies to anatomically distinct areas of the myocardium become linked. Under certain circumstances, the hydrodynamic potential for "steal syndromes" exists, in which blood flow to one region of the myocardium is supplied at the expense of another region (81). Thus, blood flow to a specific area of myocardium may decrease at a time that total coronary flow has increased, causing changes in regional perfusion that are potentially significant. The segmental nature of atherosclerotic coronary disease changes the heart from a homogeneous muscle mass that has adequate and uniform vascular reserve to one in which vascular reserve varies widely. Regions of myocardium may exhibit differential susceptibility to stress and nonuniform perfusion may result in regional dysfunction as well as angina during stress (82). Such dysfunction may, in turn, place excessive mechanical demands on the remaining normal myocardium, which may then intensify the ischemic state. Factors that increase resting myocardial oxygen demand and decrease tolerance to stress in patients with athero-

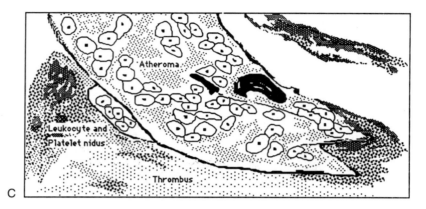

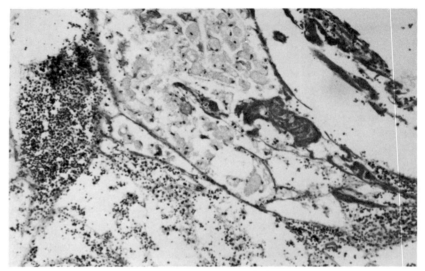

FIG. 17. *Continued.*

sclerotic coronary disease, but which are potentially remediable, include hypertension, tachycardia, tachyarrhythmias, sympathomimetic drugs, hyperthyroidism, left ventricular outflow obstruction, and congestive heart failure. A fixed reduction in the capacity of the blood to deliver oxygen must also be considered (anemia, chronic pulmonary disease, carboxyhemoglobin, hemoglobinopathy).

Fixed atherosclerotic coronary artery lesions limit blood flow to the myocardium. In stable exertional angina, exercise or emotion will predictably provoke an imbal-

ance between myocardial oxygen supply and demand, causing chest pain. However, sometimes an excessive increase in vasomotor tone or coronary artery spasm is thought to occur in the presence of fixed atherosclerotic lesions, causing limited blood flow and angina at rest. This mixture of disease processes has received considerable attention, and it probably accounts for some of the chest pain episodes experienced by patients with stable exertional angina. Thus, in the setting of stable exertional angina, medical therapy must be directed at both decreasing myocardial oxygen demand and increasing coronary blood flow by preventing excessive increases in vasomotor tone.

Medical therapy continues to play an important role in the treatment of angina pectoris and ischemic heart disease, despite the successes of coronary artery bypass graft surgery and percutaneous transluminal coronary angioplasty. As always, some patients will refuse invasive procedures, whereas others are not anatomically suitable for them. Furthermore, coronary atherosclerosis is an unrelenting disease process that occurs in the vein grafts, progresses in the native vessels distal to the graft insertions over time, or recurs at the site of previously successful angioplasty. Thus, patients may ultimately fail invasive mechanical therapy and require medical therapy.

CLINICAL DETECTION OF MYOCARDIAL ISCHEMIA: EXERCISE STRESS TESTING

Myocardial ischemia has traditionally been appreciated as a dynamic imbalance of oxygen demand and supply. Electrocardiographic monitoring during provocative maneuvers that increase oxygen demand,

i.e., bicycle pedaling or treadmill walking, has been used to evaluate patients with suspected ischemic heart disease. Exercise electrocardiography, based on repolarization changes that are traditionally defined as 0.1 mV (1 mm) of horizontal or downsloping ST segment depression occurring 80 msec after the J point as being abnormal, may be utilized as a diagnostic test (Fig. 18). In patients with known coronary artery disease, exercise testing may provide information about functional capacity, efficacy of therapy, and prognosis. After myocardial infarction, low-level exercise testing prior to discharge from the hospital provides useful information for stratifying patients with respect to subsequent morbidity and mortality. The sensitivity of clinical exercise testing is 85%, 65%, and 40% in triple-, double-, and single-vessel disease, respectively. The sensitivity and specificity may be improved by using radionuclide studies (thallium scintigraphy or radionuclide angiography) in addition to the exercise electrocardiogram. For minimally symptomatic patients with three-vessel coronary artery disease who have ST-segment depression of 1 mm or more, a decrease in ejection fraction during exercise, and a decreased exercise tolerance ($\leq$120 W), the probability of

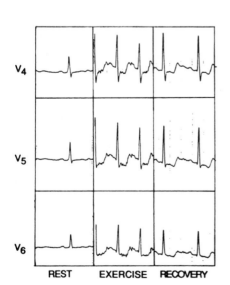

REST   EXERCISE   RECOVERY

FIG. 18. Exercise stress test. The three ECGs in the first panel on the left are chest leads V_{4-6} obtained at rest (from top to bottom, respectively). There is no ST-segment depression. The middle panel recorded during exercise shows ST-segment depression in the same leads (V_4, 1.5 mm; V_5, 2.3 mm; V_6, 1.6 mm). The right panel recorded 5 min into recovery demonstrates persistent ST-segment depression (V_4, 1.0 mm; V_5, 1.3 mm; V_6, 0.8 mm).

survival for 4 years is significantly lowered (83).

MECHANISMS OF ACTION OF ANTIANGINAL AGENTS

Nitrates

The nitrates have been the cornerstone of antianginal therapy for years because they reduce myocardial oxygen demand and increase oxygen supply. Myocardial oxygen demand is decreased in a somewhat complex fashion: peripheral veins dilate causing blood pooling in the extremities. This reduces venous return and diminishes left ventricular preload, which in turn decreases left ventricular chamber size, volume, and pressure with consequent reduction in wall tension. As myocardial wall tension decreases, so does oxygen demand. To a lesser extent, nitrates at high doses decrease left ventricular afterload. They do this by dilating the peripheral arterioles and reducing arterial pressure, which further reduces wall stress. Nitrates reduce coronary artery spasm in susceptible individuals with variant angina via a vasodilatory mechanism (84). Although controversial, nitrates appear to favorably alter blood flow to the endocardium (85,86). Nitrates may in some cases improve collateral coronary blood flow to areas of myocardium supplied by occluded or severely diseased coronary arteries (87). Recent quantitative angiographic studies have shown that nitroglycerin can dilate coronary arteries with eccentric stenosis and improve blood flow to ischemic areas (88). Nitrates do not directly affect heart rate or contractility; however, they may affect both indirectly or through reflexes (89). With the venodilating effects, arteriolar resistance and systemic blood pressure are usually also reduced. The hypotensive action of nitrates is exaggerated in the upright position. Decreased stroke volume and arterial pressure activate arterial baroreceptors that stimulate sympathetic mechanisms and result in a reflex augmentation of heart rate and contractility. Thus, a multiplicity of hemodynamic changes theoretically could increase MVO_2 (tachycardia, increased contractility) or decrease MVO_2 (decrease in heart size, decreased blood pressure) as a result of nitrates' actions.

In stable exertional angina, nitrates act by reducing myocardial oxygen demand and, to a lesser extent, by reducing coronary vasomotor tone. In unstable angina, nitrates act by reducing left ventricular wall stress and dilating eccentric coronary stenoses. In classic variant angina, the primary action of nitrates is to relieve coronary artery spasm. Nitrate-induced vasodilation occurs through interaction with nitrate receptors containing sulfhydryl groups. The fact that nitrates produce vasodilation regardless of whether the endothelium is intact suggests that these receptors are located on the vascular smooth muscle cells. Interaction between the receptor and nitrates converts nitrates to inorganic nitrate, NO, and eventually forms S-nitrosothiol. S-nitrosothiol is thought to stimulate guanylate cyclase to produce cGMP (45). The cyclic nucleotide formed is thought to cause vasodilation by several possible mechanisms: (a) inhibiting calcium ion entry, (b) interfering with actin-myosin interaction, or (c) promoting calcium exit. Physiological tolerance occurs when there is a deficiency of reduced sulfhydryl groups in vascular smooth muscle, as sulfhydryl groups are oxidized by excessive exposure to nitrates (90). In animals and humans, the administration of agents such as N-acetylcysteine, which increases the available reduced sulfhydryl groups, augments the effects of nitrates (91,92). A recent study has shown that an infusion of N-acetylcysteine potentiates the effect of nitroglycerin on coronary sinus blood flow in humans (93).

Nitroglycerin given sublingually or via buccal mucosa is rapidly absorbed and exerts a peak effect in 3 to 10 min, but its duration of action is only 20 to 30 min. As a result, it is effective in the treatment of acute episodes of angina or prophylactically prior to short-term activities that might precipitate an attack, but it is impractical for prolonged usage. There are two drugs demonstrated objectively to be of value (Fig. 19): 1,2,3-propanetriol trinitrate (0.15, 0.3, 0.4, 0.6 mg) and isosorbide dinitrate (2.5, 5.0, 10.0 mg). Patients should carry nitroglycerin at all times and be encouraged to use them to prevent or eliminate anginal pain. Patients should be warned about the possible loss of potency if unused for months. Nitroglycerin is volatile and should be kept in a stoppered vial, and it should burn under the tongue as an indication that it has not spontaneously decomposed. Adverse reactions most commonly described are transient headache immediately after use, dizziness, weakness, and palpitation. Postural hypotension may develop. Syncope has been ascribed to vasodilation. Alcohol may accentuate the symptoms due to cerebral ischemia.

Based on studies in animals in which ni-

trate preparations were metabolized quickly, there was initial skepticism regarding the efficacy of oral nitrates in humans. In general, nitrates have a very large plasma clearance, a very large volume of distribution, and a short half-life. After oral administration, plasma concentrations are very low, suggesting a large hepatic first-pass effect. There have been clinical studies that demonstrate efficacy in the long-term treatment of angina. The sustained-release or long-acting oral preparations have an onset of action in 20 to 45 min with a peak effect in 45 to 120 min and duration of 2 to 6 hr. These agents are used to prevent angina rather than for acute treatment. Subsequent clinical trials have shown that orally administered, long-acting nitrate preparations, such as isosorbide dinitrate, exert an antianginal effect for 2 to 4 hr (94,95).

Tolerance to the hemodynamic and antianginal effects of nitrates is well documented and is defined as a state in which increased drug doses are required to produce a predetermined effect or a state in which less effect is produced by the same

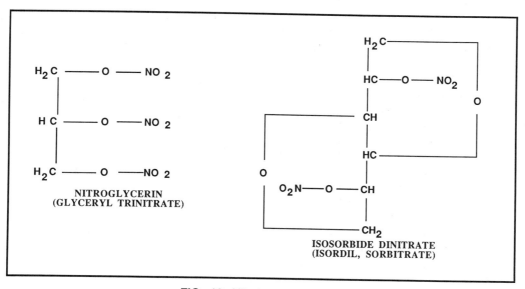

FIG. 19. Nitrate preparations.

amount of drug. During sustained oral nitrate therapy, both the magnitude and duration of nitrate effect, decrease in systolic blood pressure, and improvement in treadmill exercise duration are lessened despite the presence of high-plasma nitrate concentrations. Parker et al. (96) have suggested dosing oral nitrates so that no medication is taken in the evening. They suggested that tolerance to the clinical effects of isosorbide dinitrate develops with a sustained dosage of 30 mg four times daily, but not when the drug is given two or three times daily.

Cutaneous nitroglycerin ointment application produces a maximal hemodynamic effect in 60 to 90 min, which is followed by sustained nitroglycerin plasma levels for 4 to 6 hr, but these preparations are aesthetically difficult to manage. Transcutaneous nitroglycerin patches have been received enthusiastically because they are applied once a day and do not soil the clothing. However, in the manner in which they may be prescribed, their therapeutic benefit is controversial. They probably provoke rapid development of nitrate tolerance (97). To avoid this, the patient may be advised to remove the patch after 12 to 18 hr. All these reports support the concept that intermittent therapy prevents the attenuation of antianginal effects of nitrates. In addition, the patches are associated with occasional dermatological reactions. The product surface area ranges from 5 to 30 cm² and the nitroglycerin content from 12.5 to 120 mg with delivery in 24 hr of 2.5 to 15 mg.

Intravenous nitroglycerin (1,2,3-propanetriol trinitrate or isosorbide dinitrate) is frequently given for 24 to 36 hr; the clinical impression is that benefit is sustained, although in some patients higher and higher doses are needed to control anginal attacks. Recent observations with intravenous nitroglycerin in stable patients have shown development of tolerance, as assessed by exercise testing. Eight hours into the infusion, substantial attenuation was seen and by 24 hr there was no longer a significant effect (98). The initial dose is usually 5 to 10 μg/min, which can be titrated up to 200 μg/min or higher, depending on the clinical course. There should be an overall aim to control angina without decreasing mean blood pressure more than 10%. The agent adsorbs to plastic and polyvinyl chloride tubing, and the dose described assumes use of a special infusion set up, otherwise higher doses will be required. Again, there is an apparent large volume of distribution and rapid metabolism. The half-life is estimated at 1 to 4 min and infusions can be maintained for 36 hr or longer. It is, however, customary to have the unstable condition stabilized and the patient on oral agents within 48 hr. In addition to its use in the treatment of angina that is unresponsive to usual treatment, intravenous nitroglycerin can be used to (a) lower blood pressure during cardiovascular procedures when perioperative hypertension occurs, (b) treat congestive heart failure associated with acute myocardial infarction, (c) produce controlled hypotension during surgical procedures.

Therapeutic Mechanisms

1. Reduce venous return via peripheral venodilation, which reduces left ventricular preload decreasing left ventricular size, volume, and pressure, which consequently reduces wall tension
2. Dilate peripheral arterioles decreasing left ventricular afterload
3. Dilate coronary arteries
4. Improve endocardial blood flow

Potential Limitations

1. Hypotension and decreased stroke volume stimulate the sympathetic nervous system causing reflex tachycardia and increased contractility
2. Tolerance may develop to the hemodyamic and antianginal effects

Adverse Reactions

1. Headache
2. Dizziness
3. Weakness
4. Palpitations
5. Postural hypotension
6. Syncope
7. Angina

β-Adrenergic Blocking Agents

In 1948, Ahlquist (99) described a series of sympathomimetic amines with varied effects on organs or systems that could be used to define two types of adrenergic receptors: α and β. The α-adrenergic receptors are located in the membranes of vesicles of sympathetic neurons, which form storage sites for endogenous neurotransmitters, and are divided into two subtypes: α_1 and α_2. There are also two subtypes of β-adrenergic receptors: β_1 and β_2. The presynaptic α-adrenergic receptors are predominantly of the α_2 subtype, whereas both α_1- and α_2-adrenergic receptors are found at postsynaptic sites. Stimulation of presynaptic α-adrenergic receptor by an agonist inhibits endogenous norepinephrine release, whereas receptor blockade by α_2 or nonselective antagonists results in increased endogenous neurotransmitter release (100). Most presynaptic β-adrenergic receptors are the β_2 subtype. Agonists promote endogenous norepinephrine release and the antagonists inhibit vesicular norepinephrine release. Postsynaptic vascular α-adrenergic receptor stimulation causes vasoconstriction, which in turn increases peripheral vascular resistance. Postsynaptic α_1 receptors are located in the synapse, whereas α_2 receptors are extrasynaptic and considered noninnervated. These α_2 receptors are hormone receptors responsive to circulating catecholamines, especially epinephrine. Stimulation of postsynaptic vascular β-adrenergic receptors, which are predominantly the β_2 subtype, causes vasodilation, whereas antagonists result in vasoconstriction. These β receptors are also considered noninnervated hormone receptors. There are specific tissue receptor density changes that occur in response to changes in physiological or pharmacological conditions. For example, in chronic heart failure, down-regulation of cardiac β_1-adrenergic receptors occurs, changing the β_1/β_2 receptor ratio and preventing the expected responses to high-plasma norepinephrine levels. β_1-Adrenergic blockers cause β_1-adrenergic receptor up-regulation, which in heart failure might improve myocardial contractility in response to circulating norepinephrine. In terms of predominant physiological responses, the β_1 receptors mediate the effects of the neuronally released transmitter norepinephrine primarily to stimulate the heart, release renin, and cause lipolysis. At the same time, the β_2 receptors mediate the response to epinephrine released from the adrenal medulla causing relaxation of smooth muscles in the peripheral vasculature, bronchi, and gut and promoting glycogenolysis (101). There are, however, a small number of β_2 receptors in the heart and a significant number of β_1 receptors in the lung (102).

The majority of patients with angina secondary to atherosclerotic coronary artery disease have improved exercise tolerance and reduction in chest pain with β-adrenergic blocker treatment. β-Adrenergic blockers have been shown to be efficacious in placebo-controlled, double-blind, crossover studies and are the mainstay of therapy for stable exertional angina (103). The β-adrenergic blockers are effective antianginal agents because they reduce several determinants of myocardial oxygen demand: heart rate (at rest and especially during exercise), left ventricular contractility, and left ventricular wall tension. In addition, they are effective in reducing the incidence of sudden death and reinfarction during the years following an acute myocardial infarction, regardless of heart size (104–106). However, in these studies in which β-adrenergic blockers were administered in the acute or chronic phases of myocardial infarction, 40% to 50% of patients were excluded, often because of symptomatic congestive heart failure.

β-Adrenergic blockers are competitive inhibitors of catecholamine binding at β-adrenergic receptor sites. β-Adrenergic blockers may protect the heart from physiological or psychological stresses by limiting catecholamine-induced increases in heart rate, blood pressure, velocity and extent of myocardial contraction, and oxygen demands at any level of activity (107). The β_1 receptors in the heart mediate increases in heart rate and contractility and are blocked by both β_1 selective and nonselective β-adrenergic blockers. Newer β-adrenergic blockers with intrinsic sympathomimetic activity (partial agonist activity) do not affect resting heart rate and may not be effective in the treatment of angina at rest. However, all β-adrenergic blockers limit exercise-induced tachycardia and are useful for the treatment of exertional angina. In patients with intrinsic conducting system disease, sinus node function may be impaired by β-adrenergic blockade and atrioventricular conduction diminished to a degree that causes symptomatic bradycardia or heart block. β-Adrenergic blockers probably have a minimal effect on myocardial contractility at rest and have their greatest effect on exercise-induced (catecholamine-related) increments in contractility. Overall, the decrease in heart rate and contractility leads to a reduction in cardiac output, both at rest and during exercise, which may cause subjective fatigue or limit exercise capacity in some patients. β-Adrenergic blockers effectively reduce left ventricular wall stress by decreasing systolic blood pressure. In patients with cardiomegaly and heart failure, blocking the sympathetic tone may cause ventricular fiber lengthening with increased heart size, increased end-diastolic pressure, and increased myocardial oxygen demand, which would compromise further the decompensated heart.

Effects of β-adrenergic blockers on coronary blood flow are not well understood. The reduction in myocardial oxygen demands may increase vascular resistance via autoregulation. One potential drawback with the β-adrenergic blockers is their failure to cause coronary vasodilation and the theoretical potential to allow vasoconstriction. This is related to blockade of β_2-vasodilating receptors in the coronary circulation so that unopposed α and other vasoconstrictive influences can lead to increased coronary artery spasm (108,109). For these reasons, β-adrenergic blockers are usually not prescribed for those patients with variant angina, in which increased vasomotor tone causes angina at rest. Increased vasomotor tone also occurs in the presence of fixed atherosclerotic lesions, further limiting blood flow and causing angina at rest. This mixture of disease processes accounts for some chest pain episodes (mixed angina) in patients with stable exertional angina. Here β-adrenergic blockers are still used, often in combination with coronary vasodilating agents. In one clinical trial, the β-adrenergic blocker was as effective as the calcium channel blocker in eliminating rest angina, and more effective in preventing exertional angina (110). It has also been noted during the past decade that patients with mixed angina often experience electrocardiographic evidence of ischemia, either at rest or during exertion, without chest pain. This "silent ischemia" is probably due to intermittent decreases in coronary blood flow, possibly due to coronary artery spasm. Initially it was thought that β-adrenergic blockers should not be used in these patients. Results of clinical studies show that an increased heart rate may precede the ischemic events and that β-adrenergic blockers are effective in relieving silent ischemia (111,112). In fact, further studies have shown that β-adrenergic blockers are actually more effective in preventing ischemic episodes not initiated by a rapid heart rate (113).

β-Adrenergic blockers that selectively block the β_1 receptors should be associated with less bronchospasm, whereas unwanted β_2 blockade may permit bronchospasm in patients with reactive airways disease. Comparing atenolol, metoprolol, acebutolol, pindolol, propranolol, and oxprenolol to placebo in asthmatics showed atenolol similar to placebo in its effect on forced expiratory volume in 1 sec (FEV_1). Metoprolol and acebutolol are associated with some β_1 selectivity and cause a greater decrease in FEV_1 than atenolol but less than the other agents. Other studies (114,115) have demonstrated that atenolol can reduce resting FEV_1, but the increase in FEV_1 that normally occurs after inhaling isoproterenol or infusing terbutaline was not blunted. In many patients with obstructive airway disease, long-term atenolol treatment is well tolerated. Additionally, selective β_1-adrenergic blockers should cause less peripheral arterial vasoconstriction than nonselective agents. However, at high doses, clinically reliable selectivity has not been clearly demonstrated for those drugs that are supposed to be selective β_1-adrenergic blockers.

The relative effects of individual β-adrenergic blockers is in part related to the degree of lipid solubility. Lipophilic (lipid-soluble) β-adrenergic blockers reach the brain easily and undergo hepatic metabolism with the potential for inactivation on the first pass through the liver. They tend to be short acting. Hydrophilic (water-soluble) β-adrenergic blockers do not reach the brain easily and are not metabolized but are excreted intact by the kidney. They tend to be long acting and doses must be adjusted in patients with renal insufficiency. Measurable serum $t_{1/2}$ is generally shorter than the physiological $t_{1/2}$ of β-adrenergic blockers (Table 3). One property initially described with propranolol is inhibition of *in vitro* platelet aggregation induced by several agonists (epinephrine, collagen, thrombin, ADP [116,117]). This effect on platelets may be related to propranolol's high degree of lipid solubility or a membrane stabilizing effect. Heightened platelet activity determined *in vitro* from peripheral venous and coronary sinus blood of patients with angina can be normalized after therapeutic doses of propranolol (118). This antiaggregatory effect on platelet activity has been noted with oxprenolol and pindolol (117), but the clinical relevance of this effect is unknown. The membrane stabilizing effect is nonspecific and seen with high doses of several agents (propranolol, metoprolol, alprenolol). This effect is considered a local anesthesic effect and results in a decrease in the rate of rise of the cardiac action potential in animal studies. This

TABLE 3. β-*Adrenergic blocking agents*

Name	Blockade	Lipophilic	ISA	MSA	$t_{1/2}$ (hr)
Propranolol	$\beta_1 + \beta_2$	+	−	++	4–6
Metoprolol	$\beta_1 \gg \beta_2$	+	−	+	3–4
Timolol	$\beta_1 + \beta_2$	+	−	−	4–5
Pindolol	$\beta_1 + \beta_2$	+	+++	+	3–4
Atenolol	$\beta_1 \gg \beta_2$	−	−	−	5–7
Nadolol	$\beta_1 + \beta_2$	−	−	−	16–18
Acebutolol	$\beta_1 \gg \beta_2$	+	+	+	3–6
Labetalol	$\beta_1 + \beta_2 > \alpha_1$	−	−	+	6–8
Oxprenolol	$\beta_1 + \beta_2$	+	++	+	1–2
Practolol	$\beta_1 \gg \beta_2$	−	++	−	5–13

ISA, intrinsic sympathomimetic activity; MSA, membrane stabilizing effect; $t_{1/2}$, half-life. +, ++, +++, degree property present; −, property absent.

membrane stabilizing activity may contribute to the antiarrhythmic effects, in addition to the antiplatelet actions, of high doses of propranolol (119,120).

Some of the newer β-adrenergic blockers have intrinsic sympathomimetic activity, a term used to describe partial agonist activity or the cardioacceleration that occurs in reserpinized animals with low sympathetic tone. In humans, obvious stimulation is not observed, but resting bradycardia is uncommon. However, there is blocking activity seen during exercise. Weak intrinsic sympathomimetic activity is a property of pindolol and, to a lesser extent, of acebutolol. These agents may be thought of as blocking the agonist action of catecholamines but themselves providing weak stimulation of the receptors. These agents may lower systemic vascular resistance and have less negative inotropy in the failing ventricle than other β-adrenergic blockers. Intrinsic sympathomimetic activity is not a measurable factor in the exercise or catheterization laboratory.

Some of the adverse effects of β-adrenergic blockers represent relative contraindications for patients with resting bradycardia, cardiac conducting system disease, heart failure, asthma, or insulin-dependent diabetes mellitus with the propensity for hypoglycemic episodes. The rate of recovery from hypoglycemia is prolonged after nonselective β-adrenergic blockers compared with selective β-adrenergic blockers (121). The hemodynamic response to insulin-induced hypoglycemia involves an adrenergic component that invokes an increase in blood pressure and heart rate. Propranolol allows exaggerated hypertension and reflex bradycardia to occur. Propranolol attenuates the rise in glucose and lactate seen during exercise. The mechanism of this is unclear but may involve decreased skeletal muscle and hepatic glycogenolysis, which may in part explain one of its side effects: fatigue. Certainly propranolol also blunts the normal hemodynamic response to exercise, which may contribute to fatigue. However, cardioselective β-adrenergic blocking agents with similar hemodynamic profiles (metoprolol) cause less symptomatic fatigue. The side effects from action in the central nervous system of β-adrenergic blockers include depression, insomnia, hallucinations, impotency, and slowed mentation. These side effects occur more often with the more lipophilic β-adrenergic blockers (122).

One potential adverse affect of β-adrenergic blockers that may be overlooked is their impact on plasma lipids and lipoprotein concentrations. In hypertensive patients treated with these agents for 12 months, triglycerides increased, HDL cholesterol decreased, and total and LDL cholesterol increased (123). The postprandial lipemic response is increased by nonselective β-adrenergic blockers (124). This is important because of the relationship between elevated blood cholesterol and the development of atherosclerotic coronary artery disease. Plasma LDL cholesterol concentrations are strongly and positively related to atherosclerosis, whereas plasma HDL cholesterol is strongly and inversely related to atherosclerosis (125,126).

To date, there is no therapeutic advantage of one β-adrenergic blocker over another in the treatment of angina pectoris. In patients with stable angina, β-adrenergic blocker efficacy was assessed by improved exercise duration and decreased ST-segment depression in comparison with a placebo. Near maximal response to an acute oral dose reached peak improvement at 160 mg for propranolol and oxprenolol, 200 mg for metoprolol, and 400 mg for practolol. The improvement occurred within 1 hr and persisted for 8 hr. Noncardioselective agents (propranolol, oxprenolol), cardioselective agents (practolol, metoprolol), and drugs with intrinsic sympathomimetic activity (oxprenolol and practolol) were equally effective (127).

One final caution, β-adrenergic blocking agents should not be withdrawn abruptly except under closely monitored conditions.

After chronic administration there may be a withdrawal syndrome with tachycardia, hypertension, and exacerbation of angina pectoris (128,129). In some patients, myocardial infarction has occurred (130). The drugs should be tapered off over several days or another agent may be administered to blunt the withdrawal symptoms, i.e., clonidine or diltiazem.

Therapeutic Mechanisms

1. Limit catecholamine-induced increases in heart rate, which increases diastolic coronary perfusion time
2. Decrease in blood pressure and contractility, which reduces left ventricular afterload and wall tension, with consequential reduction in oxygen demand
3. Inhibit platelet aggregation
4. Quinidine-like membrane stabilizing effect

Potential Limitations

1. Individual variability in degree of bradycardia and hypotension induced
2. Lack of coronary vasodilating effect and potential for vasoconstriction
3. β-Sympathetic withdrawal may cause decompensation in borderline heart failure
4. β-Sympathetic antagonism may predispose to increased airways resistance (bronchoconstriction)
5. β-Sympathetic blockade may potentiate unopposed peripheral α-sympathetic agonist-induced vasoconstriction (claudication)
6. Sudden drug withdrawal syndromes with increased angina and possible myocardial infarction

Adverse Reactions

1. Bradycardia
2. Heart block
3. Hypotension
4. Worsened heart failure
5. Bronchoconstriction
6. Unrecognized hypoglycemia in diabetics
7. Cold extremities
8. Worsened claudication

Calcium Channel Blocking Agents

Calcium ions are involved in generation of the action potential in the automatic and conduction cells of the heart, in the linkage of excitation and contraction in the myocardial contractile cells, and in the control of energy storage and use. During relaxation calcium ion concentration is lower in the myocardial cytosol than the extracellular fluid. During activation calcium ion concentration rises and the ion binds to troponin, which in the presence of ATP allows interaction between myosin and actin. Subsequent reduction in cytosolic calcium ion causes calcium ion to dissociate from troponin, breaking the myosin-actin crosslinks and muscular relaxation ensues. β-Adrenergic agonists induce cAMP, which increases the rate at which calcium ion is available to contractile sites and promotes contraction. There are several mechanisms that control calcium ion concentration in the cytoplasm: (a) inward movement along a concentration gradient and across the sarcolemma, i.e., electrogenic slow inward current through the slow calcium ion channels; (b) bidirectional sodium-calcium ion exchange system across the sarcolemma, i.e., as cardiac glycosides increase intracellular sodium ion concentration, the calcium ion enters and a positive inotropic state results; (c) calcium ion ATPase of the sarcolemma lowers cellular calcium ion concentration; (d) calcium ion-stimulated magnesium ATPase in the sarcoplasmic reticulum increases calcium ion uptake into the sarcoplasmic reticulum; (e) mitochondrial controlled calcium ion uptake and release; (f) ionophore- and concentration-dependent movement of calcium ion across the sarcolemma; (g) intracellular proteins buffer calcium ion (131).

The luminal dimensions of systemic and coronary arteries are also influenced by the movement of calcium ions across the cell membranes of vascular smooth muscle. In these vascular smooth muscles, the calcium-ion binding protein is calmodulin and this complex activates myosin kinase, which phosphorylates light chain myosin permitting myosin-actin interaction, thus leading to arteriolar constriction as the smooth muscle cell contracts. β-Adrenergic agonists induce cAMP, which promotes vasodilation via two possible mechanisms: (a) cAMP-dependent protein kinase may lower intracellular calcium ion by increased efflux and decreased transmembrane influx or (b) cAMP-induced inactivation of myosin kinase may decrease phosphorylation of light chain myosin (132).

In view of the wide range of effects the calcium ion has on the cardiovascular system, it is not surprising that calcium channel blocking agents have been developed. The calcium channel blockers exert their action at very low concentrations and exhibit stereospecificity, suggesting that they bind to specific structures in the calcium ion channel decreasing slow-channel calcium influx. Nifedipine may actually plug the calcium ion channel, whereas verapamil and to a lesser extent diltiazem are use dependent, i.e., the more often the channel is open, the more drug enters, and the greater the degree of block induced. They are also voltage dependent; they will access the calcium channel and block it only if the cell is depolarized. These agents variably exert a beneficial effect on both sides of the myocardial oxygen supply-demand relationship in the treatment of ischemic heart disease. The calcium channel blockers have been effective in the treatment of ischemic heart disease, i.e., stable exertional angina, variant angina, unstable angina, postinfarction angina, in addition to the treatment of systemic hypertension, supraventricular arrhythmias, and hypertrophic cardiomyopathy. Importantly, all three agents have been shown to be effective in the treatment of stable exertional angina (133–135) and variant angina (136,137) in double-blind, randomized, placebo-controlled studies.

Nifedipine is the most potent vasodilator. Its administration is accompanied by a reflex increase in sympathetic activity, which increases heart rate and overcomes its intrinsic negative inotropic effect. Nifedipine reduces myocardial oxygen demand by decreasing left ventricular afterload (dilating peripheral arteries) and increases myocardial oxygen supply by inhibiting coronary vasoconstriction. Related side effects included hypotension (especially orthostatic changes), flushing, headache, tachycardia, and peripheral edema. When used alone or with nitrates, the tachycardia may actually increase the incidence of angina. The usual dose range is from 30 to 90 mg a day in three divided doses. Occasionally the agent is used sublingually or intravascularly for control of hypertension or arterial spasm.

Verapamil and diltiazem reduce myocardial oxygen demand by decreasing heart rate and reducing left ventricular contractility and wall tension. They increase oxygen supply by inhibiting coronary vasoconstriction and favorably affect the time course of left ventricular diastolic filling. Verapamil, as it is used clinically, has been shown to be the least potent peripheral dilator, yet the most effective in depressing sinus and atrioventricular node function and myocardial contractility. Diltiazem is intermediate between nifedipine and verapamil with respect to these characteristics. Diltiazem and verapamil undergo first-pass hepatic metabolism and are given in larger doses than nifedipine. Both are well absorbed after oral administration (80%–90%) but only 30% to 40% of the dose is bioavailable after hepatic metabolism. The metabolites are excreted in urine and bile; dose adjustments should be made in patients with hepatic or renal insufficiency. The drugs are significantly bound to plasma proteins. Adverse effects are similar and usually more remarkable with verapamil than diltiazem and include bradycardia, heart block, transient sinus node arrest, worsening congestive heart failure, hypotension, flushing, nausea, constipation, headache, dizziness, peripheral edema, and elevated transaminase activity. Concurrent use with β-adrenergic blocking agents, digoxin, or amiodarone may potentiate or increase the incidence of side effects.

Calcium channel blockers have been administered to patients after myocardial infarction in clinical trials to determine if the incidence of death and reinfarction can be reduced. Diltiazem given prophylactically during the first 2 weeks after a subendocardial myocardial infarction (non-Q-wave infarction) has been shown to decrease the incidence of reinfarction (12.9% placebo vs 6.3% diltiazem, $p = 0.03$) and the incidence of refractory angina (6.9% placebo vs 3.5% diltiazem, $p = 0.03$). However, mortality was unchanged (138). More recently, data have been presented involving the effect of diltiazem on mortality and reinfarction in patients with previous infarction. Total mortality rates were identical in the two treatment groups (diltiazem 60 mg four times a day vs placebo). However, a significant bidirectional interaction was observed between diltiazem and pulmonary congestion. Without pulmonary congestion, diltiazem was associated with a reduction in the number of cardiac events; with pulmonary congestion, it was associated with an increased number of cardiac events. This interaction was similar with respect to left ventricular ejection fraction dichotomized at 0.40 (139). Neither nifedipine nor verapamil has been shown to be beneficial for patients suffering acute myocardial infarction or for postinfarction patients with regard to reinfarction or mortality.

Therapeutic Mechanisms

1. Inhibition of cellular calcium fluxes results in coronary vasodilation, reduced contractility, slowed heart rate and impulse conduction, thus increasing myocardial oxygen delivery and decreasing oxygen demand
2. Decrease in blood pressure, which reduces left ventricular afterload and wall tension, with further reduction in oxygen demand
3. Decreased responsiveness to sympathetic stimulation

Potential Limitations

1. Individual variability in degree of bradycardia, heart block, and hypotension induced
2. Nifedipine induces a reflex increase in sympathetic activity, which increases heart rate and overcomes its intrinsic negative inotropic effect that may increase myocardial oxygen demand
3. Limited sympathetic responsiveness and negative inotropy may cause decompensation in borderline heart failure

Adverse Reactions

1. Bradycardia
2. Heart block
3. Transient sinus node arrest
4. Worsening congestive heart failure
5. Hypotension
6. Flushing
7. Nausea
8. Constipation
9. Headache
10. Dizziness
11. Peripheral edema
12. Elevated transaminase activity

Combined Therapy

Certainly monotherapy for ischemic heart disease would be ideal for several reasons: simplicity, expense, side effects, compliance. However, single-agent therapy is not always effective. Antianginal agents are often used in combination, including nitrates, β-adrenergic blocking agents, and calcium channel blocking agents. Most worrisome of the side effects that must be monitored include bradycardia, hypotension, and negative inotropy (140).

Antithrombotic and Thrombolytic Therapy

Factors responsible for the conversion of chronic stable ischemic heart disease to acute ischemic syndromes, i.e., unstable angina and myocardial infarction, most often involve platelet activation/aggregation (141,142), vasoconstriction (143), and development of thrombus in the presence of a critical stenosis or atherosclerotic plaque rupture (144–147). At least half of the cases of myocardial infarction occur in the presence of preceding unstable angina. Further support for the initial postulate comes from the protective effects of antiplatelet or anticoagulant therapy in patients with unstable angina that does not progress to infarction. The antiplatelet effect of aspirin is to permanently acetylate cyclooxygenase and inhibit thromboxane synthesis. This does not appear to affect platelet adhesion. Aspirin reduced the incidence of death and progression to definite myocardial infarction in several clinical trials: Veterans Administration Cooperative Study using 300 mg/day in men for weeks (148) and Canadian Multicenter Trial using 325 mg q.i.d. in men and women over a 2-year period (149). Heparin acts as an anticoagulant by decreasing thrombin formation and availability, which limits fibrin formation from fibrinogen. Heparin activates antithrombin III, heparin cofactor II, serine proteases that inactivate thrombin as well as coagulation factors XII, XI, X, IX, and perhaps VII. Telford and Wilson (150) reported morbidity and mortality results of a randomized, double-blind, placebo-controlled trial using heparin, atenolol, both, or placebo in patients with unstable angina. Transmural myocardial infarction developed in 17% of

patients on placebo, 13% of patients receiving atenolol, 2% on heparin, and 4% of patients on both heparin and atenolol ($p = 0.024$). Death occurred in 5 of 214 patients, none of whom had been given heparin.

Comparison of these two agents, aspirin taken orally (325 mg b.i.d.) and intravenous heparin (1,000 units/hr), in patients with acute unstable angina showed that either or both together significantly reduced the incidence of myocardial infarction compared with patients receiving placebo (151). However, only intravenous heparin was associated with a decrease in the occurrence of medically refractory angina. Although it may not be routine practice, patients with unstable angina often undergo catheterization with an intracoronary thrombus being detected (152). In such cases fibrinolytic agents may be infused into the coronary artery with subsequent thrombolysis and stabilization of the acute syndrome (153). Selected patients with unstable angina unresponsive to intensive pharmacological treatment, are sometimes found at catheterization to have critical stenosis without obvious intraluminal thrombus. Emergency percutaneous transluminal coronary angioplasty (PTCA) may be performed safely with relief of symptoms and improved cardiac functional status (154). Restenosis occurs after PTCA in at least 25% to 35% of cases. Platelet activation and thrombus formation contribute to early acute occlusion, but the mechanisms of restenosis are less well understood. Results of a recent randomized, placebo-controlled trial using antiplatelet therapy (heparin, aspirin, dipyridamole) beginning 24 hr before the procedure, found the incidence of transmural myocardial infarction during or soon after PTCA could be markedly reduced, but the incidence of restenosis 4 to 7 months later was unchanged (155).

Current treatment of acute myocardial infarction is directed toward salvaging myocardium during and after a coronary artery has been occluded. Mortality is directly related to the extent of left ventricular dysfunction, which is directly related to the amount of myocardium that becomes infarcted. Toward this goal, proper aggressive management of acute myocardial infarction is aimed at early reperfusion of the occluded artery and prevention of reocclusion after patency has been established. The fibrinolytic agents currently available or being studied in clinical trials for the treatment of acute myocardial infarction act as plasminogen activators, either directly or indirectly (Table 4). Streptokinase, urokinase, and recombinant tissue plasminogen activator are commercially available in the United States and approved by the Food and Drug Administration for the treatment of acute myocardial infarction. Clinical research with an acylated plasminogen-streptokinase activator complex is in an advanced state and likely to be available in the United States soon; trials with a recombinant form of single-chain, urokinase-type plasminogen activator are well underway. Patients who present early in the course of an evolving myocardial infarction benefit from thrombolytic therapy that effectively opens thrombosed coronary arteries (156–159). There is a reduction in mortality, improved wall motion, and reduction in infarct size. Often the disrupted atherosclerotic plaque persists, and early rethrombosis occurs in 15% to 35% of cases despite therapy with heparin and aspirin

(160–162). The risk of reinfarction during the next 12 months is increased.

In view of this, secondary revascularization with PTCA has been investigated. Guerci et al. (163) showed that suitable subjects undergoing PTCA 3 days after thrombolysis have fewer episodes of ischemia during hospitalization and improved exercise ejection fraction response than patients who did not undergo PTCA. Topol et al. (164) found that PTCA performed immediately, 90 min after lytic therapy was successfully initiated, on vessels with significant residual stenoses ($\geq$50%) was associated with an increased risk of major complication, including death, when compared with more elective PTCA performed after 7 to 10 days. The necessity of secondary revascularization is apparent, the appropriate timing in stable patients is subacutely prior to initial hospital discharge. In patients in whom thrombolytic therapy fails or cannot be used, PTCA can be used as primary therapy. Restoration of arterial patency is similar when PTCA is compared with lytic therapy (165). The subgroup of patients suffering myocardial infarction complicated by cardiogenic shock carries a high mortality rate (80%), which has not been reduced with inotropic drugs, invasive hemodynamic monitoring, or supported circulation (intraaortic balloon counterpulsation). PTCA, alone or in combination with lytic therapy and in-

TABLE 4. *Thrombolytic agents*

	Streptokinase	Urokinase	tPA	APSAC	scu-PA
Efficacy (patency <4 hr)	50%–80%	60%–70%	60%–80%	60%–70%	60%–80%
Improved LV ejection fraction (%)	Yes	?	Yes	Yes	?
Mortality decrease	Yes	?	Yes	Yes	?
Reocclusion rate	10%–20%	10%	15%–25%	10%	?
Dose	1.5 MU	2–3 MU	100 mg	30 mg	40–60 mg
Infusion duration	30–60 min	5–15 min	3 hr	2–5 min	1–3 hr
$t_{1/2}$	23 min	16 min	5 min	90 min	7 min
Cost	+	++++	++++	+++	++++

tPA, tissue plasminogen activator; APSAC, acylated plasminogen-streptokinase activator complex; scu-PA, single-chain urokinase-type plasminogen activator; LV, left ventricular; ?, unknown; +, ++, +++, relative expense.

traaortic balloon counterpulsation, restores arterial patency and improves short-term prognosis: 1 month 50% survival compared with 20% survival rate with standard treatment (166).

Until recently, there were scant data regarding antiplatelet therapy given to patients early during acute myocardial infarction. The ISIS-2 (Second International Study of Infarct Survival) trial was a randomized, placebo-controlled trial of aspirin (160 mg on admission and daily thereafter) and/or streptokinase (1.5 MU, i.v. for 1 hr) given within the first 24 hr after the onset of acute myocardial infarction in 17,187 patients (167). Streptokinase alone and aspirin alone each promoted a significant reduction in 5-week vascular mortality compared with placebo. Streptokinase was associated with an increased requirement for transfusions (0.5% vs 0.2%). With the combination of streptokinase and aspirin, there were fewer reinfarctions (1.8% vs 2.9%), strokes (0.6% vs 1.1%), and deaths (8.0% vs 13.2%) than those patients receiving neither. This difference remained significant after a median 15 month follow-up.

Long-term use of aspirin in survivors of acute myocardial infarction, based on data from six trials analyzed as pooled data (168), has been shown to reduce the risk for cardiovascular death 16% ($p<0.01$), and the combined end point of fatal and nonfatal myocardial infarction is reduced by 21% ($p<0.001$). The Food and Drug Administration has approved aspirin therapy postmyocardial infarction as effective for prevention of further coronary events.

Along the same line of reasoning, does the long-term use of aspirin serve as a primary prevention in subjects at risk for coronary events? Such a prospective study was conducted among male American physicians (22,071) assigned to 325 mg aspirin every other day or placebo (169). The risk of fatal or nonfatal myocardial infarction was reduced by 47% ($p<0.00001$), which led to premature termination of the study. The combined end point of either nonfatal

infarction, stroke, or cardiovascular death was also reduced by 23% ($p<0.006$). However, the incidence of hemorrhagic stroke was increased with aspirin compared with placebo (10 men vs 2 men, respectively, $p<0.02$).

ADJUNCTIVE THERAPY IN ACUTE MYOCARDIAL INFARCTION

Preventing Rethrombosis

Heparin and aspirin have been used in many clinical trials as adjunctive therapy for the prevention of reocclusion after thrombolysis. The value of heparin, however, has not been established in this setting (170). The use of novel anticoagulant and antiplatelet agents in experimental myocardial infarction offers great promise for clinical use in humans in the near future. Some of these newer antithrombotic approaches include the use of activated protein C, tissue factor antagonists, or monoclonal antibodies directed against platelet receptors such as the glycoprotein IIb/IIIa. The use of these antibodies results in profound antithrombotic effects *in vitro* (171) and *in vivo* (172,173). Antibodies directed against the platelet glycoprotein Ib, which effectively block platelet adhesion to von Willebrand factor (174), are also promising.

Preventing Reperfusion Injury

Experimental studies of acute myocardial infarction indicate that the process of restoring coronary blood flow (reperfusion) is potentially harmful to the myocardium that was previously ischemic. Postulated causes of this injury include the production of oxidants (including oxygen free radicals) and the accumulation of white blood cells. These inflammatory cells, the polymorphonuclear leukocytes (neutrophils), are capable of tissue destruction mediated by production of oxidant species from molecular oxygen via a membrane-bound enzyme nic-

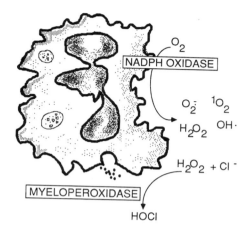

FIG. 20. Schematic drawing of a polymorphonuclear leukocyte (PMN). The membrane-bound enzyme NADPH oxidase produces superoxide ($\cdot O_2-$) and hydrogen peroxide (H_2O_2) from molecular oxygen (O_2). From these species, hydroxyl radical ($OH\cdot$) may be formed. Myeloperoxidase is a PMN granule enzyme released on PMN activation that catalyzes the formation of hypochlorous acid (HOCl) from hydrogen chloride (Cl^-).

otinamide adenine dinucleotide phosphate, reduced oxidase (NADPH) (Fig. 20). Another source of potentially harmful neutrophil-derived products are the proteases in the lysosomes of these cells that are released at sites of tissue injury.

Free radicals are highly reactive molecules that are formed as a result of the addition of an unpaired electron to the outer orbital of a molecule. Oxygen is reduced during normal metabolism in four steps with the sequential univalent addition of electrons to molecular oxygen (Table 5). Univalent reduction of oxygen leads to the formation of superoxide anion ($\cdot O_2 \overline{}$), which is a highly reactive radical molecule. Superoxide by nature can act as an oxidant or as a reductant. The addition of a second electron to superoxide (catalyzed by SOD) forms hydrogen peroxide. Addition of another electron to hydrogen peroxide via either a Fenton or Haber Weiss type reaction, which requires transition metal catalysis (between superoxide and hydrogen

peroxide), results in the formation of hydroxyl radical ($OH\cdot$). This highly reactive oxidant has been postulated to be one of the most reactive and thus one of the more harmful oxygen-derived radical species produced.

In addition to neutrophil-derived oxidants, tissue sources of these oxidants include mitochondria and the many oxidative enzymes present within tissues. These enzymes include xanthine oxidase (Fig. 21) and the enzymes involved in prostaglandin biosynthesis (Fig. 22).

Jolly and colleagues (175) first demonstrated that oxygen-derived free radicals were involved in the process of myocardial reperfusion injury *in vivo*. They demonstrated that when SOD and catalase (Fig. 23) were administered to dogs during reperfusion after a period of regional ischemia, these free radical metabolizing enzymes provided protection as measured by a significant reduction in the ultimate myocardial infarct size. Since this report, these

TABLE 5. *Reduction products of molecular oxygen*

	Electrons	Unprotonated	pH 7.0
Oxygen	0	O_2	O_2
Superoxide	1	$O_2^{\cdot-}$	$O_2^{\cdot}$
Hydrogen peroxide	2	$O_2^{=}$	H_2O_2
Hydroxyl radical	3	$O^- + O^=$	$OH\cdot + H_2O$
Water	4	$O^= + O^=$	$H_2O + H_2O$

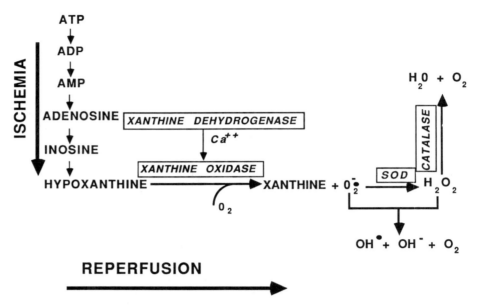

FIG. 21. During ischemia, high-energy phosphates decrease and substrates from ATP metabolism such as hypoxanthine accumulate. In addition, calcium accumulates within the cells and this enables the conversion of xanthine dehydrogenase to xanthine oxidase. During reperfusion, the other substrate (in addition to hypoxanthine) necessary for xanthine oxidase, oxygen, is introduced. The xanthine oxidase is then able to metabolize hypoxanthine to xanthine or xanthine to uric acid with the production of superoxide anion ($\cdot O_2-$). SOD can then catalyze the conversion of $\cdot O_2-$ to H_2O_2 and catalase metabolizes H_2O_2 to H_2O and O_2.

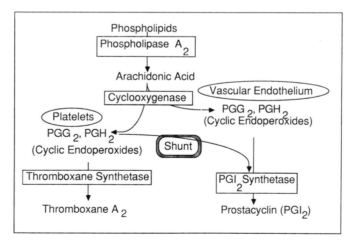

FIG. 22. Arachidonic acid is released from membrane phospholipids via the action of phospholipases. Cyclooxygenase then catalyzes the formation of cyclic endoperoxides that can then be metabolized to thromboxane A_2 (in platelets) or to prostacyclin (in other tissues). When thromboxane synthetase is inhibited, the cyclic endoperoxides can "shunt" metabolism toward other eicosanoids.

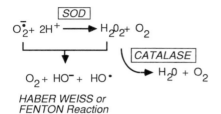

$$\boxed{SOD}$$
$$O_2^{\overline{\cdot}} + 2H^+ \longrightarrow H_2O_2 + O_2$$

$$O_2 + HO^- + HO^{\cdot}$$

$$\boxed{CATALASE}$$
$$H_2O + O_2$$

HABER WEISS or
FENTON Reaction

FIG. 23. SOD catalyzes the reduction of superoxide ($O_2^{\overline{\cdot}}$) to hydrogen peroxide (H_2O_2), which is catalyzed to water (H_2O) and molecular oxygen (O_2) by catalase.

findings have been confirmed by a number of other investigators (176,177). In addition, direct measurement of free radicals in myocardium during reperfusion has recently been reported (178).

During the process of reperfusion of previously ischemic myocardium, there is activation of an inflammatory process such that neutrophils are recruited into regions of the myocardium that have undergone some degree of injury. Experimental evidence suggests that this process of infiltration and activation of inflammatory cells in the myocardium further damages potentially compromised myocardium resulting in infarct extension. Romson and colleagues (179) demonstrated that if dogs were depleted of circulating neutrophils prior to induction of regional myocardial ischemia, the infarct size that results was smaller in the dogs that were previously depleted of neutrophils. Since that study, numerous other agents have been shown to limit myocardial infarction through mechanisms related to inhibition of neutrophil functions (Table 6) (180). Many of the protective effects of nonsteroidal anti-inflammatory agents in acute myocardial infarction are attributable to inhibitory effects on neutrophils (Table 6).

Thromboxane antagonists and thromboxane synthetase inhibitors are effective agents for reducing myocardial reperfusion injury (181–185). It has been hypothesized that the effectiveness of thromboxane synthetase inhibitors may be due to the ability of these drugs to cause a shunt of cyclic endoperoxides away from the platelet synthesis of thromboxane A_2 toward the production of protective prostaglandins such as PGI_2, PGEs, or PGD_2 (Fig. 22). It has been shown that the protective effects of prostaglandins are due to effects on inhibiting neutrophil activation (186–190). Thus, the use of thromboxane synthetase inhibitors would be protective through this same prostaglandin-dependent mechanism. However, thromboxane receptor antagonists have recently been shown to be effective for reducing myocardial injury. A recent investigation indicates that thromboxane A_2 may directly activate circulating neutrophils *in vivo* to increase the production of oxidants (184). Thus, the relevant mechanism of protection by thromboxane antagonists and thromboxane synthetase inhibitors may be due to inhibition of neutrophil activation at the site of tissue injury.

The potential for directly affecting relevant neutrophil functions during reperfusion of previously ischemic myocardium was demonstrated by Simpson et al. (191). They showed that a monoclonal antibody directed against the plasma membrane adhesive glycoprotein Mo1 (CD11b/CD18; Mac-1; Complement receptor type 3) was a very effective agent for reducing the amount of myocardium that became infarcted in a canine model of myocardial reperfusion injury. This antibody was previously shown to inhibit canine and human neutrophil adhesive interactions such as aggregation *in vitro* (192). Thus, the potential exists for preventing reperfusion injury via a direct inhibition of neutrophil adhesion with monoclonal antibodies or other molecules that interfere with neutrophil adhesive functions.

Agents that are effective for limiting myocardial infarction after reperfusion from animal experiments can be classified into two categories (Table 6) according to known or suspected mechanisms of action. These two categories include agents that scavenge

TABLE 6. *Experimental myocardial reperfusion injury: agents tested* in vivo

Agents reducing infarction by neutrophil suppression	Ref.
Ibuprofen	193
Nafazatrom	194,195
BW755C	196,197
REV-5901	198
"Neutrophil depletion"	179,197,199,200
Aprotinin	201
Perfluorochemical	202
PGE_1	187
PGI_2	188
Iloprost	189,190
Defibrotide	203,204
Monoclonal antibody 904	191
Lidocaine	205
Thromboxane antagonists	181,186
Thromboxane synthetase inhibitors	182,186

Agents reducing infarction by scavenging free radicals or other oxidents	
SOD	176,177,206
Mercaptopropionylglycine	207
2-Octadecylascorbic acid	208
Dimethylthiourea	209
Deferoxamine	210
Cytochrome c	211
Allopurinol	212
Coenzyme Q_{10}	213

Other potential mechanisms	
Nicorandil (bradycardia)	214
KT-362 (intracellular Ca^{2+} antagonist)	215,216
Inhibition of phospholipase A_2	217

Agents not effective for reducing myocardial infarct size	
Aspirin	218
Peptidoleukotriene antagonists	219

free radicals and oxidants or agents that affect neutrophil function. Thus, future directions for adjunctive treatment of acute myocardial infarction will address not only the problems of recanalization and reocclusion but will also address issues of infarct extension and the roles of free radicals and neutrophils in the process of acute myocardial infarction.

REFERENCES

1. Heberden W. Some accounts of a disorder of the breast. *M Trans R Coll Physicians* (London) 1772;2:59–67.

2. Keefer CS, Resnick WH. Angina pectoris: a syndrome caused by anoxemia of the myocardium. *Arch Intern Med* 1928;41:769–807.
3. Streeter DC, Spotnitz HM, Patel DU, Ross J, Sonnenblick EH. Fiber orientation in the canine left ventricle during diastole and systole. *Circ Res* 1969;24:339–347.
4. Sones FM, Shirey EK. Cine coronary arteriography. *Mod Concepts Cardiovasc Dis* 1962; 31:735–738.
5. Favaloro RG. Saphenous vein graft in the surgical treatment of coronary artery disease: operative technique. *J Thorac Cardiovasc Surg* 1969;58:178–185.
6. Johnson WD, Flemma RJ, Lepley T, Ellison EH. Extended treatment of severe coronary artery disease: a total surgical approach. *Ann Surg* 1969;170:460–470.
7. Scharper W. *The collateral circulation of the heart.* New York: American Elsevier, 1971.
8. Noble D. *The initiation of the heartbeat.* 2nd

ed. New York: Clarendon Press, Oxford University Press, 1979.

9. Jennings RB. Early phase of myocardial ischemic injury and infarction. *Am J Cardiol* 1969;24:753–765.

10. Sonnenblick EH, Ross J, Braunwald E. Oxygen consumption of the heart: newer concepts of its multifactorial determination. *Am J Cardiol* 1968;22:328–335.

11. St. John Sutton MG, Plappert TA, Hirshfeld JW, Reichek N. Assessment of left ventricular mechanics in patients with asymptomatic aortic regurgitation: a two-dimensional echocardiographic study. *Circulation* 1984;69:259–268.

12. Bing RJ. Cardiac metabolism. *Physiol Rev* 1965;45:171–213.

13. Mitchell JH, Blomqvist G. Maximal oxygen uptake. *N Engl J Med* 1971;284:1018–1022.

14. Feigl EO. Reflex parasympathetic coronary vasodilation elicited from cardiac receptors in the dog. *Circ Res* 1975;37:175–182.

15. Furchgott RF, Zawadzki JV. The obligatory role of endothelial cells in the relaxation of arterial smooth muscle by acetylcholine. *Nature* 1980;288:373–376.

16. Furchgott RF, Zawadzki JV, Cherry PD. Role of endothelium in the vasodilator response to acetylcholine. In: Vanhoutte PM, Leusen I, eds. *Vasodilation*. New York: Raven Press, 1981;49–66.

17. Cherry PD, Furchgott RF, Zawadzki JV, Jothianandan D. Role of endothelial cells in relaxation of isolated arteries by bradykinin. *Proc Natl Acad Sci USA* 1982;72:2106–2110.

18. Gruetter CA, Barry BK, McNamara DB, Gruetter DY, Dadowitz PJ, Ignarro LJ. Relaxation of bovine coronary artery and activation of coronary arterial guanylate cyclase by nitric oxide, nitroprusside and a carcinogenic nitrosoamine. *J Cyclic Nucleotide Protein Phosphor Res* 1979;5:211–224.

19. Murad F, Arnold WP, Mittal CK, Braughler JM. Properties and regulation of guanylate cyclase and some proposed functions for cyclic GMP. *Adv Cyclic Nucleotide Protein Phosphoryl Res* 1979;11:175–204.

20. Rapoport RM, Murad F. Agonist-induced endothelium-dependent relaxations in rat thoracic aorta may be mediated through cGMP. *Circ Res* 1983;52:352–357.

21. Diamond J, Chu ES. Possible role for cyclic GMP in endothelium-dependent relaxation of rabbit aorta by acetylcholine. Comparison with nitroglycerin. *Res Commun Chem Pathol Pharmacol* 1983;41:369–381.

22. Furchgott RF, Cherry PD, Zawadzki JV. Endothelial cells as mediators of vasodilation of arteries. *J Cardiovasc Pharmacol* 1984;6(Suppl 2):S336–S344.

23. Ignarro LJ, Burke TM, Wood KS, Wolin MS, Kadowitz PJ. Association between cyclic GMP accumulation and acetycholine-elicited relaxation of bovine intrapulmonary artery. *J Pharmacol Exp Ther* 1984;228:682–690.

24. Furchgott RF. Endothelium-dependent relaxation in systemic arteries. In: Vanhoutte PM, ed. *Relaxing and contracting factors*. Clifton, NJ: Humana, 1988;1–26.

25. Forstermann U, Mulsch A, Bohme E, Busse R. Stimulation of soluble guanylate cyclase by an acetycholine-induced endothelium-derived factor from rabbit and canine arteries. *Circ Res* 1988;58:531–538.

26. Ignarro LJ, Harbison RG, Wood KS, Kadowitz PJ. Activation of purified soluble guanylate cyclase by endothelium-derived relaxing factor from intrapulmonary artery and vein: stimulation by acetylcholine, bradykinin and arachidonic acid. *J Pharmacol Exp Ther* 1986; 237:893–900.

27. Rapoport RM, Draznin MB, Murad F. Endothelium-dependent relaxation in rat aorta may be mediated through cyclic GMP-dependent protein phosphorylation. *Nature* 1983;306:174–176.

28. Martin W, Villani GM, Jothianandan D, Furchgott RF. Selective blockade of endothelium-dependent and glyceryl trinitrate-induced relaxation by hemoglobin and by methylene blue in the rabbit aorta. *J Pharmacol Exp Ther* 1985;232:708–716.

29. Moncada S, Palmer RMJ, Gryglewski RJ. Mechanism of action of some inhibitors of endothelium-derived relaxing factor. *Proc Natl Acad Sci USA* 1986;83:9164–9168.

30. Rubanyi GM, Vanhoutte PM. Superoxide anions and hyperoxia inactivate endothelium-derived relaxing factor. *Am J Physiol* 1986; 250:H822–H827.

31. Katusic Z, Vanhoutte PM. Superoxide anion is an endothelium-derived contracting factor. *Am J Physiol* 1989;257:H33–H37.

32. Christie MJ, Lewis MJ. The pig coronary artery is more responsive to endothelium-derived relaxing factor (EDRF) than the rabbit aorta. *Br J Pharmacol* 1987;91:318.

33. Griffith TM, Henderson AH, Hughes-Edwards D, Lewis MJ. Isolated perfused rabbit coronary artery and aortic strip preparations: the role of endothelium-derived relaxant factor. *J Physiol (Lond)* 1984;351:13–24.

34. Collins P, Chappell SP, Griffith TM, Lewis MJ, Henderson AH. Differences in basal endothelium-derived relaxing factor activity in different artery types. *J Cardiovasc Pharmacol* 1986;8:1158–1162.

35. Holtz J, Forstermann U, Pohl U, Giesler M, Bassenge E. Flow-dependent, endothelium-mediated dilation of epicardial coronary arteries in conscious dogs: Effects of cyclooxygenase inhibition. *J Cardiovasc Pharmacol* 1984;6:1161–1169.

36. Pohl U, Busse R, Kuon E, Bassenge E. Pulsatile perfusion stimulates the release of endothelial autocoids. *J Appl Cardiol* 1986;1:215–235.

37. Ingarro LJ, Byrns RE, Buga GM, Wood KS. Endothelium-derived relaxing factor from pulmonary artery and vein possesses pharmacologic and chemical properties identical to those of nitric oxide. *Circ Res* 1987;61:866–879.

38. Schultz K-D, Schultz K, Schultz G. Sodium nitroprusside and other smooth muscle relaxants increase cyclic GMP levels in rat ductus deferens. *Nature* 1977;265:750–751.

39. Furlong B, Henderson AH, Lewis MJ, Smith JA. Endothelium derived relaxing factor inhibits in vitro platelet aggregation. *Br J Pharmacol* 1987;90:687–692.

40. Verbeuren TJ, Jordaens F, Zonnekeyn L, Van Hove CE, Coene M-C, Herman AG. Endothelium-dependent and endothelium-independent contractions and relaxations in isolated arteries of control and hypercholesterolaemic rabbits. *Circ Res* 1986;58:552–564.

41. Forstermann U, Mugge A, Alheid U, Haverich A, Frolich JC. Selective attenuation of endothelium-mediated vasodilation in atherosclerotic human coronary arteries. *Circ Res* 1988;62:185–190.

42. Van de Voorde J, Leusen I. Endothelium-dependent and independent relaxation of aortic rings from hypertensive rats. *Am J Physiol* 1986;250:H711–H717.

43. Shirasaki Y, Su C, Lee TJ-F, Kolm P, Cline WH, Nickols GA. Endothelial modulation of vascular relaxation to nitrovasodilators in aging and hypertension. *J Pharmacol Exp Ther* 1986;239:861–866.

44. Oyama Y, Kawasaki H, Hattori Y, Kanno M. Attenuation of endothelium-dependent relaxation in aorta from diabetic rats. *Eur J Pharmacol* 1986;131:75–78.

45. Katsuki S, Arnold W, Mittal C, Murad F. Stimulation of guanylate cyclase by sodium nitroprusside, nitroglycerin and nitric oxide in various tissue preparations and comparison to the effects of sodium azide and hydroxylamine. *J Cyclic Nucleotide Protein Phosphor Res* 1977;3:23–25.

46. Ignarro LJ, Lippton H, Edwards JC, et al. Mechanism of vascular smooth muscle relaxation by organic nitrates, nitrites, nitroprusside and nitric oxide: evidence for the involvement of S-nitrosothiols as active intermediates. *J Pharmacol Exp Ther* 1981;218:739–749.

47. Palmer RMJ, Ferrige AG, Moncada S. Nitric oxide release accounts for the biological activity of endothelium-derived relaxing factor. *Nature* 1987;327:524–526.

48. Ignarro LJ, Buga GM, Wood KS, Byrns RE, Chaudhuri G. Endothelium-derived relaxing factor produced and released from artery and vein is nitric oxide. *Proc Natl Acad Sci USA* 1987;84:9265–9269.

49. Hutchinson PJA, Palmer RMJ, Moncada S. Comparative pharmacology of EDRF and nitric oxide on vascular strips. *Eur J Pharmacol* 1987;141:445–451.

50. Ignarro LJ, Byrns RE, Buga GM, Wood KS, Chaudhuri G. Pharmacological evidence that endothelium-derived relaxing factor is nitric oxide: use of pyrogallol and superoxide dismutase to study endothelium-dependent and nitric oxide-elicited vascular smooth muscle relaxation. *J Pharmacol Exp Ther* 1988;244:181–189.

51. Ignarro LJ, Kadowitz PJ. The pharmacological and physiological role of cyclic GMP in vascular smooth muscle relaxation. *Annu Rev Pharmacol Toxicol* 1985;25:171–191.

52. Schmidt HHHW, Klein MM, Niroomand F, Bohme E. Is arginine a physiological precursor of endothelium-derived nitric oxide? *Eur J Pharmacol* 1988;148:293–295.

53. Ignarro LJ, Gold ME, Buga GM, et al. Basic polyamino acids rich in arginine, lysine, or ornithine cause both enhancement of and refractoriness to formation of endothelium-derived nitric oxide in pulmonary artery and vein. *Circ Res* 1989;64:315–329.

54. Chen W-Z, Palmer RMJ, Moncada S. Release of nitric oxide from rabbit aorta. *J Vasc Med Biol* 1989;1:2–6.

55. Amezcua JL, Dusting GJ, Palmer RMJ, Moncada S. Acetylcholine induces vasodilatation in the rabbit isolated heart through the release of nitric oxide, the endogenous nitrovasodilator. *Br J Pharmacol* 1988;95:830–834.

56. Bassenge E, Busse R, Pohl U. Abluminal release and asymmetrical response of the rabbit arterial wall to endothelium-derived relaxing factor. *Circ Res* 1988;61(suppl II):II68–II73.

57. Furchgott RF, Vanhoutte PM. Endothelium-derived relaxing and contracting factors. *FASEB J* 1989;3:2007–2018.

58. Ignarro LJ. Biological actions and properties of endothelium-derived nitric oxide formed and released from artery and vein. *Circ Res* 1989;65:1–21.

59. DeMey JG, Vanhoutte PM. Heterogenous behavior of the canine arterial and venous wall: importance of the endothelium. *Circ Res* 1982;51:439–447.

60. DeMey JG, Vanhoutte PM. Anoxia and endothelium-dependent reactivity of the canine femoral artery. *J Physiol (Lond)* 1983;335:65–74.

61. Agricola K, Rubanyi G, Paul RJ, Highsmith RF. Characterization of a potent coronary artery vasoconstrictor produced by endothelial cells in culture. *Fed Proc* 1984;43:899.

62. Hickey KA, Rubanyi G, Paul RJ, Highsmith RF. Characterization of a coronary vasoconstrictor produced by endothelial cells in culture. *Am J Physiol* 1985;248:C550–C560.

63. Yanagisawa M, Kurihara H, Kimura S, et al. A novel potent vasoconstrictor peptide produced by vascular endothelial cells. *Nature* 1988;332:411–415.

64. Itoh Y, Yanagisawa M, Ohkubo S, et al. Cloning and sequence analysis of cDNA encoding the precursor of a human endothelium-derived vasoconstrictor peptide, endothelin: identity of human and porcine endothelin. *FEBS Lett* 1988;231:440–444.

65. Yanagisawa M, Inoue A, Ishikawa T, et al. Primary structure, synthesis, and biological activity of rat endothelin, an endothelium-derived vasoconstrictor peptide. *Proc Natl Acad Sci USA* 1988;85:6964–6967.

66. Miyazaki H, Kondoh M, Watanabe H, et al. Identification of the endothelin-1 receptor

in chick heart. *J Cardiovasc Pharmacol* 1989; 13(Suppl 5):S155–S156.

67. Berne RM, Rubio R. Coronary circulation. In: Berne RM, Sperelakis N, Geiger SR, eds. *Handbook of physiology, Section 2. The cardiovascular system.* Bethesda, MD: American Physiological Society, 1979;924.

68. Drury AN, Szent-Gyorgyi A. The physiological activity of adenine compounds with special reference to their action upon the mammalian heart. *J Physiol (Lond)* 1929;68:213–237.

69. Lindner F, Rigler R. Uber die Beeinflussung der Weite der Herzkranzgefasse durch Produckte des Zellkernstoffwechsels. *Pflugers Arch* 1931;226:679–708.

70. Rubio R, Berne RM. Release of adenosine by the normal myocardium in dogs and its relationship to the regulation of coronary resistance. *Circ Res* 1969;25:407–415.

71. Bardenheuer H, Schrader J. Relationship between myocardial oxygen consumption, coronary flow and adenosine release in an improved isolated working heart preparation of guinea pigs. *Circ Res* 1983;52:263–271.

72. Nees S, Herzog V, Becker BF, et al. The coronary endothelium: a highly active metabolic barrier for adenosine. *Basic Res Cardiol* 1985;80:515–529.

73. Berne RM, Rubio R. Coronary circulation. In: Berne RN, Sperelakis N, eds. *Handbook of physiology, the coronary system.* Washington, D.C.: American Physiological Society, 1979; 873–952.

74. Berne RM. The role of adenosine in the regulation of coronary blood flow. *Circ Res* 1980;47:807–813.

75. Berne RM, Rall TW, Rubio R, eds. *Regulatory function of adenosine.* Boston: Martinus Nijhoff, 1983.

76. Kusachi S, Thompson RD, Olsson RA. Ligand selectivity of dog coronary adenosine receptor resembles that of adenylate cyclase stimulatory (Ra) receptors. *J Pharmacol Exp Ther* 1983;227:316–321.

77. Kurtz A. Adenosine stimulates guanylate cyclase activity in vascular smooth muscle cells. *J Biol Chem* 1987;262:6296–6300.

78. Fenton RA, Bruttig SP, Rubio R, et al. Effect of adenosine on calcium uptake by intact and cultured vascular smooth muscle. *Am J Physiol* 1982;242:H797–H804.

79. Amsterdam EA, Hughes JL, DeMaria AN, Zelis R, Mason DT. Indirect assessment of myocardial oxygen consumption in the evaluation of mechanisms and therapy of angina pectoris. *Am J Cardiol* 1974;33:737–743.

80. Gregg DE, Patterson RE. Functional importance of the coronary collaterals. *N Engl J Med* 1980;303:1404–1406.

81. Becker LC. Conditions for vasodilator-induced coronary steal in experimental myocardial ischemia. *Circulation* 1978;57:1103–1110.

82. Forman R, Kirk ES, Downey JM, Sonnenblick EH. Nitroglycerin and heterogeneity of myocardial blood flow. Reduced subendocardial blood flow and ventricular contractile force. *J Clin Invest* 1978;52:905–911.

83. Bonow RO, Kent KM, Rosing DR, et al. Exercise-induced ischemia in mildly symptomatic patients with coronary artery disease and preserved left ventricular function: identification of subgroups at risk of death during medical therapy. *N Engl J Med* 1984;311:1339–1345.

84. Prinzmetal M, Ekmekci A, Kennamer R, Kwoczynski J, Shubin H, Toyoshima H. Variant form of angina pectoris. Previously undelineated syndrome. *JAMA* 1960;174:102–108.

85. Winbury MM, Howe BB, Weiss HR. Effect of nitroglycerin and dipyridamole on epicardial and endocardial oxygen tension—further evidence for redistribution of myocardial blood flow. *J Pharmacol Exp Ther* 1971;176:184–199.

86. Swain JL, Parker JP, McHale PA, Greenfield JC Jr. Effects of nitroglycerin and propranolol on the distribution of transmural myocardial blood flow during ischemia in the absence of hemodynamic changes in the unanesthetized dog. *J Clin Invest* 1979;63:947–953.

87. Mehta J, Pepine CJ. Effects of sublingual nitroglycerin on regional flow in patients with and without coronary disease. *Circulation* 1978; 58:803–807.

88. Brown G, Bolson E, Petersen RB, Pierce CD, Dodge HT. The mechanism of nitroglycerin action. Stenosis vasodilation as a major component of drug response. *Circulation* 1981;64: 1089–1097.

89. Vatner SF, Higgins CB, Millard RW, Franklin D. Direct and reflex effects of nitroglycerin on coronary and left ventricular dynamics in conscious dogs. *J Clin Invest* 1972;51:2872–2882.

90. Thadani U. Current status of nitrates in angina pectoris. *Mod Concepts of Cardiovasc Dis* 1987;56:49–54.

91. Winniford MD, Kennedy PL, Wells PJ, Hillis LD. Potentiation of nitroglycerin induced coronary dilation with N-acetylcysteine. *Circulation* 1986;73:138–142.

92. Horowitz JD, Antman EM, Lorell BH, Barry WH, Smith TW. Potentiation of the cardiovascular effects of nitroglycerin by N-acetylcysteine. *Circulation* 1983;68:1247–1253.

93. May DC, Popma JJ, Black WH, et al. In vivo induction and reversal of nitroglycerin tolerance in human coronary arteries. *N Engl J Med* 1987;317:805–809.

94. Markis JE, Gorlin R, Mills RM, Williams RA, Schweitzer P, Ransil BJ. Sustained effects of orally administered isosorbide dinitrate on exercise performance of patients with angina pectoris. *Am J Cardiol* 1979;43:265–271.

95. Thadani U, Fung HL, Darke AC, Parker J. Oral isosorbide dinitrate in the treatment of angina pectoris: dose-response relationship and duration of action during acute therapy. *Circulation* 1980;62:491–502.

96. Parker JO, Farrell B, Lahey KA, Moe G. Effect of intervals between doses on the development of tolerance to isosorbide dinitrate. *N Engl J Med* 1987;316:1440–1444.

97. Crean PA, Ribeiro P, Crea F, Davies GJ, Ratcliffe D, Maseri A. Failure of transdermal nitroglycerin to improve chronic stable angina: a randomized, placebo-controlled, double-blind, double crossover trial. *Am Heart J* 1984; 108:1494–1500.

98. Zimrin D, Reichek N, Bogin K, Cameron S, Douglas P, Fung H-L. Antianginal effects of I.V. nitroglycerin. *Circulation* 1985;72(Suppl 3):III–460A.

99. Ahlquist RP. A study of the adrenotropic receptors. *Am J Physiol* 1948;153:586–600.

100. Van Zwieten PA. The role of adrenoceptors in circulatory and metabolic regulation. *Am Heart J* 1988;116:1384–1392.

101. Shand DG. Clinical pharmacology of the beta-blocking drugs: implications for the postinfarction patient. *Circulation* 1983;67(Suppl I):I2–I5.

102. Barnes PJ. Neural control of human airways in health and disease. *Am Rev Respir Dis* 1986;134:1289–1314.

103. Grant RHE, Keelan P, Kernahan RJ, Leonard JC, Nancekievilli L, Sinclair K. Multicenter trial of propranolol in angina pectoris. *Am J Cardiol* 1966;18:361–365.

104. Rodda BE. The timolol myocardial infarction study: an evaluation of selected variables. *Circulation* 1983;67(Suppl I):I101–I106.

105. β-blocker Heart Attack Trial Research Group. A randomized trial of propranolol in patients with acute myocardial infarction. I. Mortality results. *JAMA* 1982;247:1707–1714.

106. Goldman L, Sia STB, Cook EF, Rutherford JD, Weinstein MC. Costs and effectiveness of routine therapy with long-term β-adrenergic antagonists after acute myocardial infarction. *N Engl J Med* 1988;319:152–157.

107. Frishman WH. Multifactorial actions of beta-adrenergic blocking drugs in ischemic heart disease: current concepts. *Circulation* 1983; 67(Suppl I):I11–I18.

108. Maseri A, Chierchia S. Coronary artery spasm: demonstration, definition, diagnosis and consequences. *Prog Cardiovasc Dis* 1982;25:169–192.

109. Parodi O, Simonetti I, L'Abbate A, Maseri A. Verapamil vs propranolol for angina at rest. *Am J Cardiol* 1982;50:923–928.

110. Quyyumi AA, Crake T, Wright CM, Mockus LJ, Fox KM. Medical treatment of patients with severe exertional and rest angina: double-blind comparison of β-blocker, calcium antagonist, and nitrate. *Br Heart J* 1987;57:505–511.

111. Deanfield JE, Maseri A, Selwyn AP, et al. Myocardial ischemia during daily life in patients with stable angina: its relation to symptoms and heart rate changes. *Lancet* 1983; 2:753–758.

112. Rocco MB, Nabel E, Mead K, Barry J, Selwyn AP. Effects of beta versus alpha/beta blockade on transient myocardial ischemia. *Circulation* 1987;76(Suppl IV):277.

113. Chierchia S, Glazier JJ, Gerosa S. A single-blind, placebo-controlled study of effects of atenolol on transient ischemia in 'mixed' angina. *Am J Cardiol* 1987;60:36A–40A.

114. Lofdahl CG, Svedmyr N. Cardioselectivity of atenolol and metoprolol: a study in asthmatic patients. *Eur J Respir Dis* 1981;62:396–404.

115. Ellis ME, Sahay JN, Chatterjee SS, Cruickshank JM, Ellis SH. Cardioselectivity of atenolol in asthmatic patients. *Eur J Clin Pharmacol* 1981;21:173–176.

116. Weksler B, Gillick M, Pink J. Effect of propranolol on platelet function. *Blood* 1977; 149:185–196.

117. Rubegni M, Provvedi D, Bellini PG, Bandellini C, DeMauro G. Propranolol and platelet aggregation. *Circulation* 1975;52:964–965.

118. Frishman WH, Silverman R. Clinical pharmacology of the new β-adrenergic blocking drugs. Part 2. Physiologic and metabolic effects. *Am Heart J* 1979;97:797–807.

119. Woosley RL, Kornhauser D, Smith RL, et al. Suppression of chronic ventricular arrhythmias with propranolol. *Circulation* 1979;60:819–827.

120. Campbell WB, Callahan KS, Johnson AR, Graham RM. Anti-platelet activity of β-adrenergic antagonists: inhibition of thromboxane synthesis and platelet aggregation in patients receiving long-term propranolol treatment. *Lancet* 1981;2:1382–1390.

121. Deacon SP, Barnett D. Comparison of atenolol and propranolol during insulin induced hypoglycemia. *Br Med J* 1976;2:272–273.

122. Cruickshank JM. The clinical importance of cardioselectivity and lipophilicity in beta blockers. *Am Heart J* 1980;100:160–178.

123. Lehtonen A. Effects of beta-blockers on plasma lipids during antihypertensive therapy. *J Cardiovasc Pharmacol* 1985;7:S110–S114.

124. Barboriak JJ, Freidberg HD. Propranolol and hypertriglyceridemia. *Atherosclerosis* 1973;17: 31–35.

125. Grundy SM. Cholesterol and coronary heart disease—a new era. *JAMA* 1986;228:2849–2858.

126. Gordon T, Castelli WP, Hjortland MC, Kannel WB, Dawber TR. High density lipoprotein as a protective factor against coronary heart disease. The Framingham Study. *Am J Med* 1977;62:707–714.

127. Thadani U, Davidson C, Singleton W, Taylor SH. Comparison of the immediate effects of five β-adrenoreceptor blocking drugs with different ancillary properties in angina pectoris. *N Engl J Med* 1979;300:750–755.

128. Miller RR, Olson HG, Amsterdam EA, Mason DT. Propranolol withdrawal rebound phenomenon: exacerbation of coronary events after abrupt cessation of anti-anginal therapy. *N Engl J Med* 1975;293:416–418.

129. Frishman WH, Christadoulou J, Weksler B, Smithen C, Killip T, Schjeidt S. Abrupt propranolol withdrawal in angina pectoris: effects on platelet aggregation and exercise tolerance. *Am Heart J* 1978;95:169–179.

130. Alderman EL, Coltart DJ, Wettach GE. Coronary artery syndrome after sudden propranolol withdrawal. *Ann Intern Med* 1974;81:925–927.
131. Braunwald E. Mechanism of action of calcium channel blocking agents. *N Engl J Med* 1982;307:1618–1627.
132. O'Rourke RA. Calcium-entry blockade: basic concepts and clinical implications. *Circulation* 1987;75(Suppl V):V1–V194.
133. Frishman WH, Klein NA, Strom JA, et al. Superiority of verapamil to propranolol in stable angina pectoris; a double-blind randomized crossover trial. *Circulation* 1982;65(Suppl 1):I51–I59.
134. Lynch P, Dargie H., Krikler S, Krikler D. Objective assessment of antianginal treatment: a double-blind comparison of propranolol, nifedipine, and their combination. *Br Med J* 1980;281:184–187.
135. Hung J, Lamb IH, Connolly SJ, Jutzy KR, Goris ML, Schroeder JS. The effect of diltiazem and propranolol, alone and in combination, on exercise performance and left ventricular function with stable effort angina: a double-blind, randomized, and placebo-controlled study. *Circulation* 1983;68:560–567.
136. Winniford MD, Johnson SM, Mauritson DR, et al. Verapamil therapy for patients with prinzmetal's variant angina: comparison with placebo and nifedipine. *Am J Cardiol* 1982;50:913–918.
137. Schroeder JS, Feldman RL, Giles TD, et al. Multiclinic controlled trial of diltiazem for prinzmetal's angina. *Am J Med* 1982;72:227–232.
138. The Diltiazem Reinfarction Study Groups. Diltiazem and reinfarction in patients with non-Q wave myocardial infarction. *N Engl J Med* 1986;315:423–429.
139. The Multicenter Diltiazem Postinfarction Trial Research Group. The effect of diltiazem on mortality and reinfarction after myocardial infarction. *N Engl J Med* 1988;319:385–392.
140. Packer M. Drug therapy: combined beta-adrenergic and calcium-entry blockade in angina pectoris. *N Engl J Med* 1989;320:709–718.
141. Davies MJ, Thomas AC, Knapman PA, Hangartner JR. Intramyocardial platelet aggregation in patients with unstable angina suffering sudden ischemic cardiac death. *Circulation* 1986;73:418–427.
142. Meuller HS, Rao PS, Greenberg MA, et al. Systemic and transcardiac platelet activity in acute myocardial infarction in man: resistance to prostacyclin. *Circulation* 1985;72:133–1345.
143. Golino P, Ashton JH, Buja LM, et al. Local platelet activation causes vasoconstriction of large epicardial canine coronary arteries in vivo. *Circulation* 1989;79:154–166.
144. DeWood MA, Spores J, Notske R, et al. Prevalence of total coronary occlusion during the early hours of transmural myocardial infarction. *N Engl J Med* 1980;303:897–902.
145. Ridolfi RL, Hutchins GM. The relationship between coronary artery lesions and myocardial infarcts: ulceration of atherosclerotic plaques precipitating coronary thrombosis. *Am Heart J* 1977;93:468–486.
146. Ambrose JA, Winters SL, Arora RR, et al. Angiographic evolution of coronary artery morphology in unstable angina. *J Am Coll Cardiol* 1986;7:472–487.
147. Vetrovec G, Crowley MJ, Overton H, Richardson DW. Intracoronary thrombus in syndromes of unstable myocardial ischemia. *Am Heart J* 1986;102:1202–1208.
148. Lewis HD, Davis JW, Archibald DG, et al. Protective effects of aspirin against acute myocardial infarction and death in men with unstable angina. Results of a Veterans Administration Cooperative Study. *N Engl J Med* 1983;309:396–403.
149. Cairns JA, Gent M, Singer J, et al. Aspirin, sulfinpyrazone, or both in unstable angina: results of a Canadian multicenter trial. *N Engl J Med* 1985;313:1369–1375.
150. Telford AM, Wilson E. Trial of heparin versus atenolol in prevention of myocardial infarction in intermediate coronary syndrome. *Lancet* 1981;1:1225–1228.
151. Theroux P, Ouimet H, McCans J, et al. Aspirin, heparin or both to treat acute unstable angina. *N Engl J Med* 1988;319:1105–1111.
152. Sherman CT, Litvack F, Grundfest W, et al. Coronary angioscopy in patients with unstable angina pectoris. *N Engl J Med* 1986;315:913–919.
153. Gold HK, Johns JA, Leinbach RC, et al. A randomized, blinded, placebo-controlled trial of recombinant human tissue-type plasminogen activator in patients with unstable angina pectoris. *Circulation* 1987;75:1192–1199.
154. DeFeyter PJ, Serruys PW, Vanden Brand M, et al. Emergency coronary angioplasty in refractory unstable angina. *N Engl J Med* 1985;313:342–346.
155. Schwartz L, Bourassa MG, Lesperance J, et al. Aspirin and dipyridamole in the prevention of restenosis after percutaneous transluminal coronary angioplasty. *N Engl J Med* 1988;318:1714–1719.
156. Sheehan FH, Braunwald E, Canner P, et al. The effect of intravenous thrombolytic therapy on left ventricular function: a report on tissue-type plasminogen activator and streptokinase from the Thrombolysis in Myocardial Infarction (TIMI Phase I) Trial. *Circulation* 1987;75:817–829.
157. Simoons M, Brand M, Zwaans C, et al. Improved survival after early thrombolysis in acute myocardial infarction. *Lancet* 1985;2:578–581.
158. Gruppo Italiano Per lo Studio Della Streptochinasi Nell'Infarto Micardio (GISSI). Effectiveness of intravenous thrombolytic treatment in acute myocardial infarction. *Lancet* 1986;1:397–401.
159. Dalen JE, Gore J, Braunwald E, et al. Six- and twelve-month follow-up of the phase 1 throm-

bolysis in myocardial infarction. *Am J Cardiol* 1988;62:179–185.

160. Topol EJ, George BS, Kereiakes DJ, et al. A multicenter randomized controlled trial of intravenous tissue plasminogen activator and early intravenous heparin in acute myocardial infarction. *J Am Coll Cardiol* 1988;11:232A.

161. Harrison DG, Ferguson DW, Collins SM, et al. Rethrombosis after reperfusion with streptokinase: importance of geometry of residual lesions. *Circulation* 1984;69:991–999.

162. Shaer DH, Ross AM, Wasserman AG. Reinfarction, recurrent angina and reocclusion after thrombolytic therapy. *Circulation* 1987; 76(Suppl II):II57–II62.

163. Guerci AD, Gerstenblith G, Brinker JA, et al. A randomized trial of intravenous tissue plasminogen activator for acute myocardial infarction with subsequent randomization to elective coronary angioplasty. *N Engl J Med* 1987;317:1613–1618.

164. Topol EJ, Califf RM, George BS, et al. A randomized trial of immediate versus delayed elective angioplasty after intravenous tissue plasminogen activator in acute myocardial infarction. *N Engl J Med* 1987;317:581–588.

165. O'Neill WW, Timmis CG, Bourdillon PD, et al. A prospective randomized clinical trial of intracoronary streptokinase versus coronary angioplasty for acute myocardial infarction. *N Engl J Med* 1986;314:812–818.

166. Lee L, Bates ER, Pitt B, Walton JA, Laufer N, O'Neill WW. Percutaneous transluminal coronary angioplasty improves survival in acute myocardial infarction complicated by cardiogenic shock. *Circulation* 1988;78:1345–1351.

167. ISIS-2 (Second International Study of Infarct Survival) Collaborative Group. Randomized trial of intravenous streptokinase, oral aspirin, both, or neither among 17,187 cases of suspected acute myocardial infarction: ISIS-2. *Lancet* 1988;2:349–360.

168. Anonymous. Aspirin after myocardial infarction (Editorial). *Lancet* 1980;I:1172–1173.

169. The Steering Committee of the Physicians' Health Study Group. Preliminary report: findings from the aspirin component of the ongoing physicians' health study. *N Engl J Med* 1988;318:262–264.

170. Braunwald E. Thrombolytic reperfusion of acute myocardial infarction: resolved and unresolved issues. *J Am Coll Cardiol* 1988; 12:85A–92A.

171. Coller BS, Folts JD, Scudder LE, Smith SR. Antithrombotic effect of a monoclonal antibody to the platelet glycoprotein IIb/IIIa receptor in an experimental animal model. *Blood* 1986;68:783–786.

172. Gold HK, Coller BS, Yasuda T, et al. Rapid and sustained coronary artery recanalization with combined bolus injection of recombinant tissue-type plasminogen activator and monoclonal antiplatelet GPIIb/IIIa antibody in a canine preparation. *Circulation* 1988;77:670–677.

173. Hanson SR, Pareti FI, Ruggeri ZM, et al. Effects of monoclonal antibodies against the platelet glycoprotein IIb/IIIa complex on thrombosis and hemostasis in the baboon. *J Clin Invest* 1988; 81:149–158.

174. Badimon L, Badimon JJ, Chesebro JH, Fuster V. Inhibition of thrombus formation: blockage of adhesive glycoprotein mechanism versus blockage of the cyclooxygenase pathway. *J Am Coll Cardiol* 1988;11:30A.

175. Jolly SR, Kane WJ, Bailie WB, Abrams GD, Lucchesi BR. Canine myocardial reperfusion injury: its reduction by the combined administration of superoxide dismutase and catalase. *Circ Res* 1984;54:227–285.

176. Werns SW, Shea MJ, Driscoll EM, et al. The independent effects of oxygen radical scavengers on canine infarct size: reduction by superoxide dismutase but not catalase. *Circ Res* 1985;56:895–898.

177. Ambrosio G, Becker LC, Hutchins GM, Weisman HF, Weisfeldt ML. Reduction in experimental infarct size by recombinant human superoxide dismutase: insights into the pathophysiology of reperfusion injury. *Circulation* 1986;74:1424–1433.

178. Zweier JL, Flaherty JT, Weisfeldt ML. Direct measurement of free radical generation following reperfusion of ischemic myocardium. *Proc Natl Acad Sci USA* 1987;84:1404–1407.

179. Romson JL, Hook BG, Kunkel SL, Abrams GD, Schork MA, Lucchesi BR. Reduction of the extent of myocardial injury by neutrophil depletion in the dog. *Circulation* 1983;67:1016–1023.

180. Simpson PJ, Fantone JC, Lucchesi BR. Myocardial ischemia and reperfusion injury: oxygen radicals and the role of the neutrophil. In: *Oxygen radicals and tissue injury: proceedings of an Upjohn symposium.* Bethesda, MD: Federation of American Societies for Experimental Biology, 1988;63–77.

181. Mullane KM, Fornabaio D. Thromboxane synthetase inhibitors reduce infarct size by a platelet-dependent, aspirin-sensitive mechanism. *Circ Res* 1988;62:668–678.

182. Grover GJ, Schumacher WA. Effect of the thromboxane A_2 receptor antagonist SQ 30,741 on ultimate myocardial infarct size, reperfusion injury and coronary flow reserve. *J Pharmacol Exp Ther* 1989;248:484–491.

183. Bhat AM, Sacks H, Osborne JA, Lefer AM. Protective effects of the specific thromboxane receptor antagonist, BM-13505, in reperfusion injury following acute myocardial ischemia in cats. *Am Heart J* 1989;117:799–803.

184. Paterson IS, Klausner JM, Goldman G, et al. Thromboxane mediates the ischemia-induced neutrophil oxidative burst. *Surgery* 1989;106:224–229.

185. Smith EF III, Griswold DE, Egan JW, Hillegass LM, DiMartino MJ. Reduction of myocardial damage and polymorphonuclear leukocyte accumulation following coronary artery occlu-

sion and reperfusion by the thromboxane receptor antagonist BM 13.505 *J Cardiovasc Pharmacol* 1989;13:715–722.

186. Nichols WW, Mehta J, Wargovich TJ, Franzini D, Lawson D. Reduced myocardial neutrophil accumulation and infarct size following thromboxane synthetase inhibitor or receptor antagonist. *Angiology* 1989;209–221.

187. Simpson PJ, Mickelson J, Fantone JC, Gallagher KP, Lucchesi BR. Reduction of experimental canine myocardial infarct size with prostaglandin E₁: inhibition of neutrophil migration and activation. *J Pharmacol Exp Ther* 1988;244:619–624.

188. Simpson PJ, Mitsos SE, Ventura A, et al. Prostacyclin protects ischemic reperfused myocardium in the dog by inhibition of neutrophil activation. *Am Heart J* 1987;113:129–137.

189. Simpson PJ, Mickelson JK, Fantone JC, Gallagher KP, Lucchesi BR. Iloprost inhibits neutrophil function in vitro and in vivo and limits experimental infarct size in the canine heart. *Circ Res* 1987;60:666–673.

190. Simpson PJ, Frantone JC, Mickelson JK, Gallagher KP, Lucchesi BR. Identification of a time window for therapy to reduce experimental canine myocardial injury: suppression of neutrophil activation during 72 hours of reperfusion. *Circ Res* 1988;63:1070–1079.

191. Simpson PJ, Todd RF III, Fantone JC, Mickelson JK, Griffin JD, Lucchesi BR. Reduction of experimental canine myocardial reperfusion injury by a monoclonal antibody (anti-Mol, anti-CD11b) that inhibits leukocyte adhesion. *J Clin Invest* 1988;81:624–629.

192. Giger U, Boxer LA, Simpson PJ, Lucchesi BR, Todd RF III. Deficiency of leukocyte glycoproteins Mo1, LFA-1, and Leu M5 in a dog with recurrent bacterial infections: an animal model. *Blood* 1987;69:1622–1630.

193. Romson JL, Hook BG, Rigot VH, Schork MA, Swanson DP, Lucchesi BR. The effect of ibuprofen on accumulation of indium-111-labeled platelets and leukocytes in experimental myocardial infarction. *Circulation* 1982;66:1002–1011.

194. Shea MJ, Murtagh JJ, Jolly SR, Abrams GD, Pitt B, Lucchesi BR. Beneficial effects of nafazatrom on the ischemic reperfused myocardium. *Eur J Pharmacol* 1984;102:63–70.

195. Bednar M, Smith B, Pinto A, Mullane KM. Nafazatrom-induced salvage of ischemic myocardium in anesthetized dogs in mediated through inhibition of neutrophil function. *Circ Res* 1985;57:131–141.

196. Jolly SR, Lucchesi BR. Effect of BW755C in an occlusion reperfusion model of ischemic myocardial injury. *Am Heart J* 1983;106:8–13.

197. Mullane KM, Read N, Salmon JA, Moncada S. Role of leukocytes in acute myocardial infarction in anesthetized dogs: relationship to myocardial salvage by anti-inflammatory drugs. *J Pharmacol Exp Ther* 1984;228:510–522.

198. Mullane K, Hatala MA, Kraemer R, Sessa W, Westlin W. Myocardial salvage induced by Rev-5901: an inhibitor and antagonist of the leukotrienes. *J Cardiovasc Pharmacol* 1987;10:398–406.

199. Engler RL, Schmid-Schönbein GW, Pavelec RS. Leukocyte capillary plugging in myocardial ischemia and reperfusion in the dog. *Am J Pathol* 1983;111:98–111.

200. Jolly SR, Kane WJ, Hook BG, Abrams GD, Kunkel SL, Lucchesi BR. Reduction of myocardial infarct size by neutrophil depletion: effect of duration of occlusion. *Am Heart J* 1986;112:682–690.

201. Hallett MB, Shandall A, Young HL. Mechanism of protection against "reperfusion injury" by aprotinin: roles of polymorphonuclear leukocytes and oxygen radicals. *Biochem Pharmacol* 1985;34:1757–1761.

202. Bajaj AK, Cobb MA, Virmani R, Gay JC, Light RT, Forman MB. Limitation of myocardial reperfusion injury by intravenous perfluorochemicals: role of neutrophil activation. *Circulation* 1989;79:645–656.

203. Thiemermann C, Löbel P, Schrör K. Usefulness of defibrotide in protecting ischemic myocardium from early reperfusion damage. *Am J Cardiol* 1985;56:978–982.

204. Thiemermann C, Thomas GR, Vane JR. Defibrotide reduces infarct size in a rabbit model of experimental myocardial ischemia and reperfusion. *Br J Pharmacol* 1989;97:401–408.

205. Lesnefsky EJ, VanBenthuysen KM, McMurtry IF, Shikes RH, Johnston RB Jr, Horwitz LD. Lidocaine reduces canine infarct size and decreases release of a lipid peroxidation product. *J Cardiovasc Pharmacol* 1989;13:895–901.

206. Tamura Y, Chi L, Driscoll EM, et al. Superoxide dismutase conjugated to polyethylene glycol provides sustained protection against myocardial ischemia/reperfusion injury in canine heart. *Circ Res* 1988;63:944–959.

207. Mitsos SE, Fantone JC, Gallagher KP, et al. Canine myocardial reperfusion injury: protection by a free radical scavenger, N-2-mercaptopropionyl glycine. *J Cardiovasc Pharmacol* 1986;8:978–988.

208. Kuzuya T, Hoshida S, Nishida M, et al. Role of free radicals and neutrophils in canine myocardial reperfusion injury: myocardial salvage by a novel free radical scavenger, 2-octadecylascorbic acid. *Cardiovasc Res* 1989;23:323–330.

209. Portz SJ, Lesnefsky EJ, VanBenthuysen K, et al. Dimethylthiourea, but not dimethylsufoxide, reduces canine myocardial infarct size. *Free Radical Biol Med* 1989;7:53–58.

210. Reddy RR, Kloner RA, Przyklenk K. Early treatment with deferoxamine limits myocardial ischemic/reperfusion injury. *Free Radical Biol Med* 1989;7:45–52.

211. Zalewski A, Goldberg S, Krol R, Maroko PR. The effects of cytochrome C on the extent of myocardial infarction and regional function

of the ischemic myocardium. *Am Heart J* 1987;113:124–129.

212. Werns SW, Shea MJ, Mitsos SE, Lucchesi BR. Reduction of the size of infarction by allopurinol in the ischemic-reperfused canine heart. *Circulation* 1986;73:518–524.

213. Nakamura Y, Takahashi M, Hayashi J, et al. Protection of ischemic myocardium with coenzyme Q10. *Cardiovasc Res* 1982;16:132–137.

214. Endo T, Nejima J, Kiuchi K, et al. Reduction of size of myocardial infarction with nicorandil, a new antianginal drug, after coronary artery occlusion in dogs. *J Cardiovasc Pharmacol* 1988;12:587–592.

215. Pelc LR, Farber NE, Warltier DC, Gross GJ. Reduction of myocardial ischemia-reperfusion injury by KT-362, a new intracellular calcium antagonist in anesthetized dogs. *J Cardiovasc Pharmacol* 1989;13:586–593.

216. Farber NE, Gross GJ. Collateral blood flow following acute coronary artery occlusion: comparison of a new intracellular calcium antagonist (KT-362) and diltiazem. *J Cardiovasc Pharmacol* 1989;14:66–72.

217. Zalewski A, Goldberg S, Maroko PR. The effects of phospholipase A2 inhibition on experimental infarct size, left ventricular hemodynamics and regional myocardial blood flow. *Int J Cardiol* 1988;21:247–257.

218. Flynn PF, Becker WK, Vercellotti GM, et al. Ibuprofen inhibits granulocyte responses to inflammatory mediators: a potential mechanism for reduction of experimental myocardial infarct size. *Inflammation* 1982;8:33–44.

219. Egan JW, Griswold DE, Hillegass LM, et al. Selective antagonism of peptidoleukotriene responses does not reduce myocardial damage or neutrophil accumulation following coronary artery occlusion with reperfusion. *Prostaglandins* 1989;37:597–613.

Cardiovascular Pharmacology, Third Edition, edited by Michael Antonaccio. Raven Press, Ltd., New York © 1990.

Congestive Heart Failure: Pathophysiology and Therapy

Gary S. Francis and Jay N. Cohn

Cardiovascular Division, Department of Medicine, University of Minnesota Medical School; and the Veterans Administration Medical Center, Minneapolis, Minnesota 55417

The escalating costs of heart disease in the United States have increased from $40 billion in 1975 (1) to an estimated $85.2 billion in 1987 (2). Congestive heart failure (CHF) contributes significantly to this amount, being considered the most common diagnosis for patients hospitalized over the age of 65 (3). It afflicts some 2.3 million Americans, with 400,000 new cases diagnosed each year (4). The National Center for Health Care Statistics estimates that the number of hospital discharges for CHF almost tripled between 1970 and 1982, from 570,000 to 1,557,000 (5). In 1981 there were more than 4 million office-based visits for heart failure (6). Despite a marked decline in overall deaths from ischemic heart disease and a dramatic improvement in hypertension control, the mortality rate for heart failure has failed to decline (7).

Virtually all forms of heart disease can lead to heart failure. Coronary artery disease, hypertension, and diabetes mellitus are the dominant precursors of CHF in the United States. Considerable controversy exists regarding an appropriate operational definition of CHF (8). There are two essential components: cardiac dysfunction and reduced exercise tolerance. Heart failure is also characterized by a high incidence of ventricular arrhythmias and shortened life expectancy (Fig. 1). For purposes of this discussion, CHF will be subdivided into diastolic and systolic dysfunction, with the emphasis on systolic dysfunction. Treatment of both the acute and chronic phases of the syndrome will be considered.

DIASTOLIC DYSFUNCTION

When considering the diastolic properties of the intact ventricle, it is important to differentiate factors responsible for alterations in chamber stiffness, as derived from left ventricular diastolic pressure-volume relationships, from factors affecting myocardial stiffness, which are derived from stress-strain characteristics of the left ventricular wall. Myocardial muscle stiffness is the instantaneous ratio of stress to strain at any given point on the curve relating stress to strain. Left ventricular diastolic chamber stiffness refers to the stiffness of the whole ventricle and is expressed as a simple ratio of change in pressure (dP) to change in volume (dV) (Fig. 2).

When left ventricular chamber stiffness is acutely increased, as during acute myocardial infarction, there is a much higher left ventricular end-diastolic pressure at any given end-diastolic volume. The dP/dV relationship is shifted upward and to the left (Fig. 2). Very high end-diastolic pressures

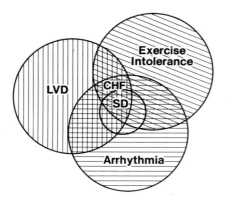

FIG. 1. Diagram showing left ventricular dysfunction (LVD), exercise intolerance, and ventricular arrhythmias as the most common manifestations of the failing heart syndrome. Clinical heart failure (CHF) represents the co-existence of LVD and exercise intolerance. Sudden death (SD) occurs in patients with arrhythmias and predominantly in those with LVD and CHF. (From ref. 8.)

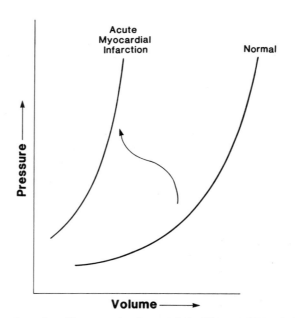

FIG. 2. Left ventricular diastolic stiffness as it refers to the stiffness of the whole ventricular chamber is expressed as the curvilinear relationship between the change in pressure and the change in volume during diastole. Normally there is a very gradual change in pressure as end-diastolic volume increases, because of the inherent compliance of the left ventricle. When the left ventricular compliance is altered to stiffen the chamber, such as occurs in acute myocardial infarction (shown schematically) or left ventricular hypertrophy, the dP/dV relationship is shifted up and to the left, allowing for a much higher end-diastolic pressure for any given diastolic volume. Pulmonary edema can occur despite normal global systolic function.

can cause dyspnea or even pulmonary edema, despite a relatively normal-sized heart and normal global systolic function. This is referred to as "diastolic heart failure," and it can occur during acute myocardial ischemia (with or without chest pain), as a result of left ventricular hypertrophy (LVH), or from chronic myocardial fibrosis related to previous myocardial infarction.

The dP/dV relationship approximates an exponential curve. The slope of dP/dV represents the elastic stiffness of the whole chamber and is useful for detecting changes in wall stiffness. The compliance of the left ventricle is determined by a complex interplay of numerous variables, including relaxation of the ventricle, elasticity, filling of the right ventricle, inertial and viscous properties, the shape of the ventricle, and pericardial constraint (9). Nevertheless, the clinical concept of diastolic dysfunction leading to chronic and/or acute breathlessness is well established and often occurs with intact left ventricular systolic function.

The increasing practice of measuring left ventricular function noninvasively has led to the observation that CHF commonly occurs with intact systolic function (10,11). Current literature suggests that 30% to 40% of patients with CHF referred for echocardiography or radionuclide left ventriculography have "diastolic heart failure." Of course, the prevalence of diastolic heart failure largely depends on how one defines heart failure. In the majority of these patients, diastolic dysfunction is attributed to evidence of LVH, a prolonged early diastolic filling period, and reduced peak diastolic dimension change (12). These measurements are usually made by echocardiography (including Doppler) or volume curves derived from radionuclide ventriculography data. However, many of these noninvasive techniques of measuring diastolic function have not been carefully validated. The precise measurement of left ventricular diastolic function is very complex and has remained clinically elusive (13). Despite these misgivings, there is no doubt that hypertension, LVH, and coronary artery disease can profoundly alter diastolic properties of the left ventricle, leading to severe dyspnea either acutely or on a chronic basis.

TREATMENT OF DIASTOLIC DYSFUNCTION

There is no uniformly agreed on therapy for CHF secondary to diastolic left ventricular dysfunction. When ischemic heart disease is documented to be an important etiologic factor, coronary revascularization may prove helpful (14). Therapies aimed at enhancing systolic function, such as positive inotropic agents or vasodilators, may be of no benefit or may even worsen symptoms (12), although nitrates may improve compliance in the acute ischemic left ventricle.

Acute pulmonary edema due to diastolic dysfunction with intact global systolic function is most likely to occur in the settings of acute myocardial infarction, severe transient myocardial ischemia with or without acute mitral regurgitation, and acute hypertensive emergency. Human studies have shown that nitroprusside and nitroglycerin, which cause venodilation and reduced left ventricular diastolic volume, can shift the pressure-volume relationship downward and to the right, back toward normal (15,16). Nifedipine has also been shown to improve the dP-dV relation in patients with hypertrophic cardiomyopathy (17). In the acute setting, when blood pressure is often increased, intravenous nitroprusside or nitroglycerin will usually control blood pressure and reduce left ventricular end-diastolic pressure sufficiently to markedly improve symptoms.

Chronic pharmacologic therapy of chronic or intermittent diastolic heart failure is currently undefined. Calcium channel blockers, β-adrenergic blockers, and nitrates have all been used as therapy for left ventricular diastolic dysfunction, but none has been rigorously investigated in placebo-controlled trials. This is partly due to the difficulty in measuring improved diastolic function in these patients. In theory, the angiotensin-converting enzyme inhibitors may provide some benefit for the prevention of chronic diastolic heart failure. Because angiotensin-converting enzyme (ACE) inhibition appears to reduce the extent of myocardial and vascular smooth muscle hypertrophy, a vicious cycle involving excessive rise in cardiac afterload leading to myocardial hypertrophy and failure may possibly be interrupted in patients with systemic hypertension by the early application of this therapy. More research is clearly necessary to determine which chronic therapy, if any, should be given to patients with chronic diastolic heart failure.

PATHOGENESIS OF SYSTOLIC CHF

CHF due to left ventricular systolic dysfunction is a well-recognized clinical syndrome. The diagnosis is made by taking a careful history, doing a physical examination, and measuring left ventricular function. Patients complain of breathlessness and fatigue and when systolic dysfunction is present usually have a dilated heart with some evidence of reduced left ventricular contractile function. Under some circumstances, it is possible to have the full syndrome of CHF and normal left ventricular function (e.g., mitral regurgitation, aortic regurgitation, mitral stenosis, aortic stenosis, pulmonic stenosis, and other various types of congenital heart disease, thyrotoxicosis, arteriovenous fistula, beriberi, sepsis), but the chronic stages of heart failure are usually characterized by a large, dilated, and poorly contracting heart, venous congestion, and inadequate blood flow to vital organs. As the circulation fails, a num-

TABLE 1. *Compensatory mechanisms in CHF*

1. Myocardial hypertrophy
2. Augmented sympathetic activity
3. Sodium and water retention
4. Ventricular dilatation

ber of compensatory mechanisms provide adaptations in an attempt to maintain perfusion pressure to vital organs and improve stroke volume (Table 1). It is these "adaptive" neuroendocrine and ventricular remodeling mechanisms that are ultimately responsible for the clinical manifestations of the syndrome of heart failure. To understand the treatment of heart failure, one must first understand the underlying mechanisms operative during the body's attempt to compensate for inadequate forward flow.

THE BASIC LESION

There is general agreement that in most forms of systolic heart failure the myocardium fails to generate an appropriate velocity of shortening for any given load. Papillary muscles removed from the right ventricles of cats in which hypertrophy and heart failure have developed following banding of the pulmonary artery demonstrate reduced maximum velocity of shortening (V_{max}) *in vitro* (18). The depression of contractility of the failing heart muscle appears to be related to a lack of contractile tissue (as occurs in myocardial infarction) or to an intrinsic defect of the muscle (as in dilated cardiomyopathy) rather than to its operation at an abnormal position on a basically normal length-tension curve. Whereas the contractile state may be depressed, the cardiac index and stroke volume are often maintained in the resting state, albeit at elevated ventricular end-diastolic volumes and pressures, as muscle mass increases and the heart dilates. The elevations in ventricular pressure and volume in accordance with the Frank-Starling mechanism stretch sarcomeres to optimal levels, but this tends to promote pulmonary and systemic venous congestion and the formation of pulmonary and peripheral edema.

MYOCARDIAL ENERGY PRODUCTION AND UTILIZATION

The depression of myocardial contractility probably is not due to a reduction of total myocardial high-energy stores. The concentration of both adenosine triphosphate (ATP) and creatine phosphate (CP) have been found to be normal in the papillary muscles removed from failing hearts and hypertrophied hearts studied *in vitro* (19). However, it is possible that ATP is depleted in a small compartment vital for muscular contraction. Also, the activity of myofibrillar ATPase activity may be reduced, and this could explain many of the functional changes in failing heart muscle, such as depression of the force-velocity curve.

EXCITATION-CONTRACTION COUPLING

Studies in a number of *in vitro* systems have indicated that there is impairment of the delivery of Ca^{2+} for activation of the contractile process in heart failure. The uptake of Ca^{2+} by sarcolemma, the sarcoplasmic reticulum, and the mitochondria, which partly depends on Ca^{2+}-activated ATPase, could play a role in the development of myocardial failure. Experimental heart failure in the rabbit produced by aortic regurgitation appears to be associated with a significant alteration in the intracellular distribution of Ca^{2+} (20). Whereas total intracellular Ca^{2+} is normal, mitochondrial Ca^{2+} is greatly increased, and the rate of binding of Ca^{2+} to the sarcoplasmic reticulum is reduced. This may limit the quantity of Ca^{2+} available to initiate contraction. Although disturbances of Ca^{2+} transport frequently accompany heart failure, the nature of the abnormality of Ca^{2+} transport differs in various forms of heart failure.

β-ADRENERGIC RECEPTOR DENSITY AND COUPLING TO G PROTEINS

Recent studies on human myocardium removed from patients undergoing heart transplantation have indicated that there is a decreased catecholamine sensitivity and reduced membrane-bound β-adrenergic receptor density in failing human hearts (21). The reductions in β-receptor density, adenyl cyclase, and the contractile response to isoproterenol suggest that human myocardium has no "spare" receptors, a situation that places β-adrenergic receptor regulation in a crucial position for modulating the contractile state of the heart. The cause of this reduction in β-receptor density is unknown but is believed to be related to the well-known concept of "down-regulation" of receptor density that occurs during heightened sympathetic activity. This is an area of intense research, but the role of this alteration in β-receptor density in initiating or sustaining heart failure is uncertain (22).

More recently, it has become apparent that myocyte β-receptors are normally coupled by regulatory proteins, called G proteins or guanine nucleotide regulatory proteins, to adenylate cyclase activity. These regulatory G proteins can either stimulate (G_s) or inhibit (G_i) the production of cyclic AMP, an important source of heightened cellular contractile function. Lymphocytes from patients with severe heart failure have reduced levels of G_s, and it is presumed that cardiac myocytes likewise have reduced G_s activity (23). It is possible that these alterations in G regulatory proteins contribute to reduced contractile function in the failing myocardium.

THE INFLUENCE OF LOADING CONDITIONS

In addition to reduced contractile function, it is now clear that alterations in preload (end-diastolic fiber length) and particularly afterload (left ventricular systolic wall tension) contribute to the diminished myocardial performance in CHF. The function of the normal left ventricle depends on preload, but the relationship between preload and contractility in CHF is both depressed and flattened. The result is that increases in preload do not result in improved stroke volume in advanced heart failure. Initially, end-diastolic volume and intravascular volume increase, probably due to sodium and water retention. Ultimately, because of the reduced response of contractility to enhanced preload, pulmonary and circulatory congestion ensues. The heart dilates, and systolic wall tension increases according to the LaPlace equation ($T = (P \times R)/h$, where P is pressure, R is ventricular radius, and h is wall thickness). The excess wall tension, or afterload, presents a further burden to the ejecting heart. The total impedance to ejection includes the systolic wall tension, systemic vascular resistance, the compliance of the large conduit and small arteriolar vessels, and the blood viscosity. In contrast to the relative independence of the failing left ventricle to changes in preload, the failing heart is exquisitely sensitive to alterations in afterload (24). Small increases in afterload may significantly worsen left ventricular function, whereas small decreases in afterload may markedly improve ventricular function in heart failure. The heightened impedance to ejection present in the syndrome of CHF is due in part to increased left ventricular systolic wall tension (increased radius) and enhanced systemic vascular resistance brought about by excessive peripheral vasoconstriction (increased pressure). Manipulation of left ventricular afterload, or impedance, is critical to the therapy of CHF. Since the advent of vasodilator therapy, dramatic improvements have been made in both the relief of symptoms and improved survival (25,26). For the first time we have been able to interrupt the natural course of a serious medical illness, extend-

ing life for many patients. These improvements in therapy have occurred as a direct result of an improved understanding of the multiple mechanisms operative in heart failure.

NEUROENDOCRINE ABNORMALITIES

CHF is a highly complex syndrome that cannot be defined by a single laboratory test. Rather there appears to be a general sequence of adaptive mechanisms that are operative early in the course of the syndrome. These adaptive mechanisms seem to occur in response to a perceived sense of inadequate effective circulating volume. When the output of the diseased heart becomes diminished, the body responds as it would to shock, severe dehydration, or exercise. It cannot distinguish the primary cause. These responses to stress or control systems evolved over some 600 million years to coordinate the needs of the entire organism. Both the endocrine and the autonomic nervous systems work to maintain circulating volume and peripheral perfusion during two of the body's most stressful situations—shock and exercise. Unfortunately, these neuroendocrine adaptations are designed more for short-term adjustments rather than for long-term compensation. Unlike volume loss or dynamic exercise, CHF presents a uniquely weak link in the adjustment cycle—the inability of the weakened myocardium to eject against a heightened impedance.

Heart failure is characterized by increased sympathetic nervous system activity, increased activity of the renin-angiotensin-aldosterone system, and the enhanced release of arginine vasopressin (AVP) (27). The use of radioimmunoassay and radioenzymatic techniques has allowed for accurate measurement of plasma AVP, plasma renin activity, and plasma norepinephrine (Fig. 3). These vasopressor-sodium retentive systems are offset to some extent by the release of vasodilator-natriuretic sub-

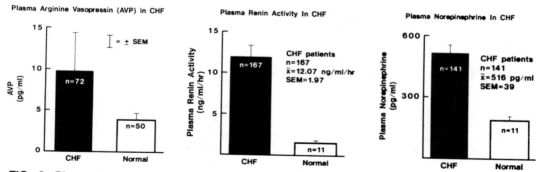

FIG. 3. Plasma levels of AVP, renin activity, and norepinephrine measured in a group of patients with varying degrees of chronic heart failure while off vasodilators and in most cases off diuretics. Blood samples were obtained from a peripheral vein with the patient supine for several minutes. Plasma renin activity and plasma AVP were determined by radioimmunoassay, and plasma norepinephrine by radioenzymatic technique. (These samples were obtained in collaboration with Steven R. Goldsmith, M.D.) (From ref. 27a.)

stances, including atrial natriuretic factor (ANF) (28), dopamine (29), and prostaglandins (30). On balance, however, there is a clear tendency for patients with heart failure to have peripheral vascular constriction and sodium retention (Fig. 4). The increased peripheral vascular resistance imposes an additional afterload stress on the failing ventricle, which sets the stage for a vicious cycle (Fig. 5), leading to a further

reduction in left ventricular performance, vascular congestion, and the full clinical expression of CHF.

THE SYMPATHETIC NERVOUS SYSTEM

The increase in sympathetic nervous system activity in patients with CHF generally

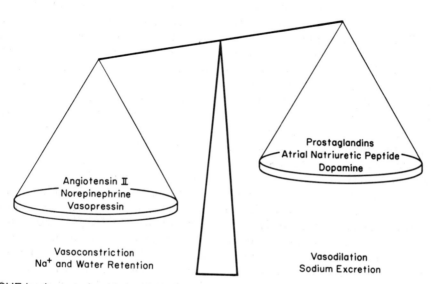

FIG. 4. CHF is characterized by an imbalance of neurohumoral adaptive mechanisms, with a net result of excessive vasoconstriction and salt and water retention. (From ref. 30a.)

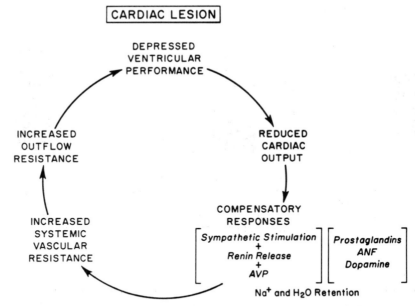

FIG. 5. The vicious cycle of CHF. A reduction in cardiac output leads to activation of series of neuroendocrine adaptive mechanisms, the result of which is sodium and water retention, increased impedance to left ventricular ejection, and further depression of left ventricular myocardial function.

parallels the severity of the disease (31). The mechanism by which sympathetic nervous system activity is enhanced in unknown (32). It is likely that both increased release and delayed clearance play a role in the elevated plasma levels of norepinephrine (33). Direct neurographic recordings indicate that central nervous system sympathetic outflow is increased (34). Baroreceptor reflex activation is blunted in patients with heart failure (35), and the degree of unresponsiveness appears to be associated with a poor prognosis (36). High basal levels of plasma norepinephrine (>600 pg/ml) in patients with CHF are associated with a shortened survival (37).

The response of the sympathetic nervous system to exercise, as measured by plasma norepinephrine, has been extensively studied in patients with CHF. There is a rapid rise in plasma norepinephrine early during exercise in patients with CHF (38), but this may be because they are exercising near

their maximal effort. If one examines the plasma norepinephrine level during exercise as a function of the percentage of maximal oxygen consumption rather than at absolute oxygen consumption, plasma norepinephrine levels are reduced compared with the levels of normal subjects (39). It is not known if the relatively blunted sympathetic response to exercise is causally related to the observed reduction in exercise capacity, but it may account for the well-known attenuated heart rate and blood pressure response to exercise observed in patients with heart failure (39).

Conventional wisdom has been that the failing circulation depends on augmented sympathetic activity for additional support (40). This is likely true for patients with very advanced CHF (41), but it is possible that enhanced sympathetic activity may be detrimental on a long-term basis. Excessive sympathetic activity may promote down-regulation of β-adrenergic receptors, thus impairing an important component of tractile function (21). Plasma catecholamines may be directly toxic to the myocardium (42,43). Peripheral vasoconstriction may be augmented by heightened sympathetic drive (44). Increased sympathetic activity may also contribute to ventricular arrhythmias (45), salt and water retention (46), and stimulation of the renin-angiotensin system (47). Preliminary reports of the beneficial effects of β-adrenergic blockade on functional status (48) and survival (49) suggest that heightened sympathetic nervous system activity may be contributing to the pathophysiology of heart failure, but only large, randomized, and controlled trials of β-blockers can determine if such therapy can actually change the natural course of the syndrome.

RENIN-ANGIOTENSIN-ALDOSTERONE SYSTEM

In 1944 Warren and Stead (50) reported that body weight and plasma volume began to increase prior to any rise in venous pressure in patients with heart failure whose treatment had been stopped. Merrill (51) subsequently demonstrated that retention of sodium occurred in association with a striking decrease in renal blood flow. This sodium retention was later shown to be due to an increase in tubular reabsorption rather than a simple decrease in glomerular filtration (52,53). In 1953 Singer and Werner (54) observed that the urine of patients with heart failure contained a sodium-retaining substance, and this was subsequently identified as aldosterone (55). By 1946 Merrill and colleagues (56) had reported that renin was increased in the venous efflux from the kidneys of patients with CHF, but the significance of this observation was not clear until 1959, when Tobian and co-workers (57) postulated that the release of renin depended on mean arterial perfusion pressure rather than blood flow. Renin is released as

the mean arterial pressure falls from 100 to 85 mm Hg (58). The responsiveness of the system is greatly increased by the sympathetic nervous system, which acts by decreasing the threshold for renin release, so that even a small decrease in arterial pressure can evoke a substantial release of renin (58). Changes in sodium and chloride ion concentration (hyponatremia) in the blood perfusing the macula densa also cause renin release (59), although renin can be released independently of this mechanism (60). Diuretic and vasodilator therapy along with dietary sodium restriction are additional stimuli for renin release in patients with CHF (Table 2).

Renin is a large enzyme (40,000 daltons) that acts on renin substrate (angiotensinogen) to produce angiotensin I, a small decapeptide (Fig. 6). Angiotensin I is converted by an enzyme to angiotensin II. It is likely that the kidney, brain (61,62), and vascular tissue (63) are important sites of angiotensin-II formation. Angiotensin II has multiple sites of action in CHF (Fig. 7). It is a powerful constrictor, which is important in maintaining glomerular filtration by increasing postglomerular vascular resistance (64). It stimulates the secretion of aldosterone, enhances adrenergic neuroeffector transmission, promotes the sensation of thirst, enhances the release of AVP, and is associated with vascular and myocardial hypertrophy (65). Angiotensin II is one of the dominant factors in the pathophysiology of CHF (66).

TABLE 2. *Stimuli for renin release in CHF*

1. Decreased stretch of renal vascular baroreceptor (diminished renal blood flow/perfusion pressure)
2. Renal β-adrenergic receptor activation (heightened sympathetic nervous system activity)
3. Reduced tubular sodium and/or chloride ion load sensed by the macula densa cells of the distal tubule
4. Diuretic and vasodilator therapy
5. Sodium restriction

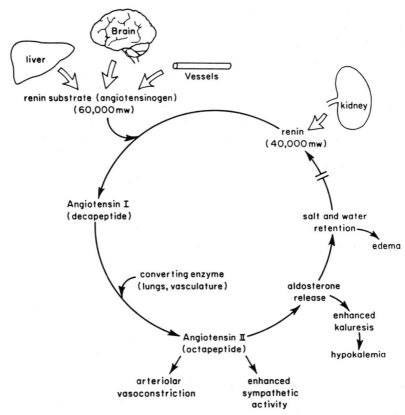

FIG. 6. The renin-angiotensin-aldosterone axis in CHF. Renin is released from the kidney in response to multiple stimuli (Table 2). Angiotensinogen, or renin substrate, is produced by the liver, brain, and endothelium, where it likely is converted to angiotensin I and angiotensin II. Much of the angiotensin-I conversion to angiotensin II takes place in the circulation, primarily in the lungs, where it then circulates to have multiple biological activities (Fig. 7).

AVP

As the mammalian organism evolved, it became necessary to develop multiple systems to replenish volume and maintain circulatory status (67,68). The chemical phylogeny of the neurohypophyseal hormones is well-known, as they are all octapeptides and vary only in substitutions at positions 3 and 8. At some point in evolution a mutation occurred resulting in a change from arginine vasotocin to AVP. The action of AVP is to increase the permeability of the renal collecting tubules to water and thereby help to concentrate the urine. Because many species use their skin for the absorption of

water, it is not surprising that AVP might contract epithelium and smooth muscle. In fact, the original effect of vasotocin seems to have been vasoconstriction. Next to endothelin (69), AVP is perhaps the most potent vasoconstrictor in the body (70). It is released in response to many stimuli, including an increase in osmotic pressure, a decrease in cardiopulmonary blood volume or blood pressure, angiotensin II and norepinephrine, emotion, nausea and vomiting, and increased temperature. Plasma AVP is increased in patients with advanced heart failure (71).

The mechanism of AVP release in CHF is not well understood. Because of various

Angiotensin II

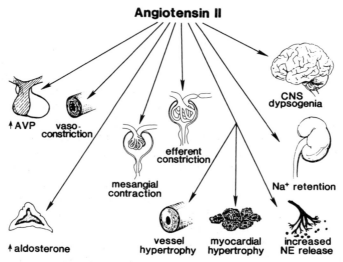

FIG. 7. Angiotensin II has multiple biological functions. In heart failure, it likely contributes to enhancement of AVP release, arteriolar vasoconstriction, increased secretion of aldosterone, mesangial contraction (which reduces glomerular filtration rate), efferent arteriole constriction (which maintains glomerular filtration rate), vascular and myocardial hypertrophy, enhanced release of norepinephrine (NE) from sympathetic nerve endings, a direct effect on sodium reabsorption, and an increased sensation of thirst. The net result of these activities is increased systemic vascular resistance, heightened sympathetic activity, peripheral edema and hyponatremia—all hallmarks of advanced CHF.

compensatory mechanisms, the chronic administration of AVP to normal subjects does not lead to any substantial increase in body water or elevation of blood pressure. However, more thorough hemodynamic assessment of AVP infusion in patients with CHF does reveal an increase in systemic vascular resistance and a redistribution of cardiac output (72). Moreover, selective inhibition of the vascular (V_1) AVP receptor in patients with very severe CHF causes vasodilation and improvement in cardiac function (44,73). It therefore seems likely that AVP may play some role in the pathophysiology of patients with CHF, but this role is likely limited to those in the late stages of the syndrome.

COUNTERREGULATORY ADAPTIVE MECHANISMS (ANF, PROSTAGLANDINS, DOPAMINE)

The neuroendocrine forces that promote vasoconstriction and sodium retention in

CHF are offset to some extent by the release of ANF (74), prostaglandin E_2 (PGE_2) (30), and dopamine (29). These endogenous substances tend to enhance renal blood flow and sodium excretion and subserve vasodilation in various regional vascular beds.

There has been a particularly strong interest in ANF since the landmark experiments of deBold et al. (75), who demonstrated that atrial extracts produced a marked increase in sodium and water excretion when infused into rats. It is now clear that mammalian atria contain secretory granules. These granules release a group of closely related 21 to 26 amino acid peptides, collectively referred to as ANF, in response to atrial distention, increased extracellular sodium, or tachycardia. Physiologic actions of ANF include natriuresis, diuresis, vasodilation, and suppression of the renin-angiotensin system (28). It is likely that ANF is important in the day-to-day adjustment of circulatory homeostasis.

Its role in the pathophysiology of edematous states is less clear.

The ANF gene codes for a prehormone containing 152 amino acids, including a signal peptide of 24 amino acids. The primary form is stored as a 126-amino-acid peptide. Large amounts of the peptide are produced, with as much as 5% of the messenger RNA in the atria coding for the peptide. In heart failure the ventricle can also produce ANF (76). Only minute quantities of ANF circulate, suggesting that it is released continuously at low levels.

Once in the circulation, ANF mediates its biological effects in part by binding to a receptor coupled to cyclic GMP. Receptors for ANF have been identified on cultured vascular cells (77) and adrenal glomerulosa cells (78). Direct renal effects of ANF include an increase in glomerular filtration and a pronounced diuresis and natriuresis. Renal blood flow usually increases transiently. Aldosterone (79) and AVP (80) are normally inhibited by ANF. These biological effects are apparent when ANF is infused into normal subjects (81) but are blunted when ANF is infused into patients with CHF (81). There is also less pronounced peripheral vasodilation when ANF is given intraarterially to patients with heart failure than when given to normal subjects (82). This may be due to a generalized lack of peripheral vasodilation response common in patients with heart failure (83). Moreover, unlike most vasodilators, ANF does not reduce systemic vascular resistance but rather lowers blood pressure by reducing venous return, possibly related to extravasation of fluid out of the capacitance veins into the interstitium. Although attempts to develop ANF as an adjunctive therapy for patients with heart failure have been somewhat disappointing, there is still much interest in ANF as a modulator of circulatory homeostasis in normal subjects.

Prostaglandins, unlike ANF, are not true circulating hormones but are autacoids; that is, they are synthesized and released and act locally. PGE_2 and PGI_2 are impor-

tant endogenous vasodilators, particularly in states of diminished renal blood flow, such as occurs in patients with CHF. PGE_2 metabolites and 6-keto-$PGF_{1\alpha}$ are increased in patients with heart failure (30,84). The stimuli for the release of renal prostaglandins likely includes reduced perfusion as well as heightened activity of angiotensin II and norepinephrine (85,86). In normal subjects, there is no clear dependence on prostaglandins to maintain intrarenal circulatory hemodynamics. On the contrary, patients with advanced CHF appear to be critically dependent on prostaglandins to maintain renal circulatory function. The use of nonsteroidal anti-inflammatory agents in patients with heart failure, which block prostaglandin production, frequently results in progressive azotemia as well as enhanced systemic vascular resistance, heightened pulmonary capillary wedge pressure, and reduced cardiac output (30). These observations emphasize the need for prostaglandins as an important counterregulatory system in patients with advanced heart failure.

Dopamine, like norepinephrine, is stored and released from sympathetic nerve endings via exocytosis. Unlike norepinephrine, dopamine subserves renal vasodilation, natriuresis, and diuresis. Plasma levels of dopamine are increased in patients with heart failure (29), presumably in a further attempt to maintain circulatory homeostasis. There are two known dopamine receptors, DA_1 and DA_2 (87). The DA_1 receptors subserve vasodilation in the renal, mesenteric, coronary, and cerebral vasculature and may also enhance renal sodium excretion. The DA_2 receptors are neuronal and presynaptic in location and subserve inhibition of norepinephrine release. Fenoldopam, a selective oral DA_1-receptor agonist, is being investigated in patients with CHF (88,89), in whom it has been demonstrated to be a potent vasodilator. These observations are consistent with a vasodilator role for endogenous dopamine in patients with CHF, but the extent that endogenous dopamine offsets the intensive vasoconstriction and sodium retention that occur in heart failure is likely somewhat limited.

TREATMENT OF ACUTE HEART FAILURE

The treatment of acute heart failure, or pulmonary edema, is highly individualized and predicated on an understanding of the mechanisms operative at the time of diagnosis (90). Commonly, severe respiratory distress does not allow one the luxury of taking a careful history. The physical exam generally reveals an acutely ill patient, breathing rapidly and laboriously, sitting upright, diaphoretic and cyanotic. Initial evaluation would generally include an electrocardiogram, chest x-ray, electrolytes, blood urea nitrogen, creatinine, and arterial blood gases.

If blood pressure is adequate, an intravenous loop diuretic (furosemide 40–100 mg) and nitroprusside 10 to 300 μg/min along with low-flow oxygen are the immediate therapeutic considerations. Intravenous furosemide usually results in a prompt diuresis within ½ to 1 hr, unless renal function is severely impaired. Nitroprusside is a potent smooth muscle dilating agent (venous and arteriole) with no direct effects on the myocardium. It has a relatively balanced effect on both afterload and preload, thereby lowering impedance to ejection and reducing end-diastolic volume and pressure. Cardiac output markedly improves and blood pressure usually changes only slightly with nitroprusside because the fall in systemic vascular resistance is usually offset by the increase in forward flow (91–93). Nitroprusside is particularly useful in patients with acute myocardial infarction and persistent left ventricular pump dysfunction (94,95). The usual practice is to begin the drug at an infusion rate of 10 to 15 μg/min and gradually titrate the dose upward to achieve a desired effect on hemo-

dynamic measurements and urine output. Doses greater than 300 μg/min are rarely necessary, with most patients responding to less than 150 μg/min.

Nitroprusside should probably not be used when directly measured arterial pressure is already low (e.g., systolic pressure less than 90 mm Hg), although nitroglycerin might still be employed in this situation for its predominant preload effect. The extraordinary utility of nitroprusside in acute heart failure or pulmonary edema is based on its quick onset of action, very short half-life, lack of tachyphylaxis, and lack of any direct effect on the myocardium or sympathetic nervous system. Toxicity, in the form of increased blood thiocyanate levels, is unusual and can be minimized by short-term use of the drug. Like intravenous nitroglycerin, nitroprusside dilates the coronary vascular bed. Its effects are more prominent on the small arteriole resistance coronary vessels, whereas nitroglycerin tends to mainly dilate the large conductance vessels (96). Nitroglycerin may have a more favorable effect on coronary blood flow to myocardial ischemic segments (97,98) when flow depends on collaterals, but experimental (99) and human (100) studies indicate that both nitroprusside and nitroglycerin may have similarly beneficial effects during acute coronary insufficiency.

When acute pulmonary edema occurs in the setting of hypotension, dopamine 3 to 20 μg/kg/min should be used to restore adequate perfusion pressure (101,102). When systolic blood pressure is greater than 90 mm Hg, nitroprusside can be added to dopamine to further augment cardiac output and reduce left ventricular filling pressure (103). Intravenous furosemide or bumetanide should be used to promote diuresis. Dopamine, rather than dobutamine, is preferred when restoration of blood pressure is the immediate goal of therapy (104). Dopamine has potent peripheral vasoconstrictor properties in addition to its inotropic action. Dobutamine lacks vasoconstrictor activity and can only raise blood pressure by increasing stroke volume, a relatively inefficient hemodynamic mechanism in cardiogenic shock (104).

Acute decompensation of stable CHF is common and frequently occurs with a systolic blood pressure in the range of 100 to 120 mm Hg. Loop diuretics, nitroprusside, and supplemental oxygen are the preferred initial therapy. Low-dose dopamine (<3 µg/kg/min) has a renal artery dilating effect and may improve sodium and water excretion in patients refractory to loop diuretics. Nitroprusside, rather than dobutamine, is used to augment pump performance because of its lack of direct effects on the myocardium (105). Moreover, nitroprusside is more likely than dobutamine to reduce pulmonary capillary wedge pressure (Fig. 8), a most desired effect of treatment.

Dobutamine is frequently added to nitroprusside when blood pressure is adequate to augment cardiac output (106). It is a synthetic catecholamine with almost pure β-adrenergic effects. It is generally administered at a constant infusion rate (2–5 µg/kg/min) and titrated upward to 20 µg/kg/min as needed to increase cardiac output. The dose is usually increased every 30 min, with tachycardia, arrhythmias, headache, nausea, and tremor being the limiting factors (107). Dobutamine enhances atrioventricular conduction and may worsen atrial flutter or fibrillation (108,109).

Kates and Leier (110) observed that dobutamine has a very short half-life (2.37 ± 0.7 min). This feature and the lack of a biologically active metabolite are attractive properties of dobutamine. It has been extensively studied as short-term (48–72 hr) therapy for patients with severe CHF, in which it will occasionally result in sustained improvement of the severely ill patient over several weeks (111–114). After 72 hr of sustained dobutamine infusion, however, tolerance will develop in some patients (115). Long-term benefit is possibly

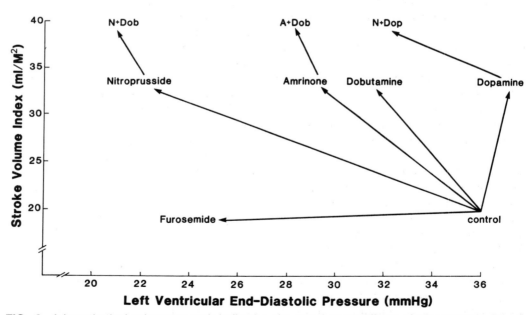

FIG. 8. A hypothetical schematograph indicating the usual acute effects of nitroprusside (N), dobutamine (Dob), amrinone (A), dopamine (Dop), and furosemide on left ventricular function in the setting of severe pump dysfunction. Combinations of drugs are often more effective than single agents. (From ref. 90.)

related to improvement in myocardial mitochondria (114).

Patients unresponsive to dobutamine and nitroprusside may occasionally be responsive to amrinone, which has mixed inotropic and vasodilator properties. Amrinone is a bipyridine derivative that increases myocardial cyclic AMP by inhibiting phosphodiesterase, thereby bypassing the β-adrenergic receptor. Its hemodynamic profile is similar to dobutamine (116) (Fig. 8), but pump performance improves with less myocardial oxygen demand. Adding amrinone to dobutamine is a useful strategy when there is an insufficient response to either agent used alone (117). Therapy with amrinone should be initiated with a 0.75 mg/kg bolus given slowly over 2 to 3 min, and maintained at 5 to 10 μg/kg/min, with titration of the infusion according to the patient's clinical and hemodynamic needs. Heart rate and blood pressure are not greatly affected by amrinone in conventional doses, but high doses can produce tachycardia and hypotension. Amrinone may actually reduce cardiac output in patients with a normal or low left ventricular filling pressure (118).

TREATMENT OF CHRONIC HEART FAILURE

A recent survey of 1,500 physicians (cardiologists, internists, family practitioners) and 1,306 academic cardiologists indicated widespread confusion about the diagnosis and treatment of chronic heart failure (119). There appear to be no generally accepted criteria for the diagnosis of heart failure. Initial treatment using diuretics alone was favored by 53%, digitalis alone by 7%, and a starting combination of diuretics and digitalis by 30% of participants. Only 9% favored using vasodilators either alone or in combination as the best initial treatment for CHF. These survey data were gathered in March 1984, before the publication of two landmark studies indicating that a combination of isosorbide dinitrate plus hydrala-

zine (25) or enalapril, a long-acting converting enzyme inhibitor (26), exerted a striking improvement on the survival of class-II and -III patients and class-IV patients, respectively, who were already on baseline therapy with digitalis and diuretics. Moreover, a recent publication (120) has indicated that captopril may be superior to digitalis and diuretics by improving exercise tolerance in patients with mild to moderate CHF. There now appears to be a current trend to begin therapy with a diuretic and a vasodilator regimen, with digitalis being used to a highly variable degree.

DIURETICS

Patients with CHF and evidence of edema should clearly be treated with a diuretic. Many physicians begin therapy with a thiazide diuretic and add or change to a loop diuretic as signs of extracellular fluid accumulation appear. The reduction in preload serves to diminish breathlessness and vascular congestion and may reduce vascular "stiffness," although the latter mechanism is not well documented. Overly aggressive use of diuretics in CHF may further reduce effective circulating volume, however, thus further reducing cardiac output and renal blood flow, resulting in worsening azotemia and causing other untoward consequences. The simplest and safest method to monitor the effects of diuretic therapy in heart failure is by careful, repeated examinations of jugular venous pressure and its response to right upper quadrant abdominal pressure.

Thiazides act on the distal convoluted tubule of the kidney to cause a maximal increase in sodium excretion of 5% to 8% of the filtered load. They are relatively ineffective in patients with glomerular filtration rates below 30 ml/min, and this limits their effectiveness in severe heart failure. Their effects may be potentiated by spironolactone or triamterene, agents that act primarily on the distal tubule to inhibit potassium loss. The quinethazone derivative metola-zone has a site of action and potency similar to those of chlorothiazide but at the usual doses (2.5 or 5 mg) it does not reduce renal blood flow or glomerular filtration rate. Metolazone also has a longer duration of action (24–48 hr), is effective even in patients with markedly reduced glomerular filtration rates, and is particularly useful when added to a diuretic acting at a different location in the kidney, such as furosemide.

In more advanced heart failure, diuretics that are capable of increasing the fractional sodium excretion to more than 20% of the filtered load are usually employed. Furosemide and ethacrinic acid act to inhibit chloride transport in the ascending limb of the loop of Henle, thereby enhancing the excretion of sodium and water. They are powerful diuretics that also act to remove the gradient for passive water movement from the descending limb of Henle's loop and may somewhat reverse the shunting of renal blood flow away from the cortex of the kidney. For very refractory cases of extracellular fluid accumulation in heart failure, a combination of metolazone plus a loop diuretic plus a distal tubular diuretic is sometimes used. The intermittent use of supplemental metolazone, depending on the patient's weight and edema status, is generally preferred to a fixed and constant dose of metolazone in order to avoid volume depletion. When severe, refractory edema occurs with persistent hypokalemia, secondary aldosteronism should be suspected. A spot urine showing a K^+/Na^+ ratio of >1 confirms the diagnosis, and the potassium-sparing agent amiloride (5 mg/day) should be considered.

DIGITALIS

Despite its clinical use for more than 200 years, controversy regarding the use of digitalis for CHF continues to thrive. Even to-day the precise mechanism of action remains elusive, although activation of the myocyte membrane bound Na-K-ATPase pump appears important. The net result is that Na^+ is replaced by Ca^{2+}, allowing for more Ca^{2+} to be available for contractile proteins (121), although this mechanism is by no means universally accepted (122).

The efficacy of digitalis in heart failure is no less controversial than its basic mechanism of inotropic action. There is little doubt that a substantial proportion of patients receiving chronic administration of digitalis do not derive obvious benefit from use of the drug, while at the same time being subjected to an appreciable risk of toxicity. This is particularly true of patients in normal sinus rhythm. Digoxin is the most commonly used preparation of digitalis. Much needed information documenting the long-term effects of digoxin administration for chronic heart failure has been provided by Arnold et al. (123), clearly demonstrating the beneficial effects in a selected group of patients. These observations were subsequently confirmed by another group of investigators (124), who demonstrated that patients who responded to digoxin had more chronic and severe heart failure, greater left ventricular dilatation, a more reduced ejection fraction, and a third heart sound. Chronic use of digoxin improves the ejection fraction even in patients with mild or moderate heart failure (120). There are no data available regarding the impact of digitalis therapy on long-term prognosis for patients with heart failure, although a trial examining this issue is currently being planned. At the present time it seems reasonable to use digitalis in patients with more advanced heart failure in hopes of deriving some improvement in clinical status, but controversy will remain until mortality data become available. The usual dose of digoxin is 0.25 mg/day as adjusted for renal function. There is no clear relation between digoxin levels and measurements of efficacy.

INOTROPIC AGENTS

Except for digitalis, there are no oral inotropic agents approved by the U.S. Food and Drug Administration for use in chronic heart failure. A number of agents are currently undergoing clinical trials, however (125). Milrinone is a potent bipyridine derivative that can be given orally and has both positive inotropic and vasodilator properties (126). It is a phosphodiesterase (PDE) III inhibitor and thereby increases cellular content of cyclic AMP. Oral therapy is usually begun at 5 mg every 4 to 6 hr, with an average dose being in the range of 50 mg/day. Enoximone (127) and piroximone (128) are also PDE III inhibitors shown to have short-term favorable effects on left ventricular function. There are no controlled data available on these agents regarding survival, and more experience in context of randomized, placebo-controlled trials will be necessary to determine their role as chronic therapy for heart failure.

Additional agents that have been studied as oral inotropic therapy for CHF include levodopa (129), ibopamine (130), and dopexamine (131). Levodopa is converted to dopamine via amino-acid decarboxylation. Dopamine then acts on β-adrenergic receptors to increase myocardial contractility. Levodopa has a rather high side-effect profile and is not widely used to treat heart failure. Ibopamine, a diisobutyric ester of epinine, is hydrolyzed by plasma esterases to epinine, which is a DA$_1$-receptor agonist and should behave similarly to low-dose dopamine. Dopexamine is a DA$_1$- and B$_2$-receptor agonist and has primarily vasodilator properties. These agents have not undergone large, long-term, rigorously controlled trials, although ibopamine is presently being studied in a multicenter trial.

Milrinone, enoximone, piroximone, and possibly levodopa, ibopamine, and dopexamine are mediated through mechanisms that depend on the generation of a cyclic nucleotide (cyclic AMP) for the production of a positive inotropic effect. Therefore, it is possible that each of these agents will lose effectiveness as heart failure progresses. They may serve as short-term or temporary therapeutic measures, useful until cyclic AMP can no longer be adequately restored in the failing myocardium (132). On the contrary, agents that primarily act to sensitize contractile proteins to calcium, such as OPC-8212 (133) and pimobendan (134), bypass the dependency to generate new cyclic nucleotides and may prove to be more effective in promoting long-term positive inotropy. Clearly, this is an area where more basic and clinical research will be focused in the near future.

β-ADRENERGIC BLOCKERS AND PARTIAL β-AGONISTS

Because sympathetic nervous system activity may be detrimental to the failing heart, it is reasonable to assume that chronic β-adrenergic blockade may be beneficial in the treatment of CHF (48,49). Unlike nearly all other agents that have been used to treat chronic heart failure, the β-blocking drugs do not generally produce immediate hemodynamic or clinical benefits (135). In fact, short-term trials have not consistently demonstrated clinical improvement (136). The results of randomized, controlled trials are not yet currently available, however. Preliminary studies suggest that as many as 60% to 70% of patients with chronic heart failure may benefit from the long-term treatment of β-blocking drugs (48,49). β-Adrenergic blockers with intrinsic sympathomimetic activity such as pindolol, although theoretically more advantageous than pure β-blockers, have not proven to be as successful (137). Patients with the most advanced heart failure and the highest plasma norepinephrine levels are most likely to have clinical deterioration during the initiation of pindolol (137). Because of possible clinical deterioration, β-blockers are generally begun very cautiously with the lowest possible dose (e.g., 6.25 mg metoprolol b.i.d.) and titrated over weeks to a maximal dose (50 mg b.i.d.). A favorable clinical response may not be apparent for 2 to 6 months. Despite some encouraging preliminary results, the use of β-blocking drugs must be considered strictly investigational at the present time.

Xamoterol is an orally active partial β-adrenergic agonist that acts as a β_1 agonist at low levels of sympathetic drive and a β_1-blocker during states of high sympathetic activity, such as during exercise. It has been used in doses of 100 mg b.i.d. to treat patients with heart failure with encouraging results (138). Although potentially a negative inotrope when administered acutely (139), it might conceivably improve exercise tolerance and left ventricular diastolic function when given chronically. More clinical experience will be needed with xamoterol in placebo-controlled trials to determine what role, if any, it may have in the chronic treatment of CHF.

VASODILATORS

Oral vasodilators have been commonly used for the past 15 years for the treatment of CHF (139). Recently two large rigorously controlled trials have demonstrated that survival can be substantially improved in class-II and -III patients with a combination of isosorbide dinitrate plus hydralazine (25), or in class-IV patients with enalapril (26). The Vasodilator Heart Failure Trial (V-HeFT) was a Veterans Administration cooperative study of 642 men with impaired cardiac function and reduced exercise tolerance who were taking digoxin and a diuretic and then randomly assigned to receive additional double-blinded treatment with a placebo, prazosin (20 mg/day), or the combination of hydralazine (300 mg/day) and isosorbide dinitrate (160 mg/day). Follow-up averaged 2.3 years. The mortality-risk reduction in the group treated with hydralazine and isosorbide dinitrate was 34% by 2 years ($p<0.028$) and 36% by 3 years. Left ventricular ejection fraction measured

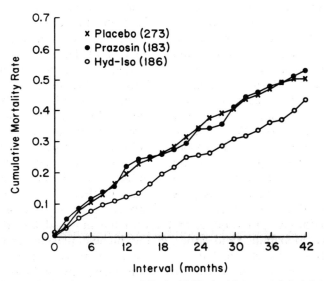

FIG. 9. Influence of vasodilator drugs on mortality in CHF: the Veterans Administration V-HefT. Hyd-Iso, hydralazine and isosorbide dinitrate. (From ref. 25.)

sequentially rose significantly at 8 weeks and at 1 year in the group treated with hydralazine and isosorbide dinitrate but not in the placebo or prazosin groups. The mortality in the placebo and prazosin groups was similar (Fig. 9). This trial, which was planned in the late 1970s, was the first to show that a specific vasodilator regimen could successfully alter the natural course of heart failure.

In June 1987 the results of the Cooperative North Scandinavian Enalapril Survival Study (CONSENSUS) were published (26). This trial evaluated the influence of the ACE inhibitor enalapril (2.5–40 mg/day) on the prognosis of severe class-IV heart failure. The investigators randomly assigned 253 patients in a double-blind study to receive either placebo ($n = 126$) or enalapril ($n = 127$) in addition to conventional therapy, including other vasodilators. The follow-up averaged 188 days. The crude mortality at the end of 6 months was 26% in the enalapril group and 44% in the placebo

group—a reduction of 40% ($p = 0.002$) (Fig. 10). The beneficial effect on mortality was due to a reduction in death from the progression in heart failure.

These two landmark studies (V-HeFT and CONSENSUS) have provided firm evidence for the role of vasodilator therapy for patients with CHF. Questions still remain, however. Is converting-enzyme inhibitor therapy preferable to hydralazine and isosorbide dinitrate? When should vasodilator therapy be initiated in the natural course of heart failure? V-HeFT II is a second Veterans Administration trial comparing enalapril with hydralazine and isosorbide dinitrate in class-II and -III patients to be completed in 1991. Studies of Left Ventricular Dysfunction (SOLVD) and Survival and Ventricular Enlargement (SAVE) are large, multicenter, placebo-controlled trials examining the question of whether enalapril (SOLVD) or captopril (SAVE) will improve survival if initiated in patients with reduced left ventricular function prior to the onset

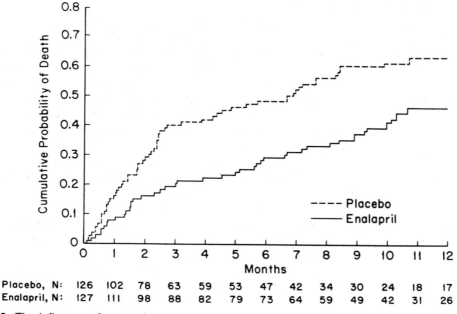

Placebo, N:	126	102	78	63	59	53	47	42	34	30	24	18	17
Enalapril, N:	127	111	98	88	82	79	73	64	59	49	42	31	26

FIG. 10. The influence of converting-enzyme inhibition with enalapril on mortality in severe chronic CHF: the CONSENSUS Trial. (Adapted from ref. 26.)

of overt CHF. Until the completion of V-HeFT II, SOLVD, and SAVE, physicians should reserve judgment as to which vasodilator regimen is preferable and refrain from treating asymptomatic patients with a low ejection fraction.

NITRATES AND NITRIC OXIDE INDUCERS

The organic nitrates exert their vasodilator effects by stimulating soluble guanylate cyclase in smooth muscles which consequently increases intracellular cyclic GMP. Molsidomine stimulates guanylate cyclase directly, whereas the mono-, di-, and tetranitrates require the formation of an S-nitrosothiol intermediate to activate the enzyme (140). These agents all principally stimulate cyclic GMP in veins (141), thereby exerting venodilation as their primary action. Current work strongly suggests that all nitrovasodilators act to ultimately generate nitric oxide (142), a potent relaxant of vascular smooth muscle. Nitric oxide is now considered to be endothelium-derived relaxing factor (EDRF) (143), a potent endogenous smooth muscle relaxant factor. Therefore, organic nitrates and molsidomine can be considered exogenous forms of EDRF.

The oral nitrates lower right and left ventricular filling pressures at rest and during exercise (144,145). Nitrates have an initially favorable hemodynamic effect in nearly all patients, but loss of pharmacological activity tends to occur in proportion to the frequency of dosing (146–148). Loss of efficacy can be prevented if the drugs are dosed intermittently, separated by an 8- to 12-hr nitrate-free period (146,147). However, resistance to isosorbide dinitrate is relatively common in patients with severe heart failure, particularly in those with markedly elevated right atrial pressure (148–150).

Nitrate tolerance is poorly understood but may be due to activation of endogenous vasoconstrictor neuroendocrine systems and a decline in the ability of these drugs to generate smooth muscle cyclic GMP (146). When vessels become tolerant, they may not be able to form the required reactive nitrosothiols. It may be possible in some cases to reverse the nitrate tolerance by giving exogenous sulfhydryl-containing compounds (146). To date, however, the most commonly employed maneuver used to avoid nitrate tolerance is the use of intermittent dosing with a nitrate-free period of 8 to 12 hr.

The long-acting oral nitrates appear to improve exercise tolerance in patients with heart failure following 2 to 3 months of treatment (145), but this is not a consistent finding (144). In the V-HeFT trial, isosorbide dinitrate combined with hydralazine modestly improved exercise tolerance (151). There are insufficient data to recommend nitrates as vasodilator monotherapy for CHF, but their role as adjunctive treatment is firmly established.

DIRECT-ACTING VASODILATORS

Only hydralazine and flosequinan are currently being widely used or actively investigated as direct-acting vasodilators for CHF. Hydralazine primarily dilates arteriolar vessels and thereby improves cardiac output and regional distribution of flow without changing left ventricular filling pressure (152). When hydralazine is used as the sole vasodilator for CHF, it does not demonstrate long-term efficacy (153,154). Tolerance can occur with hydralazine (155), and side effects are common. The usual dose of hydralazine for CHF is 300 mg in divided doses, although there is wide variation in individual requirements and drug tolerance.

Flosequinan is an orally effective drug with combined arteriolar- and venous-dilating properties (156). Short-term therapy with 100 or 125 mg once daily produces a balanced reduction in left ventricular filling pressure and increased cardiac output. Like all direct-acting vasodilators, flosequinan can promote sodium and water retention and activation of endogenous neuroendocrine systems. More experience will be required with flosequinan in placebo-controlled trials to define its therapeutic role in heart failure.

Calcium channel blockers have varying molecular configurations, but all reduce systemic vascular resistance and therefore are potentially useful in the treatment of heart failure. These agents have not been studied in rigorously controlled clinical trials, however. At least one controlled crossover trial with nifedipine failed to demonstrate sustained efficacy (157). Moreover, there has been a long-standing concern that calcium channel blocking drugs further depress myocardial contractility in proportion to the degree of baseline left ventricular dysfunction (158–160). Serious clinical deterioration, including pulmonary edema and cardiogenic shock (158,161), has occurred when these drugs are employed for overt CHF. It is possible that second-generation calcium channel blockers such as nicardipine, nitrendipine, felodipine, or isradipine will have less negative inotropic properties than verapamil, nifedipine, and diltiazem. However, until more data are available, calcium channel blockers should not be considered "first-line" therapy in the management of patients with overt heart failure.

CONVERTING-ENZYME INHIBITORS

Unlike other vasodilators, the ACE inhibitors exert their vasodilatory response by interfering with endogenous neuroendocrine mechanisms. It is now generally believed that these mechanisms contribute significantly to the pathophysiology of heart failure. Impaired cardiac function is associated with activation of the renin-angiotensin-aldosterone system and the sympathetic nervous system that, along with other less defined mechanisms, interact to promote peripheral vasoconstriction along with salt and water retention. ACE inhibitors can break this vicious cycle by blocking angiotensin-II formation and undoubtedly have other mechanisms of action that are less well understood.

Three ACE inhibitors are now approved in the United States for the treatment of CHF—captopril, enalapril, and lisinopril. At least eight others are being evaluated in clinical trials. All appear to be similar in their basic mechanism of action but vary in their chemical structure, pharmacokinetics, and pharmacodynamics. ACE inhibitors produce a sustained reduction in left ventricular filling pressure but do not markedly improve cardiac output or ejection fraction (162–164). Exercise tolerance improves with captopril (165) and enalapril (166–168). Breathlessness is improved (120,165) and the need for hospitalization is reduced (165). Tolerance to converting-enzyme inhibitors is possible but is far less common than with direct-acting vasodilators. ACE inhibitors reduce the need for diuretics and potassium supplements, often correcting underlying hypokalemia and hyponatremia (169). They may also reduce the frequency of complex ventricular arrhythmias (170). Captopril is usually begun at 6.5 mg and gradually increased to 25 to 50 mg t.i.d. Enalapril is started at 2.5 or 5 mg and increased to 20 mg b.i.d. Enalapril, being a prodrug, must be deesterified by the liver to the active moiety, enalaprilat. Captopril and enalapril appear to have similar efficacy and side-effect profiles.

Most patients with CHF will have a favorable response to ACE inhibitors, although those with renal insufficiency (serum creatinine >1.5 mg%) and a high right atrial pressure (>12 mm Hg) are less likely to benefit (171). Patients who are volume depleted and/or hyponatremic are at risk to develop hypotension following initial therapy with ACE inhibitors. This can usually be avoided by reducing or temporarily discontinuing diuretic therapy. Severely ill patients with reduced renal perfusion pressure are more dependent on angiotensin II to maintain intraglomerular pressure (172) and may develop renal insufficiency with ACE inhibitors. Once again, reduction in diuretic dose is useful in reversing this complication, but occasional patients will not tolerate ACE inhibitors because of symptomatic hypotension or progressive deterioration in renal function.

SUMMARY

There have been substantial improvements in our understanding of heart failure and the management of this syndrome since the last edition of this book. Driven by the recognition of an important emerging public health problem, investigators have successfully planned and conducted a number of controlled clinical trials that have demonstrated that there may be extension of lives for some patients with heart failure. More questions remain, however, and it is likely that further probes into the basic biology and clinical intricacies of heart failure will continue to provide advances on which practitioners will act.

ACKNOWLEDGMENT

The superb secretarial assistance of Sandy Thiesse is greatly appreciated.

REFERENCES

1. Kolata GB. Prevention of heart disease: clinical trials at what cost? *Science* 1975;190:764–765.
2. Data on file with American Heart Association. Dallas, Texas.
3. Data on file with the National Health Care Statistics. Washington, D.C.
4. Francis GS. Heart failure management: the impact of drug therapy on survival. *Am Heart J* 1988;115:699–702.
5. Furberg CD, Yusuf S, Thom T. Potential for altering the natural history of congestive heart failure: need for large clinical trials. *Am J Cardiol* 1985;55:45A–47A.
6. Gillum RF. Heart failure in the United States 1970–1985. *Am Heart J* 1987;113:1043–1045.
7. Smith WM. Epidemiology of congestive heart failure. *Am J Cardiol* 1985;55:3A–8A.
8. Cohn JN. Current therapy of the failing heart. *Circulation* 1988;78:1099–1107.
9. Glantz SA. Ventricular pressure-volume indices change with end-diastolic pressure. *Circ Res* 1976;39:772–785.
10. Dougherty AH, Naccerelli GV, Gray EL, Hicks CH, Goldstein RA. Congestive heart failure with normal systolic function. *Am J Cardiol* 1984;54:778–782.
11. Soufer R, Wohlgelernter D, Vita NA, et al. Intact systolic left ventricular function in clinical congestive heart failure. *Am J Cardiol* 1985;55:1032–1036.
12. Topol EJ, Traill TA, Fortuin NJ. Hypertensive hypertropic cardiomyopathy of the elderly. *N Engl J Med* 1985;312:277–283.
13. Ishida Y, Meisner JS, Tsujioka K, et al. Left ventricular filling dynamics: influence of left ventricular relaxation and left atrial pressure. *Circulation* 1986;74:187–196.
14. Kunis R, Greenberg H, Yeoh CB, et al. Coronary revascularization for recurrent pulmonary edema in elderly patients with ischemic heart disease and preserved ventricular function. *N Engl J Med* 1985;313:1207–1210.
15. Brodie BR, Grossman W, Mann T, McLaurin LP. Effects of sodium nitroprusside on left ventricular diastolic pressure-volume relations. *J Clin Invest* 1977;59:59–68.
16. Ludbrook PA, Byrne JD, McKnight RC. Influence of right ventricular hemodynamics on left ventricular diastolic pressure-volume relations in man. *Circulation* 1979;59:21–31.
17. Lorell BH, Paulus WJ, Grossman W, Wynne J, Cohn PF. Modification of abnormal left ventricular diastolic properties by nifedipine in patients with hypertrophic cardiomyopathy. *Circulation* 1982;65:499–507.
18. Spann JF Jr, Buccino RA, Sonnenblick E, Braunwald E. Contractile state of cardiac muscle obtained from cats with experimentally produced ventricular hypertrophy and heart failure. *Circ Res* 1967;21:341–354.
19. Pool PE, Spann JF Jr, Buccino RA, Sonnenblick EH, Braunwald E. Myocardial high energy phosphate stores in cardiac hypertrophy and heart failure. *Circ Res* 1967;21:365–373.
20. Ito Y, Suko J, Chidsey CA. Intracellular calcium and myocardial contractility. *J Mol Cell Cardiol* 1974;6:237–247.
21. Bristow MR, Ginsberg R, Minobe W, et al. Decreased catecholamine sensitivity and beta adrenergic receptor density in failing human hearts. *N Engl J Med* 1982;307:205–211.
22. Willerson JT. What is wrong with the failing heart? *N Engl J Med* 1982;307:243–245.
23. Horn EM, Corwin SJ, Steinberg SF, et al. Reduced lymphocyte stimulatory guanine nucleotide regulatory protein and β-adrenergic receptors in congestive heart failure. *Circulation* 1988;78:1373–1379.
24. Cohn JN, Broder M, Franciosa JA, Guiha NH, Limas CJ. Relative importance of preload and

afterload as determinants of left ventricular performance in acute myocardial infarction. *J Clin Invest* 1972;51:20.

25. Cohn JN, Archibald DG, Ziesche S, et al. Effect of vasodilator therapy on mortality in chronic congestive heart failure: results of a Veterans Administration Cooperative Study. *N Engl J Med* 1986;314:1547–1552.

26. CONSENSUS Trial Study Group. Effects of enalapril on mortality in severe congestive heart failure: results of the Cooperative North Scandinavian Enalapril Survival Study (CONSENSUS). *N Engl J Med* 1987;316:1429–1435.

27. Francis GS, Goldsmith SR, Levine TB, Olivari MT, Cohn JN. The neurohumoral axis in congestive heart failure. *Ann Intern Med* 1984; 101:370–377.

27a. Francis GS, Pierpont GL. Pathophysiology of congestive heart failure secondary to congestive and ischemic cardiomyopathy. In: Shaver JA, Brest AN, eds. *Cardiomyopathies: clinical presentation, differential diagnosis, and management.* Cardiovascular Clinics. Philadelphia: FA Davis, 1988;57–74.

28. Laragh JH. Atrial natriuretic hormone, the renin-aldosterone axis and blood pressure-electrolyte homeostasis. *N Engl J Med* 1985; 313:1300–1340.

29. Francis GS, Goldsmith SR, Pierpont GL, Cohn JN. Free and conjugated plasma catecholamines in patients with congestive heart failure. *J Lab Clin Med* 1984;103:393–398.

30. Dzau VJ, Packer M, Lilly LS, Swartz SL, Hollenberg NK, Williams GH. Prostaglandins in heart failure: relation to activation of the renin-angiotensin system and hyponatremia. *N Engl J Med* 1984;310:347–352.

30a. Francis GS, Goldsmith SR. Adaptive neurohumoral mechanisms in dilated cardiomyopathy. In: Engelmeier RS, O'Connell JB, eds. *Drug therapy in dilated cardiomyopathy and myocarditis.* New York: Marcel Dekker, 1988;23–48.

31. Levine TB, Francis GS, Goldsmith SR, Simon AB, Cohn JN. Activity of the sympathetic nervous system and renin angiotensin system assessed by plasma hormone levels and their relationship to hemodynamic abnormalities. *Am J Cardiol* 1982;49:1659–1666.

32. Francis GS, Cohn JN. The autonomic nervous system in congestive heart failure. In: Creager WP, ed. *Annual review of medicine,* vol 37. Palo Alto: Annual Reviews, Inc., 1986;235–247.

33. Hasking GJ, Esler MD, Jennings GL, Burton D, Johns JA, Korner PI. Norepinephrine spillover to plasma in patients with congestive heart failure: evidence of increased overall and cardiorenal sympathetic nerve activity. *Circulation* 1986;73:615–621.

34. Leimbach WN, Wallin BG, Victor RG, Aylward PE, Sundlof G, Mark AL. Direct evidence from intraneural recordings for increased central sympathetic outflow in patients with heart failure. *Circulation* 1986;73:913–919.

35. Levine TB, Francis GS, Goldsmith SR, Cohn JN. The neurohumoral and hemodynamic response to orthostatic tilt in patients with congestive heart failure. *Circulation* 1983;67: 1070–1075.

36. Olivari MT, Levine TB, Cohn JN. Abnormal neurohumoral response to nitroprusside infusion in congestive heart failure. *J Am Coll Cardiol* 1983;2:411–417.

37. Cohn JN, Levine TB, Olivari MT, et al. Plasma norepinephrine as a guide to prognosis in patients with chronic congestive heart failure. *N Engl J Med* 1984;311:819–823.

38. Francis GS, Goldsmith SR, Ziesche SM, Cohn JN. The response of plasma norepinephrine and epinephrine to dynamic exercise in patients with congestive heart failure. *Am J Cardiol* 1982;49:1152–1156.

39. Francis GS, Goldsmith SR, Ziesche S, Nakajima H, Cohn JN. Relative attenuation of sympathetic drive during exercise in patients with congestive heart failure. *J Am Coll Cardiol* 1985;5:832–839.

40. Gaffney TE, Braunwald E. Importance of the adrenergic nervous system in support of circulatory function in patients with congestive heart failure. *Am J Med* 1963;34:320–324.

41. Binkley PF, Lewe R, Leier CV. Neurohumoral profile determines hemodynamic response to beta blockade in congestive heart failure. *Clin Res* 1986;34:283A.

42. Eliot RS, Todd GL, Clayton FC, et al. Experimental catecholamine induced acute myocardial necrosis. *Adv Cardiol* 1978;25:107–118.

43. Garcia R, Jennings JM. Pheochromocytoma masquerading as a cardiomyopathy. *Am J Cardiol* 1972;29:107–118.

44. Creager MA, Faxon DP, Cutler SS, Kohlmann O, Ryan TJ, Gavras H. Contribution of vasopressin to vasoconstriction in patients with congestive heart failure: comparison with the renin angiotensin system and the sympathetic nervous system. *J Am Coll Cardiol* 1986;7:758–765.

45. Dargie HJ, Cleland JGF, Leckie BJ, Inglis CG, East BW, Ford I. Relation of arrhythmias and electrolyte abnormalities to survival in patients with severe chronic heart failure. *Circulation* 1987;75(Suppl IV):IV99–IV107.

46. Gottschalk CW. Renal nerves and sodium excretion. *Annu Rev Physiol* 1979;41:229–240.

47. Boke T, Malik KU. Enhancement by locally generated angiotensin II of release of the adrenergic transmitter in isolated rat kidney. *J Pharmacol Exp Ther* 1983;226:900–907.

48. Engelmeier RS, O'Connell JB, Walsh R, Rad N, Scanlon PJ, Gunnar RM. Improvement in symptoms and exercise tolerance by metoprolol in patients with dilated cardiomyopathy: a double-blind, randomized, placebo-controlled trial. *Circulation* 1985;72:536–546.

49. Swedberg K, Waagstein F, Hjalmarson A, Wallentin I. Prolongation of survival in congestive cardiomyopathy by beta receptor blockade. *Lancet* 1979;1:1374–1376.

50. Warren JV, Stead EA Jr. Fluid dynamics in chronic congestive heart failure. *Arch Intern Med* 1944;73:138–147.

51. Merrill AJ. Edema and decreased renal blood flow in patients with chronic congestive heart failure: evidence of "forward failure" as primary cause of edema. *J Clin Invest* 1946; 25:389–400.

52. Briggs AP, Fowell DM, Hamilton WF, Remington JW, Wheeler NC, Winslow JW. Renal and circulatory factors in the edema formation of congestive heart failure. *J Clin Invest* 1948;27:810–817.

53. Bradley SE, Blake WD. Pathogenesis of renal dysfunction during congestive heart failure. *Am J Med* 1949;6:470–480.

54. Singer B, Werner J. Excretion of sodium retaining substances in patients with chronic heart failure. *Am Heart J* 1953;45:795–801.

55. Ayelrod BJ, Cates JE, Johnson BB, Leutscher JA Jr. Aldosterone in urine of normal man of patients with edema. *Br Med J* 1955;1:196–199.

56. Merrill AJ, Morrison JF, Brannon EG. Concentration of renin in renal venous blood in patients with congestive heart failure. *Am J Med* 1946;1:468–472.

57. Tobian L, Tomboulian A, Janacek J. The effect of high perfusion pressure on the granulation of juxtaglomerular cells in an isolated kidney. *J Clin Invest* 1959;38:605–610.

58. Farhi ER, Cant JR, Barger AC. Interactions between intrarenal epinephrine receptors and the renal baroreceptor in the control of PRA in conscious dogs. *Circ Res* 1982;50:477–485.

59. Skott O, Briggs JP. Direct demonstration of macula densa related renin secretion. *Science* 1987;237:1618–1620.

60. Blair EH, Davis JO, Witty RT. Renin release after hemorrhage and after suprarenal aortic constriction in dogs without sodium delivery to the macula densa. *Circ Res* 1970;27:1081–1089.

61. Stornetta RL, Hawelu-Johnson CL, Guyenet PG, Lynch KR. Astrocytes synthesize angiotensinogen in brain. *Science* 1988;242:1444–1446.

62. Dzau VJ, Ingelfinger J, Pratt RE, Ellison KE. Identification of renin and angiotensinogen messenger RNA sequences in mouse and rat brains. *Hypertension* 1986;8:544–548.

63. Kifor I, Dzau VJ. Endothelial renin-angiotensin pathway: evidence for intracellular synthesis and secretion on angiotensins. *Circ Res* 1987;60:422–428.

64. Packer M, Lee WH, Kessler PD. Preservation of glomerular filtration rate in human heart failure by activation of the renin-angiotensin system. *Circulation* 1986;74:766–774.

65. Peach MJ. Renin-angiotensin system: biochemistry and mechanisms of action. *Physiol Rev* 1977;57:313–370.

66. Francis GS. Extracardiac features of heart failure: catecholamines and hormonal changes. *Cardiology* 1987;75(Suppl I):19–29.

67. Capelli JP, Wesson LG Jr, Aponte GE. A phylogenetic study of the renin-angiotensin system. *Am J Physiol* 1970;218:1171–1178.

68. Nighimura H, Ogawa M, Sawyer WH. Renin-angiotensin system in primitive bony fishes and a holocephalian. *Am J Physiol* 1973;224:950–956.

69. Yanagisawa M, Kurihara H, Kimura S, et al. A novel potent vasoconstrictor peptide produced by vascular endothelial cells. *Nature* 1988;332:411–415.

70. Monos E, Cox RH, Peterson CH. Direct effect of physiologic doses of arginine vasopressin on the arterial wall *in vivo*. *Am J Physiol* 1978;243:H167–H173.

71. Goldsmith SR, Francis GS, Cowley A, Levine TB, Cohn JN. Increased plasma arginine vasopressin levels in patients with congestive heart failure. *J Am Coll Cardiol* 1983;1:1385–1390.

72. Goldsmith SR, Francis GS, Cowley AW, et al. Hemodynamic effects of arginine vasopressin in congestive heart failure. *J Am Coll Cardiol* 1986;8:779–783.

73. Nicod P, Waeber B, Bussien, et al. Acute hemodynamic effects of a vascular antagonist of vasopressin in patients with congestive heart failure. *Am J Cardiol* 1985;55:1043–1047.

74. Burnett JC Jr, Kao PC, Hu DC, et al. Atrial natriuretic peptide elevation in chronic congestive heart failure. *Science* 1986;231:1145–1147.

75. deBold AJ, Borenstein HB, Veress HT, Sonnenberg H. A rapid and potent natriuretic response to intravenous injection of atrial myocardial extract in rats. *Life Sci* 1981;28:89–94.

76. Edwards BS, Ackermann DM, Wold LE, Burnett JC Jr. Identification of ventricular immunoreactive "atrial" natriuretic factor (ANF) in heart failure. *J Clin Invest* 1988;81:82–86.

77. Schenk DB, Phelps MN, Porter JG, Scarborough RM, McEnroe GA, Lewicki JA. Identification of the receptor for atrial natriuretic factor on cultured vascular cells. *J Biol Chem* 1985;26:14887–14890.

78. Schiffrin EL, Chartier L, Thibault G, St. Louis J, Cartin M, Genest J. Vascular and adrenal receptors for atrial natriuretic factor in the rat. *Circ Res* 1985;56:801–807.

79. Campbell WB, Currie MG, Needleman P. Inhibition of aldosterone biosynthesis by atriopeptins in rat adrenal cells. *Circ Res* 1985; 57:113–118.

80. Samson WK. Atrial natriuretic factor inhibits dehydration and hemorrhage induced vasopressin release. *Neuroendocrinology* 1985;40: 277–279.

81. Cody RJ, Atlas SA, Laragh JH, et al. Atrial natriuretic factor in normal subjects and heart failure patients. Plasma levels and renal, hormonal, and hemodynamic responses to peptide infusion. *J Clin Invest* 1986;78:1362–1374.

82. Cody RJ, Kubo SH, Atlas SA, et al. Direct demonstration of the vasodilator properties of atrial natriuretic factor in normal man and heart failure patients. *Clin Res* 1986;34:476A.

83. Zelis R, Nellis SH, Longhurst J, Lee G, Mason DT. Abnormalities in the regional circulations accompanying congestive heart failure. *Prog Cardiovasc Dis* 1975;18:181–199.

84. Punzengruber C, Staneck B, Sinzinger H, Sil-

berbauer K. Bicycloprostaglandin E$_2$ metabolite in congestive heart failure and relation to vasoconstrictor neurohumoral principles. *Am J Cardiol* 1986;57:619–623.

85. Horton R, Zipser R, Fichman M. Prostaglandins, renal function and vascular regulation. *Med Clin North Am* 1981;65:891–914.

86. Dzau VJ, Swartz SL, Creager MA. The role of prostaglandins in the pathophysiology and therapy for congestive heart failure. *Heart Failure* 1986;2:6–13.

87. Goldberg LI, Rajfer SI. Dopamine receptors: applications in clinical cardiology. *Circulation* 1985;72:245–248.

88. Young JB, Leon CA, Pratt CM, Suarez JM, Aronoff RD, Roberts R. Hemodynamic effects of an oral dopamine receptor agonist (fenoldopam) in patients with congestive heart failure. *J Am Coll Cardiol* 1985;6:792–796.

89. Francis GS, Wilson BC, Rector TS. Hemodynamic, renal and neurohumoral effects of a selective oral DA$_1$ agonist (fenoldopam) in patients with congestive heart failure. *Am Heart J* 1988;116:473–479.

90. Francis GS, Archer S. Management of congestive heart failure in the intensive and coronary care unit. *J Intensive Care Med* 1988.

91. Cohn JN, Mathew KJ, Franciosa JA, Snow JA. Chronic vasodilator therapy in the management of cardiogenic shock and intractable left ventricular failure. *Ann Intern Med* 1974;81:777–780.

92. Guiha NH, Cohn JN, Mikulic E, Franciosa JA, Limas CJ. Treatment of refractory heart failure with infusion of nitroprusside. *N Engl J Med* 1974;291:587–592.

93. Palmer RF, Lasseter KC. Sodium nitroprusside. *N Engl J Med* 1975;292:294–297.

94. Franciosa JA, Limas CJ, Guiha NH, Rodriguera E, Cohn JN. Improved left ventricular function during nitroprusside infusion in acute myocardial infarction. *Lancet* 1972;1:650–654.

95. Cohn JN, Franciosa JA, Francis GS, et al. Effect of short-term infusion of sodium nitroprusside on mortality rate in acute myocardial infarction complicated by left ventricular failure. Results of a Veterans Administration Cooperative Study. *N Engl J Med* 1982;306:1129–1135.

96. Macho P, Vatner SF. Effect of nitroglycerin and nitroprusside on large and small coronary vessels in conscious dogs. *Circulation* 1981;64:1101–1107.

97. Mann T, Cohn PF, Holman BL, Green LH, Markis JE, Phillips DA. Effects of nitroprusside on regional myocardial blood flow in coronary artery disease. Results in 25 patients and comparison with nitroglycerin. *Circulation* 1977;57:732–738.

98. Chiariello M, Gold HK, Leinback RC, Davis MA, Maroko PR. Comparison between the effects of nitroprusside and nitroglycerin on ischemic injury during acute myocardial infarction. *Circulation* 1976;54:766–773.

99. Kerber RE, Martins JB, Marcus ML. Effect of acute ischemia, nitroglycerin and nitroprusside on regional myocardial thickening, stress and perfusion. Experimental echocardiographic studies. *Circulation* 1979;60:121–129.

100. Feldman RL, Conti CR, Pepine CJ. Comparison of coronary hemodynamic effects of nitroprusside and sublingual nitroglycerin with anterior descending coronary arterial occlusion. *Am J Cardiol* 1983;52:915–920.

101. McCannell KL, McNay JL, Meyer MB, Goldberg L. Dopamine in the treatment of hypotension and shock. *N Engl J Med* 1966;275:1389–1398.

102. Talley RC, Goldberg LI, Johnson CE, McNay JL. A hemodynamic comparison of dopamine and isoproterenol in patients with shock. *Circulation* 1969;39:361–378.

103. Stemple DR, Kleiman JH, Narrison DC. Combined nitroprusside-dopamine therapy in severe chronic congestive heart failure. Dose-related hemodynamic advantages over single drug infusions. *Am J Cardiol* 1978;42:267–275.

104. Francis GS, Sharma B, Hodges M. Comparative hemodynamic effects of dopamine and dobutamine in patients with acute cardiogenic circulatory collapse. *Am Heart J* 1982;103:995–1000.

105. Berkowitz C, McKeever L, Croke RP, Jacobs WR, Loeb HS, Gunnar RM. Comparative responses of dobutamine and nitroprusside in patients with low output cardiac failure. *Circulation* 1977;56:918–924.

106. Mikulic E, Cohn JN, Franciosa JA. Comparative hemodynamic effects of inotropic and vasodilator drugs in severe heart failure. *Circulation* 1977;56:528–533.

107. Leier CV, Unverferth DV. Dobutamine. *Ann Intern Med* 1983;99:490–496.

108. Bianchi C, Diaz R, Gonzales C, Beregovich J. Effects of dobutamine on atrioventricular conduction. *Am Heart J* 1975;90:474–478.

109. Masoni A, Alboni P, Malacarne C, Codeca L. Effects of dobutamine on electrophysiologic properties of the specialized conduction tissue in man. *J Electrocardiol* 1979;12:361–370.

110. Kates RE, Leier CV. Dobutamine pharmacokinetics in severe heart failure. *Clin Pharmacol Ther* 1978;24:537–541.

111. Unverferth DV, Magorien RD, Lewis RP, Leier CV. Long-term benefit of dobutamine in patients with congestive cardiomyopathy. *Am Heart J* 1980;100:622–630.

112. Unverferth DV, Magorien RD, Altschuld R, Kolibash AJ, Lewis RP, Leier CV. The hemodynamic and metabolic advantages gained by a three-day infusion of dobutamine in patients with congestive cardiomyopathy. *Am Heart J* 1983;106:29–34.

113. Liang C-S, Sherman LG, Doherty JU, Wellington K, Lee VW, Hood WB Jr. Sustained improvement of cardiac function in patients with congestive heart failure after short-term infusion of dobutamine. *Circulation* 1984;69:113–119.

114. Unverferth DV, Leier CV, Magorien RD, et al. Improvement of human myocardial mitochondria after dobutamine: a quantitative ultra-

structural study. *J Pharmacol Exp Ther* 1980; 215:527–531.

115. Unverferth DV, Blanford M, Kates RE, Leier CV. Tolerance to dobutamine after a 72 hour continuous infusion. *Am J Med* 1980;69:262–266.

116. Klein NA, Siskind SJ, Frishman WH, Sonnenblick EH, LeJemtel TH. Hemodynamic comparison of intravenous amrinone and dobutamine in patients with chronic congestive heart failure. *Am J Cardiol* 1981;48:170–175.

117. Gage J, Ratman H, Lucido D, LeJemtel TH. Additive effects of dobutamine and amrinone on myocardial contractility and ventricular performance in patients with severe heart failure. *Circulation* 1986;74:367–373.

118. Firth BG, Ratner A, Grassman ED, Winniford MD, Nicod P, Hillis LD. Assessment of the inotropic and vasodilator effects of amrinone versus isoproterenol. *Am J Cardiol* 1984;54:1331–1336.

119. Hlatky MA, Fleg JL, Hinton PC, et al. Physician practice in the management of congestive heart failure. *J Am Coll Cardiol* 1986;8:966–970.

120. The Captopril-Digoxin Multicenter Research Group. Comparative effects of captopril and digoxin in patients with mild to moderate heart failure. *JAMA* 1988;289:539–544.

121. Smith TW. Digitalis: mechanisms of action and clinical use. *N Engl J Med* 1988;318:358–365.

122. Okita GT. Dissociation of Na⁺, K⁺-ATPase inhibition from digitalis inotropy. *Fed Proc* 1977;36:2225–2230.

123. Arnold SB, Byrd RC, Meister W, et al. Long-term digitalis therapy improves left ventricular function in heart failure. *N Engl J Med* 1980;303:1443–1448.

124. Lee DCS, Johnson RA, Bingham JB, et al. Heart failure in outpatients: a randomized trial of digoxin versus placebo. *N Engl J Med* 1982;306:699–705.

125. Francis GS. Inotropic agents in the management of heart failure. In: Cohn JN, ed. *Drug treatment of heart failure,* 2nd ed. Secaucus, NJ: Advanced Therapeutics Communications International, 1988;179–197.

126. Baim DS, Colucci WS, Monrad ES, et al. Survival of patients with severe congestive heart failure treated with oral milrinone. *J Am Coll Cardiol* 1986;7:661–670.

127. Uretsky BT, Generalovich T, Versalis JG, Valdes AM, Reddy PS. MDL 17,043 therapy in severe congestive heart failure. *J Am Coll Cardiol* 1985;5:1414–1421.

128. Weber KT, Janicki JS, Jain MC. Piroximone (MDL 19,205) in the treatment of unstable and stable chronic heart failure. *Am Heart J* 1987;114:805–813.

129. Rajfer SI, Anton AH, Rossen JD, Goldberg LI. Beneficial hemodynamic effects of oral levodopa in heart failure. *N Engl J Med* 1984; 310:1357–1362.

130. Rajfer SI, Rossen JD, Douglas FL, Goldberg LI, Karrison T. Effects of long-term therapy with oral ibopamine on resting hemodynamics and exercise capacity in patients with heart failure. *Circulation* 1986;73:740–748.

131. Bayliss J, Thomas L, Poole-Wilson P. Acute hemodynamic and neuroendocrine effects of dopexamine, a new vasodilator for the treatment of heart failure: comparison with dobutamine, captopril, and nitrate. *J Cardiovasc Pharmacol* 1987;9:551–554.

132. Feldman MC, Copelas L, Gwathmey JK, et al. Deficient production of cyclic AMP: pharmacologic evidence of an important cause of contractile dysfunction in patients with end-stage heart failure. *Circulation* 1987;75:331–339.

133. Asanol H, Susayama S, Iuchi K, Kameyama T. Acute hemodynamic effects of a new inotropic agent (OPC-8212) in patients with congestive heart failure. *J Am Coll Cardiol* 1987;9:865–871.

134. Fujino K, Sperelakis N, Solaro RJ. Sensitization of dog and guinea pig heart myofilaments to Ca²⁺ activation and the inotropic effect of pimobendan: comparison with milrinone. *Circ Res* 1988;63:911–922.

135. Ikram H, Chan W, Bennett SI, Bones P. Hemodynamic effects of acute beta adrenergic receptor blockade in congestive cardiomyopathy. *Br Heart J* 1979;42:311–315.

136. Ikram H, Fitzpatrick D. Double-blind trial of chronic oral beta blockade in congestive cardiomyopathy. *Lancet* 1981;2:490–493.

137. Binkley PF, Lewe R, Lima JJ, Al-Awwa A, Unverferth DN, Leier CV. Hemodynamic-inotropic response to beta-blocker with intrinsic sympathomimetic activity in patients with congestive cardiomyopathy. *Circulation* 1986;74:1390–1398.

138. The German and Austrian Xamoterol Study Group. Double-blind placebo-controlled comparison of digoxin and xamoterol in chronic heart failure. *Lancet* 1988;1:489–493.

139. Cohn JN, Franciosa JA. Vasodilator therapy of cardiac failure. *N Engl J Med* 1977;297:27–31,254–258.

140. Schmidt K, Kubovetz WR. Stimulation of soluble coronary arterial guanylate cyclase by SIN-1. *Eur J Pharmacol* 1986;122:75–79.

141. Edwards JC, Ignarro LJ, Hyman AI, Kadowitz PJ. Relaxation of pulmonary artery and veins by nitrogen-oxide containing vasodilators and cyclic GMP. *J Pharmacol Exp Ther* 1984; 228:33–42.

142. Moncada S, Palmer RMJ, Higgs EA. The discovery of nitric oxide as the endogenous nitrovasodilator. *Hypertension* 1988;12:365–372.

143. Palmer RM, Ferrige AG, Moncada S. Nitric oxide release accounts for the biological activity of endothelium-derived relaxing factor. *Nature* 1987;327:524–526.

144. Franciosa JA, Goldsmith SR, Cohn JN. Contrasting immediate and long-term effects of isosorbide dinitrate on exercise capacity in congestive heart failure. *Am J Med* 1980; 69:559–566.

145. Leier CV, Huss P, Margorien RD, Unverferth

DV. Improved exercise capacity and differing arterial and venous tolerance during chronic isosorbide dinitrate therapy for congestive heart failure. *Circulation* 1983;67:817–822.

146. Packer M, Lee WH, Kessler PD, Gottlieb SS, Yurshak M, Medina N. Prevention and reversal of nitrate tolerance in patients with congestive heart failure. *N Engl J Med* 1987;317:799–804.

147. Sharpe N, Coxon R, Webster M, Luke R. Hemodynamic effects of intermittent transdermal nitroglycerin in chronic congestive heart failure. *Am J Cardiol* 1987;59:895–899.

148. Kulic D, Rath A, McIntosh N, Rahimtoola SH, Elkayam U. Resistance to isosorbide dinitrate in patients with severe chronic heart failure: incidence and attempt at hemodynamic prediction. *J Am Coll Cardiol* 1988;12:1023–1028.

149. Packer M, Medina N, Yushak M, Lee WH. Hemodynamic factors limiting the response to transdermal nitroglycerin in severe chronic congestive heart failure. *Am J Cardiol* 1986; 57:260–267.

150. Armstrong PW, Armstrong JA, Marks GS. Pharmacokinetic-hemodynamic studies of intravenous nitroglycerin in congestive heart failure. *Circulation* 1980;62:160–166.

151. Cohn JN, Archibald DG, Johnson G. Effect of vasodilator therapy on peak exercise oxygen consumption in heart failure. V-HeFT (abst). *Circulation* 1987;75(Suppl II):II443.

152. Magorien RD, Unverferth DV, Leier CV. Hydralazine therapy in chronic congestive heart failure. Sustained central and regional hemodynamic responses. *Am J Med* 1984;77:267–274.

153. Franciosa JA, Weber KT, Levine TB, et al. Hydralazine in the long-term treatment of chronic heart failure: lack of a difference from placebo. *Am Heart J* 1982;104:587–594.

154. Conradson TB, Ryden L, Ahlmark G, Saetre H, Person S, Nyquist O. Clinical efficacy of oral hydralazine in chronic heart failure. One-year double-blind placebo controlled study. *Am Heart J* 1984;108:1001–1006.

155. Packer M, Meller J, Medina N, Yushak M, Gorlin R. Hemodynamic characterization of tolerance to long-term hydralazine therapy in severe chronic heart failure. *N Engl J Med* 1982;306:57–62.

156. Kessler PD, Packer M. Hemodynamic effects of BTS 49465, a new long-acting systemic vasodilator drug, in patients with severe chronic heart failure. *Am Heart J* 1987;113:137–143.

157. Agostoni PG, DeCesare N, Doria E, Polese A, Tamborini G, Guazzi MD. Afterload reduction: a comparison of captopril and nifedipine in dilated cardiomyopathy. *Br Heart J* 1986;55:391–399.

158. Elkayam U, Weber L, McKay C, Rahimtoola S. Spectrum of acute hemodynamic effects of nifedipine in severe congestive heart failure. *Am J Cardiol* 1985;56:560–566.

159. Fifer MA, Colucci WS, Lorell BH, Barry WH. Inotropic, vascular and neuroendocrine effects of nifedipine in heart failure: comparison with nitroprusside. *J Am Coll Cardiol* 1985;7:737–747.

160. Packer M, Lee WH, Medina N, Yushak M, Bernstein JL, Kessler PD. Prognostic importance of the immediate hemodynamic response to nifedipine in patients with severe left ventricular dysfunction. *J Am Coll Cardiol* 1987; 10:1303–1311.

161. Barjon JN, Rouleau J-L, Bichet D, Juneau C, De Champlain J. Chronic renal and neurohumoral effects of the calcium entry blocker nisoldipine in patients with congestive heart failure. *J Am Coll Cardiol* 1987;9:622–630.

162. Kramer BL, Massie BM, Topic N. Controlled trial of captopril in congestive heart failure: a rest and exercise hemodynamic study. *Circulation* 1983;67:807–816.

163. Sharp DN, Murphy J, Coxon R, Hannon SF. Enalapril in patients with chronic heart failure: a placebo controlled, randomized, double-blind study. *Circulation* 1984;70:271–278.

164. Packer M, Medina N, Yushak M, Meller J. Hemodynamic patterns of response during long-term captopril therapy for severe chronic therapy. *Circulation* 1983;68:803–812.

165. Captopril Multicenter Research Group. A placebo-controlled trial of captopril in refractory congestive heart failure. *J Am Coll Cardiol* 1983;2:755–763.

166. Franciosa JA, Wilen MM, Jordan RA. Effects of enalapril, a new angiotensin converting enzyme inhibitor, in a controlled trial in heart failure. *J Am Coll Cardiol* 1985;5:101–107.

167. Creager MA, Massie BM, Faxon DP, et al. Acute and long-term effects of enalapril on the cardiovascular response to exercise tolerance in patients with congestive heart failure. *J Am Coll Cardiol* 1985;6:163–170.

168. Cleland JGF, Dargie HJ, Ball SG, et al. Effects of enalapril in heart failure: a double-blind study of effects on exercise performance, renal function, hormones, and metabolic state. *Br Heart J* 1985;54:305–312.

169. Packer M, Medina M, Yushak M. Correction of dilutional hyponatremia in patients with severe chronic heart failure by converting enzyme inhibition. *Ann Intern Med* 1984;100:782–789.

170. Cleland JGF, Dargie HJ, Hodsman GP, et al. Captopril in heart failure: a double-blind controlled trial. *Br Heart J* 1984;52:530–535.

171. Packer M, Lee WH, Medina N, Yushak M, Kessler P. Identification of patients with severe heart failure most likely to fail long-term therapy with converting enzyme inhibitors. *J Am Coll Cardiol* (abst) 1986;7:181A.

172. Packer M, Lee WH, Kessler PD. Preservation of glomerular filtration rate in human heart failure by activation of the renin-angiotensin system. *Circulation* 1986;74:766–774.

Cardiovascular Pharmacology, Third Edition, edited by Michael Antonaccio.
Raven Press, Ltd., New York © 1990.

Antiarrhythmic Drugs

Benedict R. Lucchesi

Department of Pharmacology, The University of Michigan Medical School, Ann Arbor, Michigan 48109-0626

The classification of antiarrhythmic drugs, for the most part, has been based on the suspected primary pharmacologic mechanism of action (1,2). The classification may include a consideration of actions on membrane channels, alterations in receptor function, changes in the electrophysiologic properties of single myocardial cells, and modulation of autonomic function as well as other parameters of the cardiac cell. The most often employed classification is that of Vaughan-Williams (3) who initially described four groups in which class I drugs have as their major distinguishing characteristic the potential to decrease the rate of sodium ion entry via the fast inward sodium channel during depolarization of the myocardial cell. Class II agents include those drugs that possess as their major pharmacologic mechanism the ability to antagonize cardiac β-adrenoceptors. The members of class III are distinguished by their ability to prolong the phase of repolarization in ventricular muscle and/or Purkinje tissue. The class IV agents influence the cardiac cell membrane by interfering with the movement of calcium ion through the slow inward calcium channel. There have been several modifications of the classification of antiarrhythmic drugs as new information has been obtained regarding specific electrophysiologic characteristics of individual drugs. The class I drugs have been subdivided into classes IA, IB, and IC.

The ideal approach to treatment of cardiac rhythm disorders depends on proper identification of the arrhythmia, an understanding of the factors involved in the production of the arrhythmia, knowledge of the mechanisms of action of the wide variety of available pharmacologic agents, and an understanding of the clinical effects of the antiarrhythmic agents, particularly as they relate to the clinical setting in which they are employed. Because this text is not concerned with the problems of clinical diagnosis, we shall devote primary attention to the possible electrophysiologic mechanisms underlying the genesis of arrhythmias and the pharmacologic properties of drugs used in the control of abnormal cardiac rhythms.

NORMAL CARDIAC ACTION POTENTIAL

Two major types of electrical activity exist in cardiac cells. These two types of electrical activity are termed the "fast response" and "slow response" and are characteristic for the specialized electrical functions provided by the various cardiac conductile tissues.

The fast-response fibers of the heart are those cardiac fibers that conduct electrical activity at a relatively rapid rate (0.3–3 m/sec). This group includes working atrial

369

and ventricular muscle fibers and fibers of the specialized conducting systems of atria and ventricles. The property of rapid conduction and other related electrophysiologic characteristics that will be described here are dependent on a transmembrane action potential with a rapid rate of depolarization known as the fast-response potential.

Under physiologic conditions, the transmembrane potential of working atrial and ventricular muscle fibers and fibers of the specialized atrial and ventricular conducting system is characterized by a resting membrane potential between -80 and -95 mV. On excitation, a rapid regenerative depolarization is activated at a threshold potential of approximately -70 mV and rapidly carries the transmembrane potential to a value of $+25$ to $+35$ mV. The rapid depolarization (phase 0 of the cardiac cell action potential) is dependent on rapid influx of sodium ions, carrying a strong positive inward current through specific membrane channels. These channels controlling sodium conductance of the membrane respond rapidly to a change in transmembrane potential, resulting in a rapid depolarization or fast response (Fig. 1). Sodium conductance of the membrane is then inactivated rapidly, and the inward sodium current ceases. In addition, in these fast-response fibers, a

second inward positive current (depolarizing current) is activated when the fast depolarization phase has lowered the membrane potential to values less negative than -55 mV. This is a weaker current than the initial sodium current, and it is probably carried by calcium ions through a "slow" membrane channel that is distinct from the "fast" sodium channel. This slow current is not affected by tetrodotoxin or other inhibitors of sodium influx through the rapid-response channel. Because the slow membrane channels are activated slowly and the current density is low in comparison to the initial inward rapid sodium current, the slow current does not contribute significantly to the rapid depolarization (phase 0) of the normal cardiac action potential. However, inactivation of this secondary inward current is slow; the current still flows after the initial rapid depolarization is over and maintains the membrane in a depolarized state. Thus, the slow current is primarily responsible for the plateau phase (phases 2 and 3) of the action potential (Fig. 1).

Because of the nature of the voltage and time dependence of the mechanisms that control the fast sodium channels, fibers that generate action potentials by this fast-response mechanism have certain characteristic electrophysiologic properties. The

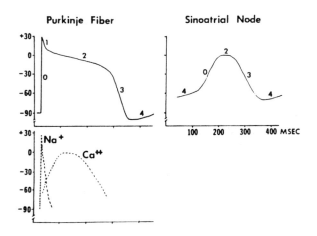

FIG. 1. Diagrammatic representation of the membrane action potential as recorded from a Purkinje fiber and the sinoatrial node. The membrane resting potential is -90 mV with respect to the exterior of the fiber. At the point of depolarization there is a rapid change (phase 0) to a more positive value. The phases of depolarization and repolarization are indicated by the numbers 0, 1, 2, 3, and 4. The sinoatrial node has a resting value of only -60 mV, and depolarization (phase 0) proceeds at a much slower rate. The lower graph shows the rates of influx of sodium and calcium during the Purkinje fiber action potential.

large resting potential (-75 to -90 mV), the value of the threshold potential (-70 mV), the rapid rate of phase-0 upstroke velocity, and the large amplitude of depolarization (100–130 mV) result in relatively rapid conduction of the cardiac impulse. Fast responses have a large safety factor for conduction, so that propagation of the impulse usually is not blocked by minor electrical and anatomic impediments to its spread. A normal response in these fibers can be elicited only when repolarization has restored the normal resting potential.

Slow cardiac fibers of the heart conduct electrical activity at a relatively slow rate (0.01–0.10 m/sec). This group includes the sinus and atrioventricular nodes, cardiac fibers of the atrioventricular ring, and mitral and tricuspid valve leaflets. The property of slow conduction is dependent on a transmembrane action potential with a slow rate of depolarization. This type of action potential has been termed the "slow response."

The electrophysiologic characteristics of the slow response are entirely different from those described for the fast-response fibers. The slow fibers have a low resting membrane potential between -70 and -60 mV, and on excitation a slow regenerative depolarization phase carries the transmembrane potential to a value of only 0 to $+15$ mV. This slow depolarization is not dependent on sodium influx through a rapid membrane channel but rather is due to a weak inward current, possibly carried by calcium through a slow membrane channel. This channel is also inactivated slowly, resulting in a prolonged phase of repolarization. There is no evidence for rapid channels in these fibers, and the depolarization phase is not affected by tetrodotoxin or other inhibitors of rapid sodium influx.

MECHANISMS FOR GENESIS OF CARDIAC ARRHYTHMIAS

Current theories of the electrophysiologic mechanisms thought to be responsible for the origin and perpetuation of cardiac arrhythmias have been derived primarily from experimental models. Of the many proposed mechanisms, the simplest approach is to consider abnormal rhythm formations as being due to either altered impulse formation (automaticity) or altered conduction or both acting simultaneously in the same location or different locations in the heart. The reader who would like to pursue this study in detail should consult one or more of the excellent publications in this area (4–7).

RHYTHM DISTURBANCES DUE TO ECTOPIC IMPULSE FORMATION

An impulse can be generated by an excitable membrane when its transmembrane potential is reduced (becomes less negative) from the normal resting potential to some critical level of potential that has been designated the "threshold potential" or the "critical firing potential." This change from the resting potential to the critical firing potential is achieved by a flow of positive charge into an area of resting membrane. At the time of excitation, the cell membrane suddenly becomes permeable to sodium. The intense inward sodium current carries sufficient positive charge into the cell to alter the transmembrane voltage to a value near the sodium equilibrium potential (transmembrane potential becomes positive). Figure 1 is a schematic representation of the transmembrane action potential of a Purkinje fiber and is represented as having five phases. The generation of the cardiac impulse is normally confined to specialized tissues in the heart that spontaneously depolarize during phase 4. Slow spontaneous depolarization proceeds to a threshold, at which an action potential is initiated and propagated through the cardiac conduction system to the myocardial cells. Cells capable of giving rise to slow diastolic depolarization have the property of automaticity (Fig. 2).

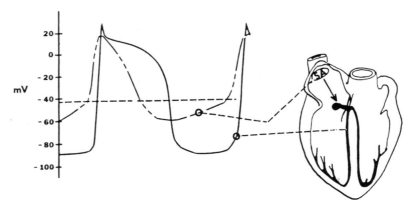

FIG. 2. Diagrammatic representation of the membrane action potential as recorded from the sinoatrial node (SA: *broken line*) and from a Purkinje fiber (*solid line*). The generation of the cardiac impulse is normally confined to the specialized cells in the sinoatrial node. Pacemaker cells possess the characteristic of spontaneous phase-4 depolarization (automaticity). When the slow spontaneous depolarization reaches the level of the threshold potential (*horizontal broken line*), an action potential is generated and propagated through the cardiac conduction system to the myocardial cells.

In the normal heart, automaticity is most prominent in the specialized cells of the sinoatrial node located in the right atrium. This region is commonly referred to as the "pacemaker," for it is this area of the heart that gives rise to the normal rhythmic beat of the heart. The spontaneous electrical activity that can be recorded from the sinoatrial node serves as the impulse that ultimately depolarizes or excites all the cardiac cells and causes the heart to contract. The spontaneous electrical depolarization of the sinoatrial pacemaker cells is independent of the nervous system and can be demonstrated to proceed in the heart removed from the body and maintained with adequate oxygen and metabolic substrates. The specialized pacemaker cells of the sinoatrial node are innervated by both sympathetic and parasympathetic nerves. The sympathetic nerve fibers (adrenergic nerves) release the catecholamine norepinephrine, which causes an increase in the rate of spontaneous diastolic depolarization in the sinoatrial nodal pacemaker cells and an increase in the heart rate. In contrast, the parasympathetic nerves (vagus nerve) to the sinoatrial node release the chemical

neurotransmitter acetylcholine, which causes a decrease in the rate of pacemaker discharge and a slowing of the heart rate. The pacemaker cells of the sinoatrial node display the property of automaticity, which, although independent of the nervous system, can be modified by the influence of the sympathetic and parasympathetic nervous systems. The neuronal influences on the pacemaker cells help the beating heart to adjust its rate in an effort to regulate the cardiac output to meet the needs of the body.

Other specialized cells in the normal heart also possess the property of automaticity. Under circumstances in which the normal pacemaker cells of the sinoatrial node fail to pace the heart, the subsidiary pacemaker cells serve the function of maintaining the heartbeat. The subsidiary pacemaker cells discharge at a slower rate than those of the sinoatrial node, and their rate of discharge is not as well modulated by the autonomic nervous system. Because the cardiac rhythm is dominated by the fastest pacemaker, the normal heart rhythm is controlled by the automaticity of the sinoatrial node. The subsidiary pacemakers influence the cardiac rhythm when the normal pacemaker is suppressed or when, because of pathologic changes or drugs, the rate of discharge is increased to the point at which it can dominate the cardiac rhythm (Figs. 3 and 4). Automaticity of subsidiary pacemakers can occur as a result of myocardial cell damage due to infarction or can be due to digitalis toxicity or excessive amounts of catecholamines released from sympathetic nerve fibers to the heart or circulating in the blood. Thus, the enhancement of automaticity in specialized cardiac cells can lead to cardiac arrhythmias. Cardiac cells other than those of the sinoatrial node that are capable of automaticity include (a) special-

ized atrial fibers, (b) atrioventricular nodal cells in the N-H region, (c) the bundle of His, and (d) Purkinje fibers.

Depression of automaticity in pacemaker fibers is a property common to all class I antiarrhythmic drugs. It is fortunate that most antiarrhythmic agents depress subsidiary pacemaker cells to a greater degree than those of the sinoatrial node, although toxic doses of some antiarrhythmic drugs can suppress all cardiac pacemaker activity and result in arrest of the heartbeat.

The differential effects of antiarrhythmic drugs on automaticity in the various tissues of the heart are, in part, due to the different mechanisms involved in impulse formation

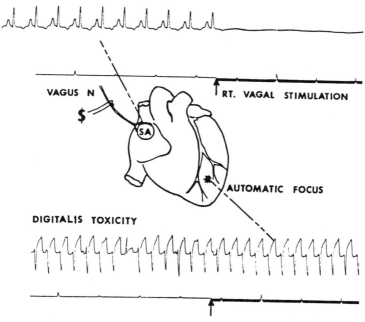

FIG. 3. Under special circumstances, automaticity in areas other than the sinoatrial node may dominate the rhythm of the heart. The electrocardiogram in the upper portion of the figure illustrates the normal sequence of events in which the cardiac pacemaker originates within the sinoatrial node and leads to activation of the atrial and ventricular fibers, thus giving rise to the electrocardiogram showing the P, QRS, and T-wave configuration. Stimulation of the right vagus nerve suppresses pacemaker activity within the sinoatrial node, leading to a loss of electrical activity from the heart as the subsidiary pacemakers fail to discharge during the brief period of vagal-induced sinoatrial arrest. Under certain conditions, such as in the presence of toxic doses of a digitalis glycoside (ouabain), the action of subsidiary pacemakers may be enhanced to the point at which they dominate the cardiac rhythm (*lower panel*). Stimulation of the right vagus nerve is ineffective in terminating the ectopic ventricular pacemaker. Thus, the enhancement of automaticity in cardiac cells outside the sinoatrial node is an important mechanism for the genesis of cardiac arrhythmias.

24 HOURS POST MYOCARDIAL INFARCTION

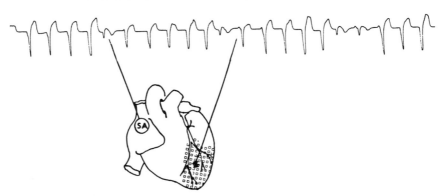

FIG. 4. Role of enhanced automaticity in the genesis of cardiac arrhythmias. Twenty-four hours after experimental infarction in the canine heart, multiple sites of pacemaker activity exist within the ventricle, simultaneously with pacemaker activity from the sinoatrial node. The objective in antiarrhythmic therapy is to suppress the ectopic pacemaker sites so that the sinoatrial node can once more control the cardiac rhythm.

in the various heart regions. Spontaneous diastolic depolarization in fast-response fibers begins immediately after repolarization, at a maximum diastolic potential of -75 to -90 mV. The inward current that depolarizes cells until threshold potential is attained results from a time- and voltage-dependent decrease in membrane potassium conductance and a coexisting steady inward sodium current. A second mechanism for spontaneous diastolic depolarization probably exists only in slow cardiac fibers. This spontaneous diastolic depolarization occurs at maximum diastolic potentials of -60 mV or less. The prototype for this second slow-fiber automaticity is the sinus node. The rapid-response fiber automaticity is very sensitive to class I antiarrhythmic agents, whereas the slow-response fiber automaticity is most sensitive to the class IV antiarrhythmic agents.

RHYTHM DISTURBANCES DUE TO ABNORMAL CONDUCTION

Premature beats or extrasystoles originate in ectopic foci in the atria, the ventricles, or the atrioventricular junctional tissue and may, in turn, initiate episodes of sustained tachyarrhythmias of either supraventricular or ventricular origin. Some of these ectopic rhythms are no doubt due to enhanced automaticity of specialized fibers in the intraatrial conduction tissue and the His-Purkinje system. Certain features of clinically encountered and experimentally induced arrhythmias suggest that ectopic rhythms may result from some mechanism other than enhanced automaticity of the specialized fibers. These abnormal mechanisms seem to be related to the phenomenon called reentrant activity or reentry, which is thought to result from nonuniformity of the cardiac tissues with respect to excitability and impulse conductivity.

To understand better the mechanisms involved in the origin and perpetuation of arrhythmias due to disturbances in conduction, it is necessary to consider the factors that determine normal conduction.

Conduction velocity is dependent on a number of interrelated factors that include (a) the maximal rate of depolarization during the rising phase of the action potential (maximal dV/dt of phase 0), (b) the magnitude of the depolarization (amplitude of the action potential), (c) the levels of threshold and membrane potentials, (d) the cable properties of the fibers (membrane resistance and capacitance), and (e) the fiber diameter. Two of the variables (maximal dV/dt during phase 0 and the amplitude of the action potential) are of singular importance in the determination of conduction velocity.

The conduction velocity of an impulse away from a given site will depend not only on the conduction velocity of the impulse as it approaches the given site but also on the ability of the given site to respond to the excitatory nature of the impulse. The most important determinant of the ability of a fiber to respond to an impulse or stimulus is the level of membrane potential at the moment of excitation. The relationship between fiber response and transmembrane potential has been determined by Weidmann (8) and Hoffman et al. (9) and has been shown to resemble a sigmoid curve. This relationship is depicted on the right side of Fig. 5, which illustrates the relationship between the maximum depolarization rate during phase 0 (V_{max}) of the canine Purkinje fiber action potential in volts per second on the ordinate and the level of membrane potential (E_m) at the moment of fiber

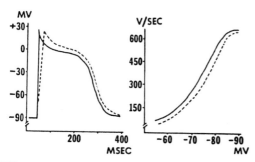

FIG. 5. Diagrammatic relationship between the transmembrane action potential (**left**) and fiber responsiveness (**right**). Membrane responsiveness is reduced by factors causing depolarization. For any given level of transmembrane potential, antiarrhythmic drugs will either reduce membrane responsiveness, as occurs with quinidine or procainamide, or improve membrane responsiveness, as is seen with lidocaine or diphenylhydantoin.

excitation in millivolts on the abscissa. The Purkinje fiber action potential is shown to the left. The role of V_{max} or maximum upstroke velocity as a major determinant of conduction velocity has been demonstrated for heart muscle by the studies of Noble (10). From the relationship between upstroke velocity and conduction velocity, it can readily be seen how impulse conduction in a given fiber will be decreased if the membrane potential at the moment of excitation is reduced (11).

Figure 6 is a schematic representation of possible mechanisms for reentrant excitation due to unidirectional block and the development of a bigeminal or coupled ventricular rhythm. Under normal circumstances, impulse conduction from terminal branches of Purkinje fibers to ventricular muscle causes ventricular depolarization (Fig. 6A). Activation of ventricular myocardium is rapid and synchronous. Impairment of impulse conduction may result because of ischemic injury, which leads to depolarization in the involved fibers and establishes the essential conditions necessary for localized reentry of myocardial electrical activity, slowed conduction, and unidirectional block. Thus, as shown in Fig. 6B, the impulse in Purkinje fiber 2 fails to propagate beyond the injured zone because of a reduced membrane potential in the ischemically injured area. However, the same impulse spreading through a normal terminal branch and reaching the ventricle may enter the depolarized zone (Fig. 6C) from the opposite direction through ventricular tissue. The impulse conducts slowly through the damaged Purkinje fiber and exits the fiber only after the normal Purkinje fiber has regained the ability to conduct this impulse to again excite ventricular muscle. Because the ventricular muscle is excited shortly after the previous event (Fig. 6B), the two resulting ventricular depolarizations are related temporally (coupled) and may account for the genesis of bigeminal rhythms. Antiarrhythmic drugs, by reducing the responsiveness of cardiac cell membranes to

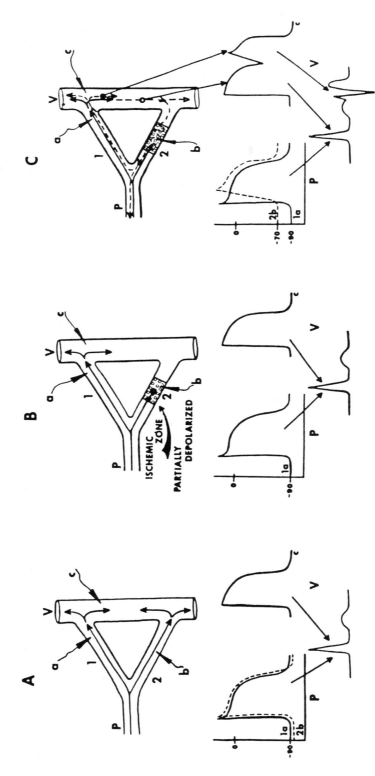

FIG. 6. Schematic representation of possible mechanisms for reentrant excitation due to unidirectional block and the development of a bigeminal or coupled ventricular rhythm. P, Purkinje fiber and its terminal branches 1 and 2 as they enter ventricular muscles; V, micro-electrode recordings from sites a, b, and c are shown below each of the diagrams along with the compound electrocardiogram. The demarcated segment in 2b of **B** and **C** represents a partially depolarized region in which unidirectional block exists.

stimulation and thus reducing conduction velocity, abolish reentry by converting unidirectional block to bidirectional block, or by altering myocardial refractoriness may prevent the entry of electrical activity to normal or damaged myocardium.

ELECTROPHARMACOLOGY OF DRUGS USED FOR TREATMENT OF VENTRICULAR ARRHYTHMIAS

Actions of Class I Drugs

Quinidine is often regarded as the prototype of antiarrhythmic drugs, and along with the other agents listed in Table 1, it makes up the class I antiarrhythmic drugs.

The characteristic actions of the members of this class are that they interfere with myocardial cell depolarization, causing a reduction in the maximum rate of depolarization without producing a change in the resting membrane potential or significant prolongation of the action-potential duration (Fig. 5). The presumed mechanism by which class I antiarrhythmic drugs decrease phase 0 of the membrane action potential is believed to result from a reduction in the rate of entry of the depolarizing sodium current. Because the inward flow of sodium during membrane depolarization is reduced, the rate of rise of phase 0 of the membrane action potential is reduced, as is the absolute height or "overshoot" of the action potential. To obtain a propagated action potential, it is necessary to obtain a minimum rate of depolarization, the latter being dependent on the resting membrane potential and the availability of a sufficient number of active sodium carriers. Without attaining this minimal rate of depolarization, conduction of the premature impulse is sufficiently poor that the premature local response fails to propagate to surrounding ventricular tissue. In the presence of class I drugs, therefore, the entry of the depolarizing current is reduced, and the process of repolarization must proceed for a longer time before an adequate rate of rise for phase 0 can be obtained in order to assure propagation of the impulse to neighboring cells. Thus, repolarization must continue for a longer time in the presence of a class I drug before a propagated event can occur. The result of this action is that class I drugs prolong the effective refractory period of fast-response cardiac fibers.

In summary, class I antiarrhythmic drugs are characterized by their ability to (a) restrict the rate of sodium entry during cardiac membrane depolarization, (b) decrease the rate of rise of phase 0 of the cardiac membrane action potential, (c) require that a greater (more negative) membrane potential be achieved before the membrane becomes excitable and can propagate to its neighbors, and (d) prolong the effective refractory period of fast-response fibers.

Class I antiarrhythmic drugs are characterized further by the fact that they possess local anesthetic actions on nerve and depress myocardial contractile force. Both actions are observed at concentrations greater than that needed to depress the rate of depolarization of phase 0 of the cardiac cell membrane action potential.

How can the electrophysiologic actions of the class I drugs be converted into a salutary effect? Electrophysiologic studies have presented evidence to suggest that slowed conduction in damaged or partially depolarized myocardial cells can contribute to the development of unidirectional block and reentrant cardiac rhythms (Fig. 6). The

TABLE 1. *Classification of antiarrhythmic drugs*

Class I	Class II	Class III	Class IV
Quinidine	Propranolol	Bretylium	Verapamil
Procainamide	Metoprolol	Amiodarone	
Disopyramide	Nadolol	Sotalol	
Phenytoin	Atenolol		
Mexiletine	Acebutolol		
Lidocaine			
Tocainide			
Propranolol[a]			

[a]Additional mechanism.

speed of impulse conduction is related to the rate of depolarization, which in turn is dependent on the level of the resting membrane potential. Antiarrhythmic drugs belonging to class I may convert unidirectional block into bidirectional block and abolish reentry by further depressing conduction through a partially depolarized region (Fig. 6). The beneficial effect would result from the depressant effects of the drugs on the inward sodium current and the production of conduction block.

As indicated earlier, cardiac rhythm disorders can arise from spontaneous impulses or altered automaticity. Two different automatic mechanisms are known to exist in heart tissue. One type of automaticity occurs at membrane potentials between -90 and -60 mV and is due to a time- and voltage-dependent decrease in outward potassium ion current. The second mechanism for the development of automaticity occurs when the membrane potential has been reduced to -65 mV or less. At this level of membrane potential, the fast inward current is inactivated, and the inward current is then dependent on the slow inward movement of calcium ions. This latter type of automaticity is enhanced by the presence of catecholamines.

The antiarrhythmic drugs in class I are known to suppress both normal Purkinje fiber and His-bundle automaticity, as well as abnormal automaticity resulting from myocardial damage that occurs at membrane potentials between -60 and -90 mV. Because the normal pacemaker activity in the sinoatrial node is more dependent on the slow inward calcium current, the antiarrhythmic drugs in class I can suppress spontaneous diastolic depolarization and automatic impulse formation that occur at membrane potentials between -60 and -90 mV at concentrations that do not suppress impulse formation in the sinoatrial node. The ability to "selectively" suppress abnormal automaticity permits the sinoatrial node to once again assume the role of the dominant pacemaker.

In summary, class I antiarrhythmic agents can exert an antiarrhythmic effect by virtue of their ability to depress myocardial conduction in damaged ventricular myocardium and, in addition, suppress abnormal ectopic pacemaker activity.

Actions of Class II Drugs

Drugs belonging to class II exert antisympathetic effects by competitive blockade of β-adrenergic receptors. It should also be noted that whereas all β-adrenergic receptors can be classified as class II drugs, a few members of this group also possess class I and/or class III actions. Thus, propranolol and acebutolol possess class I actions often referred to as "membrane-stabilizing" effects. β-adrenergic receptor antagonists also include drugs such as sotalol, metoprolol, atenolol, and nadolol.

Determining which of the actions of the β receptor blocking drugs can explain their antiarrhythmic effects has proved to be a complex problem. There is no doubt that adrenergic stimulation of the heart can lead to disorders of cardiac rhythm. It is also well known that all β receptor blocking drugs prevent catecholamine-induced alterations of the transmembrane action potential and that this action itself can lead to an antiarrhythmic effect. The arrhythmias associated with halothane or cyclopropane anesthesia have been attributed to the interaction of the anesthetic with catecholamines (12) and have been suppressed with propranolol (13,14). Similarly, catecholamine-induced arrhythmias in experimental animals are known to respond favorably to propranolol, but not to the non-β receptor blocking dextro isomer (15,16).

Davis and Temte (17) have described the effects of propranolol on Purkinje fiber preparations from canine hearts. Propranolol (3.0 mg/liter) decreased the rate of rise of phase 0 of the action potential, decreased the overshoot potential, and decreased membrane responsiveness. At somewhat lower concentrations (0.3 mg/liter), the drug increased the effective refractory period relative to the duration of the action potential. This action of the drug is one that is associated with class I antiarrhythmic agents. Most important was the observation that low concentrations (0.1 mg/liter) of propranolol, which had no effect on the transmembrane potential, blocked the usual increase in diastolic depolarization produced by epinephrine. This would suggest that this is a mechanism by which β receptor blocking agents may suppress or prevent ventricular arrhythmias induced by catecholamines. In addition, the direct effects of propranolol on membrane responsiveness and conduction, plus its direct depressant effects on spontaneous automaticity, may provide mechanisms by which propranolol counteracts ventricular arrhythmias that are not due to β-receptor-mediated events. Depending on the clinical circumstances in which the drug is used, either of the two actions of propranolol (β-adrenergic receptor blockade or direct membrane effects) can be important with respect to the mechanisms by which propranolol produces its antiarrhythmic action.

There is no doubt that many clinically encountered arrhythmias are influenced by endogenously released catecholamines, and all β receptor blocking agents would be effective in removing this component of the arrhythmia-generating mechanism. It is also a well-established fact that propranolol and other β receptor blocking agents are most effective as antiarrhythmic drugs when used for the management of supraventricular arrhythmias. For example, chronic atrial fibrillation and flutter are not usually converted to sinus rhythm, although the ventricular rate may be controlled. The mechanism is undoubtedly due to β receptor blockade, especially in the region of the atrioventricular node. Similar results can be achieved with all β receptor blocking agents at plasma concentrations that do not exert direct effects on the cardiac cells that usually are associated with class I antiarrhythmic

drugs. On the other hand, propranolol is only partially effective in suppressing ventricular arrhythmias not caused by digitalis or exercise (18). Similarly, although propranolol may convert paroxysmal ventricular tachycardia to sinus rhythm, or prevent exercise-induced episodes, the rate of ventricular tachycardia is not slowed by propranolol given in β receptor blocking doses (19,20). Once again, one could attribute the effectiveness of propranolol in paroxysmal supraventricular tachycardia to its β blocking effects within the atrioventricular node. β receptor blockade would decrease the conduction velocity and increase the refractory period within the atrioventricular node and interrupt or make it less possible to maintain or establish a reciprocating mechanism. This would be less likely to occur in ventricular tachycardia in the absence of plasma concentrations of propranolol that would be required to achieve direct membrane effects.

In summary, the class II antiarrhythmic drugs, primarily the β receptor blocking agents, are characterized by the fact that they inhibit catecholamine-induced stimulation of cardiac β-adrenergic receptors. In addition, some members of the group, in particular propranolol and sotalol, produce electrophysiologic alterations in Purkinje and myocardial fibers that resemble those observed with class I and class III antiarrhythmic drugs. These latter effects have been referred to as direct membrane effects. The direct membrane effects occur at plasma concentrations above those needed to achieve β receptor blockade.

Actions of Class III Drugs

The members of class III include bretylium, amiodarone, and sotalol. The feature common to all three is that they prolong the duration of the action potential and the effective refractory period.

When examined in canine Purkinje fibers, bretylium was found to possess electrophysiologic properties that differed markedly from those of other antiarrhythmic agents (21,22). Except at high concentrations, bretylium usually does not affect the resting potential, the rate of rise of phase 0 and the amplitude, membrane responsiveness, or conduction velocity. When examined in partially depolarized fibers, bretylium was reported to produce a transient hyperpolarization that was due to catecholamine release, because the response was not observed in Purkinje fiber preparations obtained from reserpine-pretreated dogs. Thus, bretylium does not resemble the members of class I or II in its electrophysiologic effects. Bretylium's primary electrophysiologic action is to prolong ventricular muscle and Purkinje fiber action potentials, thereby increasing the duration of the ventricular effective refractory period.

Amiodarone, a member of the class III antiarrhythmic agents, differs from bretylium in that it does not alter neuronal function by either releasing or preventing the release of the adrenergic neurotransmitter. It does resemble bretylium, however, in that it produces a significant prolongation of the intracellular cardiac action potential. This effect was observed in studies in which the drug was given both acutely (23) and chronically to animals before removal of the hearts for the purpose of conducting intracellular recordings (24).

Sotalol is a new addition to the class III antiarrhythmic agents and is distinguished by the fact that it possesses β-adrenoceptor blocking properties in addition to its ability to prolong the phase of repolarization in ventricular muscle and Purkinje fibers.

In summary, the class III antiarrhythmic drugs possess complex and unrelated pharmacologic properties, but they seem to share one common property, that of prolonging the duration of the membrane action potential without altering the phase of depolarization or the resting membrane potential. The prolongation of recovery, as well as that of the effective refractory period, is uniform in that it occurs both in ventricular muscle and in Purkinje fibers. It is most likely that the antiarrhythmic actions of class III compounds can be attributed to this singular electrophysiologic effect rather than to the secondary effects that involve alterations in responses of the heart to sympathetic innervation. The importance of the class III drugs is that bretylium, a quaternary ammonium drug, and amiodarone have been shown clinically to be effective in cases of intractable ventricular tachycardia and ventricular fibrillation. These observations alone deserve to be pursued further in the hope that it can lead to the development of an effective and safe antifibrillatory agent. The existence of such a drug would be of extreme value in patients who are at risk of sudden cardiac death and in whom the most common mechanism of death is ventricular fibrillation.

Actions of Class IV Drugs

The prototype drug of the class IV antiarrhythmic agents is verapamil. The members of this group are characterized by their ability to block the slow inward current in cardiac tissue, a current that is dependent on the inward movement of the calcium ion during phases 0–2 of the membrane action potential.

The most pronounced electrophysiologic effects of verapamil are exerted on cardiac fibers with slow-response action potentials. These slow-response fibers are found in the sinus node and atrioventricular node. Administration of verapamil slows conduction velocity and increases refractoriness in the atrioventricular node, thereby reducing the ability of the atrioventricular node to conduct supraventricular impulses to the ventricle. This action will terminate supraventricular tachycardias that utilize the atrioventricular node as a point of reentry and will reduce the number of conducted supraventricular impulses during atrial flutter or atrial fibrillation. Verapamil and other calcium antagonists do not exert marked electrophysiologic actions that depress conduction in fibers other than slow-response fibers of the sinus and atrioventricular node.

An attempt has been made to review the electropharmacology of the four classes of antiarrhythmic drugs and to relate these events to mechanisms suspected of being involved in the genesis of cardiac rhythm disorders. Although it is possible to classify the known antiarrhythmic agents according to their predominant electrophysiologic or pharmacologic action, there are many instances in which an agent can possess a multiple number of effects, each of which may exert a beneficial effect in controlling cardiac arrhythmias. Thus, whereas the grouping of antiarrhythmic drugs into four classes may be convenient, it may fall short of explaining the underlying mechanisms by which these agents exert their antiarrhythmic effects.

Assuming that we know the mechanisms for the development of cardiac arrhythmias, then it becomes possible to examine the electrophysiologic effects of drugs on cardiac cells and attempt to provide an electrophysiologic explanation for antiarrhythmic efficacy. Another difficulty occurs when one recognizes that most of our knowledge concerning the electrophysiologic effects of drugs on cardiac cells has been obtained from essentially "normal" heart muscle preparations. Thus, the challenge remains for the pharmacologist to reexamine the accepted concepts, but to do so in models that represent the pathophysiologic state as it would occur under clinical conditions. Much of the controversy surrounding the electrophysiologic mechanisms of antiarrhythmic drug actions may then be resolved. More important, such an approach may lead to the development of antiarrhythmic drugs that are effective in clearly defined arrhythmias. Antiarrhythmic drug therapy may then be approached on a scientific basis rather than on the empirical methods.

PHARMACOLOGIC BASIS FOR MANAGEMENT OF SUPRAVENTRICULAR TACHYARRHYTHMIAS

Most examples of paroxysmal supraventricular tachycardia (PSVT) have been presumed for many years to be the result of circus movement reentry or reciprocation within a portion of the atrioventricular conduction system. However, reentry has been observed in experimental animal studies to occur within the sinoatrial node (25), the atrium (26), the atrioventricular (A-V) node (27), and the His-Purkinje system (28). Of primary importance is the fact that similar sites for reentry or reciprocation have been suggested as occurring in humans (29–31). The potential reciprocating circuit is activated when it is penetrated by an extrasystole that can be supraventricular or ventricular in origin. A requisite for a reciprocating tachycardia is the combination of the two pathways with unequal conduction velocities and unidirectional block in one of the pathways, thus permitting the initiating impulse to set up a circus movement (Fig. 7). The presence of unidirectional block in one pathway and slow conduction in the second pathway provides sufficient time for the first pathway to recover from its refractory state and allow reentry of the impulse to the site of original block and return of the impulse, which may now reenter the second pathway in the form of an echo or circus movement tachycardia. Variations in the velocity of conduction and the duration of refractoriness within the atria, sinus node, A-V node, or His-Purkinje system are frequent and can result in formation of multiple functional pathways. Because of the influences of the parasympathetic and sympathetic nervous systems, this functional dissociation of conduction and formation of dual pathways occurs most commonly in the A-V node.

In addition to the foregoing mechanisms of reentry as a means of initiating and sustaining supraventricular tachyarrhythmias,

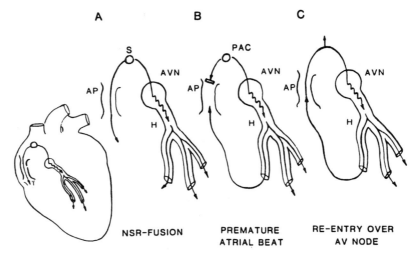

FIG. 7. A: Normal sinus beat is conducted from atria to ventricles along both the A-V node and the accessory pathway. Preexcitation occurs as the ventricles are excited prematurely through the accessory pathway and after a delay through the A-V node. **B:** Premature atrial contraction occurs before the accessory pathway has regained its excitability. However, the A-V node, with a shorter refractory period than the accessory pathway, is able to conduct the impulse to the ventricles. As the ventricles fire, the accessory pathway, having regained its excitability, is excited and conducts the ventricular impulse retrogradely to excite the atria. A circus movement pathway is set up with orthograde conduction through the A-V node and retrograde conduction through the accessory pathway. AP, accessory pathway; AVN, A-V node; H, His bundles; PAC, premature atrial contraction.

there is evidence obtained from myocardial cells from diseased atria from patients who had arrhythmias showing the presence of automatic impulse activity (32). Automaticity also has been recorded from cells within the mitral valve, the His bundle, and Purkinje fibers (33,34).

Atrial tachyarrhythmias due to enhanced automaticity usually display some degree of A-V nodal block, an observation that is incompatible with a continuous reentrant process in the A-V node. In atrial tachycardias the A-V node is not involved, except to receive rapid stimuli, which, if they exceed the maximal rate of A-V transmission, are partially blocked.

In the case of atrial flutter and atrial fibrillation there is still an unresolved question whether these arrhythmias are due to enhanced ectopic foci or reentry or both. Although the rate in atrial flutter is between 300 and 360 beats per minute, only a portion of the impulses gain access to the ven-

tricular conducting system, because of the inability of the A-V node to conduct at this rapid frequency. Thus, usually a 2:1 block with a regular ventricular rate occurs, because the conducting capacity of the A-V node has been exceeded. In atrial fibrillation, the ventricular rate becomes irregular because of variable degrees of impulse penetration that blocked conduction in the A-V node.

It should be apparent that in both atrial flutter and atrial fibrillation the ventricular rate is determined by the number of atrial impulses that are capable of traversing the A-V node and entering the His-Purkinje system. Thus, any intervention, whether it be mediated by the autonomic nervous system or by means of a pharmacologic agent acting on the A-V node, will modify the ventricular response, depending on how A-V nodal transmission is affected. The clinical objective in atrial flutter or atrial fibrillation is to adequately control the ventricular rate so that the hemodynamic status of the patient may become stabilized. Aside from converting the disorder of atrial rhythm and restoring normal sinus rhythm by means of synchronized DC countershock, the therapeutic approach is via the A-V node, which constitutes the weakest link in the conduction path between atria and ventricles. Thus, physiologic or pharmacologic maneuvers that result in a decrease in conduction through the A-V node result in a slowing of the ventricular rate regardless of the effects they have on the frequency of atrial activity.

An entirely different situation, and one that may require a different approach to its management, involves those supraventricular arrhythmias that occur in association with the Wolff-Parkinson-White (WPW) syndrome. Although various hypotheses have been proposed to explain the genesis of tachyarrhythmias in WPW syndrome (35,36), it is generally regarded as being due to the fact that the sinus or atrial impulse is conducted down both the normal and anomalous or accessory pathways to the ventricles (37). Because of the electrophysiologic characteristics of the anomalous pathway, the impulse is transmitted at a faster rate in the accessory path than it is in the normal A-V pathway. The rapid conduction velocity over the anomalous pathway permits the atrial impulse to invade a portion of the ventricular myocardium, resulting in preexcitation of the region (preexcitation syndrome). The delta wave is due to the depolarization of the ventricle around the insertion of the anomalous pathway, from which site further impulse transmission occurs slowly through the ventricular myocardium. The simultaneous slower impulse conduction through the A-V node, on exit from this region, is transmitted rapidly through the remainder of the ventricles via the His-Purkinje system. It is commonly accepted that the paroxysmal atrial tachycardias in patients with WPW are due to a reciprocal mechanism (38–40). The tachyarrhythmia may be initiated by a

properly timed premature atrial excitation due to an ectopic atrial impulse or a premature ventricular complex that conducts to the atrium in a retrograde manner. Most frequently, the supraventricular impulse travels in the anterograde direction and utilizes the A-V node and His bundle to reach the ventricular myocardium and returns to the atrium in a retrograde fashion via the anomalous pathway. The ability of the premature atrial impulse to move in the anterograde direction by way of the A-V node is due to the fact that the anomalous pathway possesses a longer refractory period, as opposed to the A-V node. Thus, the two pathways differ with regard to the relative durations of their refractory periods, so that the anomalous pathway is more likely, because of its longer refractory period, to display unidirectional block in response to a premature atrial impulse. On the other hand, the slow conduction through the normal A-V node provides sufficient time for the anomalous pathway to recover from its refractory state, so that anterograde A-V node/His-Purkinje excitation of the ventricular myocardium continues to be propagated in a retrograde manner across the accessory pathway to the atria, thereby setting the stage for a reciprocating tachyarrhythmia. Therefore, the wave of excitation enters the ventricles via the A-V node/His-Purkinje system and returns to the atria via the anomalous pathway. The initiating premature impulse can just as easily originate in the ventricles, with retrograde propagation across the anomalous pathway to the atria, whereupon it reenters the A-V nodal system and propagates to the ventricles. In both instances, a premature impulse, either atrial or ventricular, initiates the sequence in which retrograde conduction occurs through the anomalous pathway. Thus, a feature common to all cases of WPW associated tachyarrhythmias is the existence of an accessory or anomalous pathway that differs electrophysiologically from the A-V node/His-bundle system.

Therapy for supraventricular tachyarrhythmias depends on the use of physiologic maneuvers or pharmacologic interventions that prevent or alter the electrical events that predispose to initiation of the rhythm disorder (premature atrial or ventricular beats) or that maintain the reciprocating circuit once a reentry rhythm has occurred. Therefore, the therapeutic objective is to control the abnormal process by diminishing enhanced automaticity or to interrupt a reentry mechanism.

The mechanism by which drugs would be expected to provide beneficial effects would depend on their ability to (a) reduce spontaneous phase-4 diastolic depolarization, which would suppress the development of some atrial and/or ventricular premature impulses, (b) depress the rapid upstroke of phase-0 fast sodium current, which would lead to a decrease in conduction velocity of the affected myocardial cells, (c) prolong the refractory period of cardiac cells and make them less likely to serve as a pathway for conduction, and (d) affect the slow calcium current in the A-V node or abnormal cells that have low resting membrane potentials and a slow rate of depolarization.

Paroxysmal Atrial Tachycardia Due to A-V Nodal Reentry

Drugs can act on the A-V nodal or His-Purkinje system by either enhancing or delaying conduction, as reflected by the A-H and H-V intervals. Table 2 lists the effects on the A-V nodal conduction system of several of the more frequently encountered pharmacologic agents, some of which are useful in terminating episodes of A-V nodal reentrant PSVT.

Digitalis Glycosides

Digitalis glycosides usually prolong the effective refractory period of the fast or slow pathway or both. These effects of the cardiac glycosides result in greater diffi-

TABLE 2. *Effects of drugs on the A-V nodal conduction system*

Drug	A-V conduction system		
	Conduction velocity		Effective refractory period
	A-H	H-V	
Digoxin	D[a]	NC	I
Propranolol	D	NC	I
Procainamide	I[b]	D	D-I[c]
Quinidine	I[b]	D	D-I[c]
Disopyramide	NC	NC	NC
Verapamil	D	NC	I
Ajmaline	NC	D	NC
Amiodarone	D	NC	I
Atropine	I	NC	D

I, increase; D, decrease; NC, no change.
[a]Due to direct effects of digoxin plus its indirect effects mediated by vagal stimulation.
[b]Due to the vagolytic effects (blocks acetylcholine) that would enhance A-H conduction velocity.
[c]Effective refractory period is decreased initially due to vagolytic action, and it increases later because of direct effect as drug dosage is increased.

culty with induction of tachycardia as well as inability to sustain a reciprocating A-V nodal reentrant mechanism. The most vulnerable point in the system is usually with anterograde conduction in the slow pathway, and this explains why the tachycardia can be terminated by the digitalis glycosides. Although digitalis slows conduction velocity and lengthens the effective refractory periods of the fast and slow pathways within the A-V node, the important effect is the relative change in these two pathways, which determines whether PSVT can occur in a given individual. Thus, a slowing of conduction velocity alone will lengthen the cycle length of the PSVT but will not abolish it unless there is a simultaneous increase in the refractory period. The anterograde or slow pathway is highly susceptible to the influence of vagal tone. Interactions such as carotid sinus massage, a Valsalva maneuver, or administration of pharmacologic agents that can enhance vagal actions (digitalis, edrophonium, neostigmine, pressor agents such as phenylephrine) usually can result in abrupt termination of the supraventricular tachyarrhythmias. The tachyarrhythmia often ends with a P wave that blocks anterogradely because of decreased conduction velocity and an increased refractory period in the slow A-V nodal pathway. Digitalis, by virtue of its ability to enhance vagal tone, as well as its direct effects on the A-V nodal pathways, is often the agent of choice for prophylaxis against PSVT, although quinidine, procainamide, or propranolol may also be of value prophylactically, because they can suppress premature atrial and/or ventricular depolarizations that often are the precipitating factors in the development of A-V nodal reentrance and supraventricular tachycardia.

β *Receptor Blocking Agents*

β-Adrenergic receptor blocking agents, such as propranolol, can be used to interrupt paroxysmal A-V nodal reentrant supraventricular tachyarrhythmias because of their potential to alter the electrophysiologic properties in the A-V node/His-Purkinje pathways. Propranolol delays conduction within the A-V node by increasing the A-H interval, whereas conduction in the H-V region is unaltered. In addition, propranolol increases both the functional and effective refractory periods of the A-V node. Propranolol has no direct effect on either the relative or effective refractory period of the His-Purkinje system.

Therapy with a β-adrenergic receptor blocking agent appears to be of particular value in those instances where paroxysmal atrial tachycardia is precipitated by exercise or emotion. Exercise-induced PSVT frequently is not associated with other evidence of organic heart disease, and it is presumably brought about by the increased sympathetic drive of exercise (41). The tachyarrhythmia usually responds poorly to digitalis or quinidine. The beneficial effects of the β receptor blocking agents in the management of PSVT are clearly related to inhibition of adrenergic influences on the A-V node. It is safe to assume that all agents belonging to this class of drugs should result in similar actions in the acute and prophylactic management of patients with PSVT.

Verapamil

Verapamil has been noted to be a most effective treatment of A-V nodal reciprocating tachycardias (42), perhaps because its ability to interfere with the slow calcium current influences the susceptible N region of the A-V node. The electrophysiologic actions of verapamil are different from those of the more commonly used antiarrhythmic agents and can be attributed to the ability of verapamil to slow calcium conductance in the myocardial cell during membrane depolarization without altering sodium ion influx. The specific effect on calcium conductance accounts for its negative inotropic effect and is the most likely mechanism by which it exerts its antiarrhythmic actions (43–45). Electrocardiographic studies of the His bundle have shown that verapamil delays A-V conduction proximal to the His bundle without having an effect on intra-atrial or intraventricular conduction (46–48), with the effect being independent of autonomic influences (47,48). Verapamil prolongs both anterograde and retrograde conduction within the A-V node (48), an important observation in view of the fact that many cases of PSVT are known to depend on A-V nodal reentry (49,50).

Amiodarone

Amiodarone has been used extensively in Europe for the control of A-V nodal reciprocating and ectopic atrial arrhythmias. The agent produces an increase in the refractory period and slows conduction in the A-V node, as evidenced by an increase in the A-H interval (51,52). In addition, amiodarone prolongs the refractory period of the atrium as well as that of the ventricles.

Supraventricular arrhythmias showed the greatest response to amiodarone, with recurrent paroxysmal atrial flutter and fibrillation being suppressed in 29 of 30 patients (96.6%) and in 57 of 59 patients (96.6%) with PSVT.

Quinidine, Procainamide, and Disopyramide

Quinidine, procainamide, and disopyramide are each capable of antagonizing the cholinergic effects of acetylcholine on the A-V node. As indicated in Table 2, procainamide and quinidine produce variable effects on the effective refractory period of the A-V node because of the opposing actions of these agents, in which their anticholinergic effects (atropinelike, Table 2) counteract the direct effects of the drug on the A-V node. It is only at the higher dose levels that these agents can be expected to prolong the effective refractory period of the A-V node. In a similar manner, A-V conduction velocity is influenced in a variable manner, once again because of opposing effects of cholinergic blockade and direct depressant actions of the pharmacologic agents.

Disopyramide likewise possesses marked anticholinergic actions, but it has less of a direct depressant effect on A-V conduction velocity and effective refractory period (53). The net result of these opposing effects is that the drug produces no significant alteration in the electrophysiologic properties of the A-V conduction system. Because quinidine, procainamide, and disopyramide have minimal effects on the A-V node, they would not be expected to be as effective as some of the other agents listed in Table 2 with respect to being able to terminate a supraventricular tachyarrhythmia caused by an A-V reciprocating mechanism.

As previously discussed, A-V reciprocating tachyarrhythmias frequently are precipitated by atrial extrasystoles. Because procainamide, quinidine, and disopyramide can suppress atrial extrasystoles, these agents are of value in the prevention of paroxysms of supraventricular tachycardias.

Each of the three agents will prolong the effective refractory period of atrial muscle. In those instances in which the tachycardia is caused by a reentry mechanism within the atria, procainamide, quinidine, and disopyramide should be effective in terminating the arrhythmias.

We can summarize the foregoing discussion on the pharmacologic basis for treatment of supraventricular tachyarrhythmias by stating that to be effective in the prophylaxis of such rhythm disorders, a drug must (a) prevent the electrical events that predispose to A-V conduction delay required to initiate the reciprocating tachyarrhythmia (atrial premature depolarization) and (b) alter A-V conduction so that reentry is no longer a physiologic possibility.

Supraventricular Tachyarrhythmias Associated with WPW Syndrome

There exists in WPW an extranodal accessory A-V pathway with electrophysiologic properties that differ from those of the normal A-V node. Drugs acting on the two pathways may lead to electrophysiologic alterations that may favor or depress impulse transmission, so that the two pathways may become dissimilar, and conduction will be favored by one pathway over the other. The A-V nodal fibers have the characteristics of a slow conduction velocity and a short refractory period, both of which are influenced by vagal innervation. Enhanced vagal tone produces a slowing of A-V conduction and a prolongation of the refractory period. Cholinergic blockade produces the opposite effects. The extranodal accessory A-V pathway (bundle of Kent), on the other hand, possesses the properties of fast conduction velocity and a long refractory period. The bypass tract behaves like atrial muscle in response to vagal stimulation in that conduction velocity is enhanced and the refractory period is shortened. Cholinergic blockade would have the opposite effect. Therefore, an intervention that resulted in an increase in vagal tone would interfere with conduction over the normal A-V pathway and enhance impulse transmission over the extranodal accessory A-V pathway. The approach to pharmacologic management of supraventricular tachyarrhythmias associated with the WPW syndrome must consider the direct and indirect effects that any intervention will have on each of the A-V pathways. Table 3 summarizes the electrophysiologic alterations in the A-V node and accessory pathways for several of the more commonly used antiarrhythmic agents.

The paroxysmal tachycardias in WPW are of two basic types. Reciprocating tachycardia is the most common and constitutes 70% to 80% of all arrhythmias. Atrial flutter/fibrillation is the second type of arrhythmia specifically associated with the syndrome, and it carries a certain risk for the patient because it can terminate in ventricular fibrillation. The pharmacologic management of these two types of WPW-associated rhythm disorders requires special attention.

It should be recalled that in the reciprocating tachyarrhythmia of WPW, the refractory periods of the pathways are such that A-V conduction is via the A-V node and His-Purkinje system, whereas the ventriculoatrial impulse is conducted over the accessory pathway back to the atria only to reenter the A-V node. Rarely does the reentry loop operate in the opposite direction. In the latter instance, the QRS complexes are broad, as ventricular preexcitation occurs due to A-V conduction over the accessory pathway. Such QRS complexes may simulate ventricular tachycardia.

The pharmacologic management of PSVT associated with the WPW syndrome is selected to alter one or more links in the reciprocating network. Prophylaxis can be achieved by preventing the atrial and/or ventricular extrasystoles that so frequently precipitate the tachyarrhythmias. Further protection against the paroxysms can be attained by narrowing the interval during which premature beats can dissociate the normal and accessory pathways. Last, pharmacologic agents may prolong refractoriness, so that the returning impulse is blocked either in the accessory pathway or in the A-V node.

The electrophysiologic effects of the cardiac glycosides in the presence of WPW syndrome deserve special consideration because of the drug's potential detrimental effects in the patient with coexisting atrial flutter or atrial fibrillation.

The cardiac glycosides exert their electrophysiologic effects by both direct and indirect mechanisms; the latter occur as a result of enhancement of vagal tone. The cardiac glycosides shorten the refractory period of the accessory pathway—an action that results from an increase in vagal tone that causes atrial muscle (accessory pathway) to repolarize at a faster rate. In addition, conduction velocity in atrial tissue is enhanced. At the same time, digitalis, by enhancing vagal tone, prolongs the refractory period of the A-V node and delays A-V conduction. The net result of these electrophysiologic changes in the accessory

TABLE 3. *Effects of antiarrhythmic drugs on effective refractory periods of A-V node and accessory pathway in WPW syndrome*

Drug	Effective refractory period	
	A-V node	Accessory pathway
Digoxin	I[a]	D
Propranolol	I	NC
Procainamide	D-I[b]	I
Quinidine	D-I[b]	I
Disopyramide	NC	I
Verapamil	I	NC
Ajmaline	NC	I
Amiodarone	I	I
Atropine	D	I

I, increase; D, decrease; NC, no change.
[a]Due to direct effects of digoxin plus its indirect effect mediated by vagal stimulation.
[b]Due to vagolytic effect initially, which is then followed by direct effects.

pathway and the A-V node is that antero-grade impulse transmission is impeded over the A-V node and facilitated via the accessory pathway.

The digitalis glycosides, by impairing anterograde conduction through the A-V node, will limit the accessibility of an atrial premature impulse to this conduction pathway and therefore prevent the initiation of a reciprocating rhythm. The primary mechanism by which digitalis exerts a prophylactic action in the patient with reciprocating supraventricular tachyarrhythmias associated with the WPW syndrome is by decreasing the differences in the refractory periods of the two pathways and therefore abolishing the window produced by the discrepant refractory periods in the individual A-V pathways.

Patients with the preexcitation syndrome are susceptible to two types of tachyarrhythmias. The first, reciprocating tachycardia, which was mentioned earlier, can be prevented by the prophylactic use of digitalis glycosides, as well as by other agents to be discussed. The second dysrhythmia in WPW is atrial flutter or fibrillation with a rapid ventricular response due to antero-grade conduction over the accessory pathway. The accessory pathway (basically, atrial tissue) possesses a long refractory period and a rapid conduction velocity, as compared with the A-V nodal fibers, which have a slow conduction velocity and short refractory period. In the absence of an A-V bypass tract, the A-V node guards the ventricles against rapid atrial rates by failing to conduct in a 1:1 fashion above a critical rate. It is not unusual to find a patient with atrial flutter (atrial rate of 300 per min) with a ventricular rate of 150 as a result of a 2:1 block at the A-V node. In the presence of the preexcitation syndrome, however, the protective effect of the A-V node on the ventricle is bypassed because the accessory pathway is capable of conducting in a 1:1 manner, so that excessively high ventricular rates can be achieved if atrial flutter or fibrillation develops in the presence of the

WPW syndrome. In such an instance, administration of a digitalis glycoside can be hazardous. As digitalis decreases the refractory period of the accessory pathway and enhances conduction velocity in this tissue, more impulses gain access to the ventricle, and a life-threatening ventricular response and ventricular fibrillation may result (54,55). Thus, in patients who have the WPW syndrome and a relatively short refractory period in the accessory pathway, an additional shortening of the refractory pathway can be fatal.

Because of the evidence that digitalis can increase the ventricular response during atrial fibrillation in some patients, the use of cardiac glycosides in the preexcitation syndromes should be reserved for those patients in whom elective induction of atrial fibrillation has demonstrated that the patient is not at risk for developing ventricular fibrillation (55). Other pharmacologic agents will be more suitable choices if digitalis is contraindicated because of the reasons discussed. Selection of the appropriate drug will depend on an understanding of its electrophysiologic effects on each of the A-V pathways.

In a patient with the preexcitation syndrome and a rapid ventricular response in the presence of atrial fibrillation, pharmacologic intervention should be directed at depressing conduction and increasing the refractoriness of the accessory pathway. Propranolol decreases conduction via the A-V node and will favor conduction over the accessory pathway (56). Both digitalis and propranolol, by slowing A-V nodal conduction, will allow a greater time for recovery of the accessory pathway and may actually promote a reentry phenomenon (57,58).

On the other hand, a number of agents are known to prolong refractoriness and conduction in the bypass tract. Lidocaine was demonstrated to exert beneficial effects in the clinical setting of WPW and atrial fibrillation, in which the drug immediately abolished anterograde conduction down the bypass tract, thus slowing the ventricular response (59,60). Because of the ability to administer the drug rapidly by the intravenous route, lidocaine offers a means of controlling these life-threatening arrhythmias. The effect is short-lived and requires continuous intravenous administration. However, it affords an opportunity to stabilize the patient until more permanent measures can be instituted.

The effects of propranolol, as would be expected, contrast with those of lidocaine and resemble the actions of digitalis on A-V nodal impulse transmission. Propranolol does not exert any significant effect on the anomalous pathway. Because of its ability to produce β-adrenergic receptor blockade and remove sympathetic influences on the A-V node, propranolol depresses A-V nodal transmission. The electrophysiologic changes due to propranolol include prolongation of the A-V nodal refractory period and a decrease in conduction velocity. Preexcitation will tend to be accentuated as a result of the electrophysiologic changes in the A-V node (61,62).

In a patient with a very short refractory period of the accessory bundle, it is possible to initiate episodes of supraventricular tachycardia by an appropriately timed ventricular premature impulse. The premature impulse propagates to the atrium over the accessory pathway and returns to the ventricle over the normal A-V node and the His-Purkinje system, thus initiating an episode of supraventricular tachycardia. Propranolol plus procainamide or quinidine will be of value. Propranolol will prevent access of the returning impulse to the A-V node. Procainamide or quinidine will have an effect primarily on the anomalous pathway. Both drugs result in prolongation of the refractory period of the accessory pathway, and they slow both anterograde and retrograde conduction in the bypass tract (61,62). The effect of procainamide or quinidine on the sustaining mechanism of reciprocating tachycardia depends largely on the influence of the drugs on the length of the

circulatory wave, that is, the mean conduction velocity times the refractory period. As shown by Sellers et al. (62), to be effective, the drug must increase the length of the refractory period of the different components of the reciprocating circuit more than it decreases the mean conduction velocity of the circulating wave. Thus, some patients may become more symptomatic on therapy, making it impossible to predict the effectiveness of a certain drug on the tachycardia. Another mechanism by which procainamide or quinidine may function is by its influence on the initiating event, premature atrial or ventricular depolarizations. Procainamide is particularly effective in suppressing ventricular premature impulses, whereas quinidine is equally effective against both atrial and ventricular premature depolarizations. Procainamide is especially useful when atrial fibrillation supervenes in a patient with a short refractory period of the accessory pathway. Intravenous administration of procainamide results in immediate control of the ventricular rate, as it prolongs the effective refractory period and slows conduction via the anomalous pathway without depressing conduction over the A-V node.

An interesting feature of quinidine and procainamide is that both drugs have a vagolytic effect and thus inhibit the influences of cholinergic innervation to the accessory pathway (atrial muscle) and the A-V node. The influence of vagal stimulation on these structures was discussed previously. Inhibition of vagal tone will slow conduction velocity and prolong the refractory period of the accessory pathway and will enhance conduction velocity and decrease the refractory period of the A-V node. The net result is that procainamide and quinidine favor utilization by the atrial impulse of the normal A-V pathway. This becomes an important consideration when using procainamide or quinidine in WPW with associated atrial flutter and a rapid ventricular response because of 1:1 conduction over the anomalous pathway. Whereas the drugs will suppress impulse transmission over the anomalous pathway, their vagolytic effects may promote rapid atrial impulse transmission via the A-V nodal pathway.

Disopyramide is an antiarrhythmic agent that has been found effective in the management of extrasystoles and tachycardias of both supraventricular and ventricular origin. Disopyramide has minimal effects on the refractory period or conduction velocity of the A-V node. This lack of effect is due to the direct depressant effects of the drug on A-V nodal function being offset by the intense vagolytic actions of disopyramide (63). In patients with the WPW syndrome, disopyramide was shown to prolong the effective refractory period of the anomalous bypass tract and to prolong anterograde and retrograde conduction times of the accessory pathway. The electrophysiologic effects of disopyramide on the accessory pathway are a result of its direct actions as well as its indirect (vagolytic) actions on the tissue bridging the A-V junction. In many ways, disopyramide resembles quinidine in its cardiac electrophysiologic properties, except that it has minimal effects on conduction in the His-Purkinje system. Because of its depressant effects on the anomalous pathway, disopyramide may have potential therapeutic value for management of the WPW syndrome with atrial flutter or fibrillation (53).

Verapamil is receiving increased attention as an antiarrhythmic agent, particularly in the management of supraventricular tachyarrhythmias. Verapamil has the ability to inhibit the slow inward calcium current, and this results in a decrease in conduction velocity in the A-V node as well as an increase in the A-V nodal refractory period (64). Anterograde and retrograde conduction times in the anomalous bypass are unaffected in most patients (64). Since anterograde conduction of atrial premature impulse or of a reciprocating rhythm is by way of the A-V node, verapamil should be effective as a means of terminating tachyarrhythmias associated with the WPW syn-

drome (65) or in preventing initiation of the event by a premature atrial depolarization. Whereas studies by Spurrell et al. (64) suggest that verapamil is an effective drug in the treatment of reciprocal tachycardias associated with the WPW syndrome, it may, in some patients, influence the anomalous pathway in an adverse manner and result in ventricular fibrillation.

Ajmaline, a reserpinelike drug, has been used extensively in Europe for the management of patients with a variety of cardiac arrhythmias. Ajmaline has been reported to prolong the refractory period, depress conduction velocity in the accessory pathway, and have minimal effects on A-V nodal transmission, except for a slight prolongation of the H-V interval (66,67). The value of ajmaline in the management of supraventricular tachyarrhythmias is still uncertain, and further clinical studies are needed before its effectiveness relative to other existing agents can be adequately assessed.

A drug of promising potential is the agent amiodarone. Studies by Rosenbaum et al. (51) and Wellens et al. (68) have elucidated the electrophysiologic effects of amiodarone on the anomalous and normal pathways in patients with the preexcitation syndrome. Amiodarone lengthens the refractory period of the accessory pathway. But, as with other drugs, its effects on the accessory pathway are not the same when anterograde and retrograde conductions are compared. Whereas amiodarone uniformly prolongs refractoriness in the anomalous pathway in an A-V direction, prolongation in a V-A direction was observed in only half of the patients studied (68). In all patients in whom tachycardias could still be initiated after treatment with amiodarone, the heart rate during tachycardia was slower than before treatment, a result to be expected, because amiodarone decreases the conduction velocity of the circulatory wave. The electrophysiologic effects of amiodarone suggest that it would be of special value in patients with WPW syndrome and atrial fibrillation. In the latter clinical setting, parenteral administration of amiodarone has proved to be most beneficial in reverting what otherwise would be a life-threatening tachyarrhythmia (69).

From this discussion of the electrophysiologic effects of pharmacologic agents on the anomalous bypass and normal A-V pathways, it is apparent that the drugs used to manage patients with the WPW syndrome can be divided into those that predominantly affect impulse transmission in the A-V node and those that alter impulse transmission in the accessory bundle. Thus, quinidine, procainamide, disopyramide, ajmaline, and amiodarone have major effects in prolonging the refractory period of the anomalous pathway. In contrast, digitalis, β receptor blocking agents, and verapamil prolong refractoriness in the A-V node.

Aside from synchronized cardioversion in emergent situations, drug therapy for reciprocating tachyarrhythmias might best be accomplished with parenteral administration of lidocaine, procainamide or amiodarone, because each can act rapidly on the anomalous bypass and will be considered appropriate treatment for those patients with atrial flutter or fibrillation and rapid conduction over the bypass. Prevention of reciprocating tachyarrhythmias in the WPW syndrome may be accomplished by quinidine or disopyramide, which not only reduce the frequency of premature atrial and ventricular depolarizations but also depress conduction over the accessory pathway. However, because these drugs depress only one of the A-V pathways, it is possible that they could result in a paradoxical increase in the frequency of attacks of reciprocating tachycardias, because a premature impulse may dissociate the two pathways. In such cases it might be helpful to combine a second drug, propranolol, along with quinidine to delay conduction in the A-V node.

It is obvious that patients with the WPW syndrome do not compose a homogeneous group. The tachyarrhythmias are the results of different mechanisms, with varied electrophysiologic properties of the two A-V pathways. Each patient with the WPW syndrome and reciprocating tachyarrhythmias should be evaluated with electrophysiologic studies to determine the mechanism of the tachyarrhythmias and the effectiveness of one or more therapeutic interventions.

GENERAL PHARMACOLOGY

Quinidine

For centuries the quinidine alkaloids present in the bark of *Cinchona officinalis* have been used for treatment of malaria. As a result of the use of cinchona for treatment of malaria, it became apparent that cinchona was capable of converting atrial fibrillation to normal sinus rhythm. Clinical investigation showed that of the three major alkaloids present in the bark of the cinchona tree (quinine, quinidine, and cinchonine), quinidine was the most effective antiarrhythmic agent (70). The efficacy and long history of use of quinidine in the treatment of disorders of the cardiac rhythm led to the establishment of quinidine as the prototype antiarrhythmic agent. Despite the introduction of newer antiarrhythmic agents, quinidine still plays a major role in the treatment of chronic cardiac dysrhythmias.

The structure of quinidine (the dextro-rotary isomer of quinine) is shown in Fig. 8.

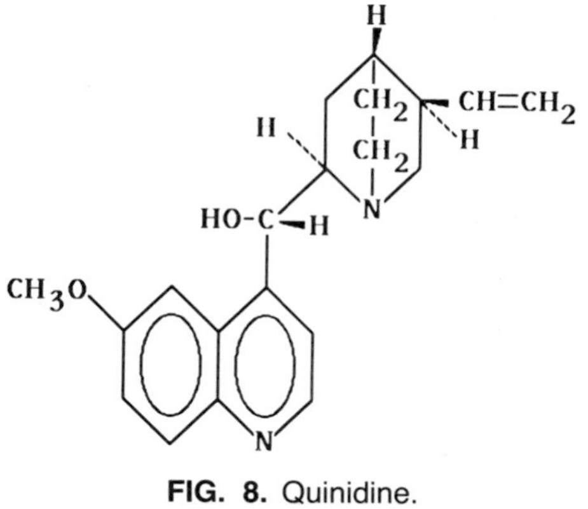

FIG. 8. Quinidine.

Quinidine shares all the pharmacologic properties of quinine, including antimalarial, antipyretic, oxytocic, and skeletal muscle relaxant actions. However, these actions also are accompanied by all the toxic manifestations observed with the administration of quinine.

Electrophysiologic Actions

The effects of quinidine on atrial myocardium and specialized conduction tissue are a composite of the direct actions of the drug on cardiac tissue electrical properties and the indirect actions of the drug mediated by competitive blockade of muscarinic cholinergic receptors. The net effect of quinidine on the electrical properties of a particular cardiac tissue is dependent on the extent of parasympathetic nervous system innervation, the level of tone exerted by the parasympathetic nervous system, and the dose of quinidine administered. Because of the relatively greater potency of quinidine as a cholinergic muscarinic antagonist versus direct electrophysiologic actions, the anticholinergic actions of quinidine predominate at the lower plasma quinidine concentrations. The anticholinergic actions of quinidine are most apparent during initial oral therapy. Later, when steady-state therapeutic plasma concentrations are achieved, the direct electrophysiologic actions of quinidine tend to predominate. The direct and indirect electrophysiologic actions of quinidine are summarized in Table 4.

Sinoatrial Node

Experimental studies have shown quinidine to increase the action-potential duration and to depress the slope of phase-4 depolarization of sinus node pacemaker cells (71). This direct depression of sinus node function also is observed in *in vitro* canine atrial preparations (72). However, when autonomic innervation is intact in conscious animals and humans, quinidine manifests either no effect or an increase in sinus heart rate (73,74). Direct depression of sinus node automaticity is counteracted by blockade of vagus-nerve-mediated depression of sinus node function, sometimes actually resulting in an increased sinus rate. Other factors may also be involved. Deterioration of hemodynamic function as a result of quinidine administration may result in increased reflex sympathetic activity. This stimulation of sympathetic tone may, in part, be responsible for an increase in sinus heart rate observed after quinidine administration in some patients.

TABLE 4. *Electrophysiologic actions of quinidine, procainamide, and disopyramide at therapeutic plasma concentrations*

Tissue	Direct action	Indirect action	Net effect
Sinus node	Decrease	Increase	No change
Atria			
Automaticity	Decrease		Decrease
Conduction velocity	Decrease	Decrease	Decrease
Refractory periods	Increase	Increase	Increase
A-V node			
Automaticity	Decrease		Decrease
Conduction velocity	Decrease	Increase	No change
Refractory periods	Increase	Decrease	No change or slight increase
His-Purkinje/ventricular muscle			
Automaticity	Decrease		Decrease
Conduction velocity	Decrease		Decrease
Refractory periods	Increase		Increase

In atrial muscle fibers, quinidine suppresses automaticity by depressing phase-4 depolarization. Atrial pacemakers are more sensitive to depression by quinidine than are ventricular pacemakers (75).

Quinidine administration results in a dose-dependent depression of membrane responsiveness in atrial muscle fibers (76). The maximum rate of phase-0 depolarization and the amplitude of the phase-0 potential are depressed equally at all membrane potentials. Quinidine also decreases atrial muscle excitability, so that a larger current stimulus is needed for initiation of an active response at the normal level of resting membrane potential (74). These actions are often referred to as the "local anesthetic properties" of quinidine. Reduction of membrane responsiveness and reduction of the action-potential amplitude, as well as the decrease in excitability, are believed to be direct results of a reduction in the rapid influx of sodium into the cell. These changes result in a reduction of conduction velocity in atrial tissue.

The action-potential duration in atrial tissue is prolonged only slightly by quinidine (76) and results in a small increase in the effective refractory period. However, because of the failure of early premature impulses to conduct from the site of stimulation as a result of depression of conduction, the effective refractory period is prolonged to a much greater extent than the action-potential duration.

The anticholinergic properties of quinidine also alter the electrophysiologic properties of atrial muscle. Stimulation of the vagus nerve or administration of acetylcholine produces both a slight depolarization of atrial muscle fibers and a shortening of the action-potential duration. These changes in the cellular electrophysiology of atrial muscle fibers result in an increase in conduction velocity and a decrease in the effective refractory periods of atrial myocardium. The actions of acetylcholine are antagonized by quinidine, thereby indirectly prolonging the action-potential duration and resulting in a decrease in conduction velocity and an increase in the effective refractory period.

Human electrophysiologic studies have confirmed the results of earlier *in vitro* and *in vivo* electrophysiologic studies. In human electrophysiologic studies, acute quinidine administration slows intraatrial conduction (77) and prolongs the effective refractory period of atrial myocardium (73). The refractory periods of A-V accessory (bypass) pathways are increased after quinidine administration and conduction velocity is decreased (67). When atrial fibrillation or atrial flutter is induced in patients with A-V accessory pathways, the resultant ventricular rate is slowed by quinidine.

A-V Node

Both the direct and indirect actions of quinidine are important in determining the ultimate effect of the drug on A-V conduction. The indirect (anticholinergic) properties of quinidine prevent vagally mediated prolongation of A-V node refractory periods and depression of A-V node conduction velocity. A-V transmission is facilitated. Quinidine's direct electrophysiologic actions on the A-V node result in a decrease in conduction velocity and an increase in the effective refractory period. The direct actions of quinidine result in depression of A-V conduction. In considering the action of quinidine on A-V transmission, one must be aware of both its direct and indirect actions. The direct effects of quinidine are manifested at therapeutic plasma concentrations. It is because of its indirect actions on the A-V node that quinidine must not be the initial drug in the treatment of atrial flutter and possibly atrial fibrillation. In both instances the atria are being stimulated at a rapid rate. The primary objective is to control the ventricular rate, and the second is to restore normal sinus rhythm. Although quinidine is often successful in restoring normal sinus rhythm, its administration in the presence of a rapid atrial rate will lead to a further, and dangerous, increase in the ventricular rate. The effect is a result of the anticholinergic properties of quinidine that result in enhancement of A-V transmission. It is for this reason that digitalis is the drug to be administered before one elects to convert atrial flutter or atrial fibrillation to sinus rhythm with quinidine. The direct and indirect effects of digitalis on the A-V node protect against the anticholinergic effects of quinidine.

In summary, quinidine has both direct and indirect effects on A-V transmission at therapeutic plasma concentrations. The anticholinergic or indirect properties of quinidine may facilitate A-V transmission and present a hazard when it is given as the initial drug in the presence of atrial flutter.

Human electrophysiologic studies have confirmed earlier electrophysiologic studies in animals that showed dangerous increases in ventricular rate to occur when quinidine was administered in the presence of atrial flutter or atrial fibrillation. Acute quinidine administration has been shown to increase conduction velocity and to decrease the effective refractory period of the A-V node (67,73). The magnitude of the increase in A-V transmission can vary widely among patients, probably because of a wide degree of variation in vagal tone.

His-Purkinje System/Ventricular Muscle

An important therapeutic action of quinidine is to depress automaticity of ventricular pacemakers by depressing the slope of phase-4 depolarization (78). Depression of pacemakers in the His-Purkinje system is more pronounced than depression of sinus node pacemaker cells. Toxic doses of quinidine, on the other hand, may increase the rate of discharge of ventricular pacemakers (79).

Quinidine administration reduces the amplitude of the action potential and produces a parallel shift to the right in the membrane responsiveness curves for Purkinje fibers and ventricular muscle (79). Membrane responsiveness (the maximum rate of phase-0 depolarization) is reduced at all levels of membrane potential without altering the resting membrane potential or intracellular sodium and potassium ion concentrations. Myocardial excitability also is depressed. The depressions of phase-0 depolarization and the action-potential amplitude combined with a decrease in myocardial excitability produce a depression of conduction velocity in the His-Purkinje system and ventricular myocardium. In the surface electrocardiogram, this reduction in conduction velocity is reflected as an increase in the QRS interval.

Quinidine prolongs repolarization in Purkinje fibers and ventricular muscle, resulting in a small increase in the action-potential duration. As in atrial muscle, quinidine administration results in prolongation of the effective refractory period by depression of conduction of premature impulses away from the site of origin.

The indirect (anticholinergic) properties of quinidine are not a factor in the actions of quinidine on ventricular muscle and the His-Purkinje system. The effects of the parasympathetic nervous system on the electrical properties of ventricular muscle and His-Purkinje fibers are of minor consequence.

Serum potassium concentrations are a major determinant of the activity of quinidine on cardiac tissue. Low extracellular potassium ion concentrations antagonize the depressant effects of quinidine on membrane responsiveness. High extracellular potassium ion concentrations increase the ability of quinidine to depress membrane responsiveness. The actions of quinidine that are dependent on potassium ion concentration may explain why hypokalemic patients are often unresponsive to its antiarrhythmic effects. Caution must be exercised, however, in that excessive extracellular potassium ion concentrations will enhance the depressant actions of quinidine on the A-V node as well as its depressant actions on pacemaker cells. Prolongation of the QRS interval and serious conduction disturbances are more likely to occur at higher plasma quinidine concentrations when hyperkalemia is present.

In clinical electrophysiologic studies, acute quinidine administration slows conduction in the His-Purkinje system and increases His-Purkinje refractory periods. The ventricular effective refractory period also is increased (61,73,77).

Electrocardiographic Changes

At normal therapeutic plasma concentrations, quinidine prolongs the PR, QRS, and QT interval of the surface electrocardiogram. QRS and QT prolongations are more pronounced with quinidine than with other antiarrhythmic agents. The magnitudes of these changes are directly related to the plasma quinidine concentration. Toxic concentrations of quinidine produce further slowing of conduction. The QRS and QT intervals are dramatically increased, and secondary repolarization waves may appear.

Hemodynamic Effects

Quinidine is well known to possess a negative inotropic effect on atrial and ventricular myocardium. This effect has been observed in humans (80) and experimental animals (16). At plasma quinidine concentrations in the normal therapeutic range, myocardial depression is not a problem in patients with normal myocardial function. However, depression of myocardial contractility in patients with compromised myocardial function may produce a significant rise in left ventricular end-diastolic pressure, resulting in overt heart failure. In addition, quinidine depresses vascular smooth muscle and results in a decrease in peripheral vascular resistance. This peripheral vasodilation is in part due to blockade of α-adrenergic receptors, with a resultant decrease in adrenergic vasoconstrictor tone

(81). The reduction in peripheral vascular resistance, combined with a reduction in cardiac output, can produce significant decreases in arterial pressure. The depressant effects of quinidine on the cardiovascular system are more likely to occur with intravenous administration. Intravenous quinidine administration should not be employed routinely for emergency treatment of arrhythmias because of the potential for producing severe cardiovascular depression.

Toxic Reactions

The cardiac toxicity of quinidine includes A-V and intraventricular block, ventricular tachyarrhythmias, and depression of myocardial contractility. The precipitation of ventricular arrhythmias by toxic doses of quinidine may be related to a marked depression of intraventricular conduction or may be due to an increase in ventricular automaticity. In most patients, toxicity can be controlled by proper adjustment of the dosage or discontinuance of the drug, if necessary.

Quinidine-induced depression of myocardial conduction and contractility can be treated by a number of interventions. Catecholamine administration may improve depressed intraventricular conduction and restore arterial pressure. Cautious administration of molar sodium lactate or sodium bicarbonate may be beneficial (82). Reversal of quinidine cardiotoxicity and hypotension by sodium lactate has been noted even during advanced stages of cardiotoxicity. The empiric use of sodium lactate or sodium bicarbonate to treat quinidine toxicity has some theoretical support, because alkalosis induces potassium shifts from extracellular to intracellular sites and increases binding of quinidine to serum albumin, reducing free quinidine plasma concentrations. On the other hand, alkalosis can result in decreased urinary excretion of the weak base, quinidine.

Large doses of quinidine can produce a

syndrome known as cinchonism, characterized by ringing in the ears, headache, nausea, visual disturbances or blurred vision, disturbed auditory acuity, and vertigo. Larger doses can produce confusion, delirium, hallucinations, or psychoses. At therapeutic doses the most commonly observed side effects are related to the gastrointestinal tract: nausea, vomiting, and diarrhea.

In some patients, thrombocytopenia may occur as a result of quinidine administration. Quinidine-induced thrombocytopenia is due to the formation of a plasma protein/quinidine complex that evokes a circulating antibody. The antibody can react with platelets in the presence of quinidine. Platelet counts return to normal on cessation of quinidine therapy. However, administration of quinidine or quinine at a later date can cause reappearance of thrombocytopenia.

Quinidine syncope and/or sudden arrhythmic death, an uncommon but major complication of quinidine therapy, is due to transient or irreversible ventricular tachycardia or ventricular fibrillation. This action of quinidine is not necessarily due to quinidine overdosage; it can occur at therapeutic or subtherapeutic plasma concentrations. The mechanism for these arrhythmias is poorly understood but may be related to a slowed intraventricular conduction.

Pharmacokinetics

Absorption

Quinidine is almost completely absorbed from the gastrointestinal tract after oral administration. Quinidine sulfate is well absorbed from solution, tablet, and capsule formulations. Peak plasma concentrations are achieved between 2 and 4 hr after oral administration. The bioavailability of oral quinidine gluconate is slightly higher (72%–87%), the balance being explained by first-pass hepatic metabolism. Intramuscular injection of quinidine gluconate is painful and

may cause significant tissue necrosis, as well as being incomplete and/or showing inconsistent absorption. Peak plasma concentrations observed after intramuscular injection are greater than those observed after oral administration and are obtained earlier after administration.

Metabolism and Excretion

Quinidine is metabolized extensively in the body, primarily by the liver. Major metabolites include 3-hydroxyquinidine and quinidine-N-oxide. Minor metabolites include 2′-oxyquinidinone and O-desmethylquinidine. The 3-hydroxy metabolite of quinidine possesses antiarrhythmic activity that may contribute to the therapeutic action of quinidine with plasma concentrations roughly one-third those of the unchanged drug. Urinary excretion of conjugated or free metabolites of quinidine accounts for 75% to 90% of the administered dose. Renal excretion of unaltered quinidine accounts for the remainder. Changes in urinary pH may markedly alter renal clearance of quinidine, a weak base with a pK_a of 8.57. Excretion of the drug increases as the urine is acidified. Dihydroquinidine, a contaminant of quinidine tablet preparations, may be detected in human serum and is an active antiarrhythmic agent.

Kinetics

After intravenous injection, quinidine disposition may be described by a two-compartment model (biphasic exponential excretion). Values for the volume of the central compartment (V_C) and steady-state volume of distribution (V_DSS) are given in Table 5. The initial rapid redistribution phase (alpha-phase) half-life is approximately 6 min. The second, slower elimination phase (beta-phase) half-life is approximately 5 to 8 hr. Renal disease may require a reduction in quinidine dosage or an increase in the dosing interval. Liver disease

TABLE 5. *Pharmacokinetic properties of quinidine*

Absorption
  Rapidly and almost completely absorbed (70%–80%) when given orally
Protein binding
  Extensively bound to plasma protein with 10% to 20% of administered dose free in the circulation
Metabolism
  Hepatic metabolism with some active metabolites
Half-life
  Approximately 6 hr
Time to peak plasma concentration
  After oral administration peak plasma concentration of quinidine gluconate is achieved in 3 to 4 hr and by
    1 to 1.5 hr for quinidine sulfate
Therapeutic plasma concentration
  Therapeutic range is 3 to 6 µg/ml; toxic effects observed at plasma concentrations above 8 µg/ml
Elimination
  Renal: primarily by the renal route with approximately 10% to 50% excreted as unchanged drug;
    excretion increased in acidic urine

also requires reduction of quinidine dosage. Renal function decreases with age, and lower doses may be necessary in elderly patients. Simultaneous administration of anticonvulsant drugs can stimulate the metabolism of quinidine and may require an increase in quinidine dosage.

In excess of 80% of plasma quinidine is bound to plasma proteins. Albumin serves as the primary source of binding protein in plasma. Neither heart failure nor renal disease alters the extent of plasma protein binding, although liver disease or hypoalbuminemia decreases plasma protein binding. Quinidine enters red blood cells and is bound to hemoglobin. At equilibrium, red blood cell concentrations are similar to plasma concentrations. In individual patients, there are wide variations in the plasma concentrations of quinidine with a given dosage regimen of the drug, with toxic manifestations correlating with serum or plasma concentration of the drug rather than with the administered dose. It must be appreciated, however, that the serum concentration may not properly reflect the myocardial tissue concentration of the drug, especially after rapid administration. After rapid administration, the serum-to-cardiac-tissue ratio may be temporarily higher than that present at steady state. Therapeutic plasma concentrations are also dependent on the analytic method used for quantitation. The earliest assays measured the quantity of quinidine plus metabolites in serum. Currently used assays are specific for quinidine and do not mistakenly measure metabolites as quinidine. Therapeutic plasma concentrations of quinidine as measured by most previously employed assay procedures ranged from 3 to 6 µg/ml. Toxic manifestations are commonly observed at plasma concentrations in excess of 8 µg/ml. Therapeutic plasma concentrations of quinidine as measured by recently developed specific assays are 2.3 to 5.0 µg/ml.

Oral Dose for Arrhythmia Conversion

One commonly used mode of administration for conversion of atrial flutter or atrial fibrillation is to give an oral dose every 2 hr for a total of five doses. The initial dose usually is 200 mg. If conversion is not attained, the oral dose is increased by 200 mg the next day, and five doses are given. On this regimen, therapeutic plasma quinidine concentrations are attained with doses of 200, 400, and 600 mg. A plasma concentration plateau is reached after the sixth dose.

Oral maintenance doses of quinidine are 300 to 600 mg every 6 hr. For intravenous dosing, 6 to 10 mg/kg quinidine gluconate may be given slowly over a period in excess of 30 min. During intravenous dosing, the patient's blood pressure, electrocardiogram, and clinical status must be monitored closely. Intravenous dosing with quinidine is a potentially dangerous procedure, especially in the setting of acute myocardial infarction or hemodynamic compromise.

Contraindications

One of the few absolute contraindications for quinidine is that of complete A-V block with an A-V pacemaker or idioventricular pacemaker that may be suppressed by quinidine. Because of the negative inotropic action of quinidine, congestive heart failure and hypotension are contraindications for quinidine therapy. Digitalis intoxication and hyperkalemia can accentuate the depression of conduction caused by quinidine, and quinidine should be used with extreme care in these conditions. Myasthenia gravis can be aggravated severely by quinidine's actions at myoneural junctions, and quinidine should not be administered.

Indications

Quinidine has withstood the test of time and continues to play an important role in therapy. Primary indications for the use of quinidine include (a) abolishing premature complexes of atrial, A-V junctional, and ventricular origin, (b) restoration of normal sinus rhythm in atrial flutter and atrial fibrillation after control of heart rate with digitalis, (c) maintenance of normal sinus rhythm after electrical conversion of atrial arrhythmias, (d) prophylaxis for arrhythmias associated with electrical countershock, and (e) termination of ventricular tachycardia and suppression of repetitive ventricular tachycardia associated with WPW syndrome. By depressing conduction through the A-V accessory pathway, quinidine favors orthograde A-V transmission and prevents the reentry mechanism, which requires the presence of an accessory pathway.

Quinidine is not primarily indicated for either prophylaxis or active treatment of ventricular flutter or ventricular fibrillation. Management of these arrhythmias often requires intravenous drug administration, and quinidine carries significant risk of toxic effects when given by this route.

Patients with atrial flutter or atrial fibrillation are often given a digitalis glycoside, such as digoxin, for the purpose of controlling the ventricular rate and subsequently are given oral quinidine in an effort to restore normal sinus rhythm. In recent years it has been appreciated that the high incidence of digitalis-induced toxicity in such patients is related to the fact that concomitant administration of the two drugs leads to an excessively high plasma concentration of the digitalis glycoside. The initial increase in plasma digoxin concentration is probably caused by displacement of the cardiac glycoside from tissue stores by quinidine (83). The prolonged rise in plasma digoxin concentrations after the administration of quinidine is most likely related to a reduction in renal clearance of the cardiac glycoside (84). Thus, through the combined effects of reducing the volume of distribution and the renal clearance of digoxin, quinidine can increase the incidence of cardiac-glycoside-induced toxicity. Therefore, a reduction in digoxin dosage is suggested when the drugs are given concurrently. In addition, frequent assessment of the plasma concentration of digoxin and careful attention to clinical symptoms of toxicity will help to prevent glycoside-induced toxicity.

Procainamide

It has been appreciated for approximately 30 years that the local anesthetic agent procaine hydrochloride was effective against cardiac arrhythmias when the drug was administered intravenously (85,86). But the use of procaine for treatment of cardiac arrhythmias had several drawbacks: (a) The drug was rapidly hydrolyzed in

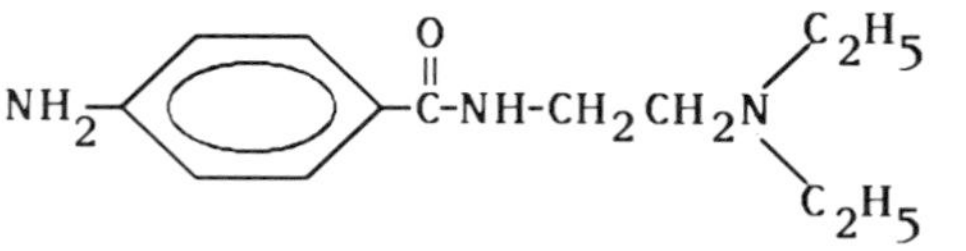

FIG. 9. Procainamide.

plasma by butyrocholinesterase and thus had a very short duration of action, making it difficult to achieve and maintain therapeutic plasma concentrations. (b) The potential to produce stimulation of the central nervous system mitigated against its use. (c) Oral administration did not prove to be effective. A systematic investigation of congeners of procaine was undertaken to identify compounds that had the therapeutic actions of procaine but did not have its drawbacks. Modification of the procaine molecule to produce procainamide yielded a compound with local anesthetic and antiarrhythmic actions that overcame the difficulties observed with the use of procaine (Fig. 9).

Procainamide was reported to be an effective antiarrhythmic drug, and subsequent investigation (86,87) led to its widespread clinical use. The amide group of procainamide prevents the drug from undergoing hydrolysis by plasma butyrocholinesterase, as occurs with procaine. Thus, procainamide is effective by oral, intramuscular, and intravenous routes, and it lacks the central nervous system effects of procaine.

Electrophysiologic Actions

The direct effects of procainamide on cardiac muscle and specialized conduction fibers are essentially the same as those of quinidine.

Sinoatrial Node

Procainamide has a direct effect on the sinoatrial node that leads to a decrease in the rate of spontaneous diastolic depolarization of specialized cells of the node. The direct actions of the drug lead to a decrease in heart rate. The direct negative chronotropic action of procainamide may be counteracted by its anticholinergic properties. At therapeutic plasma concentrations, usually no change or only a small increase in heart rate is observed. The vagolytic properties of procainamide are less pronounced than those of quinidine or disopyramide.

Atrial Muscle

Procainamide depresses automaticity in specialized atrial muscle fibers by depressing the rate of phase-4 depolarization. Atrial pacemakers are more sensitive to depression than ventricular pacemakers.

Administration of procainamide results in a dose-dependent parallel shift in atrial muscle membrane responsiveness and reduces the amplitude of the phase-0 upstroke potential. The maximum rate of phase-0 depolarization is depressed equally at all membrane potentials. Excitability of atrial muscle also is depressed, resulting in a decrease in conduction velocity in atrial muscle.

The action-potential duration of atrial muscle fibers is prolonged slightly by procainamide. This action of procainamide results in only a small increase in the atrial effective refractory period. Most of the increase in the effective refractory period can be attributed to a decrease in membrane responsiveness and failure of early premature complexes to conduct from the site of stimulation. The anticholinergic properties of the drug contribute to the depression of conduction velocity and the increase in refractoriness observed with procainamide, although its anticholinergic actions are less marked than those of quinidine.

In human electrophysiologic studies, acute procainamide administration results in an increase in atrial muscle refractory periods and a decrease in intraatrial conduction velocity (62,88). Conduction velocity in A-V accessory pathways is depressed, and the effective refractory period is increased (62). In the presence of atrial flutter or atrial fibrillation, in patients with WPW syndrome, procainamide reduces the ventricular rate by decreasing the frequency of transmission over the accessory pathway, which behaves electrophysiologically like atrial muscle (88).

A-V Node

Procainamide has both direct and indirect (anticholinergic) effects on A-V transmission. Direct effects include a decrease in A-V conduction velocity and an increase in A-V node refractoriness. Indirect or anticholinergic effects include a decrease in A-V node refractoriness and an increase in A-V nodal conduction velocity. The special considerations necessary for quinidine administration in the presence of atrial flutter and atrial fibrillation are equally applicable to procainamide administration. Procainamide administration may result in acceleration of ventricular rate due to increased transmission of atrial impulses through the A-V node because of the anticholinergic properties of the drug.

A number of investigators have studied the effects of acute procainamide on A-V conduction in humans. These studies have shown that procainamide's actions on A-V conduction velocity and A-V refractoriness are unpredictable. The effective refractory period of the A-V node can be increased, decreased, or unchanged (88,89). The same variability is seen in the action of procainamide on A-V conduction velocity. Although, in most cases, a decrease or no change in A-V transmission has been seen, in some cases there has been a dramatic increase in A-V transmission. The increase in A-V conduction observed in some patients could be potentially dangerous if atrial fibrillation or atrial flutter is also present.

In toxic doses, procainamide can produce marked depression of A-V conduc-

tion. The effects on A-V conduction are additive to those of digitalis, and extreme caution must be exercised when using the drugs in combination (90).

His-Purkinje System/Ventricular Muscle

Procainamide administration results in a decrease in membrane responsiveness and a decrease in the action-potential amplitude of Purkinje fibers and ventricular muscle (79). The phase-0 maximum rate of depolarization is depressed equally at all membrane potentials. Coupled with a decrease in excitability, these changes result in depression of conduction velocity in the His-Purkinje system and in ventricular muscle. The prolongation of ventricular action due to a decrease in conduction velocity results in prolongation of the QRS interval.

Procainamide administration also results in a slight prolongation of the action-potential duration (79). The effective refractory period is prolonged to a greater degree than the action-potential duration, a result of depression of membrane responsiveness. This action is observed in both ventricular muscle and the His-Purkinje system.

In human electrophysiologic studies, the effects of acute procainamide on conduction and refractoriness in the His-Purkinje system and ventricular muscle are more consistent than the effects on the A-V node. Consistent slowing of conduction and increases in refractoriness are observed in His-Purkinje tissue (88). Higher plasma concentrations result in a greater depression of conduction and a greater increase in refractoriness (88). Ventricular muscle effective refractory periods are increased by procainamide administration (91). Depression of conduction occurs at lower plasma concentrations than those necessary to produce increases in ventricular muscle refractory periods.

Although procainamide has been in clinical use for more than 25 years, its mechanism of action against ventricular arrhythmias is not completely understood. One reason for this is that often the mechanisms for the arrhythmias are not entirely clear. Recent observations suggest that procainamide progressively increases the coupling interval before termination of extrasystoles. The reentry of excitation within the ventricle or ventricular conducting system has been postulated as a mechanism for the production of ventricular premature depolarizations. Because procainamide depresses the maximum rate of rise and amplitude of the action potential and increases the effective refractory period, it is postulated that these actions will cause slowing of the reentrant impulse, particularly in abnormal tissue exhibiting slow conduction and unidirectional block. The reduction in responsiveness caused by procainamide could interrupt a reentrant rhythm by converting unidirectional block to bidirectional block. The proposed hypothesis is that procainamide prolongs conduction in the depressed portion of the reentrant pathway such that conduction is further delayed and conduction block finally occurs, thereby terminating the arrhythmias (92).

Procainamide decreases the spontaneous rate of firing in Purkinje fibers by depressing the slope of phase-4 depolarization. The action may account for the effectiveness of the drug in the treatment of ventricular arrhythmias occurring as a result of enhanced automaticity.

In a manner similar to that of quinidine, changes in extracellular potassium ion concentrations can alter the electrophysiologic properties of procainamide. Increased extracellular potassium concentrations potentiate depression of conduction velocity. Patients with hypokalemia may fail to respond to procainamide, and hyperkalemia will accentuate the drug's depressant actions on myocardial conduction.

Electrocardiographic Changes

Electrocardiographic changes observed with procainamide administration are simi-

lar to those observed with quinidine. At therapeutic plasma concentrations, procainamide prolongs the PR interval, the QRS interval, and the QT intervals of the surface electrocardiogram. The magnitudes of these changes are proportional to the plasma procainamide concentration. Toxic procainamide plasma concentrations may produce marked QT and QRS prolongation. Enhanced ventricular automaticity and ventricular arrhythmias are often present with excessive procainamide dosage.

Hemodynamic Effects

The hemodynamic alterations produced by procainamide are not as profound as those produced by quinidine. The route of administration, dosage, and rate of administration will determine the magnitude of the hemodynamic responses observed after procainamide administration. Alterations in circulatory dynamics will also vary according to the cardiovascular state of the individual.

Early hemodynamic studies with procainamide suggested that the drug produced both marked depression of myocardial contractility and vasodilation (93). More recent studies have suggested that depression of myocardial contractility and vasodilation are primarily a result of excessive dosage and/or too rapid administration (94). The dose-dependent relationship of these events was demonstrated by investigators studying the hemodynamic effects of procainamide administration in patients undergoing open-heart surgery (95). After a 2 mg/kg injection, systolic blood pressure and right ventricular force decreased by 10% and 12%, respectively. At a dose of 4 mg/kg, further decreases in systolic blood pressure and right ventricular force were observed (15% and 21%, respectively). The hypotensive effects are less pronounced after intramuscular administration and seldom occur after oral administration. Blood pressure can be restored by catecholamine administration, which produces vasoconstriction and augments cardiac contractility.

Toxic Reactions

Acute cardiovascular reactions to procainamide administration include hypotension, present to some degree in almost all patients receiving the drug intravenously. After oral administration, hypotensive episodes are infrequent and minor.

Procainamide, unlike procaine, has little potential to produce central nervous system toxicity (93). However, central nervous system stimulation has been observed after rapid intravenous administration of procainamide. An occasional patient may experience mental confusion or hallucinations.

Other toxic reactions to procainamide can include A-V block, intraventricular block, ventricular tachyarrhythmias, and complete heart block. The drug dosage must be reduced or even stopped if severe depression of conduction (severe prolongation of the QRS interval) or repolarization (severe prolongation of the QT interval) occurs in ventricular myocardium. Ventricular tachyarrhythmias leading to syncope or sudden unexpected ventricular fibrillation can occur with procainamide as well as quinidine administration. This toxic manifestation, however, is less common with procainamide administration. In toxic doses, procainamide may increase the slope of phase-4 depolarization in ventricular pacemakers and may produce an increase in ventricular premature complexes.

Procainamide administration may produce nausea, vomiting, and diarrhea, which are dose related and generally occur with doses in excess of 4 g/day. If the gastrointestinal symptoms remain relatively minor, it is not necessary to discontinue the drug.

An important consideration with chronic use of procainamide concerns the development of a syndrome resembling systemic lupus erythematosus, but without renal or cerebral involvement (96,97). Procainamide has a greater capacity to induce this syndrome than any other chemical. The development of the syndrome depends on both the duration of administration and the total daily dose. The most prevalent symptom is arthralgia. Other signs include skin rash, pleuropneumonic involvement, fever, and hepatomegaly. Symptomatic patients display a positive test for antinuclear factors and for lupus erythematosus cells. Other laboratory tests may differ from clinically observed systemic lupus erythematosus in that no anti-DNA antibodies are formed. The syndrome usually develops after a minimum of 1 month of therapy. Long-term use leads to increased antinuclear antibody titers in more than 80% of patients, and more than 30% of patients on long-term procainamide therapy develop a clinical lupus-erythematosuslike syndrome.

The symptoms of lupuslike syndrome disappear within a few days of cessation of procainamide therapy, although the test for antinuclear factor and lupus erythematosus cells may remain positive for several months.

Pharmacokinetics

Absorption

Oral doses of procainamide are well absorbed from the gastrointestinal tract, with bioavailability of approximately 75%. The remaining fraction can be accounted for by first-pass liver metabolism. Peak plasma concentrations are achieved 60 to 90 min after oral administration. Absorption of intramuscularly administered procainamide is more rapid, with peak plasma levels observed 12 to 45 min after injection (98).

Metabolism and Excretion

Procainamide is metabolized extensively in the liver by the enzyme N-acetyltransferase to N-acetylprocainamide. The rate of metabolism of procainamide varies widely among individuals and assumes a bimodal distribution of rapid and slow acetylators. The rate of drug acetylation is under genetic control and parallels that of isoniazid, hydralazine, and sulfonamide drugs. Rapid acetylators have higher plasma concentrations of *N*-acetylprocainamide and excrete larger amounts of *N*-acetylprocainamide in urine than slow acetylators. Acetylation of procainamide may occur predominantly as a first-pass effect after oral administration, as very little *N*-acetylprocainamide is formed after intravenous administration. *N*-acetylprocainamide possesses electrophysiologic actions similar to those of procainamide, although *N*-acetylprocainamide is less potent. Despite differences observed in the rate of procainamide metabolism by *N*-acetyltransferase in rapid and slow acetylators, the plasma clearances and therapeutic responses to procainamide are not markedly different in rapid and slow acetylators.

The renal clearance of procainamide is proportional to the creatinine clearance. However, the high rate of renal clearance suggests that both active secretion and filtration are involved in renal excretion of procainamide and *N*-acetylprocainamide. Although procainamide is a weak base, and renal excretion should be increased by urine acidification, conflicting results have been reported on the effect of urinary pH on procainamide excretion, and it is uncertain what effect alterations in urine pH have on renal elimination.

Kinetics

After intravenous injection, procainamide plasma concentrations can be described by a two-compartment model. The alpha-phase half-life is approximately 5 min, with a beta-phase half-life of 2 to 5 hr. Further pharmacokinetic data are summarized in Table 6.

Congestive heart failure alters many of the pharmacokinetic parameters that describe procainamide disposition. The steady-state volume of distribution is reduced by 20% to 25%. Renal clearance of the drug is reduced, increasing the plasma half-life. The extent and rate of oral and intramuscular absorption of the drug are reduced. Renal disease also increases the plasma half-life of procainamide. Hemodialysis can effectively increase procainamide clearance and decrease the plasma half-life. Procainamide dosage should, therefore, be altered in the

TABLE 6. *Pharmacokinetic properties of procainamide*

Absorption
  After oral administration 75% to 95% of the administered dose is absorbed rapidly
Protein binding
  Only 15% to 20% of the drug is bound to plasma proteins
Metabolism
  The drug undergoes hepatic metabolism with 25% of the dose being converted to the active metabolite, *N*-acetylprocainamide in slow acetylators and up to 40% conversion occurring in rapid acetylators
Half-life
  Approximately 2.5 to 4.5 hr for procainamide and 6 hr for *N*-acetylprocainamide
Time to peak plasma concentration
  60 to 90 min after oral administration
Therapeutic plasma concentration
  4 to 10 μg/ml of procainamide; must also consider the presence of the active metabolite *N*-acetylprocainamide
Elimination
  Renal: renal elimination is the primary route for removal of procainamide with 50% to 60% eliminated unchanged; *N*-acetylprocainamide has a slower rate of renal elimination than the parent compound and accumulated rapidly in the presence of renal failure whereas the concentration of the parent compound may be within the therapeutic range

presence of congestive heart failure and decreased renal function. Liver disease does not appear to significantly alter procainamide clearance.

Procainamide is bound poorly to plasma proteins. Approximately 85% of the drug in plasma exists in the unbound state. Myocardial tissue concentrations of procainamide are 2 to 2.5 times those in plasma.

Renal failure shifts procainamide elimination from a renal-dependent to a hepatic-dependent function. Renal disease causes N-acetylprocainamide plasma concentrations to increase dramatically, even after therapy is adjusted to maintain normal therapeutic plasma procainamide concentrations.

The effective plasma procainamide concentration for suppression of ectopic ventricular activity in patients with acute myocardial infarction has been reported to be between 4 and 6 µg/ml. Plasma procainamide concentrations of 2 to 4 µg/ml provide partial protection against ectopic impulse formation. However, recent evidence suggests that recurrent sustained ventricular tachycardia or ventricular fibrillation may be prevented only by procainamide plasma concentrations in excess of 10 µg/ml (99).

The short half-life of procainamide requires that doses be taken every 3 to 4 hr in order to maintain adequate plasma concentrations. Administration at longer intervals increases the incidence of therapeutic failures.

Oral Dose

Maintenance doses of procainamide for treatment of atrial and ventricular arrhythmias are between 500 and 1,000 mg administered every 4 to 6 hr. Shorter dosage intervals allow better control of arrhythmias, but poor patient compliance can negate this gain.

Intravenous Dose

To reduce the occurrence of hypotensive episodes, 100 mg doses may be administered every 5 min by direct slow intravenous injection, at a rate not exceeding 50 mg in any 1 min, until arrhythmia control is achieved or until a cumulative dose of 1 g has been given. To maintain therapeutic concentrations, an infusion may then be started at a rate of 2 to 6 mg procainamide per minute, depending on the person's renal status and body mass.

The following equation can be used to approximate the plasma procainamide concentration achieved by the foregoing method of administration (94):

$$Y = 0.84 + 0.73(x)$$

where Y is plasma procainamide concentration (µg/ml) and x is cumulative dose of procainamide (mg/kg). For example, if a patient weighing 70 kg were given seven 100 mg intravenous doses at 5-min intervals, the cumulative dose would be 10 mg/kg. The estimated plasma procainamide concentration would be $Y = 0.84 + 0.73(10) = 8.1$ µg/ml.

Procainamide can also be administered as an intravenous infusion, beginning with 500 to 600 mg given over a period of 25 to 30 min. This initial infusion should be followed by a maintenance infusion of 2 to 6 mg/min, based on body weight and renal function.

Intramuscular Dose

A dose of 0.5 to 1.0 g may be administered intramuscularly every 5 to 8 hr as needed.

Contraindications

The contraindications for procainamide are similar to those for quinidine. Because of its effects on A-V nodal and His-Purkinje conduction, procainamide should be administered with caution to patients with second-degree A-V block and bundle branch block. Parenteral administration may be hazardous in patients with compromised hemodynamic function, as further depression may occur as a result of procainamide's negative inotropic action. Procainamide should not be administered to patients with previous procaine or procainamide sensitivity and should be used with caution in patients with bronchial asthma. Prolonged administration should be accompanied by repeated hematologic studies, as agranulocytosis may occur.

Indications

Although the spectra of action and electrophysiologic effects of quinidine and procainamide are similar, the drugs are not interchangeable, as therapeutic response or intolerance may occur to one drug but not the other. The longer duration of action of quinidine limits procainamide use to patients who are intolerant or unresponsive to quinidine.

Clinical studies indicate that procainamide is an effective antiarrhythmic agent when given in sufficient dosage at relatively short (3–4 hr) dosage intervals. It is effective for treatment of premature atrial contractions, paroxysmal atrial tachycardia, and atrial fibrillation of recent onset. Procainamide is moderately effective in converting atrial flutter or chronic atrial fibrillation to sinus rhythm, although it is of value in preventing reoccurrences of these arrhythmias once they have been terminated by DC cardioversion.

Studies by several investigators indicate that procainamide can decrease occurrences of all types of active ventricular dysrhythmias in patients with acute myocardial infarction who are free from A-V dissociation, serious ventricular failure, and shock. It has been found that 90% of patients with ventricular premature complexes and 80% of patients with ventricular tachycardia respond to procainamide administration (100). The selection of procainamide over quinidine is in many instances a matter of personal preference. For oral administration, the longer duration of action of quinidine is advantageous. For short-term parenteral medication, intravenous or intramuscular procainamide is to be preferred because it is less likely to cause adverse hemodynamic alterations.

Disopyramide

The introduction of disopyramide, an orally effective agent capable of suppressing atrial and ventricular arrhythmias and possessing a longer duration of action than other currently available agents, has been of considerable value for treatment of disorders of cardiac rhythm. The structure of disopyramide is shown in Fig. 10.

Electrophysiologic Actions

The effects of disopyramide on the myocardium and specialized conduction tissue are a composite of the direct actions of the drug on myocardial electrical properties and indirect actions of the drug mediated by competitive blockade of cardiac cholinergic receptors. The direct actions of disopyramide are those possessed in common with other members of the class IA antiarrhythmic agents, and the indirect actions of disopyramide are virtually identical with the actions of atropine and other anticholinergic agents. These direct and indirect properties are shared with other members

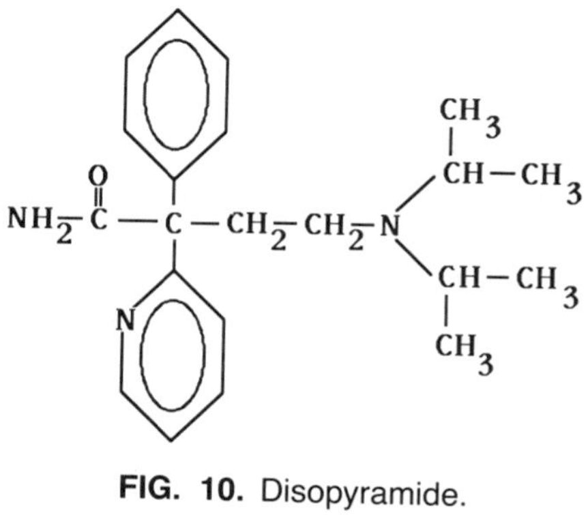

FIG. 10. Disopyramide.

of the class IA antiarrhythmic agents, quinidine and procainamide. Table 4 summarizes the electrophysiologic properties of disopyramide on atrial and ventricular myocardium and specialized conduction tissue.

Sinoatrial Node

By virtue of its direct depressant effects, disopyramide reduces the frequency of beating of isolated right atrial tissue preparations that are devoid of intact autonomic nervous system innervation (101). In conscious animals and humans, the direct depressant actions are counteracted by the anticholinergic properties, so that at therapeutic plasma concentrations of disopyramide, usually no change or a slight increase in sinus heart rate is observed (102,103). Disopyramide should be used cautiously in patients with sinus node dysfunction, as a deterioration in sinus node activity may become manifest (104).

Atrium

Disopyramide reduces membrane responsiveness in atrial muscle and thereby reduces the velocity of atrial conduction (101), a manifestation of its membrane action that places disopyramide into the category of class I antiarrhythmic agents. The action-potential duration in atrial muscle fibers is prolonged by disopyramide administration, resulting in an increase in the atrial muscle effective refractory period (101). Electrophysiologic studies performed in humans have demonstrated depression of intraatrial conduction and increased atrial muscle refractoriness at therapeutic plasma concentrations (102,103,105). These actions result from direct effects of disopyramide on cardiac membranes and are not a result of the anticholinergic properties of the drug, as they occur in patients pretreated with atropine (105).

A-V Node

Disopyramide depresses conduction velocity and increases the effective refractory period of the A-V node via a direct action. Additionally, disopyramide increases conduction velocity and decreases the effective refractory period of the A-V node as a result of its anticholinergic properties (102,103,105). The net effect on A-V transmission will be a result of the interplay of these two opposing actions, a direct depression and an indirect facilitation of A-V nodal transmission. At lower plasma concentrations, the anticholinergic actions predominate, whereas direct depression predominates at toxic concentrations. The same precautions necessary for administration of quinidine or procainamide in the presence of atrial flutter or atrial fibrillation must be exercised with disopyramide to prevent a possible acceleration of ventricular rhythm via facilitation of A-V conduction.

A number of electrophysiologic studies have been performed to examine the effects of disopyramide on A-V conduction in humans (102–105). In these studies, mean plasma disopyramide concentration ranging from 1.3 to 5.6 μg/ml produced very little change in A-V nodal conduction. No change in conduction velocity and either no change or a small decrease in the effective refractory period were observed. Large doses of disopyramide will depress A-V nodal conduction in animals (106), and this potential may exist clinically.

His-Purkinje System/Ventricular Muscle

Disopyramide reduces membrane responsiveness in canine Purkinje fibers and ventricular muscle (107,108). This action results in depression of conduction velocity in the His-Purkinje system and ventricular muscle (106,109). Disopyramide also increases the action-potential duration in canine Purkinje fibers and ventricular muscle fibers (107,108), thereby increasing the effective refractory period of ventricular myocardium (109,110). The electrophysiologic actions of disopyramide on ventricular muscle are generally analogous to those of quinidine or procainamide.

The magnitude of the depressant action of disopyramide on membrane responsiveness is dependent on the extracellular potassium concentration (107,108). Greater depression of conduction is seen at higher extracellular potassium ion concentrations. This may, in part, explain the poor response of patients with hypokalemia to class I antiarrhythmic agents. Likewise, hyperkalemia may accentuate the depression of conduction produced by disopyramide.

In electrophysiologic studies performed in humans (102–105), disopyramide has been shown to depress conduction in the His-Purkinje system and to increase the ventricular effective refractory period. These changes are associated with prolongation of the QRS and QT intervals.

Electrocardiographic Changes

The electrocardiographic changes observed after disopyramide administration are similar to those commonly observed with quinidine or procainamide. There is dose-dependent prolongation of the PR, QRS, and QT intervals.

Hemodynamic Effects

At plasma concentrations that produce an antiarrhythmic response, disopyramide produces a significant depression of myocardial contractility (106,111). This action results in an increase in left ventricular end-diastolic pressure and a decrease in cardiac output (106). Administration of disopyramide to patients with compensated heart failure may produce serious depression of cardiac function and lead to overt heart failure. Current data suggest that depression of cardiac function may be greater with disopyr-

amide than that observed at equivalent antiarrhythmic doses of procainamide or quinidine (111).

Disopyramide administration produces vasoconstriction and an increase in peripheral vascular resistance (111) via a direct action on the peripheral vasculature. The exact mechanism responsible for this vasoconstriction is not known. As a result of this increase in peripheral vascular resistance, blood pressure is well maintained despite a fall in cardiac output.

Disopyramide is presently available in the United States only for oral administration. The myocardial depressant actions of disopyramide are more marked with parenteral administration and care must be taken to avoid cardiovascular depression, especially in the setting of acute myocardial infarction. Catecholamine administration can reverse the myocardial depressant effects of the drug.

Toxic Reactions

Major toxic reactions to disopyramide include hypotension and cardiac depression. These reactions result from a dose-dependent decrease in myocardial contractility and are primarily observed in patients with poorly compensated heart failure and preexisting cardiac damage. Mild ventricular dysfunction is not an absolute contraindication. Many of the remaining side effects can be attributed to the anticholinergic action of the drug. Dry mouth and urinary hesitancy have been reported in 10% to 40% of patients. Blurred vision, nausea, constipation, and urinary retention have been reported. Central nervous system stimulation and hallucinations can occur, but they are rare. The incidence of severe adverse effects of long-term disopyramide therapy may be less than those observed with quinidine.

Disopyramide can produce depression of A-V nodal and ventricular conduction in some patients. Primary, secondary, and complete heart block have been observed.

Ventricular tachycardia or fibrillation associated with prolongation of the electrocardiographic QT interval (112) has been observed with disopyramide administration. This condition closely resembles "quinidine syncope" associated with quinidine administration. Simultaneous use of disopyramide and digoxin does not result in abnormally high plasma concentrations of the cardiac glycoside, as are known to occur with quinidine. Because of the similarity in the antiarrhythmic spectra of disopyramide and quinidine, the former agent may prove clinically advantageous in patients who are receiving digoxin and who require antiarrhythmic therapy with a class I drug.

Pharmacokinetics

Disopyramide is rapidly and almost completely absorbed from the gastrointestinal tract (83%) after oral administration. First-pass liver metabolism occurs but is not a significant factor in oral use of the drug. Peak plasma disopyramide concentrations are attained within 2 hr after an oral dose.

The clearance of disopyramide from plasma is almost equally divided between renal and hepatic clearances. The metabolism of disopyramide is not well understood; however, the major metabolite, the mono-N-dealkylated product, is active as an antiarrhythmic agent. The metabolite accumulates slowly over a period of time, and 25% to 50% of the administered drug can be found in urine in the mono-N-dealkylated form. Clearance of disopyramide and its major metabolite from plasma is dependent on renal excretion, with the remainder appearing in the feces. Plasma clearance exceeds the rate of creatinine clearance, and this implies that active tubular secretion of disopyramide may be involved in renal excretion. Renal clearance of the drug is not altered significantly by changes in urinary pH.

The clearance of disopyramide from plasma is reduced by renal insufficiency

and requires a reduction in the dosage of disopyramide to prevent systemic toxicity. Although the rate of renal clearance of disopyramide is not a linear first-order function of the plasma concentration (clearance of disopyramide is more rapid at higher doses and higher plasma concentrations because of the greater fraction of the drug in plasma being in the free, unbound form), clearance values calculated as a function of creatinine clearance can aid in adjustment of the dosage for patients with lowered renal function. Hemodialysis is effective for removal of disopyramide from plasma and can be used in cases involving renal failure or overdose.

The clearance of disopyramide from plasma can be adequately described by a two-compartment (biexponential) model providing for a rapid initial distribution phase (alpha-phase) and a slower elimination phase occurring after the drug has been distributed to body tissues (beta-phase). The initial distribution-phase (alpha-phase) half-life is approximately 2 min, with the beta-phase half-life of between 5 and 7 hr for patients with normal renal function. Pharmacokinetic values for disopyramide are given in Table 7.

The free plasma concentration, or the fraction of the drug in plasma that is not bound to plasma proteins and is therefore free to exert its pharmacologic effect, is not constant at plasma disopyramide concentrations within the normal therapeutic range. The free plasma concentration increases from 5% to 65% of the total plasma concentration as total plasma disopyramide concentrations are increased from 0.1 to 8 μg/ml. Therefore, an increase in the administered dose may produce a disproportionately large increase in the unbound plasma drug concentration and a more pronounced pharmacologic effect. As a result of this response and the ability of disopyramide to produce cardiovascular depression, the dosage of the drug must be increased slowly to avoid unwanted side effects.

The effective therapeutic plasma concen-

TABLE 7. *Pharmacokinetic properties of disopyramide*

Absorption
   After oral administration, absorption is rapid and nearly complete (83%)
Protein binding
   Moderately bound to plasma proteins approximating 50% at the therapeutic plasma concentration but may range from 35% to 95% depending on the plasma concentration
Metabolism
   Undergoes hepatic metabolism with the formation of an active metabolite
Half-life
   In the presence of normal renal function $t_{1/2}$ is 7 hr with a range of 4 to 10 hr; with renal impairment the $t_{1/2}$ may be from 8 to 18 hr
Time to peak plasma concentration
   Peak plasma concentrations may be achieved in 30 min to 3 hr
Therapeutic plasma concentration
   Range is 2 to 4 μg/ml; however, because disopyramide shows variable protein binding, the amount of free unbound drug will vary; plasma concentrations should not be used for dosage adjustment
Elimination
   Renal: approximately 80% of the drug is eliminated in the urine with 50% being unchanged and the remainder as metabolites; biliary: excretion into the bile accounts for 15% of the administered dose

tration of disopyramide as defined by early clinical trials was between 2 and 5 μg/ml (113,114). Whereas maintenance of disopyramide plasma concentrations within the range of 2 to 4 μg/ml is effective for suppression of ventricular premature complexes and maintenance of normal sinus rhythm after conversion of atrial fibrillation, significantly higher concentrations (4–8 μg/ml) are needed to suppress malignant ventricular arrhythmias (110,115,116).

As discussed earlier, quinidine alters the plasma kinetics of digoxin (83,84). On the other hand, an increase in serum digoxin concentrations is *not* observed with disopyramide administration.

Oral Dose

Patients weighing 110 pounds or more, with normal renal and hepatic function, should be given 150 mg every 6 hr. Patients weighing less than 110 pounds should receive 100 mg every 6 hr. More rapid control of arrhythmias can be obtained with an initial loading dose of 300 mg (200 mg for patients weighing less than 100 pounds), followed by the normal maintenance dose 6 hr later.

Dosage reduction is necessary for patients with hypotension, possible cardiac decompensation, reduced left ventricular function, or cardiomyopathy. The suggested initial dosage in these patients is 100 mg every 6 hr. Renal impairment requires reduction in dosage according to the following schedule (C_{cr} = creatinine clearance):

$C_{cr} > 40$ ml/min	100 mg every 6 hr
$C_{cr} = 15$–40 ml/min	100 mg every 10 hr
$C_{cr} = 5$–15 ml/min	100 mg every 20 hr
$C_{cr} = 1$–5 ml/min	100 mg every 30 hr

Severe refractory ventricular tachycardias may require larger disopyramide dosages for suppression. The dosage should be increased gradually, with electrocardiographic and blood pressure monitoring. In some cases, dosages of 250 to 400 mg every 6 hr may be necessary to effect suppression of more malignant arrhythmias.

Contraindications

Disopyramide should not be administered in the presence of cardiogenic shock, preexisting second- or third-degree A-V block, or known hypersensitivity to the drug. Disopyramide should not be administered in the presence of poorly compensated or uncompensated heart failure or in the presence of severe hypotension.

As a result of its anticholinergic properties, disopyramide should not be used in patients with glaucoma. Urinary retention and benign prostatic hypertrophy also present relative contraindications to disopyramide therapy. Patients with myasthenia gravis may present with myasthenic crisis after disopyramide administration because of the local anesthetic action of disopyramide at the neuromuscular junction.

If first-degree heart block develops during disopyramide administration, the drug dosage should be reduced. The appearance of second- or third-degree heart block (in the absence of an implanted pacemaker) requires withdrawal of the drug. Prolongation of the QRS or QT intervals in excess of 25% also requires lowering of the dosage or discontinuance of the drug.

Patients with congenital prolongation of the QT interval (Jervell-Lang-Nielsen syndrome) should not receive quinidine, procainamide, or disopyramide, because further prolongation of ventricular repolarization and a resultant increase in the QT interval may increase the incidence of ventricular fibrillation.

Indications

The indications for disopyramide are similar to those for quinidine and procainamide, except that disopyramide is not currently approved for use in the prophylaxis of atrial flutter or atrial fibrillation after DC cardioversion. The indications are as follows: (a) unifocal premature (ectopic) ventricular complexes; (b) premature (ectopic) ventricular complexes of multifocal origin; (c) paired premature ventricular couplets; (d) episodes of ventricular tachycardia (persistent ventricular tachycardia is usually treated by DC cardioversion).

As a result of the additive depression of cardiac conduction produced by disopyramide in the presence of the already depressed conduction produced by cardiac glycosides, the agent is not indicated for the treatment of digitalis-induced ventricular arrhythmias.

Lidocaine

Lidocaine was introduced into therapy in 1943 as a local anesthetic agent, and it continues to be used extensively for that purpose today. Widespread use of lidocaine was delayed until the 1960s, when it gained popularity for the treatment of ventricular arrhythmias associated with cardiac surgery, digitalis intoxication, and acute myocardial infarction. Extensive experience has demonstrated lidocaine to be an effective and safe drug for termination of ventricular arrhythmias. The chemical structure of lidocaine is shown in Fig. 11.

Electrophysiologic Actions

The therapeutic usefulness of lidocaine is in large measure due to several specific electrophysiologic properties that give it distinct advantages over other currently available antiarrhythmic agents. In contrast to quinidine and procainamide, lidocaine acts primarily on disturbances of ventricular origin and has a narrow spectrum of antiarrhythmic action.

Sinoatrial Node

In isolated tissue, high concentrations of lidocaine (greater than 10^{-4}M) produce a slowing of sinus nodal pacemaker discharge (72,117). At concentrations approximating

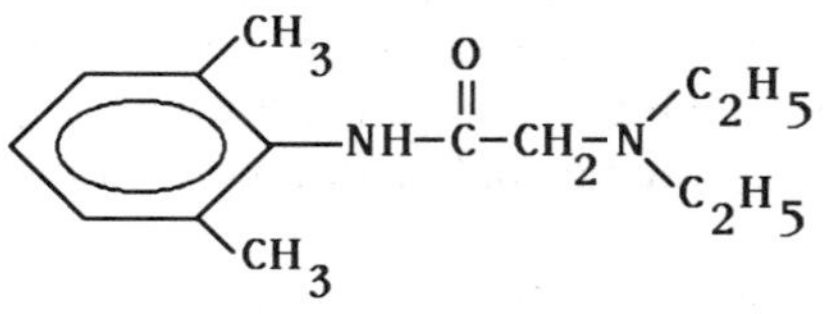

FIG. 11. Lidocaine.

therapeutic plasma concentrations, no alteration in sinus nodal pacemaker discharge is observed. Severe slowing of sinus node automaticity in isolated tissue preparations is not observed even at plasma concentrations 50 to 100 times those observed in humans. It is apparent that the striking sinoatrial nodal depression observed at moderate procainamide, quinidine, or disopyramide concentrations is not observed with lidocaine. When administered in therapeutic doses in humans, 1 to 5 mg/kg lidocaine has no effect on the sinus rate.

Atria

Early experimental studies suggested that lidocaine produced only small and variable effects on the cardiac action potential in ordinary atrial muscle fibers or specialized conduction fibers of the atria, even when toxic concentrations are used (10^{-4} M) (117). This failure to observe marked electrophysiologic effects of lidocaine may be due to the use of abnormally low extracellular potassium ion concentrations. When the extracellular potassium ion concentration is increased to that present in the extracellular fluid, the electrophysiologic properties of lidocaine in atrial muscle more closely resemble those of quinidine. Membrane responsiveness is decreased, the action-potential amplitude is decreased (118), and excitability of atrial muscle is decreased. These changes result in a decrease in atrial muscle conduction velocity. However, the depression of conduction velocity by lidocaine is less marked than that with quinidine or procainamide, even when toxic concentrations of lidocaine are used.

The action-potential duration of atrial muscle fibers is not altered by lidocaine at either normal or subnormal extracellular potassium ion concentrations (117,118). The effective refractory period of atrial myocardium either remains the same or increases slightly after lidocaine administration. Effective refractory periods are not as

greatly or consistently increased as with quinidine or procainamide.

The rate of phase-4 depolarization of atrial muscle fibers is depressed by lidocaine. Atrial muscle automaticity is depressed by lidocaine concentrations that do not affect the sinus node (117).

In human electrophysiologic studies, lidocaine failed to alter atrial refractoriness or atrial conduction velocity (119). Conduction in A-V bypass pathways is depressed, and A-V transmission is decreased in the accessory pathway (60).

In summary, lidocaine usually fails to significantly alter atrial refractoriness or conduction velocity. This is the basis for the failure of lidocaine in treatment of supraventricular arrhythmias, except for supraventricular tachycardia using an accessory pathway that may be responsive to lidocaine.

A-V Node

Lidocaine minimally alters conduction velocity and the effective refractory period of A-V node (54,119). Lidocaine does not possess anticholinergic properties and will not improve A-V transmission when atrial flutter or atrial fibrillation is present.

In electrophysiologic studies conducted in humans, lidocaine failed to alter A-V nodal refractoriness (60,119). Although lidocaine does not normally alter A-V nodal transmission, it is suggested that lidocaine *not* be administered to patients with atrial flutter or atrial fibrillation, or to patients with second- or third-degree A-V block, unless close observation of the hemodynamic and electrophysiologic status is maintained as both facilitation of A-V transmission and complete A-V block have been reported with the use of the drug.

His-Purkinje System

Lidocaine reduces the action-potential amplitude and membrane responsiveness

(120). The maximum rate of phase-0 depolarization is depressed primarily in fibers with reduced resting membrane potentials and in the presence of normal or raised extracellular potassium ion concentrations. The maximum rate of phase-0 depolarization in normal Purkinje fibers (resting membrane potential of −80 to −90 mV in the presence of physiologic extracellular potassium concentrations) is depressed less severely by lidocaine than by procainamide or quinidine. Severe depression can be observed in Purkinje fibers, with reduced resting membrane potentials (−70 to −60 mV) occurring as a result of myocardial ischemia. This depression of phase-0 upstroke can be so severe as to produce complete conduction block at lidocaine concentrations in the high therapeutic range (121,122). His-Purkinje excitability is reduced, and combined with the slight depression of phase-0 upstroke velocity, this produces a slight decrease in conduction velocity of the His-Purkinje system.

The action-potential duration in Purkinje fibers is decreased by lidocaine administration (120). Shortening of the action potential and effective refractory period occurs at lower concentrations in Purkinje fibers than in ventricular muscle. As with procainamide and quinidine, lidocaine causes the effective refractory period to lengthen relative to the action-potential duration.

Lidocaine at very low concentrations slows phase-4 depolarization in Purkinje fibers and decreases the spontaneous rate of firing (120–122). At higher concentrations, automaticity in Purkinje fibers may be suppressed and phase-4 depolarization completely eliminated. Lidocaine also suppresses automaticity in Purkinje fibers induced by stretch, hypoxia, or catecholamines.

Ventricular Muscle

Lidocaine does not alter the resting membrane potential of isolated ventricular muscle fibers. The action-potential duration and effective refractory period are decreased (120). No changes in the amplitude or the maximum rate of phase-0 depolarization can be observed with lidocaine concentrations in the normal therapeutic range. Myocardial conduction velocity and effective refractory periods are not altered by lidocaine administration.

Electrophysiologic studies in humans have confirmed the foregoing *in vitro* and *in vivo* observations. Lidocaine shortens the effective refractory period of His-Purkinje tissue and does not alter conduction velocity in the His-Purkinje system (119). Ventricular effective refractory periods are not altered by lidocaine. On the basis of lidocaine's action on normal ventricular myocardial tissue and His-Purkinje tissue, it is difficult to suggest a mechanism for its antiarrhythmic action. The effects of lidocaine on damaged myocardial tissue may determine its antiarrhythmic action. However, the effect of lidocaine on damaged myocardium is poorly understood. The ability of lidocaine to suppress automaticity in damaged myocardium may be of importance in its antiarrhythmic action, in addition to its effects on conduction velocity and refractory periods (121,122).

Electrocardiographic Changes

The PR, QRS, and QT intervals usually are unchanged, although the QT interval may be shortened in some patients. This lack of observed electrocardiographic changes with lidocaine is a result of failure of lidocaine to specifically alter conduction velocity in specialized conduction tissues and myocardium.

Hemodynamic Effects

Large doses of lidocaine produce decreases in peak force development and rate of force development in isolated ventricular muscle (123). Studies in the intact canine heart have shown either no change in ventricular performance or a slight positive inotropic effect at doses within the therapeutic range (124). At larger doses, dose-dependent decreases in myocardial contractility, cardiac output, and aortic pressure have been noted (125). Studies in the dog after experimental myocardial infarction have shown lidocaine to produce no significant hemodynamic changes at doses up to 200 μg/kg/min (124).

Lidocaine administered as an intravenous bolus at a dose of 1 mg/kg to patients undergoing cardiac surgery produced an increase in myocardial contractility. Doses of 2 mg/kg were not associated with an alteration in myocardial contractility compared with the control state (126). Infusion of either 1.5 mg/kg as an intravenous bolus or 0.3 mg/kg/min intravenous infusion produced no change in the rate of developed pressure, ejection time, time to peak pressure, or right ventricular end-diastolic pressure in a group of 10 patients with heart disease (127). Bolus injection of 100 mg of lidocaine has been shown to produce small and transient decreases in arterial pressure and cardiac output. In the setting of acute myocardial infarction, lidocaine administration fails to alter arterial pressure, right atrial pressure, heart rate, and cardiac output.

Alterations in hemodynamics occurring as a result of administration of lidocaine depend on the status of the patient and on the dose administered. Myocardial contractility and peripheral vascular resistance are depressed only slightly, if at all, by therapeutic doses of lidocaine, but they may be affected by plasma concentrations of lidocaine in excess of therapeutic concentrations.

and unless it is excessive, it may not be particularly undesirable in patients suffering from acute myocardial infarction (128). Some patients may experience paresthesias, disorientation, and muscle twitching. These undesirable effects may cause agitation or enhanced anxiety, but, of equal importance, they forewarn of more serious deleterious effects. These deleterious effects can include psychosis, respiratory depression, and seizures. Focal seizures often occur just before the appearance of generalized tonic-clonic seizures. Convulsions are a dose-related side effect and can be avoided by the simple expedient of controlling the rate of infusion and preventing plasma concentrations from exceeding 5 μg/ml. Diazepam administration will prevent these adverse central nervous system effects of lidocaine, and this is the treatment of choice for lidocaine-induced seizures. However, if signs of toxicity are present, lowering the infusion rate or stopping the drug usually will suffice to prevent further toxicity, as lidocaine has a relatively short plasma half-life.

Lidocaine may produce clinically significant hypotension, but this is exceedingly uncommon if the drug is given at moderate dosages. Depression of an already damaged myocardium may result from large doses.

Adverse electrophysiologic effects are uncommon with lidocaine administration. Lidocaine is contraindicated in the presence of second- or third-degree heart block because it may increase the degree of heart block and may abolish the idioventricular pacemaker that is maintaining cardiac rhythm. Cardiac pacing should be instituted if lidocaine or other antiarrhythmic drugs must be administered in these instances.

Toxic Reactions

The most common toxic reactions due to lidocaine are owing primarily to its actions on the central nervous system. Drowsiness is the most commonly observed side effect,

Pharmacokinetics

Absorption

Oral administration of lidocaine has been attempted, but therapeutically efficient blood levels have not been achieved by this route of administration. The failure of oral lidocaine administration is not due to poor intestinal absorption of the drug but rather to extensive first-pass liver metabolism. In excess of 70% of orally administered lidocaine is metabolized by the liver before reaching the systemic circulation. Dizziness, nausea, and vomiting may occur in humans after oral lidocaine administration, and they probably are results of the high circulating plasma concentrations of the mono-*N*-deethylated and the di-*N*-deethylated metabolites of lidocaine (monoethylglycine xylidide and glycine xylidide).

Lidocaine is absorbed rapidly after intramuscular injection. Absorption is more rapid after injection into the deltoid muscle (absorption half-life 11.7 min) than into the vastus lateralis and gluteus maximus (absorption half-life 25.7 min).

Metabolism and Excretion

Approximately 70% of the lidocaine entering the liver from the systemic circulation is metabolized on a single circulation through the liver. The rate of lidocaine metabolism is critically dependent on hepatic blood flow. Reductions in liver blood flow sharply reduce lidocaine plasma clearance. Lidocaine dosage must be reduced in the presence of decreased liver blood flow or in the presence of deficiencies in liver metabolic function.

Two major metabolites of lidocaine are found in significant concentrations in the blood of patients receiving the drug. The first metabolite, monoethylglycine xylidide, is formed by *N*-deethylation of lidocaine. Monoethylglycine xylidide is as potent an antiarrhythmic agent as lidocaine and has similar convulsant activity. Monoethylglycine xylidide has a plasma half-life of 120 min and is eliminated from plasma primarily by a second *N*-deethylation to form glycine xylidide, the second major metabolite of lidocaine. Glycine xylidide possesses

both antiarrhythmic and convulsant activity, although it is only 10% to 26% as potent as lidocaine. Glycine xylidide is both metabolized and excreted by the kidney. It has a plasma half-life of 10 hr.

Accumulation of metabolites during prolonged intravenous administration may help explain why toxicity develops despite plasma lidocaine concentrations that remain in the therapeutic range. Approximately 90% of an administered lidocaine dose appears in the urine as metabolites.

Excretion of unchanged lidocaine by the kidney is a minor route of elimination (10% of dose). Lidocaine is a weak base (pK_a 7.9), and renal clearance is facilitated by a decrease in urine pH.

Lidocaine crosses the placenta readily from mother to fetus. The drug is then broken down in the fetus or neonate at a rate comparable with that in the mother. The safety of lidocaine for use in pregnancy has not been established.

Kinetics

Lidocaine plasma concentrations after an intravenous dose can be explained by a two-compartment model. The initial distribution-phase (alpha-phase) half-life is 8 min, and the beta-phase half-life is 100 min. Other pharmacokinetic parameters are given in Table 8. A rapid equilibrium is established between tissue and plasma in organs of the body with high blood flows, such as heart, brain, lung, liver, and kidney. The prompt action of lidocaine after intravenous administration is a result of rapid delivery to and uptake in myocardial tissue. Lidocaine then slowly redistributes to other organ systems with lower blood flows. This action accounts for the initial redistribution or alpha-phase. The alpha-phase (redistribution-phase) of lidocaine is extensive and is an important factor in determining dosage regimens for lidocaine.

A number of pathologic conditions alter the disposition and clearance of lidocaine.

TABLE 8. *Pharmacokinetic properties of lidocaine*

Absorption
   Lidocaine should not be given orally because it undergoes rapid absorption and extensive first-pass metabolism giving rise to monoethylglycine xylidide and glycinexylidide, which exhibit toxic effects on the central nervous system

Protein binding
   Moderately bound to the extent of 60% to 80% depending on the drug concentration

Metabolism
   Hepatic metabolism is rapid and extensive as indicated above

Half-life
   Dose dependent and shows an initial $t_{1/2}$ of 8 min after intravenous administration and a $t_{1/2}$ of approximately 100 min after an infusion of 24 hr has been administered

Time to peak plasma concentration
   Dependent on the rate of intravenous administration and administered dose; usually achieved within 45 to 90 sec

Therapeutic plasma concentration
   Considered to be from 1.5 to 5.0 µg/ml; concentrations in excess of 5.0 µg/ml may be within the toxic range

Elimination
   Renal: 10% unchanged drug is eliminated by the kidney, with the remainder being in the form of inactive metabolites

Heart failure results in significant reductions in both the volume of distribution and plasma clearance of lidocaine. The clinical implication is that patients with congestive heart failure should receive smaller lidocaine dosages. Chronic alcoholic liver disease reduces plasma clearance of lidocaine by as much as 50%. Renal failure and age produce only small and insignificant decreases in lidocaine clearance. However, in elderly and renally compromised patients, lidocaine metabolites can accumulate and produce central nervous system toxicity. The rate of indocyanine green clearance from plasma can be used as a guide for the rate of liver lidocaine clearance.

At therapeutic plasma concentrations, 70% of the total lidocaine is plasma-protein bound. Alterations of the fraction bound to plasma proteins are minor between different plasma concentrations and are not a factor in dosing schedules.

Therapeutic plasma concentrations range from 2 to 5 µg/ml. Plasma lidocaine concentrations in excess of 7 µg/ml are frequently toxic. Plasma concentrations from 1 to 2.5 µg/ml may suppress ventricular ectopic beats, but plasma lidocaine concentrations of 2.5 µg/ml or greater may be necessary for prevention of ventricular fibrillation.

Dose

Lidocaine usually is administered intravenously. After a single intravenous bolus injection, the drug disappears rapidly from the plasma because of redistribution to other tissues (given over 1 to 3 min). The true steady-state plasma half-life of lidocaine is 100 min. Because of these pharmacokinetic properties, lidocaine is administered as an intravenous loading dose followed by a constant intravenous infusion.

A. Loading dose (objective is to administer 200 mg in 10–20 min):
   1. 100 mg given over a 2-min period at 10-min intervals, or
   2. 50 mg in 1 min, given four times, 5 min apart, or
   3. 20 mg/min infused for 10 min.

B. Continuous infusion (an infusion-regulating device should be used): 2 to 4 mg/min for 24 to 30 min.

C. To raise plasma concentration acutely if arrhythmia control is lost: 50 mg bolus over 1 min and simultaneously increase infusion rate to no more than 5 mg/min.

D. In shock, heart failure, and hepatocellular disease: reduce doses by one-half for loading and infusion rates.

Intramuscular administration of lidocaine also may be effective in the prevention of ventricular fibrillation. Absorption of lidocaine may be decreased by hemodynamic changes associated with myocardial infarction, and intravenous lidocaine is the preferred mode of administration. Intramuscular injection of 300 to 400 mg/kg gives persistent therapeutic levels lasting for 2 hr.

Contraindications

Contraindications to the use of lidocaine include the following: (a) hypersensitivity to local anesthetics of the amide type (a very rare occurrence); (b) the presence of complete heart block because lidocaine suppresses ventricular pacemakers and would result in ventricular standstill; (c) the presence of severe hepatic dysfunction; (d) a previous history of grand mal seizures due to lidocaine; (e) patients 70 years old or older. These conditions are only relative contraindications for the drug if dosage is properly altered.

Indications

In contrast to quinidine and procainamide, lidocaine is much less effective in the treatment of supraventricular arrhythmias (87). Lidocaine has been shown to be effective for terminating ventricular arrhythmias. Initially it was used primarily in postoperative patients who developed ventricular premature complexes or ventricular tachycardia, but it soon gained acceptance in the coronary care unit as a valuable agent for control of ventricular arrhythmias in patients with acute myocardial infarction. Lidocaine administration carries relatively little risk for the patient with acute myocardial infarction, because of its lack of marked depressant effects on the cardiovascular system and the reversibility and short duration of toxic side effects. Routine lidocaine administration may be indicated for all patients with acute myocardial in-

farction as a result of its ability to prevent ventricular arrhythmias and, most important, ventricular fibrillation, while being easily administered and relatively free of toxic effects. The clinical efficacy of lidocaine in prevention of ventricular fibrillation during acute myocardial infarction is unquestioned.

Lidocaine is the drug of choice for treatment of the electrical manifestations of digitalis intoxication. It also may be used to prevent arrhythmias during countershock in patients who have received digitalis.

Phenytoin

Phenytoin (diphenylhydantoin) is structurally related to the barbiturates and was introduced in 1938 for control of convulsive disorders (129). It was not until 1950 that phenytoin was used for the treatment of cardiac arrhythmias (130). The chemical structure of phenytoin is shown in Fig. 12.

Electrophysiologic Actions

Phenytoin's electrophysiologic actions differ from those of quinidine and procainamide and more closely resemble the electrophysiologic actions of lidocaine.

Sinoatrial Node

Supratherapeutic concentrations of phenytoin decrease the slope of phase-4 depolarization in sinus nodal pacemaker cells and depress the spontaneous rate of the si-

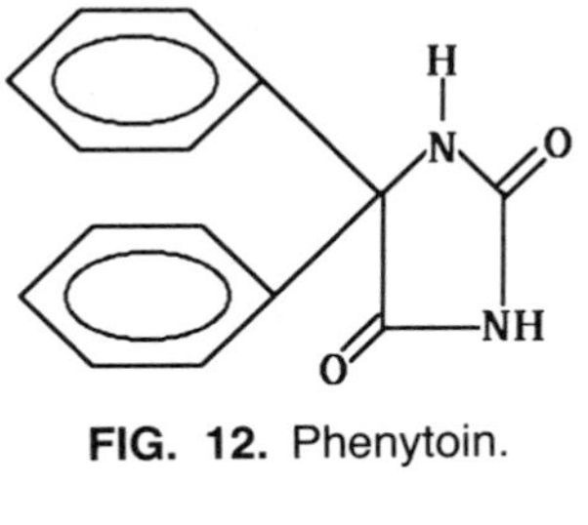

FIG. 12. Phenytoin.

nus node (131). However, therapeutic plasma concentrations of phenytoin do not alter sinus rate. When the function of the sinoatrial node or perinodal fibers is affected by disease, sinoatrial pacemaker activity may be impeded by phenytoin and other antiarrhythmic drugs. However, of the antiarrhythmic agents currently in use, phenytoin (and possibly lidocaine) produces the least alterations in sinus nodal function, even when sinus nodal function is compromised by disease. Clinically, phenytoin administration usually fails to alter sinus rate. Hypotension produced after intravenous administration may produce an increase in sympathetic tone and result in an increased sinus heart rate.

Atria

The electrophysiologic effects of phenytoin are disguised by the electrophysiologic properties of the diluent present in commercial preparations of the drug. Because of this action of the diluent, one must be careful in examining many of the earliest studies of the electrophysiologic properties of phenytoin using formulations that contained the commercial diluent.

The electrophysiologic effects of phenytoin on atrial muscle fibers resemble those of lidocaine. Except at very high concentrations, phenytoin usually does not alter the action-potential duration or effective refractory period of atrial myocardium (132,133).

The effect of phenytoin on membrane responsiveness of atrial muscle is dependent on the frequency of stimulation and the extracellular potassium ion concentration (132). When extracellular potassium ion concentrations are less than 3 mM and atrial muscle is paced at a rate below normal sinus rhythm, phenytoin may increase the rate of phase-0 depolarization of atrial muscle. When extracellular potassium ion concentrations are in the physiologic range (3–5 mM) and the atrial muscle is paced at a normal sinus rate, phenytoin depresses the rate of

phase-0 depolarization of atrial muscle fibers. Excitability of atrial muscle fibers is not altered by phenytoin. Atrial conduction velocity is either unchanged or slightly depressed after phenytoin administration.

Phenytoin depresses the rate of spontaneous phase-4 depolarization in atrial tissue and decreases the rate of discharge of atrial pacemakers. Atrial pacemakers are more sensitive to depression by phenytoin than are sinus nodal pacemakers (133).

In clinical electrophysiologic studies, phenytoin failed to significantly alter atrial refractoriness and intraatrial conduction velocity (134). The effects of phenytoin on A-V accessory pathways are unclear, although increases in the effective refractory period have been reported.

A-V Node

Phenytoin lacks the anticholinergic properties of quinidine, disopyramide, and procainamide. However, the direct actions of phenytoin on the A-V node facilitate A-V transmission.

In human electrophysiologic studies, phenytoin has been shown to decrease A-V nodal effective refractory periods and to increase A-V nodal conduction velocity (134,135). Depression of A-V conduction has not been observed. Phenytoin reverses digitalis-induced lengthening of the A-V effective refractory period and decreases in A-V conduction velocity. Phenytoin can return A-V transmission toward normal in the digitalis-intoxicated patient (135). In addition, phenytoin can reduce digitalis-induced ventricular automaticity. However, caution should be used when administering phenytoin in the presence of digitalis-induced third-degree heart block. Ventricular automaticity may be depressed before A-V conduction is restored, and the ventricular rate may decrease precipitously before being restored to normal.

Because of the increase in A-V transmission observed after phenytoin administration, phenytoin should not be administered to patients with atrial flutter or atrial fibrillation. Phenytoin probably will not be effective in restoring normal sinus rhythm and may produce an acceleration of the ventricular rate.

His-Purkinje System

The electrophysiologic effects of phenytoin on the His-Purkinje system resemble those of lidocaine. The action-potential duration and effective refractory period of the action-potential duration are increased (136).

Phenytoin's effects on membrane responsiveness have been confusing. Phenytoin can increase the maximum rate of phase-0 depolarization in Purkinje fibers after phase-0 depolarization has been depressed by digitalis overdoses or hypoxia. Restoration of depressed conduction has been observed in the His-Purkinje system after digitalis overdoses. However, normal Purkinje fibers or Purkinje fibers damaged by myocardial ischemia do not respond to phenytoin in the same manner. At physiologic extracellular potassium ion concentrations, phenytoin produces either no change or a slight decrease in phase-0 maximum rate of depolarization. In a manner similar to that of lidocaine, phenytoin decreases the maximum rate of phase-0 depolarization in diseased, depolarized Purkinje fibers with resting membrane potentials of less than -70 mV. Experiments performed in anesthetized dogs suggest that depression of conduction velocity and increases in ventricular refractoriness are the primary actions of phenytoin in myocardium damaged by myocardial ischemia (137). Improvement in cardiac conduction velocity by phenytoin may be limited to that observed in digitalis toxicity.

Phenytoin decreases the rate of phase-4 depolarization in Purkinje tissue and reduces the rate of discharge of ventricular pacemakers. This depression of automaticity is observed with procainamide, quini-

dine, disopyramide, and lidocaine, as well as with phenytoin (136).

In human electrophysiologic studies, phenytoin has been shown to decrease the effective refractory period of the His-Purkinje system, while leaving conduction velocity unaltered or slightly decreased (134). The effects of phenytoin on ventricular refractoriness are presently unknown. Phenytoin can abolish premature ventricular beats resulting from digitalis intoxication without altering His-Purkinje conduction or refractoriness.

Electrocardiographic Changes

Because phenytoin improves A-V conduction and shortens the action-potential duration of ventricular myocardium, phenytoin may decrease the PR and QT intervals of the surface electrocardiogram. The electrophysiologic properties of phenytoin are summarized in Table 9.

Hemodynamic Effects

The effects of phenytoin on the cardiovascular system may vary with the dose, mode and rate of administration, and the presence of cardiovascular abnormalities. Rapid administration of phenytoin can produce transient hypotension, a result of peripheral vasodilation and depression of myocardial contractility (138). These effects are due to direct actions of phenytoin on the vascular bed and ventricular myocardium. If large phenytoin doses are given slowly, dose-related decreases in left ventricular force, rate of force development, and cardiac output can be observed, along with an increase in left ventricular end-diastolic pressure.

In human subjects, phenytoin doses of 2.5 to 5.4 mg/kg over a 3- to 5-min period failed to produce significant changes in cardiac output, systemic or pulmonary arterial pressures, or peripheral resistance (139).

TABLE 9. *Electrophysiologic properties of lidocaine and phenytoin*

Tissue	Effect of lidocaine	Effect of phenytoin
Sinus node	No change	No change
Atria		
Automaticity	Decrease	Decrease
Conduction velocity	No change	No change
Effective refractory period	No change	No change
A-V node		
Automaticity	Decrease	Decrease
Conduction velocity	No change	No change or increase
Effective refractory period	No change	No change or decrease
His-Purkinje/ventricular muscle		
Automaticity	Decrease	Decrease
Conduction velocity	No change	No change
Effective refractory period	Decrease	Decrease

Administration of phenytoin at a rate of 50 mg/min to patients with heart disease resulted in an increase in left ventricular end-diastolic pressure, in addition to a decrease in stroke work and stroke power. There was no significant change in either cardiac index or arterial pressure (140). Phenytoin appears to be superior to quinidine, procainamide, and disopyramide when one considers their hemodynamic effects.

Toxic Reactions

The major toxic effects of phenytoin manifest themselves on the circulatory, central nervous, and hematopoietic systems.

Intravenous phenytoin administration can present a hazard, and initial enthusiasm for its use as an antiarrhythmic agent was tempered by reports of serious cardiovascular toxicity. Respiratory arrest, arrhythmias, and hypotension have been reported with the use of intravenous phenytoin. In most cases, toxicity was due to rapid administration of phenytoin (in excess of 50 mg/min) (141,142).

Even though A-V block and bradycardia are associated occasionally with phenytoin administration (143), much of the rationale for using phenytoin in preference to other antiarrhythmic agents in the treatment of digitalis toxicity lies in the fact that phenytoin usually enhances rather than depresses A-V conduction (135). Depression of conduction is rare, but it is an important factor to be aware of when administering the drug.

It is important to recognize that the diluent supplied with phenytoin is not pharmacologically inert (144), and many of the adverse hemodynamic effects attributed to phenytoin may actually be due to the diluent, which has a pH of 11 and contains 40% propyleneglycol, 10% ethyl alcohol, and water. Because of the high pH of the solution, intravenous administration of phenytoin may cause local irritation of the vein at the site of injection. To prevent pain and irritation at the site of the injection, each dose of phenytoin should be followed with an injection of sterile saline to "flush" the vein.

The central nervous system manifestations of phenytoin toxicity can include giddiness, ataxia, tremors, nystagmus on far lateral gaze, diplopia, blurring of vision, slurring of speech, sedation, and ptosis. These symptoms can generally be related to plasma phenytoin levels in patients receiving long-term phenytoin therapy. The central nervous system side effects occur at plasma concentrations of 20 μg/ml or greater, generally at concentrations that are above the therapeutic range.

Hematologic manifestations of phenytoin

toxicity include anemia, pancytopenia, and reticuloendothelial disorders that regress when the drug is discontinued. The drug may also produce a megaloblastic anemia, which responds to folate therapy.

Pharmacokinetics

Absorption

Phenytoin is absorbed almost completely after an oral dose. First-pass liver metabolism does not limit oral bioavailability to an appreciable extent. Phenytoin is poorly and erratically absorbed after intramuscular injection and is not recommended for administration by this route. Peak plasma concentrations after a single oral dose occur approximately 12 hr after ingestion.

Metabolism and Excretion

Phenytoin is metabolized to 5-phenyl-t-parahydroxy-phenylhydantoin by hepatic microsomal enzymes. The metabolite is conjugated in the liver with glucuronic acid and excreted in the urine. Approximately 50% to 75% of a single phenytoin dose is excreted in the urine as the parahydroxy glucuronide metabolite. Several other metabolites have been recovered from urine. Less than 5% of a single dose appears unchanged in the urine.

Kinetics

The kinetics of phenytoin disappearance from plasma are nonlinear and follow Michaelis-Menten kinetics. The nonlinearity and Michaelis-Menten kinetics of phenytoin disposition may be explained by saturation of microsomal enzymes responsible for its metabolism. Most patients can metabolize 10 mg/kg/day by an essentially zero-order kinetic process. The pharmacokinetic parameters of phenytoin are summarized in Table 10.

Approximately 93% of plasma phenytoin concentrations are plasma-protein bound. Small decreases in plasma-protein binding may enhance the clinical effect or toxicity of phenytoin by increasing the free plasma concentration of phenytoin without altering its total plasma concentration. Salicylates, sulfonamides, phenylbutazone, and bilirubin all displace phenytoin from plasma proteins and increase free phenytoin concentrations. In uremic patients, two- to threefold increases in free (unbound) phenytoin concentrations can be observed even though total phenytoin plasma concentrations re-

---

TABLE 10. *Pharmacokinetic properties of phenytoin*

Absorption
  Slow and variable after oral administration
Protein binding
  Very high, >90%
Metabolism
  Hepatic, with inactive metabolites being formed; genetic factors will influence pattern of metabolism and the plasma half-life of the drug
Half-life
  Varies (8–60 hr) but is approximately 22 hr
Time to peak plasma concentration
  After oral administration, 1.5 to 3 hr
Therapeutic plasma concentration
  10 to 20 μg/ml; steady-state plasma concentrations may require 7 to 10 days of administration of a daily oral dose of 300 mg
Elimination
  Renal: primarily renal as inactive metabolites; also eliminated in feces and excreted in breast milk; <5% of the dose is eliminated unchanged

main in the "therapeutic" range. Plasma-protein binding is also reduced with some hepatocellular diseases. These conditions require reductions in phenytoin doses to maintain free plasma concentrations in the therapeutic range.

Considerable variation in phenytoin plasma concentrations can occur in patients receiving identical phenytoin doses. Part of this variation may be a result of marked differences in the rate of hepatic metabolism. Some patients have a genetic deficiency in the activity of microsomal enzymes responsible for phenytoin metabolism, whereas others metabolize phenytoin at rates much faster than the normal population. Hepatocellular disease decreases phenytoin clearance.

Therapy with other drugs may alter phenytoin elimination from plasma. Isoniazid interferes with microsomal metabolism of phenytoin, whereas drugs that stimulate microsomal metabolism (barbiturates, etc.) may increase phenytoin clearance. Phenytoin itself may stimulate its own metabolism, so that hepatic phenytoin clearance may increase with the duration of therapy. These factors make individualized therapy and monitoring of plasma phenytoin concentrations mandatory.

Three-fourths of responsive cardiac arrhythmias are abolished at phenytoin plasma concentrations of 10 to 18 µg/ml. Because of a nonlinear relationship between dose and steady-state plasma concentrations, maintenance of consistent plasma concentrations is difficult.

Oral Dose

To achieve plasma concentrations of 10 to 18 µg/ml within 24 hr, an initial loading dose of 1,000 mg must be given. The dose on the second day is 500 to 600 mg, with maintenance doses of 300 to 400 mg/day thereafter. On the average, a daily dose of 300 mg gives a plasma concentration of 10 µg/ml, and a dose of 500 mg doubles that to 20 µg/ml.

Intravenous Dose

Intravenous doses of 100 mg can be given every 5 min until the arrhythmia is abolished or until 1,000 mg have been given. Oral maintenance therapy should then be started. The plasma half-life is sufficiently long to obviate the needs for continuous maintenance infusions.

Contraindications

The contraindications to the use of phenytoin are similar to those for other antiarrhythmic drugs. Thus, the drug should not be used or should be used cautiously in patients with hypotension, severe bradycardia, high-grade A-V block, severe heart failure, and hypersensitivity to the drug. Caution should be exercised when using phenytoin in conjunction with other drugs that alter the metabolism of phenytoin.

Indications

Phenytoin, like lidocaine, has been found to be more effective for treatment of ventricular arrhythmias than supraventricular arrhythmias, and it has been most effective in treating ventricular arrhythmias associated with digitalis toxicity, acute myocardial infarction, open-heart surgery, anesthesia, cardiac catheterization, cardioversion, and angiographic studies.

Phenytoin finds its most effective use in the treatment of ventricular arrhythmias associated with digitalis intoxication. It is extremely effective for the treatment of both supraventricular and ventricular arrhythmias occurring as a result of cardiac glycosides. Phenytoin's ability to improve digitalis-depressed A-V conduction is a special feature and is in contrast to other antiarrhythmic agents.

The experience of most investigators has indicated that phenytoin is not effective in the conversion of atrial flutter or atrial fibrillation to sinus rhythm, nor is it effective in the treatment of other supraventricular arrhythmias not associated with digitalis toxicity. It should be appreciated that phenytoin, by virtue of its ability to enhance A-V conduction, may increase the ventricular rate in the presence of atrial flutter or atrial fibrillation.

An important application of phenytoin has been as a prophylactic agent to prevent postconversion arrhythmias, particularly in the digitalized patient. Phenytoin administered to the digitalis-sensitized animal has a tendency to increase the threshold for producing ventricular tachycardia.

Phenytoin has been shown to be ineffective in preventing sudden coronary death (ventricular fibrillation) in patients during prolonged therapy in the healing phase of myocardial infarction. For this reason, phenytoin is not a drug of choice for treatment of patients with complicated ventricular arrhythmias due to coronary artery disease.

Tocainide

Tocainide is an orally effective antiarrhythmic agent possessing structural and pharmacologic similarities to those of lidocaine. Tocainide is an amine analog of lidocaine, and as such, is effective when used by the oral route. Like lidocaine, tocainide is classified as belonging to the class IB group of antiarrhythmic agents. The drug is approved currently for use in the management of patients with ventricular arrhythmias, and its major attribute, aside from having an antiarrhythmic spectrum similar to that of lidocaine, is that it is effective when administered orally. The chemical structure for tocainide is shown in Fig. 13.

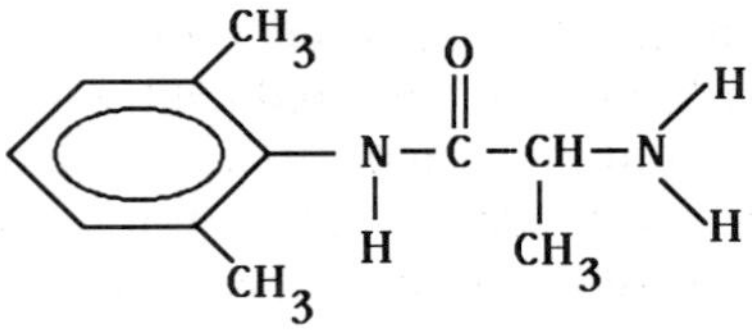

Electrophysiologic Actions

Tocainide, like lidocaine, produces a dose-dependent decrease in sodium and potassium ion conductance. The depression

FIG. 13. Tocainide.

of ion conductance is dose related and is more prominent on ischemically injured cells as compared with normal myocardial cells. The electrophysiologic actions of tocainide have been evaluated in healthy volunteers and in patients with cardiovascular disorders who had received the drug by the intravenous route at the time of cardiac catheterization. The cardiac electrophysiologic effects, after intravenous administration, are generally modest and of short duration. In normal volunteers, an intravenous dose of 450 mg given over a period of 45 min produced a slight depression in His-Purkinje conduction, as well as a delay in A-V conduction during atrial pacing. The administered dose did not alter heart rate, sinus node recovery time, His-bundle electrograms, right ventricular effective refractory period, or the excitation thresholds of atrial or ventricular muscle (145). Somewhat similar electrophysiologic effects were reported by Anderson et al. (146) who studied the drug in patients with cardiac pathology but reported that some patients exhibited decreases in atrial refractory period, A-V node, and right ventricle without affecting A-V conduction.

As with other class I agents, tocainide has membrane stabilizing effects and decreases the excitability of myocardial cells by reducing sodium conductance. Tocainide would be expected to decrease the rate of rise, phase 0, of the membrane action potential as recorded from ventricular muscle and Purkinje tissue. The effects of tocainide on the upstroke velocity of the action potential are influenced by the extracellular concentration of the potassium ion $[K^+]_o$.

At a low $[K^+]_o$ there is a minimal effect of the drug on the rapid inward current, whereas at a $[K^+]_o$ within the normal physiologic range, therapeutic concentrations of tocainide depresses V_{max} and the amplitude of the action potential, without an apparent change in the resting membrane potential (147). In superfused Purkinje fibers, tocainide decreased the action potential duration at 50% repolarization, but not at 100% repolarization and the effective refractory period was decreased slightly. The effects of the drug on these parameters tended to be in the opposite direction as concentrations in the bathing medium increased. The ventricular fibrillation threshold is increased in both normal and ischemic myocardial tissue. Automaticity within the sinus node and A-V conduction are unaltered by conventional doses of the drug and the electrocardiogram is essentially unchanged (148,149).

In studies with experimental animals made toxic with ouabain, tocainide abolished the induced ventricular arrhythmias. Similarly, tocainide showed a dose-related suppression of ventricular tachycardia and premature ectopic depolarizations in the postinfarcted heart when given parenterally or orally (150).

Hemodynamic and Cardiovascular Effects

Therapeutic plasma concentrations of tocainide, whether achieved by oral or intravenous administration of the drug, are not associated with any characteristic hemodynamic effects. Even in the presence of cardiac decompensation, tocainide is tolerated without undue concern for adverse cardiovascular effects (151). There are usually no changes in cardiac output or clinical evidence of increasing congestive heart failure in the well-compensated patient given tocainide. Depression of cardiac function is apparent, however, when tocainide is used in conjunction with a β-adrenoceptor blocking agent.

Toxic Reactions

Extended clinical studies have suggested that tocainide is tolerated well with relatively few adverse or toxic effects. Toxicity with tocainide most often involves the central nervous system and the gastrointestinal tract. Adverse effects were noted in 36% to 75% of patients given intravenous tocainide. Transient neurologic and gastrointestinal effects are the primary side effects noted most often and coincide with the peak rise in the plasma concentration with each dosing interval. These side effects often result in limiting the maximum dose that can be administered. Nausea, vomiting, dizziness, blurred vision, tremors, palpitations, paresthesias, anorexia, constipation, and confusion are the most commonly reported symptoms associated with the use of tocainide. It is apparent that the majority of the side effects can be minimized by preventing large rises in the plasma concentration with each dose. Appropriate measures would include giving the drug in divided doses and administering the drug with food. Other rare but severe manifestations of tocainide-induced toxicity that have been reported include convulsions, lupus-erythematosuslike illness, pulmonary fibrosis, and hematologic alterations among which the most alarming include leukopenia, agranulocytosis, hypoplastic anemia, and thrombocytopenia (151–153). The initial and most important signs of overdose with tocainide are related to the central nervous system. Convulsions, cardiopulmonary depression, or arrest should be managed by maintaining an airway and administering mechanical respirations along with supplemental oxygen. The continued development of seizure activity would suggest that agents such as benzodiazepine or an ultrashort-acting barbiturate be administered.

Agranulocytosis, bone marrow depression, leukopenia, neutropenia, hypoplastic anemia, thrombocytopenia, and sequelae such as septicemia and septic shock have been reported in patients receiving tocainide in recommended therapeutic dosages. Most of the adverse hematologic events occur within the first 12 weeks of therapy. It is recommended that physicians employ weekly blood studies during the first 3 months of therapy and periodically thereafter. Complete blood counts should be performed immediately if signs of infection, bruising, or bleeding become evident. The drug should be discontinued and appropriate measures instituted.

Pulmonary fibrosis, interstitial pneumonitis, fibrosing alveolitis, pulmonary edema, and pneumonia have been associated with tocainide therapy. The appearance of bilateral infiltrates on x-ray examination should lead the physician to consider alternative therapy. The development of exertional dyspnea, coughing, or wheezing should cause attention to be focused on the possible development of pulmonary involvement secondary to the use of tocainide.

Due to its tendency to facilitate rather than delay A-V transmission, tocainide may accelerate the ventricular rate in patients who have atrial flutter or atrial fibrillation.

Contraindications to the use of tocainide include patients who are hypersensitive to local anesthetics of the amide type. The presence of second- or third-degree heart block in the absence of an implanted pacemaker would constitute a contraindication to the use of the drug.

Pharmacokinetics

The pharmacokinetic properties of tocainide are summarized in Table 11. Tocainide is absorbed rapidly and fully after oral administration. The peak plasma concentration is achieved within 30 to 120 min and is delayed when the drug is administered with food. Unlike lidocaine, tocainide undergoes negligible first-pass hepatic metabolism. After oral administration, the bioavailability of tocainide is nearly 100% and is affected minimally by the presence of food. The drug is 10% bound to plasma protein. The average plasma half-life is 15 hr. The plasma concentration associated with the desired therapeutic effect is in the range of 4 to 10 μg/ml and can be obtained with an oral dosing regimen of 400 to 600 mg given every 8 hr (154). Approximately 40% of the administered dose is excreted unchanged in the urine, and there are no known cardioactive metabolites of the drug. Although the urinary excretion of tocainide

---

TABLE 11. *Pharmacokinetic properties of tocainide*

Absorption
  Bioavailability is close to 100% and is unaffected by food; tocainide crosses the blood-brain barrier
Protein binding
  Low, <10%
Metabolism
  Negligible first-pass hepatic metabolism; no cardioactive metabolites; approximately 60% of the administered dose is metabolized by hepatic mechanisms
Half-life
  Approximately 15 hr
Time to peak plasma concentration
  0.5 to 2 hr after oral administration
Therapeutic plasma concentration
  4 to 10 μg/ml
Elimination
  Renal: approximately 40% of the dose is eliminated unchanged and the percentage is reduced in the presence of an alkaline urine

is decreased by alkalinization of the urine, acidification of the urine has little effect on urinary excretion of the drug.

Dose

The dosage of tocainide must be individualized according to the patient's response in terms of controlling the arrhythmic activity of the heart and the development of side effects, both of which are dose related. Adverse effects that occur shortly after administration of the drug suggest the need to divide the dose and to decrease the interval between doses. Should arrhythmias appear during the period between doses, it would suggest that the dosing interval needs to be decreased.

The initial dose is 400 mg every 8 hr, or 1,200 to 1,400 mg/day in three divided doses. It is seldom necessary to exceed a dose of 2,400 mg/day.

Indications

Tocainide is indicated for the management of patients with life-threatening ventricular arrhythmias as well as patients with symptomatic ventricular arrhythmias. The drug is not indicated for the management of patients with tachyarrhythmias of supraventricular origin. Acceleration of the ventricular rate may occur when tocainide is administered in the presence of atrial flutter or fibrillation.

Recognition of the potential for tocainide to produce serious hematologic disorders, especially leukopenia or agranulocytosis, has led to the recommendation that the drug be reserved for patients in whom the benefits to be derived from the use of tocainide are believed to outweigh the risks associated with the use of the drug.

Tocainide has not been demonstrated to prevent sudden death in patients considered to be at high risk for the development of lethal arrhythmias. Like many other antiarrhythmic agents, tocainide is associated with the development of potentially serious side effects that include the potential to be proarrhythmic. It is necessary, therefore, that each patient who is to receive tocainide, be evaluated electrocardiographically and clinically before and during the period of treatment with the drug in order to detect a possible worsening in the status of the cardiac rhythm.

Mexiletine

Mexiletine (1-(2′, 6′-dimethylphenoxy)-2-aminopropane) (Fig. 14) is a primary amine, with local anesthetic activity. The drug originally was intended for use as an anticonvulsant agent but was noted to possess antiarrhythmic properties and has been used clinically for this purpose since 1969. Mexiletine is classified as a class IB antiarrhythmic agent that has pharmacologic properties and antidysrhythmic effects similar to those of lidocaine and tocainide.

Electrophysiologic Actions

Consistent with what is known about other members of the class IB group of antiarrhythmic agents, mexiletine slows the maximal rate of depolarization of the cardiac membrane action potential and has negligible effects on repolarization. These actions resemble those of lidocaine. Mexi-

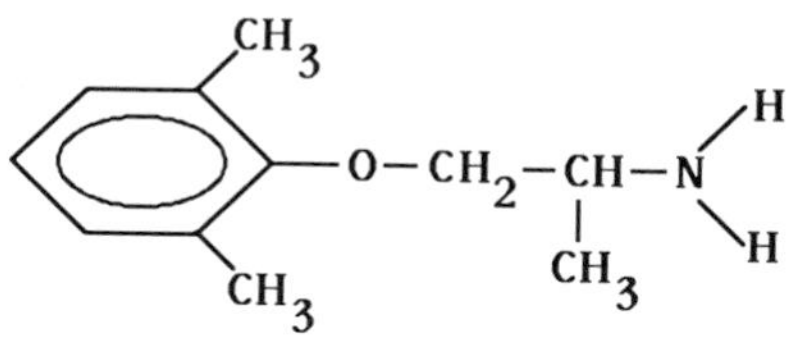

FIG. 14. Mexiletine.

letine has no effect on the resting potential of atrial, ventricular, and Purkinje fibers even when studied over a wide range of concentrations. The decrease in the up-stroke velocity of phase 0 of the membrane potential is associated with a decrease in the conduction velocity of premature impulses.

Sinoatrial Node

Mexiletine does not modify the influence of the autonomic nervous system on pace-maker activity in the heart and thus would not exert an indirect effect on spontaneous depolarization. On systemic administration, mexiletine does not have a consistent effect on sinus rate or sinus node recovery time, an observation that is in agreement with the *in vitro* effects of the drug when studied on spontaneous diastolic depolarization in iso-lated atrial preparations (155,156). Sinus node recovery times may be prolonged in patients with preexisting disease.

Atria

Like lidocaine, mexiletine has no effect on the atrial action-potential duration or the atrial refractory period (155,156). Accordingly, mexiletine is known to be without benefit in the management of patients with atrial flutter or fibrillation.

A-V Node

Mexiletine does not appear to alter the electrophysiologic properties of the A-V node in normal individuals. However, increases in A-V conduction time may be noted in patients in whom A-V nodal function may be impaired (157). Reported instances of adverse alterations in A-V conduction are rare in the case of mexiletine. Complete heart block has been reported to be associated with an overdose of mexiletine, accompanied by a very slow escape idioventricular rhythm, which ended in asystole and a failure of the ventricle to respond to electrical pacing (158).

His-Purkinje System/Ventricular Muscle

Mexiletine has little effect on His-ventricular conduction time in normal subjects but may delay conduction in the presence of cardiac disease. In Purkinje fibers, mexiletine decreases the duration of the action potential similar to the response observed to occur with lidocaine. Spontaneous dia-stolic depolarization in Purkinje fibers is suppressed at normal levels of membrane potential. Similarly, automaticity induced by digitalis at low levels of membrane potential, as well as triggered activity caused by delayed afterdepolarizations, are suppressed by mexiletine (159). Recordings from the His bundle indicate that mexiletine is without important effects as the electrogram remains unchanged. Mexiletine increases the relative and effective refractory periods of the His-Purkinje system in humans, an effect that may become more pronounced in the presence of disease leading to conduction disturbances (157,160). The electrophysiological observations in humans do not agree entirely with those made *in vitro* on canine cardiac Purkinje fibers in which V_{max} of phase 0 is reduced in conjunction with a reduction in the action-potential duration and in the effective refractory period (161). In concentrations between 1 and 5 μg/ml, mexiletine decreases V_{max} of phase 0 of the action potential resulting in an increase in the threshold of excitability, decreases conduction velocity, and prolongs the effective refractory period with little effect on the resting membrane potential (155,156,159,161,162). The decrease in the duration of the action potential in Purkinje fibers appears to be of a greater magnitude than the associated decrease in the effective refractory period. Therefore, the ratio of the effective refractory period to the action-potential duration increases under the influence of mexiletine.

In ischemic myocardium, mexiletine produces an increase in the effective refractory period, an action that is in keeping with the observation that the drug has a greater affinity for binding to sodium channels in tissue that is partially depolarized (163,164). Clinically, mexiletine does not result in a prolongation of the QRS duration, which corresponds with its relative lack of effect on ventricular muscle conduction velocity when studied *in vivo*. Mexiletine displays a rate-dependent blocking action on the sodium channel that has a rapid onset and recovery (165), suggesting that the drug may be of greater efficacy in the control of rapid as opposed to slow ventricular tachyarrhythmias. The effect is in agreement with the clinical findings that lidocaine and related members of class IB drugs selectively depress early diastolic extrasystoles in contrast to class IA fast channel blockers such as quinidine, which suppress extrasystoles in all coupling intervals. Mexiletine does not appear to affect the slow inward calcium current.

Hemodynamic Effects

The clinical use of oral mexiletine has been remarkably free of reports relating to adverse hemodynamic effects of the drug. In clinical studies, no cardiovascular toxicity was noted, or if it did occur, it was considered to be of minimal consequence (166–168). Patients with impaired ventricular contractility who were receiving oral mexiletine did not display further deterioration in their cardiovascular status as determined with radionuclide estimates of ventricular function (169).

Toxic Reactions

The most frequent unwanted effects associated with the use of mexiletine are related to the gastrointestinal tract and to the nervous system. Nausea, dyspepsia, and vomiting are the most often mentioned gastrointestinal side effects and can be reduced by administration of the drug with food. The central nervous system effects of mexiletine include dizziness, tremor, blurred vision, lightheadedness, ataxia, slurred speech, memory loss, insomnia, alterations in personality, and, on rare occasions, seizures. The central nervous system side effects are related to high plasma concentrations of the drug and can be minimized by giving the drug in smaller doses at more frequent intervals so as to avoid wide swings in the plasma concentration with the administration of each dose.

Cardiovascular toxicity is rarely observed with conventional doses of mexiletine, although exacerbation of existing arrhythmias has been reported.

Other side effects associated with the use of mexiletine are asymptomatic increases in the antinuclear antibody titer, cutaneous rash, and abnormalities in hepatic function.

Most of the side effects related to the use of mexiletine occur during the initial period of administration. Because the drug has a large volume of distribution, in excess of 500 liters, and a long plasma half-life, achieving a steady state may require several days or relatively large initial intravenous dosages. Thus, the side effects on initiation of therapy often are related to the period when blood and tissue concentrations fluctuate before reaching equilibrium, especially when the intravenous route is used.

The first signs of toxicity are manifest by a fine tremor of the hands, followed by dizziness, and blurred vision. Hypotension, sinus bradycardia, and widening of the QRS complex have been noted as the most common unwanted cardiovascular effects. The side effects are less common with long-term oral maintenance. Reducing or delaying the next dose usually reduces the severity of the undesirable side effects. The oral dosing regimen for mexiletine has been with dosages of 200 to 300 mg every 8 hr. It is estimated that 12 mg/kg/day in divided doses will be adequate to maintain therapeutic plasma concentrations.

Pharmacokinetics

The pharmacokinetic properties of mexiletine are summarized in Table 12. Like tocainide, mexiletine is effective by oral administration, being almost completely absorbed, with peak plasma concentrations being achieved within 2 to 4 hr. The majority of the administered dose is absorbed from the upper portion of the small intestine due to the basic nature of the drug. Absorption of mexiletine will be slowed under circumstances in which gastric emptying is delayed. This becomes especially noticeable in patients with acute myocardial infarction in whom there is a lag time of almost 5 hr between the time of the administered dose and the attainment of a peak plasma concentration. Mexiletine undergoes less than 10% first-pass hepatic metabolism. Because absorption is relatively complete along with the minimal first-pass hepatic metabolism, the bioavailability of mexiletine is approximately 90%.

The volume of distribution for mexiletine is large and variable, thereby suggesting that tissue uptake of the drug is extensive (170). Mexiletine undergoes hepatic metabolism, and the fraction eliminated via the kidneys is influenced by the urinary pH.

Acidification of the urine (pH 5.0) results in a plasma elimination half-life of 2.8 hr, with approximately 50% of the administered dose appearing in the urine in 48 hr. In the presence of an alkaline (pH 8.0) urine, the half-life is increased to 8.6 hr, with a negligible fraction of the dose appearing in the urine. None of the metabolites of mexiletine is known to have antiarrhythmic properties.

Therapeutic plasma concentrations of mexiletine are in the narrow range of 1 to 2 μg/ml. Thus, the drug has a limited toxic-therapeutic ratio. The unwanted side effects associated with the use of mexiletine are related to excessive plasma concentrations of the drug. The use of single oral doses of 400 to 600 mg of mexiletine, although effective in achieving a therapeutic plasma concentration within a short period after administration, it imposes the risk of increasing toxic manifestations. The daily dose of 750 mg of mexiletine needed to maintain a therapeutic plasma concentration should be divided into multiple doses so as to minimize the wide swings in the plasma concentration associated with large single oral doses. A therapeutic response can be maintained with doses of 200 to 300 mg every 6 to 8 hr. Daily doses range be-

---

TABLE 12. *Pharmacokinetic properties of mexiletine*

Absorption
  Well absorbed to the extent of 90% and shows little first-pass hepatic metabolism
Protein binding
  60% to 70% to plasma protein
Metabolism
  Hepatic metabolism with several metabolites being formed; one metabolite, *N*-methylmexiletine, shows some antiarrhythmic activity; approximately 85% of the administered dose is metabolized to inactive metabolites
Half-life
  10 to 12 hr in individuals with normal renal and hepatic function; half-life is increased to 25 hr in the presence of heart failure, hepatic dysfunction, and impairment of renal function (15–25 hr)
Time to peak plasma concentration
  2 to 3 hr
Therapeutic plasma concentration
  0.5 to 2.0 μg/ml with central nervous system toxicity becoming prominent at plasma concentrations >2.0 μg/ml
Elimination
  Renal: approximately 10% of the administered dose is eliminated unchanged and excretion is enhanced in acid urine and decreased in alkaline urine; breast milk: excretion occurs in a concentration equal to that of plasma; biliary: some of the administered dose is excreted into the bile

tween 600 and 1,000 mg. The plasma half-life is estimated at 12 hr, although in patients with myocardial infarction, the mean half-life was found to be 16.7 hr, probably because of reduced hepatic blood flow, which would impair drug metabolism.

In a number of clinical trials, mexiletine has been reported to be effective in the management of patients with acute and/or chronic ventricular arrhythmias. Initial reports suggest that plasma concentrations between 0.75 and 2.0 μg/ml are effective in the control of dysrhythmias, although mild toxicity has been observed with plasma concentrations of 0.83 to 3.0 μg/ml, and severe toxicity has occurred within the range of 1.0 to 4.4 μg/ml (171).

Dose

Oral mexiletine is employed for the suppression of ventricular arrhythmias. The dose for oral administration is 200 to 400 mg, three times a day. An initial dose of 100 or 200 mg, three times a day, can be increased or decreased by 50 to 100 mg, at intervals of at least 2 to 3 days. An initial dose of 400 mg of mexiletine given to normal volunteers produced dizziness and disorientation within 1 to 2 hr after administration even though plasma concentrations were below 1.6 μg/ml. Severe side effects occur with plasma concentrations in excess of 2 μg/ml.

Indications

Mexiletine is considered to be useful as an antiarrhythmic agent against ventricular arrhythmias with a wide variety of cardiac diseases. Its oral efficacy and low incidence of serious side effects suggest that the drug should find patient acceptance. The drug has been used in the treatment of ventricular arrhythmias associated with diverse cardiac abnormalities. The efficacy of orally administered mexiletine has been studied in the chronic treatment of patients with ven-

tricular arrhythmias secondary to acute myocardial infarction or ischemic heart disease or no apparent cardiac disease (172).

In a large series of patients with recent myocardial infarction, mexiletine was administered to reduce the frequency of "malignant" ventricular arrhythmias (i.e., ventricular premature complexes in excess of five per minute; multiform or R-on-T rhythm), ventricular tachycardia, or recurrent ventricular fibrillation. Thirty-two of the patients had persistent ST-segment elevation and were considered to be at risk for developing ventricular fibrillation. Even though mexiletine reduced the frequency of premature ventricular depolarizations, it did not prevent the recurrence of ventricular tachycardia and/or ventricular fibrillation. Whereas mexiletine may prove useful in those patients who appear to be refractory to lidocaine, its potential as an agent for long-term management of patients with electrical instability of the myocardium secondary to ischemia and for the prevention of lethal arrhythmias has not been demonstrated. The data to date do not permit the conclusion that oral administration of mexiletine will reduce the incidence of sudden coronary death in patients who survive acute myocardial infarction.

Contraindications

The main contraindications to the use of mexiletine are severe left ventricular failure, cardiogenic shock, and other conditions in which cardiac decompensation is present. Because the depressant electrophysiologic effects of the drug are more pronounced in patients with sick sinus syndrome, unstable A-V block, and severe bradycardia, these conditions are contraindications to the use of mexiletine.

Encainide

The pharmacokinetic properties of encainide are summarized in Table 13. En-

TABLE 13. *Pharmacokinetic properties of encainide*

Absorption
   Nearly complete; absorption prolonged in the presence of food without alteration in the bioavailability
Protein binding
   Encainide and ODE are highly bound, 75% to 80%; MODE is bound to an extent of 92%
Metabolism
   Metabolized by hepatic mechanisms; most patients (90%) metabolize the drug rapidly and extensively,
     forming two active metabolites, ODE and MODE; the remaining 10% of the population metabolized
     encainide slowly with the formation of little if any MODE or ODE
Half-life
   In fast metabolizers, encainide: 1 to 2 hr, ODE: 3 to 4 hr, MODE: 6 to 12 hr; in slow metabolizers,
     encainide: 6 to 12 hr
Time to peak plasma concentration
   30 to 90 min
Time to achieve steady-state plasma concentration
   After multiple dosing over 3 to 5 days
Therapeutic plasma concentration
   Difficult to determine due to the formation of active metabolites, which differ among individuals
     depending on patterns of metabolism
Elimination
   Renal and fecal routes of elimination with slow metabolizers showing predominantly renal elimination of
     the unchanged drug

cainide (Fig. 15) is a benzanilide derivative possessing local anesthetic activity. The development of encainide derived from an attempt to synthesize analogs of lysergic acid that had antiarrhythmic activity. The compound that emerged from the effort was MJ 9067, or encainide. Structurally, encainide resembles procainamide but has remarkably different electrophysiologic actions on the heart. Due to its efficacy as a blocker of the sodium channel, encainide is a member of the class IC group of antiarrhythmic agents. Encainide dissociates slowly from the sodium channel receptors and promotes marked changes in intracardiac conduction with minimal effects on repolarization. The efficacy of encainide as an antiarrhythmic agent is associated with prolongation of normal intracardiac conduction giving rise to the potential for proarrhythmic effects. An interesting feature of encainide is that the parent compound undergoes hepatic metabolism to give rise to two active metabolites, O-demethylencainide (ODE) and 3-methoxy-O-demethyl encainide (MODE), both being more active than encainide on a per-milligram basis. Encainide has a short half-life of 3 hr, but its two active metabolites have longer durations of action. The use of encainide is associated with minimal side effects, which are dose related. The drug has been used in the treatment of patients with symptomatic ventricular arrhythmias as well as in the management of patients with supraventricular tachyarrhythmias.

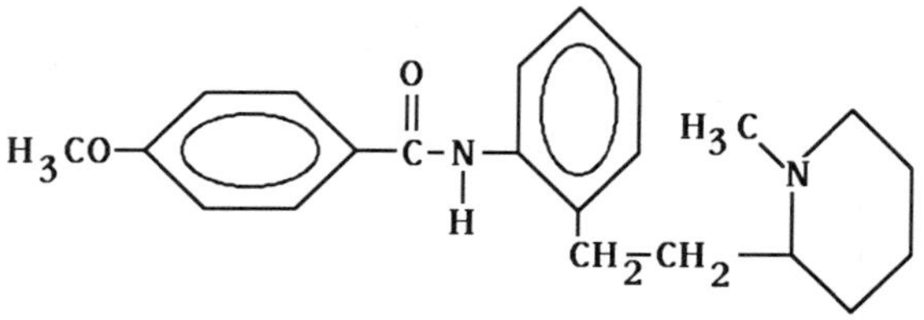

FIG. 15. Encainide.

Electrophysiologic Actions

Encainide is a class IC agent possessing a broad spectrum of antiarrhythmic actions in animals as well as in humans. Encainide increases the ventricular fibrillation threshold in the perfused rabbit heart and in the *in situ* canine heart. The drug suppresses experimentally induced atrial fibrillation in the anesthetized dog and ventricular fibrillation induced by chloroform asphyxiation in the mouse and is said to be 7 to 18 times more effective on a per-milligram basis than quinidine. The major metabolites ODE and MODE have been shown to have quantitatively different, but qualitatively similar, profiles of pharmacodynamic effects (173).

Sinoatrial Node

When administered by the intravenous route, encainide has no effect on the sinoatrial node and thus does not alter the heart rate. The oral administration of encainide and the associated appearance of ODE and MODE do not appear to affect the electrophysiologic properties of the sinoatrial node.

Atria

Encainide has no effect on the resting membrane potential of atrial fibers but depresses the rate of rise of the action potential. Encainide given intravenously has no influence on the effective refractory period of atrial muscle. In contrast, the oral administration of encainide for 3 to 5 days results in a prolongation of the atrial refractory period, suggesting an important electrophysiologic action attributable to ODE and MODE.

A-V Node

Intravenous administration of encainide has no effect on the A-V node. In contrast, oral therapy for more than 3 days results in a slowing in A-V conduction. The AH interval is prolonged as is the HV interval. Similar electrophysiologic responses could be obtained with the intravenous administration of ODE (174).

His-Purkinje System

When studied *in vitro*, encainide produces a direct depressant effect on Purkinje fibers resulting in a reduction of both the amplitude of the action potential and the maximum upstroke velocity of phase 0 of the action potential. The duration of the action potential is decreased with little effect on the refractory period (175). ODE was found to be more potent than the parent compound in decreasing the maximum upstroke velocity in both canine Purkinje fibers and ventricular muscle (176).

When studied *in vivo*, the acute effect of encainide given as an intravenous infusion results in a prolongation of the His-Purkinje conduction time (HV interval). Other measured parameters, such as the sinus node recovery time, A-V nodal conduction, QT interval and refractoriness of the atria, A-V node, and ventricle, were unaltered (177). ODE and MODE were found to be more potent than the parent compound in prolonging the HV interval (178).

Ventricular Muscle

Consistent with the findings in other tissues of the heart, the parent compound, encainide, differs from its active metabolites when examined in ventricular muscle. Encainide has no effect on the ventricular effective refractory period, but conduction velocity is depressed as is the upstroke of the membrane action potential. After 3 to 5 days of oral therapy, the ventricular effective refractory period is prolonged as is that of accessory tracts of the heart, once again suggesting the role of the active metabolites of encainide as being more effective in altering the electrophysiologic properties of the heart (179).

Electrocardiographic Changes

The effects of intravenous encainide, as reflected on the electrocardiogram, differ markedly from the changes observed to occur after oral dosing for 3 to 5 days. Intravenous dosing with encainide results in a prolongation of the HV interval and in the duration of the QRS complex. The AH interval and the ventricular refractory period are unchanged (177). Oral administration for several days was associated with increases in each of these parameters (179).

An interesting feature of encainide is the dose-dependent increase in the duration of the QRS complex, a change associated with therapeutic plasma concentrations of the drug. Under conditions in which extensive metabolism of encainide occurs with the production of ODE, there is a good correlation between arrhythmia suppression and the prolongation of the QRS duration. Prolongation of the QRS is most likely a result of the inhibition of the fast inward sodium channel by encainide and/or ODE and MODE. Inhibition of the fast inward sodium current is associated with a decrease in conduction velocity in ventricular myocardium. MODE may be more active an inhibitor of the fast inward current and, like ODE, possesses antiarrhythmic activity and is associated with QRS prolongation. MODE may be associated with variable effects on the QT interval (180). Whereas both metabolites prolong the ventricular refractory period, MODE may be more potent (174). An abnormal metabolism of encainide may be the underlying mechanism by which some patients would manifest an unusual prolongation of the QT interval without prolongation of the QRS during therapy with encainide (181).

Hemodynamic Effects

Assessment of cardiac function using radionuclide ejection fraction studies in patients who were undergoing treatment for the suppression of ventricular ectopic activity did not reveal any deleterious effects during rest or exercise in the absence or the presence of preexisting ventricular impairment (182). The drug was reported to have no detrimental effects on cardiac function in a group of patients with complex ventricular ectopy and depressed ejection fraction (183). The hemodynamic effects of oral encainide are insignificant in patients with well-preserved left ventricular function. Despite minimal myocardial depression in patients with left ventricular dysfunction, there is the potential for worsening of heart failure. Although few in number, there have been reports of a worsening of cardiac function in patients with varying degrees of cardiac decompensation who were treated with encainide (182,184). An additional consideration is the recognition that patients with left ventricular impairment may be at greater risk for the development of proarrhythmic effects of encainide.

Toxic Reactions

The side effects associated with the use of encainide are dose related and involve the central nervous system or effects on the gastrointestinal tract. The profile of drug-related adverse effects in a study of 349 patients (185) consisted of visual disturbances, dizziness, headaches, nausea, and vertigo. A large data base of 1,245 patients given encainide for the suppression of ventricular arrhythmias demonstrated an overall incidence of proarrhythmia that averaged 9.2%, but was as frequent as 16% in patients with cardiomyopathy. Proarrhythmia manifests itself as sustained ventricular tachycardia in 1.8% of patients. The incidence of proarrhythmic effects has decreased over the past years as reduced doses and gradual titration of the dose have been employed. High initial doses, previous myocardial infarction, and heart failure contribute to the possibility of sudden death being associated with the use of encainide. Death rate was also related to the severity of the arrhythmia being treated (184).

Pharmacokinetics

The pharmacokinetic properties of encainide are summarized in Table 13. The pharmacokinetics of encainide must take into consideration the presence of at least two genetic phenotypes that have distinctly different capacities to metabolize the drug. One phenotype, representing more than 90% of patients, is characterized by extensive metabolism of the parent compound in which active metabolites are formed. Under such conditions the effect of first-pass metabolism decreases the systemic bioavailability of encainide to 14% to 38%. The elimination half-life of the parent drug may range from 30 min to 4 hr. The wide range of clearances accounts for the unpredictable and marked range of plasma concentrations. Peak plasma concentrations of encainide are achieved within 1.5 hr after oral administration and those of ODE and MODE are obtained at 1.4 and 5.7 hr, respectively. Under steady-state conditions (3–5 days of oral dosing), the encainide metabolite ratio is 1:5; with the mean plasma concentration of encainide being 55 ng/liter, whereas that of ODE is 215 ng/liter and that of MODE 185 ng/liter. Extensive tissue binding occurs as reflected by the large volume of distribution for encainide, which approximates 270 liters. There is good reason to suspect that the antiarrhythmic efficacy of encainide may be enhanced by its metabolites (174,186,187). On discontinuation of the encainide, the antidysrhythmic effects persist longer than the presence of encain-

ide in the plasma, thus there is no apparent relationship between blood concentrations of encainide and its metabolites and efficacy due to the complexity of the three active compounds (188).

Approximately 7% of the population possesses the autosomal recessive trait of poor metabolism of encainide. Individuals who have a low capacity to metabolize the drug show a systemic bioavailability of encainide that ranges from 83% to 88%. Elimination is slower in this group of subjects as opposed to those who have a greater capacity to metabolize the drug. The half-life for encainide in the slow metabolizers ranges from 8 to 22 hr. Renal excretion of encainide is the major route of elimination in the slow metabolizers, and little if any MODE and only small amounts of ODE are present in the plasma of these patients.

Metabolism and Excretion

The metabolic conversion of encainide is a function of genetic polymorphism. The majority of subjects are considered to be "extensive metabolizers" in whom encainide undergoes a major first-pass hepatic metabolism to the active metabolites ODE and MODE. The plasma concentrations of these metabolites are higher than those of the parent compound, and the pharmacologic effects correlate better with the plasma metabolite concentrations than they do with those of encainide itself (189,190). The remaining individuals who make up approximately 7% of the patient population are "poor metabolizers" in whom the first-pass hepatic metabolism of the drug does not take place. These individuals show low to undetectable concentration of the two major metabolites. In such individuals the effects of encainide therapy correlate with plasma concentrations of the parent drug. Although "poor" and "extensive" metabolizers show markedly different patterns in the disposition of encainide, the dosages that produce pharmacologic effects as determined by QRS prolongation and arrhythmia suppression, are similar in both groups (189). In the presence of hepatic disease, the biotransformation of encainide would be impaired; however, no major dosage changes are required. The presence of renal disease delays the excretion of encainide and its metabolites, and starting dosages should be decreased under such conditions. Steady-state concentrations of ODE and MODE in the extensive metabolizers and of encainide itself in the poor metabolizers is achieved in 3 to 5 days in both groups. The adjustment in dosage, therefore, should be made no more frequently than every 3 to 5 days.

Oral Dose

The initial oral dose of encainide in patients with normal renal function should be 25 mg given every 8 hr. Upward adjustments of the dose may be made by increasing the dose to 35 mg and then to 50 mg every 8 hr, every 3 or more days. The lowest dose consistent with the suppression of cardiac arrhythmia should be used because the potential proarrhythmic effect of encainide increases with the dose (191,192). Rapid increases in the dose and doses in excess of 200 mg/day are discouraged. Side effects are relatively few when the daily dose is less than 150 mg/day.

The effective antiarrhythmic dose of encainide does not differ between those who metabolize the drug to its active metabolites versus patients who are poor metabolizers of the drug. Monitoring of the plasma concentration of encainide or its metabolites has not been found to be a useful guide in adjusting the oral dose of the drug, due to the wide differences to be found among patients with respect to the concentration of encainide in the blood and the variability in the antiarrhythmic actions of the metabolites. Plasma concentrations of encainide reach steady state within 3 days in patients

who are extensive metabolizers of encainide, but the plasma concentration of the active metabolites continues to increase. Therefore, the determination of the plasma concentration of encainide in the early course of treatment will have little meaning as an index of having achieved a therapeutic concentration. It is best to allow a 3-day interval between increments in the drug dose so as to permit the attainment of steady-state plasma concentrations of the parent compound before increasing the dose of encainide.

In a review (193) of several well-controlled studies involving 331 patients, encainide produced a dose-related decrease in the absolute number of ventricular arrhythmias as well as an increase in the percentage of responders (greater than 75% decrease in arrhythmia frequency). A dose of 75 mg/day was needed to obtain at least a 50% reduction in ventricular arrhythmias, or 50% of patients responding, or both. Doses in excess of 200 mg/day gave little or no increase in apparent efficacy.

Contraindications

Relative contraindications to the use of encainide would relate to patients with prolongation of the QRS complex in whom the risk of exacerbation of proarrhythmic effects would be enhanced. Treatment of such patients, if no other alternative exists, should be carried out under supervision and with monitoring. Encainide should not be given to patients with preexisting disorders of ventricular conduction or disturbances in A-V conduction unless a pacemaker is in place.

Animal studies have suggested that the presence of high concentrations of the active metabolite ODE, as well as encainide, makes electrical defibrillation of the ventricle more difficult. Similar difficulty has been experienced clinically. The mechanisms for this response to encainide is not understood, and it might constitute a contraindication to the use of the drug in patients with implanted automatic cardiac defibrillators, which may be rendered useless in the presence of the drug.

Indications

Encainide has been used most often in the management of patients with ventricular arrhythmias. Almost complete suppression of both ventricular ectopic depolarizations and repetitive periods of nonsustained ventricular tachycardia could be achieved with encainide in a number of studies (182,184,194,195). Although earlier studies with encainide overlooked the significance of active metabolites being formed with prolonged administration of the drug, subsequent trials with lower doses of encainide substantiated earlier findings with respect to the efficacy of the drug in ventricular arrhythmias (196,197). Encainide in a dose of 100 to 200 mg/day given in two to four divided doses is effective in suppressing 75% to 100% of chronic nonsustained ventricular arrhythmias in 88% of patients, a degree of efficacy exceeding that observed with quinidine.

In patients with recurrent episodes of life-threatening arrhythmias or refractory tachyarrhythmias, encainide has proved effective in reducing the incidence of such events (198–200). Despite these encouraging results it must be noted that in some patients, encainide administration is associated with proarrhythmic events, easier induction of ventricular tachycardia in response to programmed electrical stimulation, and facilitation of exercise-induced ventricular tachycardia or ventricular fibrillation (201). In contrast to its effectiveness in controlling frequent, but nonlife-threatening ventricular arrhythmias, encainide has proved less reliable in the management of patients with recurrent life-threatening ventricular tachyarrhythmias.

A number of studies have examined the use of encainide in the management of patients with supraventricular arrhythmias

(202–206). There is evidence to suggest that the drug has beneficial effects in some patients, especially those with preexcitation and rapid ventricular responses in the presence of atrial fibrillation. This observation is in concert with the ability of the drug to markedly prolong the anterograde and retrograde refractory periods of the accessory bypass tracts.

Flecainide

Flecainide, N-(2-piperidylmethyl)-2,5-*bis* (2,2,2-trifluoroethoxy)benzamide monoacetate (Fig. 16), a fluorobenzamide derivative of procainamide, represents a relatively new addition to the group of class IC antiarrhythmic drugs and possesses many of the same electrophysiologic properties of encainide. Flecainide has a wide range of electrophysiologic and antiarrhythmic actions and may be of considerable clinical importance as a drug with a broad spectrum of activity in the management of patients with cardiac rhythm disorders of supraventricular and/or ventricular origin. The drug is generally reserved for those patients who display more serious and life-threatening ventricular arrhythmias. Flecainide is absorbed rapidly and completely from the gastrointestinal tract and has a 13-hr half-life. Flecainide is tolerated with minimal side effects, which most often involve the central nervous system.

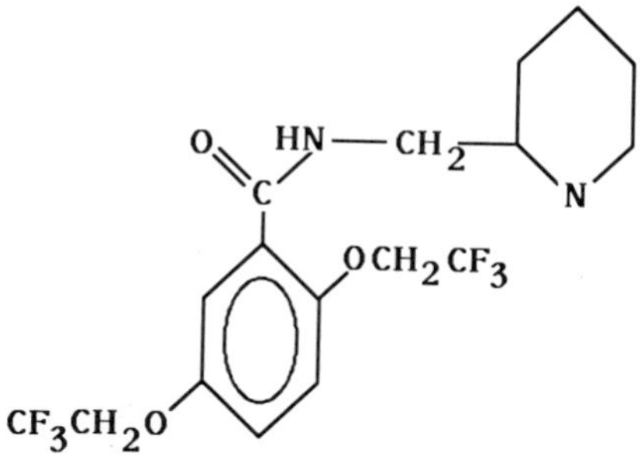

FIG. 16. Flecainide.

Electrophysiologic Actions

The electrophysiologic effects of flecainide have been studied in detail (207,208). The most significant electrophysiologic alteration on mammalian cardiac tissue is the dose-dependent decrease in the maximum velocity of membrane depolarization. The action is consistent with the inhibition of the fast inward sodium current (209). Examination of flecainide on the intact mammalian heart indicates that the drug slows impulse conduction throughout the myocardium, with the major effects being manifest in the distal regions of the His-Purkinje system and in the ventricular myocardium. Flecainide has a greater effect on conduction than on repolarization and only slight effects on hemodynamic parameters.

Sinoatrial Node

The effect of flecainide on the sinoatrial node, as would be expected with all class I antiarrhythmic agents, is best observed under conditions in which a disorder of sinus node function exists. In the absence of sinus node dysfunction, flecainide is without effect on the electrophysiology of the sinoatrial node. The derived variable such as sinoatrial conduction time and sinus node recovery time may be prolonged. Thus, patients with disorders of sinoatrial nodal function may develop prolonged pauses in sinoatrial node activity and sustained bradycardias (210). These effects would be common to all members of the class I antiarrhythmic agents.

Atria

Flecainide prolongs conduction within the atria when the drug is administered intravenously. The effects on atrial refractoriness are inconsistent and may suggest that prolongation of this parameter is to be expected. The oral administration of flecainide fails to produce consistent effects on the electrophysiologic properties of atrial muscle with the tendency being one of prolongation of the atrial refractory period (210–212).

A-V Node

The electrophysiologic properties of the normal A-V node are not affected by flecainide. In patients with dual A-V nodal pathways, the effective and functional refractory periods of the fast and slow pathways are not influenced by flecainide. However, when examined with respect to the anterograde and retrograde conduction within the A-V node, it is noted that flecainide produces a marked prolongation in retrograde refractoriness thereby causing retrograde block (211). It is presumed that the delay in retrograde conduction occurs in the His-Purkinje system.

In the presence of anomalous pathways, flecainide slows the conduction velocity in the retrograde direction as evidenced by the prolongation of ventriculoatrial conduction time (211,213,214). Total block of retrograde conduction is more likely to occur as opposed to blockade in the anterograde direction. The increase in the anterograde refractoriness is an important component in the slowing of the ventricular rate response during atrial fibrillation in patients with the preexcitation syndrome (215).

His-Purkinje System

Flecainide produces a major alteration in conduction within the His-Purkinje system and is associated with a dose-dependent increase in the H-V interval. Studies with the use of intracellular recordings (208) demonstrate that the maximum rate of rise of the action potential is reduced as is the amplitude of the action potential. The decrease in the V_{max} is rate dependent. The effective refractory period of Purkinje tissue is decreased at the lower concentrations of flecainide and returns toward control values with increasing concentrations of the drug. The duration of the action potential in Purkinje tissue is shortened in the presence of flecainide. Flecainide slows the rate of automaticity induced in Purkinje fibers by exposure to isoproterenol.

Ventricular Muscle

A prominent feature associated with flecainide is a marked slowing of conduction velocity within ventricular myocardial tissue. Both ventricular refractoriness and repolarization times have been reported to be prolonged by flecainide. Using standard microelectrode methods of study, flecainide was shown to produce a concentration-dependent decrease in V_{max}, action-potential amplitude, and overshoot potential with an increase in the effective refractory period in ventricular muscle. The effect on ventricular refractoriness is opposite to what is observed to occur in Purkinje tissue. The data suggest that the electrophysiologic effects of flecainide as determined in isolated cardiac muscle are complex, with depression being prominent on V_{max} and variable effects being produced on refractoriness in the different tissue types of the ventricle. It is possible that the differential effects of the drug on the action potential duration and refractoriness of ventricular muscle and Purkinje fibers may contribute to the arrhythmogenic potential of flecainide.

Electrocardiographic Changes

Flecainide slows cardiac conduction in a dose-related manner, thereby increasing PR, QRS, and QT intervals. The PR interval may increase to the point of new first-degree A-V block in approximately one-third of patients. The QRS complex increases on the average of 25% and as much as 150% in some patients, an action that is in keeping with the ability of the drug to depress conduction velocity in ventricular myocardium. It is not unusual to observe

QRS durations of 0.12 sec or more. It is important to note that the degree of lengthening of the PR and QRS intervals does not coincide with either the efficacy or the adverse cardiac effects of flecainide. The lowest possible dose of flecainide consistent with antiarrhythmic efficacy should be employed so as to reduce the effects on conduction within the various regions of the heart.

Flecainide increases endocardial pacing thresholds and may suppress ventricular escape rhythms. The drug must be used with caution in patients with permanent pacemakers or temporary pacing electrodes. Determinations of pacing thresholds should be done before starting therapy with flecainide and a repeat determination carried out after 1 week of therapy. An additional caution relates to the effect of flecainide on electrical thresholds needed for cardioversion. It is noted that flecainide causes an increase in the atrial defibrillation threshold in patients with chronic atrial fibrillation or atrial flutter. To achieve prompt cardioversion to sinus rhythm in these patients, it may be necessary to employ shock intensities of at least 200 joules (216).

Hemodynamic Effects

Flecainide produces dose-related decreases in cardiac contractility and cardiac output. Thus, flecainide, unlike encainide, has a negative inotropic effect that can either worsen existent heart failure or produce new congestive heart failure in approximately 5% of patients. When administered orally, the drug is tolerated without any major alterations in blood pressure or changes in exercise tolerance in patients who are in a cardiac-compensated state. However, due to its potential to exert a negative inotropic action, flecainide should be used with caution in patients who are known to display myocardial dysfunction and who would be likely to experience an incremental loss in cardiac function on administration of the drug. Flecainide should not be used in patients with ejection fractions of less than 30% because the incidence of inducing congestive heart failure approximates 50%.

Toxic Reactions

The side effects noted with the use of flecainide include blurred vision and dizziness. Headache, nausea, constipation, fatigue, nervousness, tremor, chest pain, dyspnea, paresthesias, and rash make up the list of the more commonly reported untoward responses.

Because of its potential to increase the sinus node recovery time, flecainide should be used with caution in the patient with sick-sinus syndrome or sinus node dysfunction. Flecainide has, on occasion, resulted in the development of bundle branch block or A-V block and therefore should be avoided in patients with advanced conduction disturbances.

The most serious adverse response to flecainide is the worsening of cardiac arrhythmias. New or exacerbated ventricular arrhythmias occur in 7% of patients, and new or worsened congestive heart failure in 5% of patients. As noted with encainide, flecainide has been associated with episodes of unresuscitatable ventricular tachycardia or ventricular fibrillation. Slowing of conduction velocity in the ventricular myocardium along with the incongruous alterations in Purkinje fiber and myocardial fiber refractory periods may result in inhomogeneous repolarization and reentrant circuits for the initiation and support of ventricular tachyarrhythmias.

Pharmacokinetics

The pharmacokinetic properties of flecainide are summarized in Table 14.

Absorption

Flecainide is absorbed after oral administration and is 90% bioavailable. Peak plasma concentrations are achieved within 3 hr of oral administration; the half-life is variable and ranges from 12 to 27 hr. Therefore, it is anticipated that several days of oral dosing would be required in order to approach a steady-state plasma concentration of the drug.

Metabolism and Excretion

Approximately 70% of flecainide is metabolized by the liver. Two major metabo-

TABLE 14. *Pharmacokinetic properties of flecainide*

Absorption
  Nearly complete and not altered by food or antacids
Protein binding
  Moderately bound, 40%
Metabolism
  Hepatic
Half-life
  Approximately 20 hr with a range of 12 to 27 hr; half-life is increased in the presence of renal failure or low cardiac output
Time to peak plasma concentration
  Approximately 3 hr after a single dose with a range of 1 to 6 hr
Time to achieve steady-state plasma concentration
  3 to 5 days with multiple doses
Therapeutic plasma concentration
  0.2 to 1.0 μg/ml
Elimination
  Renal: approximately 30% as unchanged drug with a range of 10% to 50%; fecal: 5%; hemodialysis removes approximately 1% of a dose as the unchanged drug

lites are formed, one that is active as an antiarrhythmic agent and the other inactive, with the remainder of the administered dose being excreted in the urine as unchanged drug. Elimination is decreased in patients with impaired renal function and dosage adjustment is necessary under such conditions. Because both metabolites of flecainide exist in the conjugated form in the plasma and the concentration of the free metabolite is low, it is unlikely that the conjugated form of the metabolic products would contribute significantly to the primary antiarrhythmic action of the parent compound. Flecainide is not bound extensively to plasma proteins, and interaction with other drugs is not significant with respect to displacement from protein binding sites.

Dose

The initiation of therapy with flecainide should be at 100 mg every 12 hr and may be increased up to 400 mg/day. The drug is administered 100 to 200 mg twice daily. The initial dose is reduced to 50 mg twice daily in patients with serious arrhythmias, or with left ventricular impairment, or in patients with poor renal function. Increase in the dose of flecainide should be done slowly at intervals of no less than 4 days and with increments of 50 mg twice daily. The plasma concentrations considered to be therapeutic are 0.2 to 1.0 $\mu g/ml$. The maximum dose of flecainide in patients with congestive heart failure is 200 mg twice daily.

Contraindications

Flecainide is contraindicated in patients with preexisting second- or three-degree A-V block or with bundle branch block when associated with left hemiblock. The drug should not be administered to patients in cardiogenic shock and should be used cautiously in patients with impaired left ventricular function.

Indications

Flecainide is used by the oral route of administration for the suppression of chronic ventricular ectopy and bouts of ventricular tachycardia. The agent was demonstrated to be more effective than quinidine or disopyramide in preventing ventricular ectopy and complex arrhythmic events. Flecainide has also proved to be of value for the long-term prevention of reentrant tachyarrhythmias involving the A-V node or accessory pathways. The intravenous form of the drug has been used experimentally for the termination of A-V nodal reentrant tachyarrhythmias associated with the Wolff-Parkinson-White syndrome.

Flecainide possesses a wide spectrum of electrophysiologic actions on the heart. The beneficial effects in reentrant A-V nodal or supraventricular tachyarrhythmias associated with accessory pathways can be attributed to one or more of the electrophysiologic changes on refractoriness and conduction velocity with the different regions of the myocardium. Likewise, the proarrhythmic actions of flecainide may be associated with the disparate electrophysiologic actions of flecainide on ventricular muscle as contrasted with that of Purkinje fibers.

Special Note: The recent results of the Cardiac Arrhythmia Suppression Trial (CAST) conducted by the National Institutes of Health, Heart, Lung, and Blood Institute has resulted in the recommendation that both encainide and flecainide undergo changes in their labeling to reflect the fact that the drugs are to be reserved for patients with life-threatening arrhythmias such as ventricular tachycardia. The drugs should not be used in patients with less severe arrhythmias even if they are symptomatic. The CAST randomized postmyocardial infarction patients with asymptomatic abnormal rhythms known to be responsive to encainide, flecainide, or a third drug, as well as to a placebo-control group. The CAST data and the safety monitoring board found that

56 of 730 patients given encainide or flecainide (average treatment period of 10 months) had died as compared with 22 fatalities among the 725 patients in the placebo-treated group. The mortality was twofold greater than that in the control population. On the basis of this finding, investigators were told to stop the two drugs.

Originally, encainide and flecainide were approved for use in two situations: (a) immediately life-threatening arrhythmias such as sustained ventricular tachycardia, and (b) less severe arrhythmias that are symptomatic if the physician considers the benefits of either drug sufficient to outweigh their potential proarrhythmic actions. The first indication for encainide or flecainide is not altered by the suggested change in the labeling. However, the second indication is no longer appropriate in view of the results of the multicenter NIH trial.

Propafenone

Propafenone (2'-3 propylamino)-2-(hydroxy)-propoxy-3 propiophenone HCl (Fig. 17) possesses properties similar to those of β-adrenoceptor antagonists as well as exhibiting class IC properties, as described by the modified electrophysiologic classification of antiarrhythmic agents established by Vaughan-Williams. Propafenone also has a slight potential to depress the slow inward calcium current. The effect of propafenone on β-adrenoceptor function may be of clinical significance, whereas its potency as a calcium channel entry blocker may be relatively insignificant. The pharmacology and clinical application of propafenone have been reviewed recently (217).

Electrophysiologic Actions

The electrophysiologic actions of propafenone have been reported by Dukes and Vaughan-Williams (218). Propafenone is a class IC antiarrhythmic with local anesthetic effects. As with all members of its class, propafenone has its major effect on the fast inward sodium current. The IC agents depress V_{max} over a wide range of heart rates and shift the resting membrane potential in the direction of hyperpolarization. The IC agents bind slowly to the sodium channel and dissociate slowly. Therefore, they exhibit what is referred to as a "rate-dependent block." During rapid rates of depolarization as occur in tachyarrhythmias, there is insufficient time for dissociation of the drug from the sodium channel, thus leading to an accumulation in the number of channels that fail to allow sodium entry. There are an increase in the number of sodium channels blocked and a slowing of conduction velocity. Inhibition of the sodium channel throughout the cardiac cycle will result in a decrease in the rate of ectopy and the trigger for the initiation of ventricular tachycardia. On the other hand, the marked slowing in the conduction velocity may lead to the establishment of a reentry circuit, thereby supporting the mechanism for a sustained ventricular tachyarrhythmia. Propafenone, like other members of the class IC agents, may at times be limited in its application due to a proarrhythmic action.

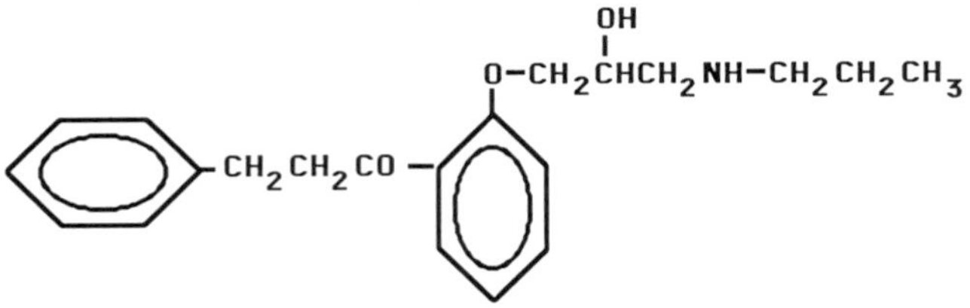

FIG. 17. Propafenone.

Sinoatrial Node

Coumel et al. (219) reported that propafenone caused sinus node slowing, which could lead to sinoatrial block. Propafenone may lengthen the sinus node recovery time with minimal effects on sinus cycle length.

Atria

The action-potential duration and effective refractory period of atrial muscle are both prolonged by propafenone. The electrophysiologic effects were of long duration and persisted beyond the time when the drug was removed from the tissue.

A-V Node

The intravenous administration of propafenone prolongs the AH and AV intervals.

His-Purkinje System

A number of studies have documented the major effect of propafenone on His-Purkinje fibers and ventricular muscle as involving a blockade of the fast inward sodium channel (218,220,221). In clinically relevant concentrations, propafenone had little effect on the resting membrane potential but increased the excitability threshold and effective refractory period. The latter, however, was not altered to the same extent as conduction velocity, which was depressed markedly. A feature common to the members of the class IC group of antiarrhythmic agents is their ability to exert a resting or tonic block of the sodium channel, as well as a phasic block on sodium entry (218,220). The slow rate of dissociation from the sodium channel contrasts with the mode of action of mexiletine or lidocaine, which dissociate rapidly during the resting phase of the membrane action potential. Although mexiletine and lidocaine will suppress

closely coupled extrasystoles, propafenone will influence cardiac excitability and refractoriness regardless of the cycle length. Propafenone depresses delayed afterdepolarizations in ischemic Purkinje fibers. The antiarrhythmic action of propafenone on digitalis and reoxygenation arrhythmias is probably due to an electrophysiologic mechanism different from that of class IB agents, such as mexiletine. Mexiletine, by reducing the amplitude of oscillatory afterpotentials, prevents the attainment of the threshold; propafenone, by reducing the excitability of the cell, increases the threshold and consequently an oscillatory afterpotential of the same amplitude will not generate arrhythmias (222).

The main metabolite of propafenone, 5-hydroxypropafenone (5-OH-P), was studied in guinea pig papillary muscles obtained from untreated animals and animals administered the metabolite in a dose of 3 mg/kg/day for 24 days (223). The effects of 5-OH-P were similar to those previously described with propafenone, and it was concluded that 5-OH-P is an active metabolite that exhibits class I antiarrhythmic effects and may be responsible for some of the cardiodepressant and antiarrhythmic effects previously described for the parent compound.

Electrocardiographic Changes

Propafenone causes dose-dependent increases in the PR interval and QRS duration. Nonsignificant increases occur in the QT_c interval, and occasional slowing of the heart rate has been observed.

Hemodynamic Effects

Several investigators have evaluated the hemodynamic effects of propafenone in patients with and without cardiac dysfunction (224–226). The intravenous administration of propafenone is accompanied by an increase in right atrial, pulmonary arterial, and pulmonary artery wedge pressures in addition to an increase in vascular resistance and a decrease in the cardiac index. In patients with preexisting left ventricular dysfunction, propafenone caused a significant decrease in ejection fraction as determined with M-mode echocardiography. In the absence of cardiac abnormalities, propafenone was without significant effects on cardiac function. Thus, propafenone has a negative inotropic action, which in part may be attributable to its ability to produce β-adrenoceptor blockade. Although the potential to decrease cardiac function is more pronounced with the intravenous administration of the drug, caution should be exercised with the oral use of propafenone.

Toxic Reactions

Concurrent administration of propafenone with digoxin, warfarin, or metoprolol increases the serum concentrations of the latter three drugs. Cimetidine slightly increases the propafenone serum concentrations. Additive pharmacologic effects can occur when lidocaine, procainamide, and quinidine are combined with propafenone. Overall, 21% to 32% of patients experience adverse effects, with 3% to 7% of these serious enough to warrant discontinuing therapy.

The most common adverse effects are dizziness or lightheadedness, metallic taste, and nausea and vomiting; the most serious adverse effects are proarrhythmic events.

Several reports (227–230) have emphasized the development of a high incidence of proarrhythmic effects in patients receiving propafenone. A worsening of the arrhythmic condition has been reported in one-third of patients undergoing electrophysiologic evaluation by programmed electrical stimulation. In some instances the arrhythmias accompanying the use of propafenone may be controlled by lidocaine. As discussed with encainide and flecainide, propafenone may make electrical conversion of tachyarrhythmias more difficult.

Pharmacokinetics

The pharmacokinetic properties of propafenone are summarized in Table 15. Propafenone is well absorbed after oral administration with maximum plasma concentrations being achieved within 2 to 3 hr. The systemic bioavailability of the drug is only 12% after a 300-mg dose (231). Patients may be classified as fast (90%) or slow (10%) metabolizers of propafenone. This variability in metabolism is thought to be due to a genetically determined deficiency in one pathway. Among the group of patients classified as extensive metabolizers (90% of the U.S. population), the bioavailability of pro-

TABLE 15. *Pharmacokinetic properties of propafenone*

Absorption
  Absorption is 100% but its bioavailability is usually <20% due to extensive first-pass metabolism
Protein binding
  >95%
Metabolism
  The drug undergoes extensive oxidative metabolism to yield 5-hydroxy and hydroxymethoxy metabolites; 5-hydroxypropafenone is known to possess antiarrhythmic properties
Half-life
  2.4 to 11.8 hr
Time to peak plasma concentration
  After 2 to 3 hr
Therapeutic plasma concentration
  Varies widely and has been reported to be from 64 to 1,044 ng/ml
Elimination
  Renal: <1% is eliminated as the unchanged compound

pafenone varies nonlinearly with the dose and increases when taken with food; these effects are not seen in poor metabolizers. This departure from dose linearity occurs when single doses above 150 mg are given. A 300-mg dose gives plasma concentrations that are six times that of a 150-mg dose. Elimination is primarily hepatic, with a mean elimination half-life after oral administration of 5.5 hr in extensive metabolizers, and 17.2 hr in poor metabolizers. The relationship between plasma propafenone concentration and clinical response varies extensively among individual patients; therefore, plasma concentrations have limited usefulness in predicting the efficacy of the drug or the anticipated electrophysiologic effects. Propafenone is metabolized extensively and undergoes oxidative metabolism to form 5-hydroxy and hydroxy-methoxy metabolites that are then conjugated to form glucuronides and sulfates. The majority of individuals are extensive metabolizers and form the active 5-hydroxy metabolite. The conjugates represent the major forms in which the drug is eliminated either by way of urinary excretion or through its appearance in the feces. The pharmacokinetics of propafenone and 5-OH-P and their relationship with the antiarrhythmic action and side effects have been studied in patients with stable, frequent, premature ventricular complexes (232). Observations were made after a single oral dose of propafenone 300 mg and after 1 and 3 months of therapy. After 1 month of treatment the plasma elimination half-life of propafenone (6.7 hr) was almost twice as long as after a single dose (3.5 hr), and the area under the plasma propafenone concentration-time curve was significantly larger than after the single dose; this was also true for the metabolite. The ratio of the area under the curves of 5-OH-P and propafenone decreased from the single dose (0.63) to 1 month (0.32). Eight patients had a ≥75% reduction of premature ventricular complexes after 3 days of therapy, and in seven patients, they were completely suppressed;

the response was maintained over 1 to 3 months. The kinetics of propafenone were time dependent. Its active metabolite did not accumulate greatly during chronic treatment.

Dose

The dose of propafenone must be individualized on the basis of the patient's response. The monitoring of plasma concentrations of the drug has not been determined to be of value. A dose-titration regimen can be used for both the fast and slow metabolizers.

The initial dose is 150 mg given every 8 hr (450 mg/day). The dose may be increased at intervals of 3 to 4 days to 300 mg every 12 hr (600 mg/day), or if additional drug is required, it may be given at a maximum dose of 300 mg every 8 hr (900 mg/day). The dose should be reduced if there is an increase in the PR interval or a widening of the QRS complex. It is recommended that the drug be administered along with food so as to increase its absorption. Because propafenone undergoes significant hepatic metabolism, the dose must be adjusted in patients with hepatic impairment. Extreme caution is recommended when propafenone is used in patients with impaired renal function.

Contraindications

Propafenone is contraindicated in the presence of severe or uncontrolled congestive heart failure; cardiogenic shock; sino-atrial, A-V, and intraventricular disorders of conduction; and sinus node dysfunction such as sick-sinus syndrome. Other contraindications include severe bradycardia, hypotension, obstructive pulmonary disease, and hepatic and renal failure. Due to its weak β-blocking action, propafenone can cause possible dose-related bronchospasm. This problem is greatest in those patients who are slow metabolizers.

Indications

Propafenone is indicated for the suppression of ventricular tachycardia and/or the suppression of ectopic ventricular rhythms such as premature ventricular complexes of unifocal or multifocal origin, couplets, or R-on-T phenomena when of sufficient severity to require treatment.

Propafenone appears to have utility in pediatric patients with supraventricular tachycardia (233). When administered three to four times daily, the drug was effective in controlling the tachyarrhythmia associated with the preexcitation syndrome. During orthodromic tachycardia, propafenone increases conduction time in both the anterograde and retrograde limbs of the tachycardia (234). Long-term oral propafenone has been evaluated in patients with recurrent episodes of symptomatic atrial fibrillation or flutter or both, and who had failed one to five previous drug trials (235). At a mean dose of 750 mg/day the percentage of patients free of recurrences of symptomatic atrial fibrillation/flutter during propafenone treatment ranged from 40% to 54%.

Propafenone is considered to be effective in reducing the frequency of premature ventricular complexes and is of special value in the management of patients with supraventricular tachyarrhythmia when the disorder is associated with the preexcitation syndrome. The efficacy and safety of propafenone in patients with life-threatening arrhythmias have not been demonstrated. Like other members of the class IC group, propafenone has not been shown to prevent sudden death in patients with serious ventricular ectopic activity. Furthermore, the potential to exert a proarrhythmic action makes it essential that each patient given propafenone be evaluated electrocardiographically and clinically before and during therapy to determine whether the response to the drug warrants its continued administration.

Propranolol

In addition to their ability to abolish certain disorders of cardiac rhythm, propranolol and other members of class II will prevent the effects of the adrenergic nervous system or adrenergic drugs (norepinephrine, epinephrine, isoproterenol, dopamine) on the heart. It is therefore a β-adrenergic receptor blocking agent, and, as such, it will produce a wide variety of effects, both hemodynamic and metabolic, by virtue of the antagonism of adrenergically mediated responses.

Several of the more important physiologic responses mediated by activation of β-adrenergic receptors include (a) increases in heart rate and cardiac contractile force in response to exercise, stress, excitation, etc., (b) an increase in A-V conduction velocity, (c) relaxation of bronchial smooth muscle and a decrease in airway resistance, and (d) release of insulin from β cells in the islets of Langerhans in response to adrenergic stimulation. After propranolol administration, the adrenergic system can no longer initiate the responses indicated.

The clinical use of propranolol or other β receptor blocking agents must take into consideration the effects of β-adrenergic receptor blockade and the consequences of such on the overall regulation of the cardiovascular system. Patients with normally functioning cardiovascular systems may be able to tolerate a blockade of adrenergic transmission to the heart; however, those with compensated heart failure will be dependent on adrenergic tone to maintain adequate cardiac output. Removal of background adrenergic tone by administration of a β-adrenergic receptor blocking agent may precipitate acute congestive heart failure or pulmonary edema.

The chemical structures of propranolol and related β-adrenoceptor antagonists are shown in Fig. 18. Each of these β-adrenergic receptor blocking agents contains a chiral center. This asymmetric center in the

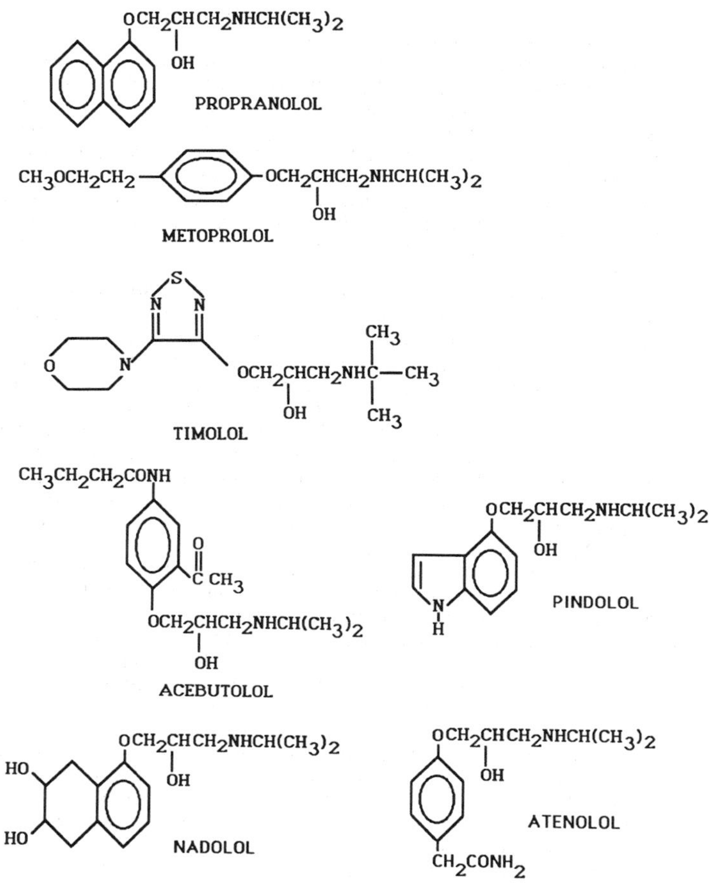

FIG. 18. Chemical structures of β-adrenoceptor antagonists.

side chain of these compounds gives rise to dextro- and levo-rotary compounds, which can differ greatly in their pharmacologic actions. Only one of the two isomers possess β-adrenergic receptor blocking activity. However, because the drug is administered as a racemate (containing both *d* and *l* forms), the actions of the non-β-adrenergic blocking components may also be important. The *d* isomer of propranolol (only the *l* isomer possesses β-adrenergic blocking activity) has direct electrophysiologic actions that resemble those of quinidine and are termed "membrane-stabilizing" properties (236,237). The direct electrophysiologic actions of propranolol together

with the ability to alter β-adrenoceptor responsiveness may be of importance in clinical management of cardiac arrhythmias. The direct membrane-stabilizing action is lacking in nadolol and present with metoprolol only at very high doses. The pharmacologic characteristics of currently approved β-adrenoceptor antagonists are summarized in Table 16.

Electrophysiologic Actions

Unlike the other antiarrhythmic agents previously discussed, propranolol has two separate and distinct actions. The first action involves the consequences of compet-

TABLE 16. β-Adrenoceptor antagonists

Propranolol	Propranolol (Inderal) is a prototype β-adrenoceptor antagonist that is nonselective in that it blocks both the β_1- and β_2-adrenoceptors. In addition, propranolol has *membrane-stabilizing* properties that can contribute to its antiarrhythmic action. Because the latter action is obtained at plasma concentrations beyond those that may be encountered clinically, it is the β-receptor blocking property that may best explain the antiarrhythmic action of propranolol.
Acebutolol	Acebutolol (Sectral) is a cardioselective β-adrenoceptor blocking agent with partial agonist activity (intrinsic sympathomimetic activity or ISA). It is approved for use in the management of patients with premature ventricular complexes and in treating essential hypertension.
Atenolol	Atenolol (Tenormin) is a β_1 selective (cardioselective) adrenoceptor blocking agent. It lacks membrane-stabilizing effects and does not exhibit ISA. Cardioselectivity is not absolute and β_2-adrenoceptors are blocked at higher doses. Atenolol does not undergo appreciable metabolism and has an elimination half-life of 6 to 7 hr.
Metoprolol	Metoprolol (Lopressor) is a selective β_1-adrenoceptor blocking agent. The cardioselectivity is not absolute and at higher doses β_2-adrenoceptors are blocked as well. The drug does not possess ISA. Metoprolol undergoes extensive hepatic metabolism and has a plasma half-life of 3 to 7 hr. It is used primarily in the management of patients with essential hypertension and angina pectoris.
Nadolol	Nadolol (Corgard) is a nonselective β-adrenoceptor blocking agent that lacks membrane-stabilizing and ISA properties. Nadolol is not metabolized and is excreted unchanged. Therefore, the drug has a long duration of action with a pharmacologic half-life of 20 to 24 hr, which permits once daily administration. It is eliminated by renal mechanisms as the unchanged drug. Nadolol is used primarily for the management of patients with angina pectoris.
Pindolol	Pindolol (Visken) is a nonselective β-adrenoceptor antagonist with considerable ISA and devoid of membrane-stabilizing activity. The drug is metabolized extensively and has a plasma half-life of 3 to 4 hr. It is indicated primarily for the management of patients with hypertension. The ISA possessed by pindolol may exacerbate symptoms in patients with ischemic heart disease.
Timolol	Timolol (Blocadren) is a nonselective β-adrenoceptor blocking agent without ISA, membrane-stabilizing, and local anesthetic properties. The drug is metabolized partially by hepatic mechanisms and has a plasma half-life of 4 hr. It is indicated for the management of patients with essential hypertension as well as for long-term prophylactic management of patients who have survived the acute phase of myocardial infarction and who are given 10 mg twice daily.
Esmolol	Esmolol (Brevibloc Injection) is an ultrashort-acting, cardioselective β-adrenoceptor blocking agent. It is indicated for use in patients with supraventricular tachyarrhythmias in which short-term management is indicated. The drug is given intravenously.

itive β-adrenergic receptor blockade and the removal of adrenergic influences on the heart. The second action of propranolol involves the direct myocardial effects (membrane stabilization) that can account for its antiarrhythmic effect against arrhythmias in which enhanced β receptor stimulation does not play a significant role in the genesis of the rhythm disturbance.

Sinoatrial Node

Propranolol administration produces a decrease in the spontaneous rate of rabbit isolated atrial preparations (238). This action of propranolol is far more significant in the intact heart, which is under the influence of the sympathetic nervous system as well as circulating catecholamines. The ability of propranolol to block β-adrenergic receptors in the sinoatrial node and prevent the effects of adrenergic influences on this structure is the primary mechanism by which it produces a bradycardia. In addition, doses in excess of those required to produce β receptor blockade can exert a direct negative chronotropic action on sinoatrial nodal pacemaker cells (238).

Atria

Propranolol has local anesthetic properties and has actions on the membrane action potential of atrial muscle similar to those of quinidine (239). Membrane responsiveness and action-potential amplitude are reduced, and excitability is decreased. Conduction velocity is reduced. Because the concentrations required to produce these effects have significant β receptor blocking actions, it is impossible to determine if the drug acts by specific receptor blockade or through an action that some have referred to as a "quinidinelike" or "membrane-stabilizing effect." However, both the *d* isomer of propranolol and its *l* isomer produce these membrane depressant actions.

Propranolol prolongs slightly the action-potential duration and the effective refractory period of atrial tissue. However, at low doses, propranolol has little effect on atrial refractoriness or conduction velocity in humans. Atrial bypass tract conduction and refractoriness are not altered.

A-V Node

Propranolol's effects on A-V node conduction velocity and effective refractory period can be attributed to both β-adrenergic receptor blockade and direct membrane depressant properties (240,241). The effects of propranolol on the A-V node are additive to those produced with digitalis administration. Thus, both drugs are of value, either alone or in combination, in slowing the ventricular rate during atrial flutter or fibrillation. In the presence of digitalis toxicity, propranolol may be contraindicated because of the possibility that it could produce complete A-V block and ventricular asystole. The depressant effects of propranolol on the A-V node are more pronounced than the direct depressant effects of quinidine because of propranolol's dual mechanism: β-adrenergic receptor blockade and direct depressant actions. Propranolol does not have the anticholinergic actions of quinidine and other antiarrhythmic agents.

In humans, propranolol administration results in a decrease in A-V conduction velocity and an increase in the A-V nodal refractory period. This effect is seen at doses of 0.1 mg/kg administered intravenously (240). When the drug is administered in the absence of atrial pacing, the simultaneous decrease in sinus rate indirectly enhances A-V conduction. The PR interval, therefore, may not be prolonged after propranolol administration.

His-Purkinje System

Propranolol decreases Purkinje fiber membrane responsiveness and reduces the action-potential amplitude (17). The maximum rate of phase-0 depolarization is depressed at all resting membrane potentials. His-Purkinje tissue excitability is also reduced. These electrophysiologic alterations are observed at propranolol concentrations that are in excess of those obtained clinically.

Propranolol administration produces decreases in the action-potential duration and the effective refractory period of Purkinje fibers. However, increases in the effective refractory period are observed only at plasma concentrations that exceed those observed in the clinical use of the drug.

The most striking electrophysiologic property of propranolol at representative therapeutic concentrations is a depression of catecholamine-stimulated automaticity. Epinephrine and isoproterenol increase phase-4 depolarization of Purkinje fibers and thereby increase the rate of spontaneous diastolic depolarization. This action of catecholamines is mediated by β-adrenergic receptors and is blocked by the β-adrenergic blocking properties of propranolol and related agents. The β-adrenergic blocking action of propranolol is probably responsible for the decrease in ventricular premature complexes observed with low or moderate propranolol dosages.

Ventricular Muscle

In ventricular muscle fibers, propranolol decreases membrane responsiveness and decreases myocardial excitability (17). The action-potential duration is not prolonged until very high propranolol dosages are used. The necessary concentrations are much higher than those obtained clinically and may be in excess of 100 ng/ml.

Summary

The antiarrhythmic action of propranolol is a result of two separate effects: (a) the β-adrenergic receptor blocking action of the drug and (b) the direct membrane depressant (membrane-stabilization or quinidine-like) properties of propranolol. At low plasma concentrations, less than 100 ng/ml, the antiarrhythmic action is a result of β-adrenergic blockade. The β-adrenoceptor blockade produced by propranolol and related drugs is responsible for reducing A-V transmission and will slow the ventricular rate in the presence of atrial flutter or fibrillation. This action may also reduce the incidence of premature ventricular complexes in patients with ischemic heart disease by reducing catecholamine-induced ventricular automaticity. However, plasma concentrations of propranolol above 100 ng/ml may be needed to reduce the ventricular rate in some patients with atrial flutter or fibrillation. At this plasma concentration, in addition to β-adrenergic blockade, the direct depressant actions of propranolol on A-V transmission are manifested, and a further reduction in ventricular rate will occur. The high plasma concentrations are necessary in order to observe the direct membrane-stabilizing properties of propranolol, and it is only at the higher plasma propranolol concentrations that the antiarrhythmic properties of propranolol in the treatment of ventricular arrhythmias are manifested (242). β-Adrenoceptor agents that possess intrinsic sympathomimetic activity (pindolol) may worsen rhythm disorders mediated as a result of β-adrenoceptor activation.

Electrocardiographic Changes

Either no change or an increase in the PR interval can be observed. No change in the QRS interval is observed unless large doses are given. The QRS interval may then be prolonged slightly. The QT interval is usually shortened with propranolol administration (243).

Hemodynamic Effects

The majority of studies dealing with the hemodynamic effects of β-receptor blockade have been conducted with propranolol. Other β-receptor blocking agents have properties that may cause them to produce effects significantly different from those of propranolol, both qualitatively and quantitatively (244). The following discussion applies primarily to propranolol.

The blockade of cardiac β-adrenergic receptors prevents or reduces the usual positive inotropic and chronotropic actions due to catecholamine administration or cardiac sympathetic nerve stimulation. In anesthetized dogs with intact cardiac innervation and intrinsic sympathetic tone, propranolol has been reported to decrease the resting heart rate, myocardial contractile force, and blood pressure (245). The effects of β-adrenergic receptor blockade on the racing performance of normal greyhounds and greyhounds with chronic intrinsic cardiac denervation have been reported (246). β-Adrenergic receptor blockade resulted in an increase in racing time in the normal animal, with only a slight reduction in maximal heart rate. In animals with chronically denervated hearts, racing time was prolonged, cardiac acceleration was severely limited, and the animals finished in a state of collapse. Maximal performance, therefore, depends on the cardiac stimulatory action of both sympathetic nerves and circulating catecholamines. Analogous studies in humans (247) were carried out to assess the effects of β-adrenergic receptor blockade on cardiovascular responses to treadmill exercise in normal subjects and subjects with heart disease. In normal subjects, propranolol produced a fall in the endurance time to maximal exercise, which was 40% less on average than the control. This was associated with decreases in cardiac output, mean arterial pressure, left ventricular minute work, and maximal oxygen uptake. Increases in the arteriovenous oxygen difference and the central venous pressure were noted after β receptor blockade. Similar results were obtained in patients with heart disease who were able to exercise normally. Under conditions of submaximal exercise, propranolol produced similar circulatory responses, with the exception that oxygen uptake was not altered. The decrease in cardiac output was compensated for by an increase in the arteriovenous oxygen difference.

The response of heart size to exercise measured before and after β-adrenergic receptor blockade is an increase in ventricular end-diastolic dimensions, whereas exercise in the normal subject results in a decrease in ventricular dimensions (248,249). Intravenous administration of propranolol produces decreases in the velocity of shortening of myocardial fibers, stroke index, and left ventricular minute work. β-Adrenergic receptor blockade prolongs systolic ejection periods at rest and during exercise and increases ventricular dimensions during exercise. Both alterations tend to increase myocardial oxygen consumption. However, these alterations are offset by factors that tend to reduce oxygen consumption: decreased heart rate and decreased force of contraction. The decrease in oxygen demand produced by decreases in heart rate and in force of contraction is

TABLE 17. *Hemodynamic effects of propranolol*

Decrease in resting heart rate
Decrease in myocardial contractility
   Decrease in stroke volume
   Decrease in ventricular pressure development
  Decrease in rate of ejection
  Increase in ventricular end-diastolic size
Decrease in inotropic and chronotropic responses to exercise

usually greater than the increase in oxygen demand produced by increased heart size and ejection time. The net result is that oxygen demand is decreased. The hemodynamic effects of propranolol are summarized in Table 17.

Toxic Reactions

The adverse effects associated with propranolol and other β-adrenergic receptor blocking agents are for the most part related to the primary pharmacologic action, that of β receptor blockade.

Cardiac failure has been the most serious adverse effect associated with β receptor blockade. Three possible mechanisms may be involved: (a) β receptor blockade will decrease the heart rate, which in the normal heart is no serious consequence, but this can lead to a fall in cardiac output in those patients who have a limited stroke volume and who depend on an increased heart rate to maintain an adequate cardiac output; (b) the increased durations of systole and diastole that accompany β receptor blockade may decrease cardiac output in patients with valvular regurgitation due to increased regurgitant flow; (c) patients in borderline failure maintain cardiac compensation partly through an increase in cardiac adrenergic tone. The sudden removal of cardiac adrenergic support by β receptor blockade removes the inotropic and chronotropic effects of adrenergic stimulation. In addition to those effects attributable to β receptor blockade, it is important to remember that propranolol possesses direct cardiac depressant effects that become manifest when the drug is administered rapidly by the intravenous route.

Heart failure due to administration of propranolol cannot be managed in the conventional manner with the use of adrenergic inotropic agents because of the presence of β-adrenergic receptor blockade, which will prevent the response of the heart to conventional doses of norepinephrine, isoproterenol, or dopamine. It is true, however, that the effects of β receptor blockade may be overcome by large doses of the adrenergic agents because of the competitive nature of the receptor blockade by propranolol. Such an approach is not convenient or easy to manage and in the case of norepinephrine may prove to be hazardous. The latter drug, when administered in the presence of β receptor blockade, will still be capable of producing peripheral vasoconstriction (an alpha-mediated effect) at a time when myocardial β receptors are blocked and the heart is unable to respond to the acute increase in outflow impedance (aortic diastolic pressure), leading to the development of acute left ventricular failure. A similar response may be anticipated from dopamine if used under similar circumstances.

The digitalis glycosides are capable of exerting a positive inotropic effect in the presence of β receptor blockade; however, the action of digitalis on the A-V node may be additive to the effect of propranolol, with the result that A-V block will develop. Furthermore, the inotropic effect of digitalis is not manifest immediately, and the delay in onset of action may be a drawback in an emergent situation.

Aminophylline would be a most suitable inotropic agent for the reversal of heart failure induced by propranolol. The drug has an immediate positive inotropic effect, but its action may be accompanied by marked hypotension if given rapidly by the intravenous route. An alternative agent would be amrinone, which, like aminophylline, is

a phosphodiesterase inhibitor, thus being able to augment myocardial contractility in the presence of β-adrenoceptor blockade. The polypeptide hormone, glucagon, will immediately reverse all of the cardiac depressant effects of propranolol, and its use is associated with a minimum of side effects when used acutely.

Electrical asystole due to depressed pacemaker activity or effects on the A-V node by propranolol may lead to ventricular asystole. It should be remembered that the heart will still respond to mechanical or electrical stimulation in the event that propranolol produces electrical asystole or complete A-V block. Catecholamines will be of little value in restoring cardiac rhythm in the presence of β receptor blockade. Intravenous atropine may be of some value and should be tried in those instances in which propranolol produces marked bradycardia.

Hypotension may occur with rapid intravenous administration of propranolol due to direct effects on the vascular smooth muscle leading to vasodilation. In addition, the cardiac actions due to β receptor blockade and direct myocardial depression further augment the fall in blood pressure.

Hypoglycemia has been reported in diabetic patients on insulin, in children during recovery from anesthesia, and in patients following partial gastrectomy. The mechanism may be related to the fact that β receptor blockade prevents adrenergic stimulation of glycogenolysis in skeletal muscle, which ordinarily would result in an increase in plasma lactate. Lactate is subsequently converted by the liver to glucose, which is added to the plasma pool.

Bronchospasm may occur in asthmatics and in normal subjects. Increased airway resistance has been observed after administration of propranolol as well as other β receptor blocking agents. Aminophylline, intravenously, will counteract the bronchospasm, but isoproterenol will not relax the bronchial smooth muscle in the presence of β-adrenoceptor blockade. β receptor blocking agents are contraindicated in patients with bronchial asthma or other chronic obstructive lung diseases.

Pregnancy is not interfered with by chronic administration of propranolol, but because the drug does cross the placenta and enters the fetal circulation, fetal cardiac responses to the stresses of labor and delivery will be blocked, as well as those of the mother (250).

It is important to remember that abrupt withdrawal of β-adrenoceptor blocking agents may be potentially dangerous for patients with ischemic heart disease. Increased incidences of angina, coronary spasm, and myocardial infarction can occur in patients who have been abruptly withdrawn from chronic β receptor blockade. The reason for this is unclear. Chronic β-adrenergic blockade may have been masking a deterioration in ischemic heart disease, or long-term β blockade may result in an upregulation of β-adrenoceptors.

Pharmacokinetics

Absorption

Propranolol is almost completely absorbed from the gastrointestinal tract after a single oral dose. Peak plasma concentrations are observed approximately 2 hr after an oral dose.

Metabolism and Excretion

Propranolol is eliminated almost entirely by metabolism. Only 1% to 4% of a dose is recovered as unchanged drug. There are four primary pathways for the metabolism of propranolol: O-dealkylation, side-chain oxidation, glucuronic acid conjugation, and ring oxidation.

The major ring-hydroxylated metabolite, 4-hydroxy-propranolol, is observed in plasma only after oral administration. Other ring-hydroxylated metabolites have been identified in human plasma and urine as conjugated sulfates or glucuronides. The ring-hydroxylated metabolites of propranolol are active as β-adrenergic blocking agents, but it is not known to what extent they contribute to β-adrenergic blockade. O-Dealkylation and side-chain oxidation account for approximately 20% of single oral doses and 40% of single intravenous doses.

Although propranolol is nearly completely absorbed from the intestinal tract, the systemic availability of propranolol is limited as a result of extensive first-pass extraction by the liver. When small doses of propranolol (5–30 mg) are given orally, only extremely low plasma concentrations of propranolol are detected. Larger doses (40 mg or greater) result in much higher plasma propranolol concentrations. It is uncertain if this hepatic extraction is a result of metabolism or bile excretion or another process. In oral doses greater than 40 mg, the hepatic extraction is approximately 70% and does not change markedly with propranolol dosage.

Kinetics

A two-compartment (biexponential) model can be used to describe plasma propranolol elimination. Pharmacokinetic parameters of propranolol and related agents are given in Table 18.

Propranolol clearance is primarily a function of the liver. In patients with normal hepatic function, clearance is limited by hepatic blood flow. Patients with hepatocellular disease have a decreased rate of propranolol metabolism and resultant decrease in hepatic clearance. Bioavailability may also be increased as a result of decreased first-pass extraction of propranolol by liver. Hepatocellular disease also decreases the plasma-protein-bound propranolol fraction and increases free propranolol concentration at a given total plasma propranolol concentration. Hyperthyroidism may increase hepatic propranolol clearance.

TABLE 18. *Pharmacokinetics of β-adrenoceptor antagonists*

Drug	Oral bioavailability	Protein binding	Metabolism	Half-life (hr)	Elimination
Propranolol	90%, first-pass metabolism results in significant decrease in bioavailability	Very high, 93%	Hepatic	3–5	Renal
Acebutolol	70%	Low, 26%	Hepatic, active metabolite diacetolol more cardioselective than parent compound	3–4	Renal 30%–40%, biliary/fecal 50%–60%
Atenolol	50%	Very low, 6%–16%	Hepatic (slight)	6–7	Renal 85%–100%
Metoprolol	95%	Low, 12%	Hepatic	3–7	Renal 3%–10%
Nadolol	30%	Low, 30%	None	10–24	Renal 70%
Pindolol	90%–100%	Moderate, 40%	Hepatic	3–4	Renal 40%
Timolol	90%	Very low, <10%	Hepatic	4	Renal 20%

Propranolol is highly bound to plasma proteins in humans (85%–96%). Plasma-protein binding is reduced by uremia and hepatic disease.

Therapeutic plasma propranolol concentrations vary widely and are individualized. β-Adrenergic receptor blockade is achieved at plasma concentrations of 5 to 50 ng/ml. Early work suggested that plasma concentrations of 40 to 85 ng/ml were necessary for suppression of ventricular ectopic complexes in patients with ischemic heart disease, but later work has suggested that suppression of ventricular arrhythmias may not occur in some patients until plasma concentrations of 100 ng/ml or more are achieved.

The plasma concentrations resulting from oral administration of propranolol to a given individual are remarkably similar on repeated administrations. Between individuals, however, there is wide variation of plasma concentrations after oral administration, with a sevenfold range in the peak plasma levels after the same dose, whereas in the same subject, interindividual plasma concentrations after intravenous administration are remarkably similar. These results were interpreted as suggesting the plasma concentrations differ after oral administration because of quantitative differences among individuals in the amount or rate of drug passing from the intestinal tract to the systemic circulation.

Oral Dose

For treatment of supraventricular arrhythmias, 10 to 30 mg three or four times daily usually is sufficient. Treatment of ventricular arrhythmias may require very large doses (320 mg/day or greater) and the effect is highly variable depending on the etiology of the cardiac rhythm disorder.

Intravenous Dose

Intravenous administration of propranolol is reserved for life-threatening arrhyth-mias or those occurring under anesthesia. The usual dose of 1 to 3 mg is administered under careful hemodynamic and electrocardiographic monitoring. The rate of administration should not exceed 1 mg (1 ml)/min, to diminish the possibility of hypotension and cardiac standstill. Sufficient time should be allowed for the drug to reach the heart from the site of injection before administering another dose. No less than 2 min should pass between doses. Additional drug should not be given in less than 4 hr.

Contraindications

The most significant complication of propranolol therapy is depression of cardiac contractility, particularly in patients with congestive heart failure, and, presumably, an increased level of circulating catecholamines. The depression in contractility is thought to result from the β receptor blocking effects of the drug that cause immediate removal of adrenergic support to the heart. In addition, when propranolol is used at doses greater than those required to produce β receptor blockade, further cardiac depression may result from the direct effects of the drug on the contractile properties of the heart. Similar depressant effects can occur from rapid intravenous administration of the drug.

The hemodynamic status of the patient is of primary importance when the use of β receptor blocking drugs is under consideration. In the presence of myocardial infarction, extreme caution should be used when propranolol is being administered intravenously. It has been suggested that a β receptor blocking agent with intrinsic sympathomimetic properties would be a suitable alternative drug because it would have less of a myocardial depressant action.

The presence of any degree of A-V block prior to the onset of a tachyarrhythmia is a contraindication to the use of propranolol, because of its ability to further depress A-V transmission. This contraindication will not apply in the presence of a demand ventricular pacing system, in which case one can guard against ventricular standstill.

Propranolol is contraindicated in therapy for patients with frequent ventricular extrasystoles in whom the basic sinus rate is already less than 60/min. The β receptor blockade induced by propranolol plus its direct effect on sinoatrial pacemaker cells would further decrease the sinus rate or might induce sinoatrial arrest.

The presence of chronic obstructive airway disease is a contraindication to the use of propranolol. The resulting β receptor blockade would intensify the degree of airway obstruction.

Patients receiving anesthetic agents that tend to depress myocardial contractility (ether, enflurane, halothane) should not receive propranolol. The presence of β receptor blockade would unmask the myocardial depressant effects of the anesthetic agents. The depressant effects of the anesthetic drugs usually are counteracted by a compensatory increase in adrenergic stimulation of the heart.

Indications

Propranolol may be indicated for management of a variety of cardiac rhythm abnormalities that are totally or in part due to enhanced adrenergic stimulation. In selected cases of sinus tachycardia due to anxiety, pheochromocytoma, or thyrotoxicosis, β receptor blockade will reduce the spontaneous heart rate.

Propranolol alone or in conjunction with digitalis is of value in controlling the ventricular rate in patients with atrial flutter or fibrillation. The mechanism by which propranolol produces its beneficial effect is through blockade of β-adrenergic receptor stimulation at the level of the A-V node. In addition, propranolol can produce a direct depressant effect on A-V transmission if it is administered in large doses or too rapidly by the intravenous route.

By virtue of its ability to delay A-V trans-

mission, propranolol is an important antiarrhythmic agent in patients with recurrent supraventricular tachyarrhythmias associated with the WPW syndrome.

Patients with supraventricular extrasystoles and intermittent paroxysms of atrial fibrillation may benefit from the institution of β receptor blockade with propranolol.

The arrhythmias associated with halothane or cyclopropane anesthesia have been attributed to the interaction of the anesthetic with catecholamines and have been suppressed by intravenous administration of 1 to 3 mg of propranolol (251).

An increase in circulating catecholamines has been observed in patients with acute myocardial infarction and has been correlated with the development of arrhythmias (252,253). Orally administered propranolol has neither improved the survival rate nor decreased the incidence of recorded arrhythmias in patients with acute myocardial infarction.

Clinically, tachyarrhythmias associated with digitalis excess, including supraventricular and ventricular extrasystoles and tachycardia, as well as ventricular fibrillation, have been suppressed by intravenously and orally administered propranolol (254–256). In spite of the experimental evidence implicating catecholamines in the genesis of digitalis-related arrhythmias (257,258), there is sufficient experimental and clinical evidence to suggest that the suppression of this group of arrhythmias is not entirely a result of β receptor blockade (242). The dose of *dl*-propranolol or *l*-propranolol required to suppress ouabain and acetylstrophanthidin arrhythmias has consistently been greater than that required to prevent epinephrine-induced arrhythmias (236). In addition, *d*-propranolol suppresses digitalis-induced arrhythmias in experimental animals and humans, and not all β-adrenergic receptor blocking agents are capable of suppressing digitalis-induced arrhythmias, although they antagonize catecholamine-induced rhythm disturbances, a finding that emphasizes that β-adrenergic blockade alone is unable to antagonize digitalis-induced arrhythmias and that some other property must explain the effectiveness of propranolol against this arrhythmia.

Propranolol has not proved effective in preventing the recurrence of atrial fibrillation after cardioversion, but the combination of propranolol and quinidine may be more effective than quinidine alone. Combined use of propranolol and procainamide has proved effective in patients with persistent ventricular fibrillation.

Propranolol has not been effective in converting chronic atrial fibrillation and flutter. It is likewise ineffective in suppressing ventricular arrhythmias not due to digitalis or to exercise.

Although propranolol has been recommended for treatment of digitalis toxicity, it is not the drug of choice because of its ability to depress myocardial contractility, depress A-V transmission, and produce bradycardia. Even though propranolol is highly effective in the treatment of digitalis-induced arrhythmias, diphenylhydantoin and lidocaine would be preferred.

Bretylium

Bretylium tosylate, (*o*-bromo-benzyl)ethyl-dimethylammonium *p*-toluenesulfonate (Fig. 19), was introduced in 1959 as an agent for treatment of hypertension (259). It soon proved ineffective for clinical management of hypertension because of rapid tolerance to its antihypertensive effect.

Bretylium's antihypertensive effect is a result of inhibition of norepinephrine release from postganglionic nerve terminals

of the sympathetic nervous system (260). Bretylium is concentrated in the postganglionic nerve terminals of adrenergic nerves and interferes with norepinephrine release without significantly altering the ultrastructural integrity of adrenergic neuronal vesicles, depressing preganglionic or postganglionic sympathetic nerve conduction, impairing sympathetic ganglionic transmission, depleting neuronal norepinephrine stores, or diminishing the responsiveness of adrenergic receptors to adrenergic agonists. The inhibition of norepinephrine release is preceded by an initial release of catecholamines from adrenergic nerve endings into the general circulation (260).

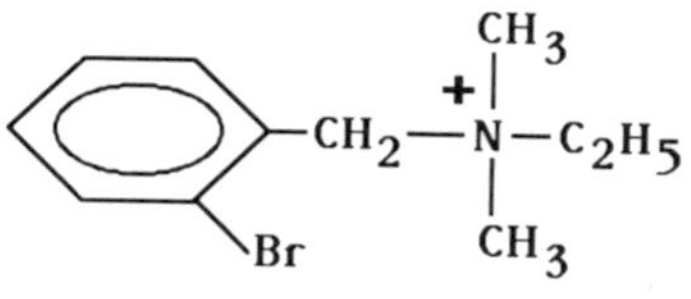

The antiarrhythmic action of bretylium was suggested initially by the observation that it prevented atrial fibrillation induced by acetylcholine in dogs made hypokalemic by administration of glucose and insulin (261). Subsequently it was reported that bretylium raised the electrical threshold necessary to induce ventricular fibrillation in the canine heart (262) and reduced the vulnerability of the human heart to develop ventricular fibrillation under a number of pathologic conditions (263). More important, bretylium was noted to suppress ventricular fibrillation associated with acute myocardial infarction (264–267).

Electrophysiologic Actions

The net effects of bretylium on the electrical and mechanical properties of the heart are a composite of the direct actions of the drug on cardiac tissues and indirect actions mediated via the drug's actions on the sympathetic nervous system. These actions are summarized in Table 19.

Sinoatrial Node

Bretylium administration produces an initial brief increase in sinus node automaticity (268–270). This initial increase in heart rate is blocked by cardiac denervation

FIG. 19. Bretylium.

TABLE 19. *Electrophysiologic properties of bretylium*

Tissue	Indirect action[a]	Direct action
Sinus node	Increase	Decrease
Atria		
Conduction velocity	Increase	No change
Refractory period	Decrease	Increase
Automaticity	Increase	No change
A-V node		
Conduction velocity	Increase	Decrease
Refractory period	Decrease	Increase
His-Purkinje/ ventricular muscle		
Conduction velocity	Increase	No change
Refractory period	Decrease	Increase
Automaticity	Increase	No change

[a]Results from bretylium-induced release of norepinephrine from adrenergic nerve terminals.

(270) and corresponds temporally with the release of catecholamines from sympathetic nerve terminals. No change (271) or a slight decrease (270,272) in sinus heart rate is observed after the initial phase of catecholamine release.

Atria

At therapeutic concentrations, the only significant action of bretylium is to prolong the action-potential duration (273). This results in prolongation of the effective refractory period in atrial tissue (269,270). The action-potential amplitude, excitability, and membrane responsiveness are not altered (273), and there does not appear to be any alteration in intraatrial conduction times (274). Quinidinelike actions (depression of membrane responsiveness and a decrease in conduction velocity in cardiac tissue) that characterize class I antiarrhythmic drugs such as quinidine, procainamide, or disopyramide are not observed with bretylium *in vivo* (269,270) and are observed in *in vitro* tissue preparations only at concentrations that are far in excess of those attained in plasma at therapeutic doses (273). Surgical denervation incompletely reverses the

increase in the atrial effective refractory period observed after bretylium administration and suggests that the increase in the atrial effective refractory period is a direct action of the drug on atrial muscle (270).

In clinical studies, the only prominent electrophysiologic effect of bretylium in atrial muscle in prolongation of the atrial effective refractory period (269). The effect of bretylium on conduction and refractoriness in A-V accessory pathways is unknown.

A-V Node

The direct action of bretylium on the A-V node is to slow A-V nodal conduction velocity and increase the A-V nodal refractory period (269,270). However, this action is observed primarily with large doses of bretylium. In humans, moderate bretylium doses increase conduction velocity and decrease the A-V nodal refractory period (269). This action may result from the initial catecholamine release, and the net effect of bretylium on A-V transmission with chronic therapy is unknown. Improvement of A-V transmission as a result of the initial catecholamine release excludes bretylium from clinical use in the presence of atrial fibrillation or flutter because a dangerous acceleration of ventricular rate may occur. Bretylium should not be administered in the presence of A-V block resulting from digitalis glycoside toxicity. Although the initial phase of catecholamine release will improve A-V transmission, catecholamine release will also potentiate digitalis-induced ventricular automaticity and may lead to ventricular fibrillation (275).

His-Purkinje System/Ventricular Muscle

Quinidinelike actions (decreased membrane responsiveness and decreased conduction velocity) associated with class I antiarrhythmic agents are not observed with bretylium (21,22,270) and not responsible for the antifibrillatory actions of the drug. At therapeutic concentrations, the predominant effect of bretylium on the canine Purkinje cell and ventricular muscle is an increase in the action-potential duration (21,22), resulting in an increase in the effective refractory period (270). The increase in the effective refractory period in Purkinje cells and ventricular muscle is greater than that observed with other currently approved antiarrhythmic agents and is the property that distinguishes bretylium as a member of the class III antiarrhythmic agents. Prolongation of the action-potential duration and effective refractory period cannot be explained by the actions of the drug on the sympathetic nervous system, as the action-potential duration and effective refractory periods are prolonged in denervated hearts (270), reserpine-pretreated animals (21), and hearts lacking intact sympathetic nervous system innervation (276).

The initial catecholamine release brings about an increase in automaticity in Purkinje fiber (21,22) and will increase the rate of a ventricular escape rhythm (270). The increase in the rate of ectopic impulse formation is most prominent in Purkinje tissue that has been damaged by myocardial ischemia (277). Reserpine pretreatment prevents the increase in Purkinje cell automaticity (21).

The most prominent electrophysiologic action of bretylium is to raise the intensity of electrical current necessary to induce ventricular fibrillation (262,278–281). This action is more prominent with bretylium than with other currently available antiarrhythmic agents belonging to class I or II and can be observed in both normal (262,278,280,281) and ischemic hearts (279,281). Spontaneous conversion of ventricular fibrillation to sinus rhythm in humans has been observed after bretylium administration (282). Chemical defibrillation is a property possessed by bretylium and other members of class III agents (282,283). The antifibrillatory actions of bretylium are not believed to result from bretylium's actions on the sympa-

thetic nervous system, as guanethidine, a compound that exerts similar actions on the sympathetic nervous system, fails to exert antifibrillatory effects in canine myocardium (278,284). Bretylium is equally as effective in reserpinized hearts (284) and hearts lacking intact adrenergic innervation (280).

Currently approved class I and II antiarrhythmic agents (quinidine, lidocaine, phenytoin, disopyramide, procainamide, and propranolol) raise the current necessary to defibrillate canine hearts (285). In contrast to this action, bretylium lowers the electrical threshold for successful defibrillation (286). This beneficial action of bretylium was previously reported by Holder et al. (264), who showed an increased rate of successful defibrillations after bretylium administration.

Hemodynamic and Cardiovascular Effects

A unique property of bretylium as an antiarrhythmic agent is its positive inotropic action (287–289). This action is related to the initial release of neuronal stores of norepinephrine associated with bretylium administration.

Bretylium's actions on the sympathetic nervous system include (a) an initial release of neuronal stores of norepinephrine and (b) an inhibition of norepinephrine release resulting from sympathetic nerve stimulation. The initial phase of catecholamine release may be associated with transient hypertension (268,271), although the most commonly observed side effect of bretylium is hypotension associated with the later development of adrenergic neuronal blockade (262,263,266–268,287). The onset of hypotension is delayed 1 to 2 hr, as the initial catecholamine release maintains arterial pressure prior to this time. Hypotension is most commonly postural, but marked reductions in supine blood pressure have been reported (271,272). Despite decreases in peripheral resistance and arterial pressure, cardiac output is maintained, and pulmonary capillary wedge pressure is not altered (287).

The hazards involved with bretylium administration, especially in the patient with acute myocardial infarction, include its positive inotropic and chronotropic effects, which may aggravate existing myocardial ischemia by further increasing myocardial oxygen requirements. Because bretylium has the potential to interfere with adrenergic tone to the heart and peripheral vasculature, it may cause further deterioration of an already compromised hemodynamic status.

Bretylium has been reported to eliminate heart block and to augment pacemaker activity (266). The low incidence of heart block of 1.6% in patients treated with bretylium, as compared with 12% in an earlier study, has suggested that bretylium prevents the emergence of heart block.

Toxic Reactions

The most important side effect associated with the use of bretylium is hypotension, as a result of peripheral vasodilation caused by adrenergic blockade. Hypotension, when it does occur, is reversed readily by intravenous fluid to increase circulating blood volume and by cautious administration of intravenous norepinephrine. Bradycardia resulting from adrenergic neuronal blockade has been observed in some patients receiving bretylium. Nausea, vomiting, and diarrhea have been reported with intravenous administration and can be minimized by slow infusion. Longer term problems include swelling and tenderness of the parotid gland, particularly occurring at meal time.

Pharmacokinetics

Bretylium, a quaternary ammonium compound with a fixed positive charge, has poor systemic availability after oral administration. Plasma concentrations after oral administration are erratic, reaching peak concentrations in approximately 3 hr with only 10% to 30% of an oral dose reaching the general circulation. Bretylium is well absorbed after intramuscular injection, with peak plasma concentrations being attained within 1 hr.

No metabolites of bretylium have been observed in any animal species, and the drug is excreted almost entirely by renal mechanisms. More than 90% of oral, intramuscular, and intravenous doses are excreted unchanged in the urine over a period of 48 hr. The remaining 10% is excreted over the next 3 days. Renal clearance is rapid and approaches that of total renal blood flow at lower bretylium plasma concentrations. This suggests that active secretion of bretylium takes place in the renal tubules. Clearance of bretylium by the kidney is reduced by renal disease, but it is not known to what extent drug dosage must be altered in such clinical conditions. Renal clearance of bretylium depends on the amount in the plasma and is more rapid at lower plasma bretylium concentrations.

Pharmacokinetic values for bretylium are given in Table 20. The concentration of bretylium in plasma has not been correlated with the intensity of its antiarrhythmic response and cannot be used as a guide for therapy. There is a complex relationship (281) between plasma bretylium concentrations, myocardial bretylium concentrations, and antifibrillatory activity. The electrophysiologic actions (262,278,281) and clinical efficacy (266,267,271) of bretylium are not apparent immediately, and a delay in onset of 3 to 6 hr may occur. Despite the rapid elimination of bretylium from plasma, the antiarrhythmic action of bretylium may persist for 8 to 14 hr or more after intravenous administration (266,267,271).

Dose and Administration

Bretylium is to be used clinically for treatment of patients with life-threatening

TABLE 20. *Pharmacokinetic properties of bretylium*

Absorption
  Administered by intravenous or intramuscular injection; oral absorption is poor
Protein binding
  Negligible; the drug accumulates in sympathetic ganglia and postadrenergic neurons
Metabolism
  None
Half-life
  Average 5 to 10 hr with a range of 4 to 17 hr
Time to peak plasma concentration
  Depends on rate of administration; the drug should be administered as a slow intravenous infusion over 15 to 30 min
Therapeutic plasma concentration
  The quaternary ammonium compound is difficult to assay and plasma concentrations show little relationship to antiarrhythmic efficacy
Elimination
  Renal: >90% of the administered dose is excreted in the urine as the unchanged drug; in the course of 24 hr, 70% to 80% of the drug is eliminated; the dose should be reduced in patients with impaired renal function

ventricular arrhythmias. Because there is a delay in the onset of its antiarrhythmic action, bretylium is not to be considered or used as a replacement for rapidly acting antiarrhythmic agents currently in use. Patients should either be kept supine during the course of bretylium therapy or be observed closely for hypotension. There is comparatively little experience with dosages greater than 30 mg/kg/day, although such doses have been used without apparent adverse effects. The following schedule is suggested.

For immediately life-threatening ventricular arrhythmias, as in ventricular fibrillation. Administer undiluted bretylium at a dosage of 5 mg/kg/body weight by rapid intravenous injection. Other usual cardiopulmonary resuscitative procedures, including electrical cardioversion, should be employed prior to and following the injection in accordance with good medical practice. If ventricular fibrillation persists, the dosage may be increased to 10 mg/kg and repeated at 15- to 30-min intervals until a total dose of not more than 30 mg/kg/body weight has been given.

For prevention of recurrent ventricular tachycardia and/or fibrillation (intravenous use). Administer a dosage of 5 to 10 mg bretylium/kg/body weight by intravenous infusion over a period greater than 8 min. More rapid infusion may cause nausea and vomiting. A second dose may be given in 1 to 2 hr if tachyarrhythmia recurs.

For intramuscular injection. Inject 5 to 10 mg bretylium/kg/body weight. Dosage may be repeated in 1 to 2 hr if the arrhythmias persist. Thereafter, maintain with same dosage every 6 to 8 hr. Intramuscular injection should not be made directly into or near a major nerve, and the sites of injection should be varied on repeated injection.

Maintenance dosage. The diluted bretylium solution may be administered by intermittent intravenous infusion or by constant infusion.

Intermittent infusion. Infuse the diluted solution at a dosage of 5 to 10 mg bretylium/kg/body weight over a period greater than 8 min, every 6 hr. More rapid infusion may cause nausea and vomiting.

Constant infusion. Infuse the diluted solution at a dosage of 1 to 2 mg bretylium/min. Dosage of bretylium should be reduced and discontinued in 3 to 5 days under electrocardiographic monitoring. Other appropriate antiarrhythmic agents should be substituted, if indicated.

Contraindications

The pharmacologic properties of bretylium should dictate in which instances the drug will be contraindicated. The associated release of catecholamines could result in an excessive pressor rise and stimulation of cardiac force and pacemaker activity. The resulting increase in myocardial oxygen consumption in a patient with ischemic heart disease could lead to the development of ischemic pain (angina pectoris).

Patients in a state of circulatory shock should probably not be administered bretylium because of its delayed sympatholytic action, which would cause further deterioration of the hemodynamic state of the individual.

Indications

Bretylium is not to be considered a first-line antiarrhythmic agent. However, because of its ability to prolong the refractory period of Purkinje fibers and elevate the electrical threshold to ventricular fibrillation, bretylium has been studied and found useful in the treatment of life-threatening ventricular arrhythmias, principally recurrent ventricular tachycardia and/or fibrillation, especially when conventional therapeutic agents such as lidocaine or procainamide prove to be ineffective. In addition, bretylium is known to facilitate the ease with which precordial shock reverses ventricular fibrillation (264,286). In the latter instance, because of the emergent nature of the patient's clinical state, the drug is administered intravenously in dosages of 5 to 20 mg/kg as a rapid bolus, followed by external cardiac massage and repeated attempts at electrical defibrillation. It is not unusual for bretylium, when administered in the presence of ventricular fibrillation and accompanied by external cardiac massage, to result in defibrillation and a return to coordinated cardiac rhythm. Bretylium is there-

fore capable of producing chemical defibrillation when its administration is accompanied by cardiopulmonary resuscitative procedures.

It is important to recognize that the use of bretylium for the prevention of recurrent ventricular tachycardia and/or ventricular fibrillation may lead to apparent disappointing results because of the fact that the onset of its antifibrillatory effect may be delayed for as long as 6 hr. Thus, the drug has a delayed onset of action when given as a slow intravenous infusion. The delay in its onset of action is undoubtedly related to the fact that the drug must achieve a critical concentration in myocardial tissue before it can favorably alter the electrophysiologic properties of the heart. Furthermore, the release of norepinephrine from cardiac nerve endings during the administration of bretylium may actually increase the frequency of ventricular premature complexes, an event that is worsened by rapid intravenous administration of the drug.

It was long assumed that the antifibrillatory effects of bretylium were associated with the ability of the drug to produce adrenergic neuronal blockade as a result of uptake into sympathetic nerve fibers. It is appreciated now that the adrenergic neuronal blocking action is unnecessary for bretylium to produce its protective effects against the recurrence of ventricular tachycardia and/or ventricular fibrillation. Previous administration of a tricyclic antidepressant drug, such as protriptyline or doxepin, which effectively blocks the amine uptake mechanism in adrenergic neurons, will prevent bretylium from gaining access to the adrenergic nerves. Thus, the catecholamine release and subsequent sympatholytic effects of bretylium can be prevented without affecting the electrophysiologic effects of the quaternary amine of the heart, therefore retaining the potential to confer an antifibrillatory effect. This form of pharmacologic antagonism can be put to good use when it becomes necessary to avoid excessive hypotension in a patient in need of the protective effects of bretylium.

Present indications for the use of bretylium limit its administration to no longer than 5 days. The drug is available for parenteral use only. However, a limited number of patients known to be at risk of developing recurrent ventricular fibrillation have been managed successfully for long terms by first being administered an intravenous dosing regimen for 24 to 48 hr and then being placed on oral drug (300–600 mg every 6 hr) (267,290,291). Repeated determinations of plasma and urine bretylium concentrations have confirmed the ability of the drug to be absorbed after oral administration (291). The low incidences of side effects following chronic administration make bretylium and other quaternary ammonium agents attractive drugs for future study in an attempt to reduce the incidence of sudden coronary death.

Amiodarone

Amiodarone hydrochloride (2-butyl-3-benzofuranyl)-[4-[2-diethylamino]ethoxy]-3,5-dilodophenyl methanone) was introduced originally as a coronary vasodilator and antianginal agent and subsequently became recognized as having unique pharmacologic properties with the potential to exert a wide range of antiarrhythmic actions. The development of amiodarone, its pharmacology, and therapeutic applications have been reviewed extensively (292–296). Amiodarone (Fig. 20) is an iodinated benzofuran derivative, first introduced in 1967 in Belgium and France and approved for use in the United States in December of 1985 as an oral agent for the management of patients with life-threatening cardiac arrhythmias. The agent possesses unusually complex pharmacodynamic and pharmacokinetic characteristics and significant toxic effects so as to make its use difficult and best undertaken by those familiar with its therapeutic application. Its use in the United States is restricted to patients with serious ventricular tachyarrhythmias not controlled by other pharmacologic measures. The drug has been used successfully for both supraventricular and ventricular arrhythmias. Despite having been available for more than 20 years, the underlying mechanism(s) for its antiarrhythmic action remains unknown. The overall pharmacologic effects of amiodarone may derive from both direct and indirect actions on cardiac tissues.

Electrophysiologic Actions

The most notable electrophysiologic effect of amiodarone after long-term administration is a prolongation of repolarization and refractoriness in all cardiac tissues; an action that is characteristic of those members of the class III group of antiarrhythmic agents. The electrophysiologic changes observed clinically as well as its efficacy as an antidysrhythmic agent are delayed in their onset. The exact mechanism of action of amiodarone is unknown. Some structural resemblance to thyroid hormone and the fact that the electrophysiologic changes resemble those seen after thyroidectomy have suggested to some that the drug may

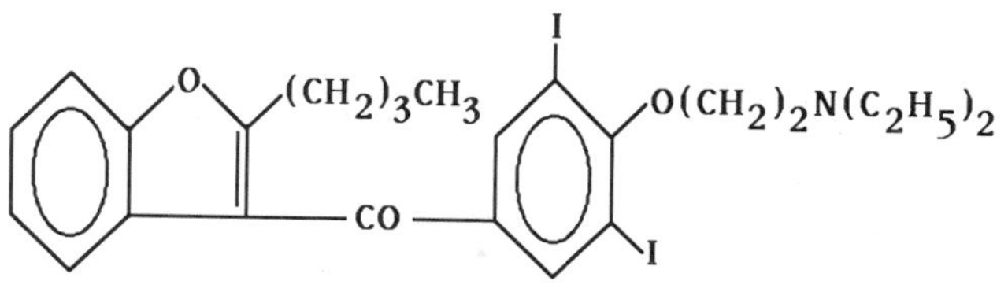

FIG. 20. Amiodarone.

in some manner interfere with the action of thyroxine or triiodothyronine on heart muscle. It has been suggested that the drug may prevent the conversion of T4 to T3 at the tissue level (297).

Amiodarone shows a wide spectrum of clinical efficacy in the management of cardiac arrhythmias consistent with its electrophysiologic actions on atrial and A-V nodal refractoriness and conduction velocity and on the electrophysiologic alterations in Purkinje and ventricular tissues.

Sinoatrial Node

Amiodarone was shown to decrease the action-potential amplitude and the slope of phase 4 of the membrane action potential recorded from the sinoatrial node (298). The cycle length of the sinoatrial node is increased by amiodarone as well as by its metabolite, desethylamiodarone (299). There are data to suggest that the depressant action of amiodarone on sinoatrial pacemaker function may be related to an inhibition of the slow inward current carried by the calcium ion (300).

Atria

Amiodarone causes prolongation of the action potential in atrial muscle as well as an increase in the absolute and effective refractory periods. Amiodarone was administered to rabbits for 1 to 6 weeks after which cardiac tissues were subjected to electrophysiologic examination (297). The drug did not alter the resting membrane potential or the action potential amplitude in atrial tissue. V_{max} was reduced slightly. The major effect observed was a prolongation in action potential duration. The effects of amiodarone on atrial muscle resembled those observed to occur in rabbit atrial tissue obtained from hypothyroid animals (301). An important feature noted with the chronic administration of amiodarone to

rabbits was the fact that the electrophysiologic alterations in atrial muscle were continuing to increase as a function of time, suggesting the role of a metabolite or an alteration in cellular metabolism. Of further interest was the finding that the progressive electrophysiologic changes could be prevented by the simultaneous administration of thyroid hormone. It was suggested that the action of amiodarone after its chronic administration may be related to an inhibitory effect on a thyroid-dependent metabolite pathway. After 6 weeks of therapy in humans, the electrophysiologic alteration in the atria was characterized by a marked prolongation in action-potential duration as recorded with suction electrodes (302). Amiodarone is an effective suppressant of atrial premature activity, which serves as a potential-triggering mechanism for the induction of supraventricular tachyarrhythmias.

A-V Node

Amiodarone, as well as its major metabolite desethylamiodarone, increases A-V nodal conduction time and refractory period. The electrophysiologic alterations in A-V nodal function depend on the rate of atrial stimulation and are consistent with use-dependent blockade of the slow inward calcium current. Junctional automaticity is reduced in vitro and in vivo by the parent compound as well as by the active metabolite. The actions on the A-V node may be related in part to the ability of amiodarone to alter β-adrenoceptor function. After chronic oral therapy with amiodarone there is a greater effect on the A-V nodal effective and functional refractory periods than after acute administration of the drug (292).

In patients with WPW syndrome, amiodarone prolongs the refractory period in the A-V nodal-His pathway and in the accessory A-V pathway. These actions most likely contribute to the efficacy of the drug in the prevention of reentrant supraventricular tachyarrhythmias.

His-Purkinje System and Ventricular Myocardium

As with many antiarrhythmic agents, the actions of amiodarone on the electrophysiology of the His-Purkinje system may be related to its direct as well as its indirect actions. Data derived with the acute application of amiodarone may not coincide with information derived from studies in which the drug is administered for a prolonged period. The acute and chronic effects of amiodarone on the electrophysiology of the cardiac tissue must be distinguished. From the standpoint of its clinical application, the effects of the long-term administration of the drug would appear to be most important in an understanding of the mechanism by which it may effectively control disorders of heart rhythm.

In vitro studies involving the acute application of amiodarone or its metabolite to cardiac tissues have demonstrated that the electrophysiologic effects are no greater at higher concentrations compared with lower concentrations. A definite period of exposure to the drug or its metabolite, desethylamiodarone, is required for the full expression of the electrophysiologic effects. The most prominent electrophysiologic alterations observed with amiodarone and its metabolite occur when the drug is administered chronically. The dominant effect on ventricular myocardium in hearts obtained from rabbits chronically treated with either amiodarone or desethylamiodarone was a prolongation in the action-potential duration with an associated increase in the refractory period and a modest decrease in V_{max} as a function of stimulus frequency (303). Amiodarone has been reported to decrease the delayed outward potassium current, a finding consistent with the observation of a prolonged action potential duration (304). Aomine et al. (305) and Yabek et al. (299) observed that both amiodarone and its metabolite significantly decreased the action-potential duration and shortened the effective refractory period in Purkinje fibers while at the same time causing a prolongation of action potential in ventricular muscle. Under normal conditions the action-potential duration in Purkinje fiber is longer than that in ventricular myocardium. The differential effects of amiodarone on Purkinje fiber action-potential duration versus that of the ventricular muscle may be of significance with respect to its antiarrhythmic action. Studies in guinea pig myocardium and Purkinje tissue have demonstrated effective sodium channel blockade with amiodarone (306). The drug is unique among agents that block the sodium channel in that the blockade occurs during phases 2 and 3 of the action potential at a time when the sodium channels are inactivated. Therefore, amiodarone would be expected to have a more prominent effect on depolarized tissue as occurs in the presence of myocardial ischemia.

Electrocardiographic Changes

As in the experimental studies discussed above, significant differences exist between the electrophysiologic changes produced by long-term oral amiodarone therapy as compared with acute intravenous administration of the drug. The major consistent actions of chronic, oral amiodarone therapy in humans are a prolongation of the sinus cycle length, prolongation of the duration of repolarization, increase in A-V nodal conduction time, and prolongation of the atrial, His-Purkinje, ventricular, and A-V nodal refractoriness. Low doses of amiodarone do not affect infranodal conduction time and QRS duration. These parameters are prolonged with higher doses. In the presence of an accessory pathway, amiodarone will increase the refractory period of the bypass tissue.

The predominant electrocardiographic changes observed with the administration of amiodarone consist of a decrease in the sinus rate of 10% to 15%, a prolongation of the PR and QT intervals, the development of U waves and changes in T-wave contour. In rare instances QT prolongation has been associated with a worsening of arrhythmias.

Hemodynamic Effects

Amiodarone relaxes vascular smooth muscle with one of its most prominent effects being on the coronary circulation thereby reducing coronary vascular resistance and improving regional myocardial blood flow. In addition, its effects on the peripheral vascular bed lead to a decrease in left ventricular stroke work and myocardial oxygen consumption. Therefore, amiodarone has a beneficial effect on the relationship between myocardial oxygen demand and oxygen supply. After oral administration, amiodarone does not induce significant changes in left ventricular ejection fraction, even in patients with impaired left ventricular function. A negative inotropic action may be observed, however, when amiodarone is administered intravenously. This response may in part be associated with the ability of the drug to induce β-adrenoceptor blockade.

Toxic Reactions

The use of amiodarone is associated with numerous adverse reactions. Those of most concern are hepatitis, exacerbation of arrhythmias, worsening of congestive heart failure, and pneumonitis.

Pulmonary toxicity results in clinically manifest disease in 10% to 15% of patients who receive 400 mg/day of the drug. The development of alterations in pulmonary diffusion capacity without symptoms occurs with a much greater frequency. Approximately 10% of patients who manifest pulmonary toxicity go on to a fatal course. If pulmonary toxicity is suspected, the drug must be withdrawn and clinical improvement may be anticipated within several weeks. The histologic findings on light microscopy are characterized by intraalveolar accumulation of foamy macrophages, alveolar septal thickening, and hyperplasia of type II pneumocytes. Multilaminar inclusion bodies within lysosomes of alveolar cells are revealed on ultrastructural examination.

Hepatic toxicity manifested as elevations in liver enzyme levels is seen frequently in patients taking amiodarone. Discontinuation of the drug is recommended if the liver enzyme concentrations exceed three times normal.

The majority of adults receiving amiodarone will develop corneal microdeposits. The changes are usually observed only by slit-lamp examination. As many as 10% of patients will observe halos or blurred vision. The corneal microdeposits are reversible on stopping the drug.

Photosensitization occurs in approximately 10% of patients taking amiodarone. With continued treatment the skin assumes a blue-gray coloration. The risk is increased in patients of fair complexion. The discoloration of the skin regresses slowly, if at all, after discontinuation of amiodarone.

Significant alterations in thyroid function occur with the continued use of amiodarone. Amiodarone inhibits the peripheral and, possibly, intrapituitary conversion of thyroxine (T4) to triiodothyronine (T3) by inhibiting 5'-deiodination. There is an increase in the serum concentration of T4 due to a decrease in its clearance and an increase in thyroid synthesis due to a reduced suppression of the pituitary thyrotropin by T3. The concentration of T3 in the serum decreases and reverse T3 appears in increased amounts. Despite these changes, the majority of patients appear to be maintained in a euthyroid state. Manifestations of both hypo- and hyperthyroidism have been reported.

Neuromuscular side effects have been reported in association with the use of amiodarone. Tremors of the hands, sleep disturbances in the form of vivid dreams, nightmares, insomnia, ataxia, and staggering and impaired ambulation have been noted. Peripheral sensory and motor neuropathy or severe proximal muscle weakness develop infrequently. Both neuropathic and myopathic changes are observed on biopsy. Neurologic symptoms resolve or improve within several weeks of dosage reduction.

Pharmacokinetics

The pharmacokinetic properties of amiodarone are summarized in Table 21. Amiodarone is absorbed slowly after oral administration. Bioavailability varies widely and is estimated to be between 35% and 65%. After a single dose, the maximum plasma concentration is reached in 3 to 7 hr. The onset of antiarrhythmic action may take from 2 to 3 days but more commonly is achieved only after 1 to 3 weeks even with the use of a loading dose.

The volume of distribution of amiodarone is extremely large (60 liters/kg) because of the extensive deposition in adipose tissue and highly perfused organs. The plasma clearance is low with negligible renal elimination. The major metabolite is desethylamiodarone, which achieves a plasma ratio of one with respect to the parent compound after chronic administration.

Hepatic excretion into the bile is the primary route of elimination of amiodarone and its major metabolite. Neither the parent compound nor the metabolite is dialyzable. After discontinuation of amiodarone, the plasma half-life varies from 26 to 107 days, with a mean of approximately 53 days. The elimination half-life of desethylamiodarone is longer than that of the parent drug.

There is no apparent relationship between the plasma concentration of amiodarone and its clinical efficacy. It has been observed that concentrations below 1 mg/liter are associated with lack of efficacy, whereas plasma concentrations of less than 2.5 mg/liter are needed.

Dose

Amiodarone should be administered by physicians who are experienced in the treatment of life-threatening arrhythmias and versed in the risks and benefits of the therapeutic agent.

Loading doses are essential to achieve a

TABLE 21. *Pharmacokinetic properties of amiodarone*

Absorption
  Slow and variable with approximately 20% to 55% of an oral dose being absorbed; the drug is widely distributed in the body with the highest concentration being found in adipose tissue, liver, spleen, and lungs, and accounts for slow achievement of steady state and long period of elimination
Protein binding
  Very high, approximating 96%
Metabolism
  Metabolized extensively with one active metabolite; desethylamiodarone being formed; possibly undergoes deiodination so that a dose of 300 mg will release approximately 9 mg of elemental iodine
Half-life
  Elimination is biphasic with an initial $t_{1/2}$ of 2.5 to 10 days and a terminal elimination phase of 26 to 107 days with a mean of 53 days (40–55 days in most patients)
Time to peak plasma concentration
  May be achieved after 3 to 7 hr; however, the onset of action may be within 2 to 3 days to 2 to 3 months; plasma concentration may be detectable up to 9 months after discontinuing the drug
Therapeutic plasma concentration
  1 to 2.5 μg/ml at steady state, which may occur after 2 months of therapy; there is a poor correlation between the plasma concentration and antiarrhythmic efficacy
Elimination
  Renal: <1% of the dose is excreted in the urine as unchanged drug; biliary elimination occurs and 25% of administered dose is excreted in breast milk

therapeutic effect within a reasonable period. For life-threatening arrhythmias, loading should be performed in a hospital setting. Loading doses of 800 to 1,600 mg/day are required for 1 to 3 weeks or longer until an initial therapeutic response is achieved. The reduction in the frequency of ectopic complexes and the elimination of recurrent ventricular tachycardia or fibrillation usually occurs within 1 to 3 weeks. The dose is reduced to 600 to 800 mg/day after 1 month with the chronic maintenance dose being on the order of 400 mg/day.

Contraindications

Amiodarone is contraindicated in patients with sick-sinus syndrome and may cause severe bradycardia and second- and third-degree A-V block.

Indications

Amiodarone is indicated for the management of patients with documented life-threatening recurrent ventricular arrhythmias that are not controlled by other therapeutic interventions.

The approved indicated uses are for recurrent ventricular fibrillation and recurrent hemodynamically unstable ventricular tachycardia. There is no evidence that amiodarone influences survival in patients subject to sudden coronary death.

Amiodarone is effective for maintaining sinus rhythm in most patients with paroxysmal atrial fibrillation and in many patients with persistent atrial fibrillation. It is effective in preventing recurrences of A-V nodal reentry and atrial tachyarrhythmias. The drug is effective in the prevention of reentrant rhythms and atrial fibrillation in patients with WPW syndrome. Amiodarone favorably alters the electrophysiologic properties of the different components involved in maintaining reentrant tachyarrhythmias associated with WPW syndrome in addition to preventing the initiation of the tachyarrhythmias by suppressing atrial premature depolarizations.

Verapamil

Verapamil 5-[(3,4-dimethoxyphenethyl) methylamino] - 2 - (3,4 - dimethoxyphenyl) - 2-isopropylvaleronitrile monohydrochloride (Fig. 21) was intended initially as a synthetic substitute for the smooth muscle relaxant papaverine. The drug was studied for its peripheral and coronary vasodilator properties in preclinical and clinical settings. Because of its ability to affect coronary vascular smooth muscle, much attention has been focused on the use of verapamil as a therapeutic intervention in the management of patients with variant an-

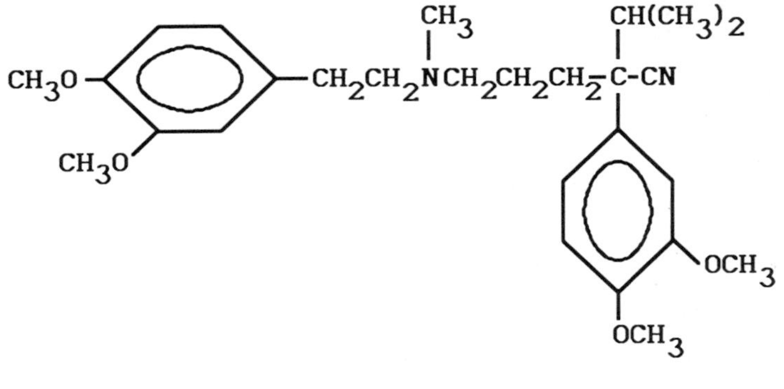

FIG. 21. Verapamil.

gina pectoris (Prinzmetal's angina), as well as patients with effort-induced angina pectoris.

Although it was first thought to be a specific inhibitor of β-adrenergic receptors, subsequent experimental studies revealed that verapamil, in addition to possessing antiarrhythmic properties, produced selective inhibition of transmembrane calcium fluxes in myocardial cells by affecting a secondary inward depolarizing current that flows through a slow channel. This current is carried primarily by calcium ions, and voltage changes due to this current are referred to as slow channel depolarizations or slow responses.

The transmembrane action potentials obtained from cells in the sinoatrial and A-V nodes show potentials with the characteristics of slow channel calcium currents. Thus, depolarization within the sinoatrial and A-V nodal regions may depend on an inward current through the slow channel and one that is susceptible to the inhibitory effects of verapamil and other slow channel calcium antagonists, thereby accounting for the use of the agent in supraventricular A-V nodal reentrant arrhythmias (307,308).

Electrophysiologic Actions

When studied in myocardial tissues in clinically relevant concentrations, verapamil fails to elicit effects characteristic of those produced by the class I, II, or III antiarrhythmic drugs. Evidence that excitation-contraction coupling in mammalian heart muscle could be blocked *in vitro* and *in vivo* by pharmacologic means was first presented by Fleckenstein (309). This calcium antagonism by verapamil is considered to be a specific action, as opposed to nonspecific calcium-antagonistic effects obtained with high dosages of barbiturates or certain β-adrenergic receptor blocking agents. Thus, the specific calcium antagonists produce their effects at concentrations at which other pharmacologic actions are negligible. Exposure of

guinea pig isolated papillary muscle to increasing concentrations of verapamil (2×10^{-6} M to 1×10^{-5} M) results in a progressive loss of contractility without affecting the membrane resting potential or the action-potential parameters, such as upstroke velocity and height of the overshoot (310). These findings indicate that the transmembrane sodium flux across the fast channel is unchanged by verapamil. The inhibitor effects of verapamil on calcium influx and contractile tension can be overcome by addition of calcium or isoproterenol.

Sinoatrial Node

Pacemaker activity in the sinoatrial node has an ionic mechanism completely different from action potentials generated in Purkinje fibers or ordinary atrial muscle cells. Spontaneous phase-4 depolarization, a characteristic of normal sinoatrial nodal cells, relies on deactivation of an outward current that is selective for potassium ions and a slow inward current that is carried by sodium and calcium ions. Thus, from the standpoint of verapamil's effect on inward calcium ion fluxes, it is understandable that the drug depresses phase-4 depolarization in the sinoatrial node. Verapamil produces reductions in the rate of rise and the slope of diastolic slow depolarization, the maximal diastolic potential, and the membrane potential at the peak of depolarization in the sinoatrial node (311,312). These findings provide additional support for the belief that the slow channel calcium current is of primary importance in the genesis of sinoatrial nodal pacemaker activity. *In vivo*, the direct effect of verapamil on sinoatrial nodal function will be manifest as a decrease in heart rate (negative chronotropic effect). However, cardiovascular reflexes in response to the changes in cardiac output and peripheral vascular resistance will result in enhancement of cardiac sympathetic tone, thereby masking the direct negative chronotropic effects of verapamil.

Atria

Verapamil fails to exert any significant electrophysiologic effects on atrial muscle. Although contractile force is depressed, the only change in the action potential of atrial muscle fibers is a shortening of the early phase of repolarization. This is not unexpected, because of the early phase of repolarization or phase 2 depends on the slow inward calcium current that is antagonized by verapamil. Electrophysiologic recordings from diseased atrial tissue obtained during surgery have demonstrated that verapamil can inhibit spontaneous diastolic activity, therefore suggesting the participation of the slow channel calcium current in the genesis of human atrial rhythm disorders (313). These findings are of significance in view of the potential role of verapamil in the clinical management of supraventricular arrhythmias.

A-V Node

Action potentials from the nodal region of the A-V junction resemble slow responses, although automaticity is not a property of the true nodal region of the A-V junction. The speed of conduction in the nodal region is quite slow. Conduction block is common, and graded electrical responses are frequent. In addition, refractoriness in A-V nodal tissue outlasts the action-potential duration. These observations suggest that depolarization in A-V nodal cells, like that in sinoatrial nodal tissue, is dependent on an inward current through the slow channel. It is well known that A-V nodal conduction is depressed by pharmacologic agents that block the slow channel calcium current. Verapamil would therefore be expected to impair conduction across the A-V node and prolong the A-V nodal refractory period at plasma concentrations that show no effect on the His-Purkinje system. A-V nodal reentry, one mechanism for maintaining reciprocating tachycardia, is prevented by verapamil, and this accounts for the effectiveness of verapamil in the treatment of supraventricular tachyarrhythmias (314). This action agrees with the role of the slow-channel calcium current in A-V nodal transmission and the proposed cellular mechanism of action of verapamil.

His-Purkinje System/Ventricular Muscle

In clinically relevant concentrations, verapamil does not have electrophysiologic effects of the class I antiarrhythmic drugs. When examined in canine Purkinje fiber action potentials, verapamil had no effect on the action-potential amplitude of V_{max} or on resting membrane potential. However, the slope of phase-2 repolarization is increased by verapamil. These changes are consistent with the block of a slow inward current such as that carried by the calcium ion (313). Further evidence for a lack of effect on the His-Purkinje system was obtained from data showing that verapamil failed to produce any change in the QRS and QT_c intervals. The only significant electrocardiographic change was a prolongation of the PR interval, a response consistent with the known effects of the drug on A-V nodal transmission (315).

His-bundle studies have provided further evidence that verapamil is without effect on intraatrial and intraventricular conduction. The predominant electrophysiologic effect is on A-V conduction proximal to the His bundle.

Hemodynamic Effects

Studies on isolated cardiac muscle preparations have shown verapamil to possess a negative inotropic action, a response consistent with its ability to reduce influx of calcium during the rapid phase of depolarization as well as phase 2 of the action-potential plateau. The negative inotropic effect can be counteracted by calcium, catecholamines, glucagon, and digitalis glycosides. When administered to intact animals or humans, verapamil shows a dose-dependent negative inotropic effect that is modified by reflex sympathetic responses. Verapamil produces peripheral vasodilation by a direct relaxant effect on vascular smooth muscle. The peripheral vasodilation results in changes in preload and afterload and changes in cardiac sympathetic tone that exert a complex interplay of factors affecting stroke volume and cardiac output. The negative inotropic action exerted by verapamil and the expected reduction in cardiac output are minimized by the effects of the drug on left ventricular afterload. The usual intravenous dose of verapamil employed for antiarrhythmic effects (10 mg) is not associated with marked alterations in arterial blood pressure, peripheral vascular resistance, heart rate, left ventricular end-diastolic pressure, or contractility. The changes that do occur on intravenous administration are short-lived. It must be recalled that the presence of an intact cardiac sympathetic nervous system markedly attenuates the cardiac depressant effects of the calcium antagonist. On the other hand, profound cardiac depression and disturbances in A-V conduction are more likely to occur when verapamil is administered concomitantly with propranolol or other β-adrenergic receptor blocking agents. The same concerns regarding the negative inotropic effects of verapamil might apply to the patient with severe cardiac decompensation or acute myocardial infarction.

Because of its capacity to modify calcium ion fluxes in vascular smooth muscle and thus interfere with excitation-contraction coupling, verapamil elicits relaxation of peripheral vessels as well as those supplying the myocardium. The coronary vasodilator effects of verapamil and its ability to decrease myocardial contractility and afterload and thus reduce myocardial oxygen consumption have suggested its use in the management of patients with effort-induced angina pectoris and variant angina. In the latter instance, in which myocardial ischemia is related to coronary vasospasm, the vasodilator effect of verapamil appears to have major importance in preventing the recurrence of ischemic episodes.

The antianginal properties of verapamil have been attributed to its coronary vasodilator effects. However, selective coronary vasodilators have not proved effective in abolishing ischemic symptoms associated with effort-induced angina pectoris. The coronary vasodilator effects of verapamil have been revealed in studies in animals or in isolated perfused hearts. When administered to patients with coronary artery disease, verapamil fails to dilate the diseased coronary vascular segments and does not improve regional coronary blood flow (316,317).

Administration of verapamil to patients with coronary artery disease resulted in a decrease in coronary blood flow at rest and during pacing stress that was of sufficient magnitude to always cause angina pectoris in the period before drug administration (318). Intravenous administration of verapamil results in decreases in mean aortic blood pressure and myocardial oxygen consumption.

Therefore, in patients with exertional or effort-induced angina pectoris, the beneficial effect of verapamil is not primarily due to its coronary vasodilator actions. Instead, verapamil decreases myocardial oxygen consumption, which most likely accounts for its ability to improve exercise tolerance by restoring the balance between myocardial oxygen supply and demand. In the presence of vasospastic or variant angina, the vasodilator effect undoubtedly plays a major role in preventing myocardial ischemia. This effect can be attributed to verapamil's inhibition of the slow channel calcium flux in coronary vascular smooth muscle and is seen with other slow channel antagonists as well (319).

Toxic Reactions

The administration of oral verapamil is well tolerated by the majority of patients. Most complaints are with respect to the gastrointestinal side effects of constipation and gastric discomfort. Other complaints include vertigo, headache, nervousness, and pruritis.

The intravenous route of administration is associated with transient and mild decreases in blood pressure. However, because the drug has such a prominent effect on cellular fluxes of calcium, rapid intravenous administration or excessive dosage could lead to cardiac depression, both mechanically and electrically, along with peripheral vasodilation and hypotension. Cardiac depression and ventricular asystole are more prone to develop in patients given verapamil while concomitantly receiving propranolol.

Verapamil should not be administered or should be given with great caution to patients with sick-sinus syndrome, disturbances in A-V conduction, or severe congestive heart failure, unless the low output state can be attributed to a persistent rapid atrial tachyarrhythmia, in which case the reversion to sinus rhythm produced by verapamil will lead to improvement in cardiac function.

The combined actions of digitalis and verapamil seem to impose no special deleterious effects unless A-V conduction is already compromised, in which case further impairment of conduction can occur as a result of verapamil's effect on the A-V node, which will add to the effects of digitalis. The negative inotropic effect of verapamil could negate some of the benefits to be derived from the positive inotropic actions of digitalis. Likewise, digitalis glycosides could overcome the negative inotropic effects of verapamil. The potential use of verapamil in patients with acute myocardial infarction from the control of arrhythmias or as a means of preserving jeopardized ischemic myocardium has not been established.

Pharmacokinetics

Examination of the hemodynamic effects after a single intravenous dose of verapamil would suggest that the drug possesses a relatively short pharmacologic half-life. The maximum cardiovascular actions are observed within 3 to 5 min, with almost complete return to baseline values within 10 to 20 min. Similar observations with respect to pharmacologic effects have been made in patients with atrial fibrillation, in whom the ventricular rate in response to verapamil was noted to decrease within a few minutes after drug administration, only to resume the initial rate within a short time. On the other hand, measurements of the A-H intervals of His-Purkinje electrocardiograms indicated that a single intravenous dose of verapamil exerted electrophysiologic effects that became apparent within 1 to 2 min, reaching a maximum effect at 10 min, with residual effects being recorded for up to 6 hr.

Studies using oral verapamil have shown that the drug is active by this route of administration, with initial effects being apparent within 2 hr and a maximum effect being obtained within 5 hr, as determined by the ability of the agent to modify the electrophysiologic properties of the A-V node in humans. Thus, in evaluating pharmacokinetic data and the pharmacologic actions of verapamil, one might conclude that the two may not correlate with respect to their temporal relationships. One possibility is that verapamil or an active metabolite accumulates in cardiac tissue and continues to exert electrophysiologic effects independent of the plasma concentration of the drug. On the basis of electrophysiologic studies, there seems to be a preferential uptake by the A-V nodal tissues, because the duration of the depressant effect of verapamil on the A-V node appears to considerably outlast the duration of the hemodynamic actions of the drug.

Although verapamil exhibits almost complete absorption from the gastrointestinal tract, the drug undergoes a substantial degree of metabolism during its first pass through the hepatic portal circulation, so that overall bioavailability is approximately 10% to 20%. Furthermore, the drug is highly bound by plasma proteins, and only 10% of the drug in the plasma exists in the free form.

Because of the extensive first-pass metabolism of verapamil, only low concentrations of drug can be measured in the plasma, and only negligible amounts are excreted unchanged in the urine and feces. The concentrations of the *N*-demethylated and *N*-dealkylated metabolites rise gradually with continued administration of verapamil. Because the pharmacologic activities of the metabolites might contribute to the overall therapeutic response, it is not possible to predict the therapeutic plasma concentration of verapamil. Further study

must be conducted to clarify this matter, and renewed approaches to examining the pharmacokinetics of verapamil and its metabolites seem warranted. Table 22 presents a summary of current pharmacokinetic data on verapamil.

Dose

The studies to date with verapamil have focused primarily on its use in the management of patients with supraventricular tachyarrhythmias, although the drug has potential use in the treatment of patients with effort-induced angina pectoris and variant angina.

In the management of atrial tachyarrhythmias, the most frequently used intravenous dose has been 10 mg or 0.145 mg/kg given as a single injection over 10 to 15 min or longer in order to reduce the potential hazard of inducing left ventricular failure and/or A-V block. A second dose can be repeated in 30 min if the initial response is unsatisfactory. The drug has been given as a

---

TABLE 22. *Pharmacokinetic properties of verapamil*

Absorption
>90% of an oral dose is absorbed rapidly; bioavailability is reduced 20% to 35% due to first-pass metabolism but may increase with chronic administration
Protein binding
Approximately 90%
Metabolism
Verapamil is metabolized extensively in the liver with 12 metabolites having been identified; the major ones being *N*- and *O*-dealkylated products, including norverapamil, which has vascular actions but does not affect cardiac function
Half-life
After repeated oral doses, ranges from 4.5 to 12 hr; norverapamil has a longer half-life of 10.3 to 16.5 hr; half-life increases with repetitive dosing due to saturation of hepatic enzyme system; the half-life after intravenous infusion shows a bioexponential rate of elimination with a rapid early distribution phase of 4 min and a slower terminal distribution phase of 2 to 5 hr
Time to peak plasma concentration
After oral administration, achieved in 1 to 2 hr; shows wide individual variation
Time to achieve steady-state plasma concentration
Usually achieved within the first 24 to 48 hr but will vary due to the changes in the plasma $t_{1/2}$ during repetitive dosing
Therapeutic plasma concentration
125 to 400 ng/ml
Elimination
Renal: 50% eliminated as conjugated metabolites within the first 24 hr, 70% within 5 days; approximately 3% to 4% excreted unchanged; fecal: 9% to 16%

continuous infusion at the rate of 0.1 mg/min. Experience in children, although limited, has suggested that an intravenous dose of 3.5 to 5.0 mg has been successful in converting paroxysmal supraventricular tachycardia.

Because of the extensive first-pass hepatic metabolism, the oral dose of verapamil is 8 to 10 times greater than the intravenous dose. Thus, long-term oral dosage for prophylaxis against supraventricular arrhythmias has required doses up to 120 or 160 mg two or three times daily. The usual starting dosage is 40 to 80 mg every 8 hr. The dosage can be increased over 2 to 3 days if needed, and in the absence of known contraindications, a dosage of 720 mg/day is possible. A slow-release form of verapamil is under investigation, and it is likely that a single daily dose of 240 mg may suffice.

Contraindications

Verapamil must be used with extreme caution or not at all in patients who are receiving β-adrenergic receptor blocking agents. Because verapamil has the ability to antagonize the movement of calcium ion via the slow channel, it will exert its primary depressant effects on the sinoatrial and A-V nodes. Thus, the heart rate and A-V conduction velocity will be decreased. In the absence of other therapeutic interventions, the negative chronotropic and dromotropic effects of verapamil will, in part, be overcome by an increase in reflex sympathetic tone. The latter would be prevented by simultaneous administration of a β receptor blocking agent, thus exaggerating the depressant effects of verapamil on heart rate and A-V conduction. Needless to say, the negative inotropic effects of verapamil would be greater in the presence of a β receptor blocking agent, thus adding to the potential of the calcium antagonist to depress ventricular function.

The direct negative chronotropic effects

of verapamil preclude its use in patients with sick-sinus syndrome. Because of the dependence of the A-V nodal cells on the slow-channel calcium current, verapamil is contraindicated in those instances in which A-V conduction is impaired.

It is noteworthy that the depressant effects of verapamil on sinoatrial and A-V nodal functions, as well as on ventricular muscle contraction, can be overcome by the use of cardiac β-adrenergic receptor agonists such as norepinephrine, dopamine, dobutamine, and isoproterenol. The pancreatic hormone glucagon will likewise reverse the depression of ventricular contraction induced by verapamil, especially if it occurs in the presence of a β receptor blocking agent, in which instance cardiac β receptor agonists are likely to be of minimal value. Whereas digitalis glycosides will reverse the negative inotropic effects of verapamil, they may produce a further decrease in A-V node function. In patients with congestive heart failure, verapamil must be used with caution, if at all, and further experience is needed in this area. Because of the dependence on renal function for elimination of verapamil and/or its metabolites, the drug should be used cautiously and at reduced dosage in patients with impaired renal function.

Indications

Clinical studies indicate that verapamil has a narrow spectrum of antiarrhythmic effectiveness. It appears to be most valuable as an antiarrhythmic drug in the management of patients with atrial tachyarrhythmias, in which the negative dromotropic effects on the A-V node lead to control of the ventricular rate or abolish the reentrant mechanism within the A-V node, thus restoring normal sinus rhythm.

Reentrant paroxysmal supraventricular tachycardia involving the sinoatrial or A-V nodes has responded favorably to verapamil, both for the acute attack and for prevention of recurrences of the tachyarrhythmias. There has been some success in reversion of atrial flutter and fibrillation to sinus rhythm, but more often the drug exerts its benefits by virtue of its ability to decrease the ventricular response to the atrial tachyarrhythmia.

A distinct advantage of verapamil in supraventricular tachyarrhythmias is its rapid onset of effect. In paroxysmal supraventricular tachycardia, the drug is 80% to 100% effective in restoring sinus rhythm and offers an advantage over current therapy, which may require the use of digitalis glycosides when vagal maneuvers have failed.

The use of verapamil in tachyarrhythmias associated with WPW syndrome offers another therapeutic application. Intracardiac recordings have shown that verapamil does not alter the electrophysiologic properties of the atrial bypass tract and thus would be of little value in atrial fibrillation in the presence of an anomalous pathway in which the fibrillatory impulses enter the ventricles via the accessory pathway. However, the ability of verapamil to alter A-V nodal conduction may allow the drug to exert a beneficial effect in WPW tachyarrhythmias in which the A-V node serves as the pathway for anterograde conduction. Verapamil would prolong the refractoriness of the A-V node and interrupt the reentrant rhythm, even though the electrophysiologic properties of the accessory path were unaffected.

In addition to its use in the management of atrial rhythm disorders, verapamil and other slow channel antagonists (nifedipine, diltiazem) are known to be effective therapeutic agents in the management of patients with vasospastic angina pectoris (Prinzmetal's angina, variant angina), as well as in effort-induced angina. A wide variety of clinical entities (Table 23) have been reported to be benefited by verapamil, clinical experience will undoubtedly determine the full extent to which this new class of drugs can be employed.

REFERENCES

1. Vaughan-Williams EM. A classification of antiarrhythmic actions reassessed after a decade of new drugs. *J Clin Pharmacol* 1984;24:129–147.
2. Arnsdorf MF. Electrophysiologic properties of antidysrhythmic drugs as a rational basis for therapy. *Med Clin North Am* 1976;60:213–232.
3. Vaughan-Williams EM. Research on a rational basis for the origin and treatment of arrhythmia. *Acta Cardiol* 1977(Suppl 22):13–32.
4. Elharrar V, Zipes DP. Cardiac electrophysiologic alterations during myocardial ischemia. *Am J Physiol* 1977;233:H329–H345.
5. Wit AL, Bigger JT. Possible electrophysiological mechanisms for lethal arrhythmias accompanying myocardial ischemia and infarction. *Circulation* 1975;51–52(Suppl III):III96–III114.
6. Bigger JT, Dresdale RJ, Heissenbuttel RH, Weld FM, Wit AL. Ventricular arrhythmias in ischemic heart disease: mechanism, prevalence, significance, and management. *Prog Cardiovasc Dis* 1977;19:255–295.
7. Lazzara R, El-Sherif N, Hope RR, Scherlag BJ. Ventricular arrhythmias and electrophysiological consequences of myocardial ischemia and infarction. *Circ Res* 1978;42:740–749.
8. Weidmann S. The effect of the cardiac membrane potential on the rapid availability to the sodium carrier system. *J Physiol* 1955:127:213–224.
9. Hoffman BF, Kao CY, Suckling EE. Refractoriness in cardiac muscle. *Am J Physiol* 1957;190:473–482.
10. Noble D. Application of Hodgkin-Huxley equations to excitable tissues. *Physiol Rev* 1966;46:1–50.
11. Van Dam RT, Moore EN, Hoffman BF. Initiation and conduction of impulses in partially depolarized cardiac fibers. *Am J Physiol* 1963:204:1133–1144.

TABLE 23. *Potential clinical uses of verapamil and other slow channel calcium antagonists*

Arrhythmias
  Sinoatrial and A-V nodal reentrant
    tachyarrhythmias (PAT)
  Atrial flutter
  Atrial fibrillation
  Tachyarrhythmias associated with WPW
    syndrome
Angina pectoris
  Effort-induced angina
  Prinzmetal's angina
Essential hypertension
Obstructive cardiomyopathy
Cardioplegic protection of ischemic heart

12. Katz RL, Epstein RA. The interaction of anesthetic agents and adrenergic drugs to produce cardiac arrhythmias. *Anesthesiology* 1968;29:763.

13. Besterman EMM, Friedlander DH. Clinical experiences with propranolol. *Postgrad Med J* 1965:41:526–535.

14. Johnstone M. Propranolol during halothane anesthesia. *Br J Anaesth* 1966;38:516–529.

15. Lucchesi BR, Whitsitt LS, Stickney JL. Antiarrhythmic effects of beta-adrenergic blocking agents. *Ann NY Acad Sci* 1967;139:940–951.

16. Parmley WW, Braunwald E. Comparative myocardial depressant and antiarrhythmic properties of *d*-propranolol, *d,l*-propranolol, and quinidine. *J Pharmacol Exp Ther* 1967;158:11–21.

17. Davis LD, Temte JV. Effects of propranolol on the transmembrane potentials of ventricular muscle and Purkinje fibers of the dog. *Circ Res* 1968;22:661–677.

18. Gibson D, Sowton E. The use of beta-adrenergic receptor blocking drugs in dysrhythmias. *Prog Cardiovasc Dis* 1969;12:16–39.

19. Schamroth L. Immediate effects of intravenous propranolol on various cardiac arrhythmias. *Am J Cardiol* 1966;18:434.

20. Gettes LS, Surawicz B. Long-term prevention of paroxysmal arrhythmias with propranolol therapy. *Am J Med Sci* 1967;254:257–265.

21. Wit AL, Stiener C, Damto AN. Electrophysiologic effects of bretylium tosylate on single fibers in canine specialized conducting system and ventricle. *J Pharmacol Exp Ther* 1970; 173:344–356.

22. Bigger JT, Jaffe CC. Effect of bretylium tosylate on electrophysiologic properties of ventricular muscle and Purkinje fibers. *Am J Cardiol* 1971;27:82–91.

23. Singh BN, Vaughan-Williams EM. The effect of amiodarone, a new antianginal drug, on cardiac muscle. *Br J Pharmacol* 1970;39:657–667.

24. Singh BN, Jewitt DE, Downey JM, et al. Effects of amiodarone and L8040, novel antianginal and antiarrhythmic drugs, on cardiac and coronary hemodynamics and on cardiac intracellular potentials. *Clin Exp Pharmacol Physiol* 1976;3:427–442.

25. Han J, Malozzi AN, Moe GK. Sino-atrial reciprocation in the isolated rabbit heart. *Circ Res* 1968;22:355–362.

26. Alessi MA, Bonke FJM, Schopman FJG. Circus movement in rabbit heart atrial muscle as a mechanism of tachycardia. *Circulation* 1974; 33:54–62.

27. Mendez D, Moe GK. Demonstration of a dual AV nodal conduction system in the isolated rabbit heart. *Circ Res* 1966;19:378–393.

28. Bailey JR, Andersen GJ, Pippenger D. Reentry within the isolated canine bundle of His: possible mechanism for reciprocating rhythm. *Am J Cardiol* 1973;32:808–813.

29. Narula OS. Sinus node reentry: a mechanism of supraventricular tachycardia. *Circulation* 1974;50:1114–1128.

30. Wu D, Amat-Y-Leon F, Denes P, et al. Demonstration of dual A-V nodal pathways in patients with paroxysmal supraventricular tachycardia. *Circulation* 1973;48:549–555.

31. Varghese PH, Damato AH, Curacta AT, et al. Intraventricular conduction delay as a determinant of atrial echo beats. *Circulation* 1974; 49:805–810.

32. Singer DH, Ten-Eick RE, DeBoer AA. Electrophysiologic correlates of human atrial tachyarrhythmias. In: Dreifus LS, Likoff W, eds. *Cardiac arrhythmias*. New York: Grune and Stratton, 1973;97–119.

33. Hoffman BF, Cranefield PF. Physiologic basis of cardiac arrhythmias. *Am J Med* 1964;37:670–684.

34. Wit AL, Cranefield PF. Physiologic basis of cardiac arrhythmias. *Am J Med* 1976;37:670–684.

35. Lau SH, Stein E, Rosowsky DB, et al. Atrial pacing and atrioventricular conduction in anomalous atrioventricular excitation (Wolff-Parkinson-White syndrome). *Am J Cardiol* 1967;19:354–359.

36. Scherf D, Bornemann C. Two cases of the preexcitation syndrome. *J Electrocardiol* 1967;2:177–184.

37. Hunter A, Papp C, Parkinson J. The syndrome of short P-R interval, apparent bundle branch block, and associated paroxysmal tachycardia. *Br Heart J* 1940;2:107–122.

38. Castellanos A, Chapunoff E, Castillo C. His bundle electrograms in two cases of Wolff-Parkinson-White (pre-excitation) syndrome. *Circulation* 1970;41:399–411.

39. Boineau JP, Moore EN. Evidence for propagation of activation across an accessory atrioventricular connection in types A and B pre-excitation. *Circulation* 1970;41:375–379.

40. Durrer D, Schoo L, Schuilenburg RM, et al. The role of premature beats in the initiation and termination of supraventricular tachycardia in the Wolff-Parkinson-White syndrome. *Circulation* 1967;36:644–662.

41. Gibson D, Sowton E. The use of beta-adrenergic receptor blocking drugs in dysrhythmias. In: Friedberg CK, ed. *Current status of drugs in cardiovascular disease*. New York: Grune and Stratton, 1969;160–179.

42. Heng MK, Singh BN, Roche AHG, et al. Effects of intravenous verapamil on cardiac arrhythmias and on the electrocardiogram. *Am Heart J* 1975;90:487–498.

43. Singh BN, Hauswirth O. Comparative mechanisms of action of antiarrhythmic drugs. *Am Heart J* 1974;87:367–382.

44. Singh BN, Vaughan-Williams EM. A fourth class of anti-dysrhythmic action? Effect of verapamil on ouabain toxicity, on atrial and ventricular intracellular potentials and on other features of cardiac function. *Cardiovasc Res* 1972;6:109–119.

45. Cranefield PF, Aronson RS, Wit AL. Effect of verapamil on the normal action potential and

on a calcium dependent slow response of canine cardiac Purkinje fibers. *Circ Res* 1974; 34:204–213.

46. Neuss H, Schlepper M. Der Einfluss von verapamil auf die atrioventrickulare Uberleitung. Lokalisation des Wirkungsortes mit His bundel Elecktrogrammen. *Verh Dtsch Ges Kreislaufforsch* 1971;37:433–441.

47. Husaini MH, Kvasnicka J, Ryden L, et al. Action of verapamil in sinus node, atrioventricular and intraventricular conduction. *Br Heart J* 1973;35:734–737.

48. Roy PR, Spurrell RAJ, Sowton GE. The effect of verapamil on the cardiac conduction system in man. *Postgrad Med J* 1974;50:270–275.

49. Goldreyer BN, Bigger JT. The site of reentry in paroxysmal supraventricular tachycardia in man. *Circulation* 1971;43:15–26.

50. Goldreyer BN, Damato AN. The essential role of atrioventricular conduction delay in the initiation of paroxysmal supraventricular tachycardia. *Circulation* 1971;43:679–687.

51. Rosenbaum MB, Chiale PA, Ryba D. Control of tachyarrhythmias associated with Wolff-Parkinson-White syndrome by amiodarone hydrochloride. *Am J Cardiol* 1974;34:215–223.

52. Touboul P, Porte J, Huerta F, et al. Electrophysiological effects of amiodarone in man. *Am J Cardiol* 1975;35:173A.

53. Spurrell RAJ, Thorburn CW, Camm J, et al. Effects of disopyramide on electrophysiological properties of specialized conduction system in man and on accessory atrioventricular pathway in Wolff-Parkinson-White syndrome. *Br Heart J* 1975;37:861–870.

54. Wellens HJJ, Durrer D. Wolff-Parkinson-White syndrome and atrial fibrillation. Relation between refractory period of the accessory pathway and ventricular rate during atrial fibrillation. *Am J Cardiol* 1974;34:777–782.

55. Sellers TD Jr, Bashore TM, Gallagher JJ. Digitalis in the preexcitation syndrome. Analysis during atrial fibrillation. *Circulation* 1977; 56:260–267.

56. Rosen KM, Barwolf C, Ehsani A. Effects of lidocaine and propranolol on the normal and anomalous pathways in patients with pre-excitation. *Am J Cardiol* 1972;30:801–809.

57. Wu D, Syndham C, Amat-Y-Leon F, et al. The effects of ouabain on induction of atrioventricular nodal re-entrant paroxysmal supraventricular tachycardia. *Circulation* 1975;52:201–207.

58. Wu D, Denes P, Dhingra R, et al. The effects of propranolol on induction of A-V nodal reentrant paroxysmal tachycardia. *Circulation* 1974;50:665–667.

59. Josephson ME, Kastor JA, Kitchen JG III. Lidocaine in Wolff-Parkinson-White syndrome with atrial fibrillation. *Ann Intern Med* 1975; 84:44–45.

60. Rosen KM, Lau SH, Weiss MB, D'Amato AN. The effect of lidocaine on atrioventricular and intraventricular conduction in man. *Am J Cardiol* 1970;25:1–5.

61. Mandel W, Laks M, Obayaski K, et al. Electrophysiological features of the WPW syndrome: modification by procainamide. *Circulation* 1973;50:665–667.

62. Sellers TD Jr, Campbell WF, Bashore TM, et al. Effects of procainamide and quinidine sulfate in the Wolff-Parkinson-White syndrome. *Circulation* 1977;55:15–22.

63. Birkhead JS, Vaughan-Williams EN. Dual effect of disopyramide on atrial and atrioventricular conduction and refractory periods. *Br Heart J* 1977;36:256–264.

64. Spurrell RAJ, Krikler DM, Sowton E. Effects of verapamil on electrophysiological properties of anomalous atrioventricular connection in Wolff-Parkinson-White syndrome. *Br Heart J* 1974;36:256–264.

65. Schamroth L, Krikler DM, Garrett C. Immediate effects of intravenous verapamil in cardiac arrhythmias. *Br Med J* 1972;1:660–662.

66. Chiale PA, Przybyiski J, Halpern MS, et al. Comparative effects of ajmaline on intermittent bundle branch block and the Wolff-Parkinson-White syndrome. *Am J Cardiol* 1977;39:651–657.

67. Wellens HJJ, Durrer D. Effect of procaine amide, quinidine and ajmaline in the Wolff-Parkinson-White syndrome. *Circulation* 1974; 50:114–120.

68. Wellens HJJ, Lie KI, Bar FW, et al. Effect of amiodarone in the Wolff-Parkinson-White syndrome. *Am J Cardiol* 1976;38:189–194.

69. Daubert JC, Couffault J. Etude clinique de *l*-amiodarone injectable. *Coeur Med Interne* 1977;16:415–421.

70. Wenckebach KF. *Die unregelmassige Herztatigkeit und ihre klinische Bedeutung*. Leipzig: W. Engelmann, 1914.

71. West TC, Amory DW. Single fiber recording of the effect of quinidine at atrial and pacemaker activity and contractility of the isolated blood-perfused atrium of the dog. *Eur J Pharmacol* 1960;57:13–19.

72. Chiba S, Kobayashi M, Furrekawa Y. Effects of disopyramide on SA nodal pacemaker activity and contractility of the isolated blood-perfused atrium of the dog. *Eur J Pharmacol* 1979;57:13–19.

73. Josephson ME, Seides SF, Batsford WP, et al. The electrophysiological effects of intramuscular quinidine on the atrioventricular conducting system in man. *Am Heart J* 1974;87:55–64.

74. Wallace AG, Cline RE, Sealy WC, Young WG, Froyer WG. Electrophysiologic effects of quinidine. *Circ Res* 1966;19:960–969.

75. Nye CE, Roberts J. The reactivity of atrial and ventricular pacemakers to quinidine. *J Pharmacol Exp Ther* 1966;152:67–74.

76. Vaughan-Williams EM. Mode of action of quinidine on isolated rabbit atria interpreted from intracellular records. *Br J Pharmacol* 1958; 13:276–287.

77. Hirschfeld DS, Ueda CT, Rowland M, Schein-

man MM. Clinical and electrophysiological effects of intravenous quinidine in man. *Br Heart J* 1977;39:309–316.

78. Weidmann S. Effects of calcium ions and local anesthetics on electrical properties of Purkinje fibers. *J Physiol (Lond)* 1955;129:568–582.

79. Hoffman BF. Action of quinidine and procaine amide on single fibers of dog ventricle and specialized conduction system. *An Acad Bras Cienc* 1958;29:365–386.

80. Stern S. Hemodynamic changes following separate and combined administration of beta blocking drugs and quinidine. *Eur J Clin Invest* 1971;1:432–436.

81. Schmid PG, Nelson LD, Mark AL, Herstad DD, Abboud FM. Inhibition of adrenergic vasoconstriction by quinidine. *J Pharmacol Exp Ther* 1974;188:124–134.

82. Bellet A, Hamdan G, Somlyo A, Lara R. The reversal of cardiotoxic effects of quinidine by molar sodium lactate. An experimental study. *Am J Med Sci* 1959;237:165–189.

83. Doherty JE, Straub KD, Murphy ML, de-Soyza N, Bissett JK, Kane JJ. Digoxin-quinidine interaction: changes in canine tissue concentrations from steady state with quinidine. *Am J Cardiol* 1980;45:1196–1200.

84. Leaky EB, Carson JA, Bigger JT, Butler VP. Reduced renal clearance of digoxin during chronic quinidine administration. *Circulation* 1979;60(Suppl II):II16 (abstract).

85. Burstein CL. Treatment of acute arrhythmias during anesthesia by intravenous procaine. *Anesthesiology* 1946;7:113–121.

86. Mark LC, Kayden HJ, Steele JM, et al. The physiological disposition and cardiac effects of procaine amide. *J Pharmacol Exp Ther* 1951; 102:5–15.

87. Bigger JT, Heissenbuttal RH. The use of procainamide and lidocaine in the treatment of cardiac arrhythmias. *Prog Cardiovasc Dis* 1961; 11:515–534.

88. Sellers TD, Campbell RWF, Bashore TM, Gallagher JJ. Effects of procainamide and quinidine sulfate in the Wolff-Parkinson-White syndrome. *Circulation* 1977;55:15–27.

89. Ogunkelu JB, Damato AN, Akhtar M, Reddy CP, Caracta AR, Lau SH. Electrophysiologic effects of procainamide in subtherapeutic to therapeutic doses on human atrioventricular conducting system. *Am J Cardiol* 1976;37:724–731.

90. Helfant RH, Scherlag BJ, Damato AN. The electrophysiological properties of diphenylhydantoin sodium (Dilantin) as compared to procaine amide in the normal and digitalis intoxicated heart. *Circulation* 1967;36:108–118.

91. Kastor JA, Josephson ME, Guss SB, Horowitz LN. Human ventricular refractoriness. II. Effects of procainamide. *Circulation* 1977; 56:462–467.

92. Giardina EGV, Bigger JT. Procaine amide against re-entrant ventricular arrhythmias. *Circulation* 1973;48:959–970.

93. Kayden HJ, Brodie BB, Steele JM. Procaine amide. *Circulation* 1957;15:118–126.

94. Giardina EG, Heissenbuttel RH, Bigger JT. Intermittent intravenous procaine amide to treat ventricular arrhythmias. *Ann Intern Med* 1973; 78:183–193.

95. Harrison D, Sprouse H, Morrow AG. The antiarrhythmic properties of lidocaine and procainamide. *Circulation* 1963;28:486–491.

96. Ladd AT. Procainamide induced lupus erythematosus. *N Engl J Med* 1962;267:1357–1358.

97. Colman RW, Sturgill BC. Lupus-like syndrome induced by procainamide. *Arch Intern Med* 1965;115:214–216.

98. Karlsson E. Clinical pharmacokinetics of procainamide. *Clin Pharmacokinet* 1978;3:97–107.

99. Greenspan AM, Horowitz LN, Spielman SR, Josephson ME. Large dose procainamide therapy for ventricular tachyarrhythmia. *Am J Cardiol* 1980;46:453–468.

100. Koch-Weser J, Klein SW, Foo-Canto LL, Kastor JA, DeSanctis RW. Arrhythmia prophylaxis with procainamide in acute myocardial infarction. *N Engl J Med* 1969;281:1253–1260.

101. Sekiya A, Vaughan-Williams EM. A comparison of the antifibrillatory actions and effects on intracellular cardiac potentials of pronethalol, disopyramide, and quinidine. *Br J Pharmacol* 1963;21:473–481.

102. Josephson ME, Caract AR, Lau SH, Gallagher JJ, Damato AN. Electrophysiological evaluation of disopyramide in man. *Am Heart J* 1973;86:771–778.

103. Befeler B, Castellanos A, Wells DE, Vagueiro MC, Yeh BK. Electrophysiologic effects of the antiarrhythmic agent disopyramide phosphate. *Am J Cardiol* 1975;35:382–389.

104. LaBarre A, Strauss HC, Scheinman MM, et al. Electrophysiologic effects of disopyramide phosphate on sinus node function in patients with sinus node dysfunction. *Circulation* 1979; 59:226–235.

105. Birkhead JS, Vaughan-Williams EM. Dual effect of disopyramide on atrial and atrioventricular conduction and refractory periods. *Br Heart J* 1977;39:657–660.

106. Yeh BK, Sung PK, Scherlag BJ. Effects of disopyramide on electrophysiological and mechanical properties of the heart. *J Pharm Sci* 1973;62:1924–1929.

107. Danilo P, Hordof AJ, Rosen MR. Effects of disopyramide on electrophysiologic properties of canine cardiac Purkinje fibers. *J Pharmacol Exp Ther* 1977;201:701–710.

108. Kus T, Sasyniuk BI. The electrophysiological effects of disopyramide phosphate on canine ventricular muscle and Purkinje fibers in normal and low potassium. *Can J Physiol Pharmacol* 1978;56:139–149.

109. Levites R, Anderson GJ. Electrophysiological effects of disopyramide phosphate during experimental myocardial ischemia. *Am Heart J* 1979;98:339–344.

110. Patterson E, Gibson JK, Lucchesi BR. Electro-

physiologic effects of disopyramide phosphate on reentrant ventricular arrhythmias in conscious dogs after myocardial infarction. *Am J Cardiol* 1980;46:792–799.

111. Walsh RA, Horwitz LD. Adverse hemodynamic effects of intravenous disopyramide compared with quinidine in conscious dogs. *Circulation* 1979;60:1053.

112. Meltzer RS, Robert EW, McMorrow M, Martin RP. Atypical ventricular tachycardia as a manifestation of disopyramide toxicity. *Am J Cardiol* 1978;42:1049–1053.

113. Deano DA, Wu D, Mautner RK, Sherman RH, Ehsani AE, Rosen KM. The antiarrhythmic efficacy of intravenous therapy with disopyramide phosphate. *Chest* 1977;71:597–606.

114. Vismara LA, Mason DT, Amsterdam EA. Disopyramide phosphate: clinical efficacy of a new oral antiarrhythmic drug. *Clin Pharmacol Ther* 1974;16:330–335.

115. Josephson ME, Horowitz LN. Electrophysiologic approach to therapy of recurrent sustained ventricular tachycardia. *Am J Cardiol* 1979;43:631–642.

116. Benditt DG, Pritchett ELC, Wallace AG, Gallagher JJ. Recurrent ventricular tachycardia in man: evaluation of disopyramide therapy by intracardiac electrical stimulation. *Eur J Cardiol* 1979;9:255–276.

117. Mandel WJ, Bigger JT. Effect of lidocaine on sinoatrial node and atrial fibers. *Am J Cardiol* 1970;25:113–124.

118. Singh BN, Vaughan-Williams EM. Effects of altering potassium concentrations in the action of lidocaine and diphenylhydantoin on rabbit atrial and ventricular muscle. *Circ Res* 1971;29:286–295.

119. Josephson ME, Caracta AR, Lau SH, Gallagher JJ, Damato AN. Effects of lidocaine on refractory periods of man. *Am Heart J* 1972;84:778–786.

120. Davis LD, Temte JV. Electrophysiologic actions of lidocaine on canine ventricular muscle and Purkinje fibers. *Circ Res* 1979;24:639–655.

121. Lazzara R, Hope RR, El-Sherif N, Scherlag BJ. Effects of lidocaine on hypoxic and ischemic cardiac cells. *Am J Cardiol* 1978;41:872–879.

122. Allen JD, Brennan FJ, Wit AL. Actions of lidocaine on transmembrane potentials of subendocardial Purkinje fibers surviving in infarcted canine hearts. *Circ Res* 1978;43:470–481.

123. Nelson DH, Harrison DC. A comparison of the negative inotropic effects of procaine amide, lidocaine, and quinidine. *Physiologist* 1965;8:241A.

124. Robinson SL, Schroll M, Harrison DC. The circulatory response to lidocaine in experimental myocardial infarction. *Am J Med Sci* 1969;258:260–269.

125. Austen WG, Moran JM. Cardiac and peripheral vascular effects of lidocaine and procaine amide. *Am J Cardiol* 1965;16:701–707.

126. Collinsworth KA, Summer MK, Harrison DC. The clinical pharmacology of lidocaine as an antiarrhythmic drug. *Circulation* 1974;50:1217–1230.

127. Grossman JJ, Cooper JA, Frieden J. Cardiovascular effects of infusion of lidocaine on patients with heart disease. *Am J Cardiol* 1969;24:191–197.

128. Jewitt DE, Kishon Y, Thomas M. Lignocaine in the management of arrhythmias after acute myocardial infarction. *Lancet* 1968;1:266–270.

129. Merritt HH, Putnam TJ. Sodium diphenylhydantoinate in the treatment of convulsive disorders. *JAMA* 1938;111:1068–1073.

130. Harris AS, Kokernot RH. Effects of diphenylhydantoin sodium and phenobarbital sodium upon ectopic ventricular tachycardia in acute myocardial infarction. *Am J Physiol* 1950;163:505–516.

131. Strauss HC, Bigger JT, Bassett AL, Hoffman BF. Actions of diphenylhydantoin on the electrical properties of isolated rabbit and canine atria. *Circ Res* 1968;23:463–477.

132. Singh BN, Vaughan-Williams EM. Effect of altering potassium concentration on the action of lidocaine and diphenylhydantoin on rabbit atrial and ventricular muscle. *Circ Res* 1971;29:286–294.

133. Rosati RA, Alexander JA, Schaal SF, Wallace AG. Influence of diphenylhydantoin on electrophysiological properties of the canine heart. *Circ Res* 1967;21:757–765.

134. Caracta AR, Damato AN, Josephson ME, Ricciutti MA, Gallagher JJ, Lau SH. Electrophysiologic properties of diphenylhydantoin. *Circulation* 1973;47:1234–1241.

135. Scherlag BJ, Helfant RH, Damato AN. The contrasting effects of diphenylhydantoin and procaine amide on A-V conduction in the digitalis intoxicated and the normal heart. *Am Heart J* 1968;75:200–205.

136. Bigger JT, Bassett AL, Hoffman BF. Electrophysiologic effects of diphenylhydantoin on canine Purkinje fibers. *Circ Res* 1968;22:221–236.

137. El-Sherif N, Lazzara R. Reentrant ventricular arrhythmias in the late myocardial infarction period. 5. Mechanism of action of diphenylhydantoin. *Circulation* 1978;57:465–472.

138. Mixter CG, Moran JM, Austen WG. Cardiac and peripheral vascular effects of diphenylhydantoin. *Am J Cardiol* 1966;17:332–338.

139. Conn RD, Kennedy JW, Blackman JR. The hemodynamic effects of diphenylhydantoin. *Am Heart J* 1967;73:500–505.

140. Lieberson AD, Schumacher RR, Childress RH, Boyd DL, Williams JF. Effects of diphenylhydantoin on left ventricular function in patients with heart disease. *Circulation* 1967;36:692–699.

141. Karliner JS. Intravenous diphenylhydantoin sodium in cardiac arrhythmias. *Dis Chest* 1967;51:256–269.

142. Russell MA, Bousvaros G. Total results from

diphenylhydantoin administered intravenously. *JAMA* 1968;206:218–223.

143. Conn RD. Diphenylhydantoin sodium in cardiac arrhythmias. *N Engl J Med* 1965;272:277–282.

144. Louis S, Kutt H, McDowell F. The cardiocirculatory changes caused by intravenous dilantin and its solvent. *Am Heart J* 1967;74:523–529.

145. Swedberg K, Pehrson J, Ryden L. Electrophysiologic and hemodynamic effects of tocainide (W-36095) in man. *Eur J Clin Pharmacol* 1978;14:15–19.

146. Anderson JL, Mason JW, Winkle RA, et al. Clinical electrophysiologic effects of tocainide. *Circulation* 1978;57:685–691.

147. Oshita S, Sada H, Kojima M, Ban T. Effects of tocainide and lidocaine on the transmembrane action potentials as related to external potassium and calcium concentrations in guinea pig papillary muscles. *Naunyn Schmiedebergs Arch Pharmacol* 1980;314:62–82.

148. Moore EN, Spear JF, Horowitz LN, et al. Electrophysiologic properties of a new antiarrhythmic drug, tocainide. *Am J Cardiol* 1978;41:703–709.

149. Schnittger J, Griffin JC, Hall RJ, et al. Effects of tocainide on ventricular fibrillation threshold: comparison with lidocaine. *Am J Cardiol* 1978;42:76–81.

150. Investigators Brochure for Tocainide HCl. Astra Pharmaceutical Products Inc., 1977.

151. Winkle RA, Anderson JL, Peters F, Meffin PJ, Fowler RE, Harrison DC. The hemodynamic effects of intravenous tocainide in patients with heart disease. *Circulation* 1978;57:787–792.

152. Klein MD, Levine PA, Ryan TJ. Antiarrhythmic efficacy, pharmacokinetics and clinical safety of tocainide in convalescent myocardial infarction. *Chest* 1980;77:726–730.

153. Soff GA, Kadin ME. Tocainide-induced reversible agranulocytosis and anemia. *Arch Intern Med* 1987;147:598–599.

154. Winkle RA, Meffin PJ, Harrison DC. Long-term tocainide therapy for ventricular arrhythmias. *Circulation* 1978;57:1008–1016.

155. Singh BN, Vaughan-Williams EM. Investigations of the mode of action of a new antidysrhythmic drug (Ko 1173). *Br J Pharmacol* 1978;44:1–9.

156. Yamaguchi I, Singh B. Electrophysiological actions of mexiletine on isolated rabbit atria and canine ventricular muscle and Purkinje fiber. *Cardiovasc Res* 1979;13:288–296.

157. Roos JC, Paalman DCA, Dunning AJ. Electrophysiological effects of mexiletine in man. *Postgrad Med J* 1977;53(Suppl I):92–94.

158. Jequier P, Jones R, Mackintosh A. Fatal mexiletine overdose. *Lancet* 1976;1:429.

159. Weld FM, Bigger JT, Swistel D, Bordiuk J, Lau YH. Electrophysiological effects of mexiletine (Ko 1173) on bovine cardiac Purkinje fibers. *J Pharmacol Exp Ther* 1979;210:222–228.

160. McComish M, Robinson C, Kitson D, Jewitt DE. Clinical electrophysiological effects of mexiletine. *Postgrad Med J* 1977;53(Suppl I):85–91.

161. Vaughan-Williams EM. Mexiletine in isolated tissue models. *Postgrad Med J* 1977;53(Suppl I):30–34.

162. Arita M, Goto M, Nagomoto Y, et al. Electrophysiologic actions of mexiletine (Ko 1173) on canine Purkinje fibers and ventricular muscle. *Br J Pharmacol* 1979;67:143–152.

163. Burke GH, Berman ND. Differential electrophysiologic effects of mexiletine on normal and hypoxic canine Purkinje fibers. *J Cardiovasc Pharmacol* 1985;7:1096–1100.

164. Hohnloser S, Weirich J, Antoni H. Effects of mexiletine on steady state characteristics and recovery kinetics of V_{max} and conduction velocity in the guinea pig myocardium. *J Cardiovasc Pharmacol* 1982;4:232–239.

165. Campbell TJ. Kinetics of onset of rate-dependent effects of Class I antiarrhythmic drugs are important in determining their effects on refractoriness in guinea-pig ventricle, and provide a theoretical basis of their subclassification. *Cardiovasc Res* 1983;17:344–352.

166. Heger JJ, Nattel S, Rinkenberger RL, Zipes DP. Mexiletine therapy in 15 patients with drug-resistant ventricular tachycardia. *Am J Cardiol* 1980;45:627–632.

167. Campbell RWF, Talbot RG, Dolder MA, Murray A, Prescott LF, Julian DG. Comparison of procainamide and mexiletine in prevention of ventricular arrhythmias after acute myocardial infarction. *Lancet* 1975;1:1257–1260.

168. Waspe LE, Waxman HL, Buxton AE, Josephson ME. Mexiletine for control of drug-resistant ventricular tachycardia: clinical and electrophysiologic results in 44 patients. *Am J Cardiol* 1983;51:1175–1181.

169. Stein, J. Podrid P, Lown B. Effects of oral mexiletine on left and right ventricular function. *Am J Cardiol* 1984;54:575–578.

170. Pottage A, Campbell RWF, Achuff SC, Murray A, Julian DG, Prescott LF. The absorption of oral mexiletine in coronary care patients. *Eur J Clin Pharmacol* 1978;13:393–399.

171. Zipes DP, Troup PJ. New antiarrhythmic agents. *Am J Cardiol* 1978;41:1005–1024.

172. Talbot RG, Julian DG, Prescott LF. Longterm treatment of ventricular arrhythmias with oral mexiletine. *Am Heart J* 1976;91:58–65.

173. Gomoll AM, Byrne JE, Antonaccio MJ. Electrophysiology, hemodynamic and antiarrhythmic efficacy model studies on encainide. *Am J Cardiol* 1986;58:10C–17C.

174. Duff JJ, Dawson AK, Roden DM, Oates JA, Smith RF, Woosley RL. Electrophysiologic actions of O-demethyl encainide: an active metabolite. *Circulation* 1983;68:385–391.

175. Gibson JK, Somani P, Bassett AL. Electrophysiologic effects of encainide (MJ 9067) on canine Purkinje fibers. *Eur J Pharmacol* 1978;52:161–169.

176. Elharrar V, Zipes DP. Effects of encainide and metabolites (MJ 14030 and MJ 9444) on canine

Purkinje and ventricular fibers. *J Pharmacol Exp Ther* 1982;220:440–447.

177. Sami M, Mason JW, Oh G, Harrison DC. Canine electrophysiology of encainide, a new antiarrhythmic drug. *Am J Cardiol* 1979;43:1149–1154.

178. Capos JJ, Samuelsson RG, Kates RE, Yee YG, Marks DJ, Harrison DC. Comparative electrophysiology of encainide and metabolites. *Clin Res* 1982;30:4A.

179. Jackman WM, Zipes DP, Nacarelli GV, Rinkerberger RL, Heger JJ, Prystowsky EN. Electrophysiology of oral encainide. *Am J Cardiol* 1982;49:1270–1279.

180. Carey EL Jr, Duff HJ, Roden DM, et al. Encainide and its metabolites. *J Clin Invest* 1984;73:539–547.

181. Davies W, Jazayeri M, Tchou P. Marked Q-T prolongation due to encainide therapy. *Cardiovasc Drugs Ther* 1988;2:283–286.

182. DiBianco R, Fletcher RD, Cohen AI, et al. Treatment of frequent ventricular arrhythmia with encainide assessment using serial ambulatory electrocardiograms, intracardiac electrophysiologic studies, treadmill exercise tests, and radionuclide cineangiographic studies. *Circulation* 1982;65:1134–1147.

183. Sami MH, Derbekyan VA, Lisbona R. Hemodynamic effects of encainide in patients with ventricular arrhythmia and poor ventricular function. *Am J Cardiol* 1983;52:507–511.

184. Soyka LF. Safety of encainide for the treatment of ventricular arrhythmias. *Am J Cardiol* 1986;58:96C–103C.

185. Soyka LF. Safety considerations and dosing guidelines for encainide in supraventricular arrhythmias. *Am J Cardiol* 1988;62:63L–68L.

186. Roden DM, Wood AJJ, Wilkinson GR, et al. Disposition kinetics of encainide and metabolites. *Am J Cardiol* 1986;58:4C–9C.

187. Winkle RA, Peters F, Kated RE, et al. Possible contribution of encainide metabolites to the long term antiarrhythmic efficacy of encainide. *Am J Cardiol* 1983;51:1182–1188.

188. Harrison DC, Kates RE, Quiart BD. Relation of blood level and metabolites to the antiarrhythmic effectiveness of encainide. *Am J Cardiol* 1986;58:66C.

189. Roden DM, Woosley RL. Clinical pharmacokinetics of encainide. *Clin Pharmacokinet* 1988; 14:141–147.

190. Barbey JT, Thompson KA, Echt DS, Woosley RL, Roden DM. Antiarrhythmic activity, electrocardiographic effects and pharmacokinetics of the encainide metabolites O-desmethyl encainide and 3-methoxy-O-desmethyl encainide in man. *Circulation* 1988;77:380–391.

191. Chesnie B, Podrid P, Lown B, Raeder E. Encainide for refractory ventricular tachyarrhythmia. *Am J Cardiol* 1983;52:495–500.

192. Rickenberger RL, Prystowsky EN, Jackman WM, Caccarelli GV, Heger JJ, Zipes DP. Drug conversion of nonsustained ventricular tachycardia to sustained ventricular tachycardia during serial electrophysiologic studies: identification of drugs that exacerbate tachycardia and potential mechanisms. *Am Heart J* 1982; 103:177–184.

193. Antonaccio MJ, Verjee S. Dosing recommendations for encainide. *Am J Cardiol* 1986; 58:114C–116C.

194. Roden DM, Reele SB, Higins SB, et al. Total suppression of ventricular arrhythmias by encainide: pharmacokinetics and electrocardiographic characteristics. *N Engl J Med* 1980; 302:877–882.

195. The CAPS Investigators. The Cardiac Arrhythmia Pilot Study. *Am J Cardiol* 1986;57:91–95.

196. Morganroth J, Pool P, Miller R, et al. Dose-response range of encainide for benign and potentially lethal ventricular arrhythmias. *Am J Cardiol* 1986;57:769–774.

197. Morganroth J, Somberg JC, Pool PE, et al. Comparative study of encainide and quinidine in the treatment of ventricular arrhythmias. *J Am Coll Cardiol* 1986;7:9–16.

198. Heger JJ, Nattel S, Rinkenberger R, Zipes D. Encainide therapy in patients with drug-resistant ventricular tachycardia. *Circulation* 1979; 60(Suppl II):II185.

199. Rahilly GT, Prystowsky EN, Zipes DP, Nacarelli GV, Jackman WM, Heger JJ. Clinical and electrophysiological findings in patients with repetitive monomorphic ventricular tachycardia and otherwise normal electrocardiogram. *Am J Cardiol* 1982;50:459–468.

200. Duff HJ, Roden DM, Carey EL, Wang T, Primm RK, Woosley RL. Spectrum of antiarrhythmic response to encainide. *Am J Cardiol* 1985;56:887–891.

201. Anderson JL, Stewart JR, Johnson TA, Lutz JR, Pitt B. Response to encainide of refractory ventricular tachycardia: clinical application of assays for parent drug and metabolites. *J Cardiovasc Pharmacol* 1982;4:812–819.

202. Abdollah H, Brugada P, Green M, Wehr M, Wellens HJJ, Paulussen G. Clinical efficacy and electrophysiologic effects of intravenous and oral encainide in patients with accessory atrioventricular pathways and supraventricular arrhythmias. *Am J Cardiol* 1984;54:544–549.

203. Kunze K-P, Kuck K-H, Schluter M, Bleifeld W. Effect of encainide and flecainide on chronic ectopic atrial tachycardia. *J Am Coll Cardiol* 1986;7:1121–1126.

204. Brugada P, Abdollah H, Wellens HJJ. Suppression of incessant supraventricular tachycardia by intravenous and oral encainide. *J Am Coll Cardiol* 1984;4:1255–1260.

205. Rinkenberger RL, Naccarelli GV, Miles WM, et al. Encainide for atrial fibrillation associated with Wolff-Parkinson-White syndrome. *Am J Cardiol* 1988;62:26L–30L.

206. Naccarelli GV, Jackman WM, Akhtar M, et al. Efficacy and electrophysiologic effects of encainide for atrioventricular nodal reentrant tachycardia. *Am J Cardiol* 1988;62:31L–36L.

207. Cowan JC, Vaughan-Williams EM. Characterization of a new oral antiarrhythmic drug, fle-

cainide (R818). *Eur J Pharmacol* 1981;73:333–342.

208. Ikeda N, Singh BN, Davis ID, Hauswirth O. Effects of flecainide on the electrophysiologic properties of isolated canine and rabbit myocardial fibers. *J Am Coll Cardiol* 1985;5:303–310.

209. Hondeghem LM. Validity of Vmax as a measure of the sodium current in cardiac and nervous tissue. *Biophys J* 1978;23:147–152.

210. Vik-Mo H, Ohm OJ, Lund-Johansen P. Electrophysiologic effects of flecainide acetate in patients with sinus node dysfunction. *Am J Cardiol* 1982;50:1090–1094.

211. Hellestrand KJ, Bexgon RS, Nathan AW, et al. Acute electrophysiological effects of flecainide acetate on cardiac conduction and refractoriness in man. *Br Heart J* 1982;48:140–148.

212. Pop T, Tresse N. Effect of flecainide on atrial vulnerability in man. *Drugs* 1985;29:1–6.

213. Hellestrand KJ, Nathan AW, Bexton RS, Camm AJ. Electrophysiological effects of flecainide on sinus node function, anomalous atrioventricular connections and pacemaker thresholds. *Am J Cardiol* 1984;50:30B–38B.

214. Hoff PI, Tronstad A, Oli B, Ohm OJ. Electrophysiologic and clinical effects of flecainide for recurrent paroxysmal supraventricular tachycardia. *Am J Cardiol* 1988;62:585–589.

215. Kappenberger LJ, Fromer MA, Shenasa M, Gloor HO. Evaluation of flecainide acetate in rapid atrial fibrillation complicating Wolff-Parkinson-White syndrome. *Clin Cardiol* 1985; 8:321–326.

216. Gelder ICV, Crijns HJGM, Gilst WHV, De Langen CDJ, Wijk LMV, Lie KI. Effects of flecainide on the atrial defibrillation threshold. *Am J Cardiol* 1989;63:112–114.

217. Somberg JC, Tepper D, Landau S. Propafenone: a new antiarrhythmic agent. *Am Heart J* 1988;115:1274–1279.

218. Dukes IV, Vaughan-Williams EM. The multiple modes of action of propafenone. *Am Heart J* 1984;5:115–125.

219. Coumel P, Leclercq J, Assayag P. European experience with the antiarrhythmic efficacy of propafenone for supraventricular and ventricular arrhythmias. *Am J Cardiol* 1984;54:60D–66D.

220. Kohlhardt M, Seifert C. Inhibition of Vmax of the action potential by propafenone and its voltage-time and pH-dependence in mammalian ventricular myocardium. *Naunyn Schmiedebergs Arch Pharmacol* 1980;315:55–62.

221. Ledda F, Mantelli L, Manzini S, et al. Electrophysiologic and antiarrhythmic properties of propafenone in isolated cardiac preparations. *J Cardiovasc Pharmacol* 1981;3:1162–1173.

222. Amerini S, Bernabei R, Carbonin P, Cerbai E, Mugelli A, Pahor M. Electrophysiological mechanism for the antiarrhythmic action of propafenone: a comparison with mexiletine. *Br J Pharmacol* 1988;95:1039–1046.

223. Valenzuela C, Delgado C, Tamargo J. Electrophysiological effects of 5-hydroxypropafenone on guinea pig ventricular muscle fibers. *J Cardiovasc Pharmacol* 1987;10:523–529.

224. Salerno D, Granrud G, Sharkey P, Asinger R, Hodges M. A controlled trial of propafenone for treatment of frequent and repetitive ventricular premature complexes. *Am J Cardiol* 1984;53:77–83.

225. Podrid P, Lown B. Propafenone, a new agent for ventricular arrhythmias. *J Am Coll Cardiol* 1984;4:117–125.

226. Baker BJ, Dinh H, Kroskey D, deSoyza N, Murphy M, Franciosa J. Effect of propafenone on left ventricular ejection fraction. *Am J Cardiol* 1984;54:20–22.

227. Beck OA, Hochrein H. Indications and risks of antiarrhythmic treatment with propafenone. *Dtsch Med Wochenschr* 1978;103:1261–1265.

228. Chilson D, Heger J, Zipes D, Browne K, Prystowsky E. Electrophysiologic effects and clinical efficacy and oral propafenone therapy in patients with ventricular tachycardia. *J Am Coll Cardiol* 1985;5:1407–1413.

229. Doherty J, Waxman H, Kienzle M, et al. Limited role of intravenous propafenone hydrochloride in the treatment of sustained ventricular tachycardia: electrophysiologic effects and results of programmed ventricular stimulation. *J Am Coll Cardiol* 1984;4:378–381.

230. Stavens CS, McGovern B, Garan H, Ruskin JN. Aggravation of electrically provoked ventricular tachycardia during treatment with propafenone. *Am Heart J* 1985;110:24–29.

231. Chow MS, Lebsack C, Hilleman D. Propafenone: a new antiarrhythmic agent. *Clin Pharm* 1988;7:869–77.

232. Giani P, Landolina M, Giudici V, et al. Pharmacokinetics and pharmacodynamics of propafenone during acute and chronic administration. *Eur J Clin Pharmacol* 1988;34:187–194.

233. Dressler F, Gravinghoff L, Grutte E, Jungst BK, Liersch R, Nomayn H, Puls I, Rautenburg HW, Schmaltz A, Schumacher G. The treatment of arrhythmias in infants and children using propafenone. *Monatsschr Kinderheilkd* 1985; 133:154–157.

234. Dubuc M, Kus T, Campa MA, Lambert C, Rosengarten M, Shenasa M. Electrophysiologic effects of intravenous propafenone in Wolff-Parkinson-White syndrome. *Am Heart J* 1988;117:370–376.

235. Antman EM, Beamer AD, Cantillon C, McGowan N, Goldman L, Friedman PL. Long-term oral propafenone therapy for suppression of refractory symptomatic atrial fibrillation and atrial flutter. *J Am Coll Cardiol* 1988;12:1005–1011.

236. Lucchesi BR, Whitsitt LS, Stickney JL. Antiarrhythmic effects of beta-adrenergic blocking agents. *Ann NY Acad Sci* 1967;139:940–951.

237. Parmley WW, Braunwald E. Comparative myocardial depressant and antiarrhythmic properties of *d*-propranolol, *d,l*-propranolol, and quinidine. *J Pharmacol Exp Ther* 1967;158:11–21.

238. Pitt WA, Cox AR. The effect of the beta-adrenergic antagonist propranolol on rabbit atrial

cells with the use of the ultramicroelectrode technique. *Am Heart J* 1968;76:242–248.

239. Vaughan-Williams EM. Mode of action of beta-receptor antagonists on cardiac muscle. *Am J Cardiol* 1966;18:399–405.

240. Berkowitz WD, Wit AL, Lau SH, Steiner C, Damato AN. The effects of propranolol on cardiac conduction. *Circulation* 1969;40:855–862.

241. Whitsitt LS, Lucchesi BR. The effects of beta-adrenergic receptor blockade and glucagon on the atrioventricular transmission system. *Circ Res* 1969;23:585–595.

242. Woosley RL, Kornhauser D, Smith R, et al. Suppression of chronic ventricular arrhythmias with propranolol. *Circulation* 1979;60:819–827.

243. Stern S, Eisenberg S. The effect of propranolol (Inderal) on the electrocardiogram of normal subjects. *Am Heart J* 1969;77:192–195.

244. Gibson DG. Pharmacodynamic properties of beta-adrenergic receptor blocking drugs in man. *Drugs* 1974;7:8–38.

245. Nakano J, Kusakari T. Effect of beta-adrenergic blockade on the cardiovascular dynamics. *Am J Physiol* 1966;210:833–837.

246. Donald DE, Terguson PA, Milburn SE. Effect of beta-adrenergic receptor blockade on racing performance of greyhounds with normal and denervated hearts. *Circ Res* 1979;22:127–137.

247. Epstein S, Robison BF, Kahler RL, Braunwald E. Effects of beta-adrenergic blockade on cardiac response to maximal and submaximal exercise in man. *J Clin Invest* 1965;44:1745–1753.

248. Sonnenblick EH, Braunwald E, Williams JFJ, Glick G. Effects of exercise on myocardial force velocity relations in intact unanesthetized man: relative roles of changes in heart rate, sympathetic activity, and ventricular dimensions. *J Clin Invest* 1965;44:2051–2062.

249. Sowton E, Hamer J. Hemodynamic changes after beta-adrenergic blockade. *Am J Cardiol* 1966;18:317–320.

250. Reed RL, Cheney CB, Fearon RE, Hook R, Hehre FW. Propranolol therapy during pregnancy: a case report. *Anesth Analg* 1974;53:214A.

251. Johnstone M. Propranolol during halothane anesthesia. *Br J Anaesth* 1966;38:516–529.

252. Norris RM, Coughey DE, Scott PJ. Trial of propranolol in acute myocardial infarction. *Br Med J* 1968;2:398–400.

253. Sowton E. Beta-adrenergic blockade in cardiac infarctions. *Prog Cardiovasc Dis* 1968;10:561–572.

254. Gibson D, Sowton E. The use of beta-adrenergic receptor blocking drugs in dysrhythmias. *Prog Cardiovasc Dis* 1969;12:16–39.

255. Naggar CZ, Alexander S. Propranolol treatment of VPB's. *N Engl J Med* 1976;294:903–904.

256. Nixon JV, Pennington W, Bitter W, Shapiro W. Efficacy of propranolol in the control of exercise-induced or augmented ventricular ectopic activity. *Circulation* 1978;57:115–122.

257. Erlij D, Mendez R. The modification of digitalis intoxication by excluding adrenergic influ-

ences on the heart. *J Pharmacol Exp Ther* 1964;144:97–103.

258. Roberts J, Ryuta I, Reilly J, Cairoli VJ. Influence of reserpine and BTM-10 on digitalis induced ventricular arrhythmias. *Circ Res* 1963;13:149–158.

259. Boura ALA, Green AF, McCoubrey A, Laurence DR, Moulton R, Rosenheim ML. Darenthin: hypotensive agent of a new type. *Lancet* 1959;2:17–21.

260. Boura ALA, Green AF. The actions of bretylium: adrenergic neurone blocking and other effects. *Br J Pharmacol* 1959;14:536–548.

261. Leveque PE. Antiarrhythmic action of bretylium. *Nature* 1965;207:203–204.

262. Bacaner M. Bretylium tosylate for suppression of induced ventricular fibrillation. *Am J Cardiol* 1966;17:528–534.

263. Bacaner M. Treatment of ventricular fibrillation and other acute arrhythmias with bretylium tosylate. *Am J Cardiol* 1968;21:530–543.

264. Holder DA, Sniderman AD, Fraser G, Fallen EL. Experience with bretylium tosylate by a hospital cardiac arrest team. *Circulation* 1977;55:541–544.

265. Terry G, Vellani CW, Higgins MR, Doig A. Bretylium tosylate in treatment of refractory ventricular arrhythmias complicating myocardial infarction. *Br Heart J* 1970;32:21–25.

266. Day HW, Bacaner M. Use of bretylium tosylate in the management of acute myocardial infarction. *Am J Cardiol* 1974;27:177–189.

267. Bernstein JG, Koch-Weser J. Effectiveness of bretylium tosylate against refractory ventricular arrhythmias. *Circulation* 1972;45:1024–1034.

268. Anderson JL, Patterson E, Wagner JG, Stewart JR, Behm HL, Lucchesi BR. Oral and intravenous bretylium disposition. *Clin Pharmacol Ther* 1980;28:468–478.

269. Touboul P, Porte J, Huera F, Belahaye JF. Etude des propriétés électrophysiologiques du tosylate de brétylium chez l'homme. *Arch Mal Coeur* 1976;69:503–511.

270. Waxman MB, Wallace AG. Electrophysiologic effects of bretylium tosylate on the heart. *J Pharmacol Exp Ther* 1972;183:264–274.

271. Romhilt DW, Bloomfield SS, Lipicky RJ, Welch RM, Fowler NO. Evaluation of bretylium tosylate for the treatment of premature ventricular contractions. *Circulation* 1972;45:800–807.

272. Cohen HC, Gozo EG, Langendorf R, et al. Response of resistant ventricular tachycardia to bretylium. *Circulation* 1973;47:331–340.

273. Papp JG, Vaughan-Williams EM. The effect of bretylium on intracellular cardiac action potentials in relation to its anti-arrhythmic and local anesthetic activity. *Br J Pharmacol* 1969;37:380–399.

274. DeAzevedo IM, Watanabe Y, Dreifus LS. Electrophysiologic antagonism of quinidine and bretylium tosylate. *Am J Cardiol* 1974;33:633–638.

275. Gillis RA, Clancy MM, Anderson RJ. Deleterious effects of bretylium in cats with digitalis-

induced ventricular tachycardia. *Circulation* 1973;47:974–983.

276. Namm DH, Wang CM, El-Sayad S, Copp FC, Maxwell RA. Effects of bretylium on rat cardiac muscle: the electrophysiological effects and its uptake and binding in normal and immunosympathectomized rat hearts. *J Pharmacol Exp Ther* 1975;193:194–207.

277. Cardinal R, Sasyniuk BI. Electrophysiological effects of bretylium tosylate on subendocardial Purkinje fibers from infarcted hearts. *J Pharmacol Exp Ther* 1978;204:159–174.

278. Bacaner MB. Quantitative comparison of bretylium with other antifibrillatory drugs. *Am J Cardiol* 1968;21:504–512.

279. Bacaner MB, Schrienemachers D. Bretylium tosylate for suppression of ventricular fibrillation after experimental myocardial infarction. *Nature* 1968;220:494–496.

280. Kniffen FJ, Lomas TE, Counsell RE, Lucchesi BR. Bretylium and its *o*-iodobenzl ammonium analog, UM-360. *J Pharmacol Exp Ther* 1975;192:120–128.

281. Anderson JL, Patterson E, Conlon M, Pasyk S, Pitt B, Lucchesi BR. Kinetics of antifibrillatory effects of bretylium: correlation with myocardial drug concentrations. *Am J Cardiol* 1980;46:583–591.

282. Sanna G, Arcidiacono R. Chemical ventricular defibrillation of the human heart with bretylium tosylate. *Am J Cardiol* 1973;32:982–987.

283. Steinberg MI, Malloy BB. Clofilium—a new antifibrillatory agent that selectively increases cellular refractoriness. *Life Sci* 1979;25:1397–1406.

284. Cervoni P, Ellis CH, Maxwell RA. The antiarrhythmic action of bretylium in normal, reserpine-pretreated, and chronically denervated dog hearts. *Arch Int Pharmacodyn Ther* 1971;190:91–102.

285. Babbs CF, Yim GKW, Whistler SJ, Tacker WA, Geddes LA. Elevation of ventricular defibrillation threshold in dogs by antiarrhythmic drugs. *Am Heart J* 1979;98:345–350.

286. Tacker WA, Niebauer MJ, Babbs CF, et al. The effect of newer antiarrhythmic drugs on defibrillation threshold. *Crit Care Med* 1980;8:177–180.

287. Chatterjee K, Mandel WJ, Vyden JK, Parmley WW, Forrester JS. Cardiovascular effects of bretylium tosylate in acute myocardial infarction. *JAMA* 1973;223:757–760.

288. Markis JE, Koch-Weser J. Characteristics and mechanisms of inotropic and chronotropic actions of bretylium tosylate. *J Pharmacol Exp Ther* 1971;178:94–102.

289. Graham JD, Chandler BM. The effects of lidocaine, propranolol, procainamide, and bretylium tosylate: a unique property of an antiarrhythmic agent. *Can J Physiol Pharmacol* 1973;51:763–773.

290. MacAlpin RN, Zalis EG, Kivowitz CF. Prevention of recurrent ventricular tachycardia with oral bretylium tosylate. *Ann Intern Med* 1970;72:909–912.

291. Anderson JL, Patterson E, Wagner JG, Johnson T, Lucchesi BR, Pitt B. Clinical pharmacokinetics of intravenous and oral bretylium tosylate in survivors of ventricular tachycardia or fibrillation. *J Cardiovasc Pharmacol* 1972;1:660–662.

292. Singh BN. Amiodarone: historical development and pharmacologic profile. *Am Heart J* 1983;106:788–797.

293. Mason JW. Amiodarone. *N Engl J Med* 1987;316:455–466.

294. Singh BN, Venkatesh N, Nademanee K, Josephson MA, Kannan R. The historical development, cellular electrophysiology and pharmacology of amiodarone. *Prog Cardiovasc Dis* 1989;31:249–280.

295. Greene HL. The efficacy of amiodarone in the treatment of ventricular tachycardia or ventricular fibrillation. *Prog Cardiovasc Dis* 1989;31:319–354.

296. Rotmensch HH, Belhassen B. Amiodarone in the management of cardiac arrhythmias. *Med Clin North Am* 1988;72:321–358.

297. Singh BN, Vaughan-Williams EM. The effect of amiodarone, a new antianginal drug on cardiac muscle. *Br J Phamacol* 1970;39:675–687.

298. Goupil N, Lenfant J. The effects of amiodarone on the sinus node activity of the rabbit heart. *Eur J Pharmacol* 1976;39:23–31.

299. Yabek S, Kato R, Singh BN. Acute electrophysiologic effects of amiodarone and desethylamiodarone in isolated cardiac muscle. *J Cardiovasc Pharmacol* 1986;8:197–207.

300. Nattel S, Talajuc M, Quantz M, et al. Frequency-dependent effects of amiodarone on atrio-ventricular nodal function and slow-channel action potentials: evidence for calcium blocking activity. *Circulation* 1987;76:442–449.

301. Freeberg AS, Papp GJ, Vaughan-Williams EM. The effects of altered thyroid state on atrial intracellular potentials. *J Physiol* 1970;207:357–369.

302. Olsson JB, Brorson L, Varnauskas E. Antiarrhythmic action in man: observations from monophasic action potential recordings and amiodarone treatment. *Br Heart J* 1973;35:1255–1259.

303. Kato R, Venkatesh N, Yabek S, et al. Electrophysiologic effects of desethylamiodarone an active metabolite of amiodarone: comparison with amiodarone during chronic administration in rabbits. *Am Heart J* 1988;115:351–359.

304. Neliat G. Effects of butoprozine on ionic currents in frog atrial and ferret ventricular fibers. Comparison with amiodarone and verapamil. *Arch Int Pharmacodyn Ther* 1982;255:237–255.

305. Aomine M, McCullough J, Mayuga R, et al. Cellular electrophysiologic effects of acute exposure to amiodarone on guinea pig heart. *Fed Proc* 1984;43:961.

306. Mason JW, Hondeghem LM, Katzung BG. Amiodarone blocks inactivated cardiac sodium channels. *Pflugers Arch* 1983;396:79–81.

307. Schamroth L, Krikler DM, Garrett C. Immediate effects of intravenous verapamil in cardiac arrhythmias. *Br Med J* 1972;1:660–662.

308. Feigl D, Ravid M. Electrocardiographic observations on the termination of supraventricular tachycardia by verapamil. *J Electrocardiogr* 1979;12:129–136.

309. Fleckenstein A. Die bedentung der energiereidren phosphate fur knotracktilitat und tonus des myokards. *Verh Dtsch Ges Inn Med* 1964;70:81–99.

310. Fleckenstein A. Prog. Vth Eur. Congr. Cardiol., Athens, 1968;255–269.

311. Zipes DP, Fischer JC. Effects of agents which inhibit the slow channel on sinus node automaticity and atrioventricular conduction in the dog. *Circ Res* 1974;34:184–192.

312. Okada T. Effect of verapamil on electrical activities of SA node, ventricular muscle, and Purkinje fibers in isolated rabbit hearts. *Jpn Circ J* 1976;40:329.

313. Rosen MR, Wit AL, Hoffman BF. Electrophysiology and pharmacology of cardiac arrhythmias. IV. Cardiac effects of verapamil. *Am Heart J* 1975;89:665–673.

314. Rinkenberger RL, Prystowsky EN, Heger JJ, Troup PJ, Jackman WM, Zipes DP. Effects of intravenous and chronic oral verapamil administration in patients with supraventricular tachyarrhythmias. *Circulation* 1980;62:996–1010.

315. Heng MK, Singh BN, Roche, AHG, Norris RM, Mercer CJ. Effects of intravenous verapamil on cardiac arrhythmias and on the electrocardiogram. *Am Heart J* 1975;90:487–498.

316. Luebs ED, Cohan A, Zaleski EJ, Bing RJ. Effect of nitroglycerin, intensain, isoptin and papaverine on coronary blood flow in man. Measured by coincidence counting technic and rubidium[84]. *Am J Cardiol* 1966;17:535–541.

317. Singh BN, Ellrodt G, Peter CT. Verapamil: a review of its pharmacological properties and therapeutic uses. *Drugs* 1978;15:169–197.

318. Terlinz J, Furbow ME. Antianginal and myocardial metabolic properties of verapamil in coronary artery disease. *Am J Cardiol* 1980: 56:1019–1025.

319. Gunther S, Muller JE, Mudge GH, Grossman W. Therapy of coronary vasoconstriction in patients with coronary artery disease. *Am J Cardiol* 1981;47:157–162.

Cardiovascular Pharmacology, Third Edition,
edited by Michael Antonaccio.
Raven Press, Ltd., New York © 1990.

Pathophysiology and Therapy of Hyperlipidemia

Henry N. Ginsberg, Yadon Arad, and Ira J. Goldberg

*Department of Medicine, Columbia University College of Physicians and Surgeons,
New York, New York 10032*

Atherosclerotic cardiovascular disease is the leading cause of death in the Western world, and coronary artery disease (CAD) is its major manifestation (1). Atherosclerosis is the end result of a multifactorial process that includes deposition of lipids, particularly cholesteryl ester, in the subintimal area of arteries. Although numerous factors associated with increased risk for CAD have been identified in prospective studies of populations around the globe, elevated fasting levels of plasma total and low-density lipoprotein (LDL) cholesterol, and reduced levels of plasma, high-density lipoprotein (HDL) cholesterol have been clearly identified as major risk factors (2). In some prospective studies, an increased fasting plasma concentration of triglycerides, the majority of which, in the fasting state, is found in very low density lipoproteins (VLDL), has also been demonstrated to be an independent risk factor for CAD (3).

Although the relationship between postprandial levels of plasma lipids and CAD has been studied in much less detail, available evidence suggests that the rise in plasma triglycerides (found mainly in chylomicrons and chylomicron remnants) during the several hours after ingestion of a fat load correlates with the risk of developing CAD. The triglyceride-rich chylomicron and the relatively cholesteryl ester-enriched chylomicron remnant have been shown to interact with cells of the arterial wall, including the most significant cellular component of early atherosclerotic lesions, the monocyte-derived macrophages (4).

In addition to the epidemiologic data relating plasma levels of lipids with CAD, laboratory studies using a variety of *in vitro* and *in vivo* techniques have demonstrated the role of lipoproteins in the delivery of lipids to cells of the vessel wall. Certain abnormal lipoproteins, particularly those enriched in cholesteryl ester such as beta-VLDL, may quite effectively cause the accumulation of cholesterol in smooth muscle cells and/or monocyte-derived macrophages in the subintimal space. Beta-VLDL may be present during the postprandial period, when they are comprised of chylomicron remnants, and during the fasting state in a rare type of hyperlipidemia called dyslipoproteinemia. Interactions between platelets and LDL and between both endothelial cells and macrophages and LDL have been observed to modify the LDL so that they are able to interact with monocyte-derived macrophages and produce cholesteryl ester-enriched foam cells (5).

In view of the available data, it would seem that appropriate pharmacologic modulation of either increased plasma levels of lipoproteins and their lipids or of abnormal or modified lipoproteins should have beneficial effects on individuals at high risk for developing CAD. Large, carefully controlled clinical trials such as the World Health Organization (WHO) Trial (6), the Lipid Research Clinics Coronary Primary Prevention Trial (LRC-CPPT) (7), the niacin component of the Coronary Drug Project (8), and the Helsinki Heart Study (9) have all indicated that ischemic heart disease events can be reduced in hyperlipidemic individuals by pharmacologic intervention. In order to approach pharmacotherapy of hyperlipidemia in a logical manner, a clear understanding of both normal and abnormal lipoprotein metabolism is needed. We will, therefore, present a brief review of these topics.

NORMAL LIPOPROTEIN METABOLISM

Both genetic and environmental factors have an impact on the plasma concentrations of VLDL, intermediate density lipoproteins (IDL), LDL, and HDL. Plasma concentrations of triglycerides and cholesterol are regulated by the rates of productions of the lipoproteins that carry these lipids, the efficiency with which these lipoproteins are removed from the plasma (fractional removal), and the rates of hydrolysis and transfer of the lipoprotein lipids by enzymes and special lipid-transfer proteins.

The plasma lipoproteins are macromolecular complexes of lipids, mainly cholesteryl ester, free cholesterol, triglycerides, and phospholipids, and a family of proteins called apolipoproteins (apo). There are eight major apolipoproteins: apo AI, apo AII, apo AIV, apo B-48, apo B-100, apo CII, apo CIII, and apo E. Each of these proteins has unique functions as regulators of lipoprotein metabolism. The characteristics of the major postprandial and fasting lipoprotein classes, chylomicrons, VLDL, IDL, LDL, and HDL, and the major apolipoproteins are presented in Tables 1 and 2.

Chylomicrons are assembled in and secreted from the mucosal cells of the small intestine after absorption of dietary triglycerides and cholesterol (10). Apo B-48 is an integral component of chylomicrons and is necessary for assembly and secretion of this intestinal lipoprotein. Chylomicrons enter the mesenteric lymph and make their way to the systemic circulation via the thoracic duct. Once in the circulation, chylomicrons interact with the enzyme, lipoprotein lipase (LPL). LPL is a glycoprotein of molecular weight 55 kdaltons that is synthesized mainly in adipose and muscle tissue and that, after secretion from those tissues, is bound to the luminal surface of capillary endothelial cells (11). LPL is responsible for the hydrolysis of chylomicron triglycerides and, therefore, delivery of dietary fatty acids to adipocytes and muscle cells. APO CII is the required activator of LPL (12). Available evidence suggests that apo CIII is an inhibitor of that enzyme's ability to hydrolyze chylomicron triglycerides (13). Triglyceride hydrolysis generates the chylomicron remnant, which is relatively enriched in cholesteryl ester and apo E.

TABLE 1. *Physical-chemical characteristics of the major lipoprotein classes*

Lipoprotein	Density (g/dl)	MW (daltons)	Diameter (nm)	Lipid (%)[a] TG	Chol	PL
Chylomicrons	0.95	400×10^6	75–1,200	80–95	2–7	3–9
VLDL	0.95–1.006	$10–80 \times 10^6$	30–80	55–80	5–15	10–20
IDL	1.006–1.019	$5–10 \times 10^6$	25–35	20–50	20–40	15–25
LDL	1.019–1.063	2.3×10^6	18–25	5–15	40–50	20–25
HDL	1.063–1.21	$1.7–3.6 \times 10^6$	5–12	5–10	15–25	20–30

TG, triglycerides; Chol, cholesterol; PL, phospholipids.
[a]Percentage of composition of lipids; apolipoproteins make up the rest.

TABLE 2. *Characteristics of the major apoliproteins*

Apolipoprotein	MW	Lipoproteins	Metabolic functions
apo AI	28,016	HDL, chylomicrons	Structural component of HDL; LCAT activator
apo AII	17,414	HDL, chylomicrons	Unknown
apo AIV	46,465	HDL, chylomicrons	Unknown: possibly facilitates transfer of other apos between HDL and chylomicrons
apo B48	264,000	Chylomicrons	Necessary for assembly and secretion of chylomicrons from the small intestine
apo B100	545,000	VLDL, IDL, LDL	Necessary for assembly and secretion of VLDL from the liver; structural protein of VLDL, IDL, LDL; ligand for LDL receptor
apo CII	8,900	All major lipoproteins	Activator of lipoprotein lipase
apo CIII	8,800	All major lipoproteins	Inhibitor of lipoprotein lipase; may inhibit hepatic uptake of chylomicron and VLDL remnants
apo E	34,145	All major lipoproteins	Ligand for binding of several lipoproteins to the LDL receptor and possibly to a separate hepatic apo E receptor

Apo E appears to be the ligand mediating removal of chylomicron remnants by the liver, via either the well-characterized apo B,E (LDL) receptor or a unique and as yet uncharacterized apo E plasma membrane receptor (14). Hepatic uptake of chylomicron remnants results in delivery of dietary cholesterol to the liver where it plays a significant role in regulating endogenous synthesis of cholesterol by the liver. There is evidence that apo CIII may oppose the action of apo E in mediating the uptake of chylomicron remnants by the liver (15). Of particular relevance to atherogenesis is the possibility that chylomicron remnants may be taken up by arterial wall smooth muscle cells or monocyte-derived macrophages (4). A scheme representing chylomicron and chylomicron remnant metabolism in plasma is depicted in Fig. 1.

VLDL are assembled and secreted by hepatocytes (16). The VLDL core and surface lipids are, in the main, synthesized in hepatocytes from smaller carbon molecules and free fatty acids that have been recycled from peripheral tissues. Dietary triglycerides and cholesterol may be resecreted in VLDL as well (17). Apo B-100 is necessary for the assembly and secretion of VLDL (18). There is one apo B-100 per VLDL, and this protein stays with the particle as VLDL is converted to IDL and LDL. Once

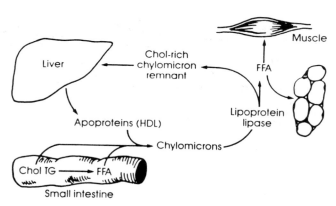

FIG. 1. Chylomicron and chylomicron remnant transport in plasma. Chol, cholesterol; TG, triglyceride; HDL, high density lipoproteins; FFA, free fatty acids.

in the plasma, VLDL, like chylomicrons, must deliver their triglycerides to peripheral tissues, and this function is accomplished through the actions of LPL and apo CII. Apo CIII appears to play an inhibitory role in this process similar to that described for chylomicrons.

Depletion of VLDL triglycerides generates a family of lipoprotein particles that may be described as VLDL remnants or IDL. The term VLDL remnants may be more appropriately reserved for those particles that, like the chylomicron remnant, are removed from the plasma via apo E-mediated uptake into the liver or other tissues. The IDL more likely represent intermediates in the generation of LDL from VLDL, although there is evidence that IDL may also interact with cell surface receptors and be removed from plasma via the binding of apo E, and possibly apo B-100, to cell surface receptors. The mechanisms regulating the conversion of VLDL to remnants marked for removal from plasma, or to IDL and possibly LDL, remain undefined. Although there is strong evidence indicating that LPL activity (19) and apo E (20) are needed for the orderly conversion of VLDL to remnants and IDL/LDL, a second lipolytic enzyme, hepatic triglyceride lipase (HTGL) is also crucial to these processes. HTGL is a glycoprotein of 52 kdal-

tons that is synthesized by the liver and secreted into the space of Disse where it is bound to the luminal surface of endothelial cells (21). HTGL appears to hydrolyze triglycerides in small VLDL and IDL (22) and to also play a role in HDL metabolism (see below). As noted for the chylomicron remnant, the role of VLDL remnants and/or IDL in the atherogenic process is under intense investigation.

After several enzymatic and cell surface interactions, some of the triglyceride-enriched lipoproteins are converted to LDL, the cholesteryl ester-enriched member of the endogenous lipoprotein family. The role of LDL is to deliver its cholesterol to peripheral tissues for incorporation into cell membranes and, in the case of the adrenals and gonads, into hormones. LDL interacts with cells via the binding of apo B-100 with the apo B,E (LDL) receptor, causing internalization of the LDL particle and the ultimate delivery of free cholesterol to the cytosol (23). The delivery of free cholesterol is associated with suppression of both endogenous cholesterol synthesis and synthesis of LDL receptors in that cell. LDL can be internalized and metabolized by cells via nonreceptor-mediated uptake as well. A scheme representing plasma transport of VLDL, IDL, and LDL is presented in Fig. 2.

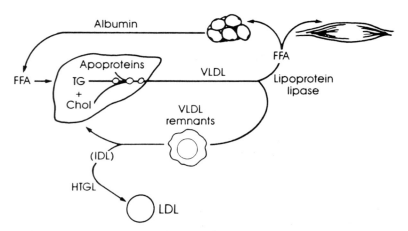

FIG. 2. Transport and metabolism of endogenous plasma lipoproteins.

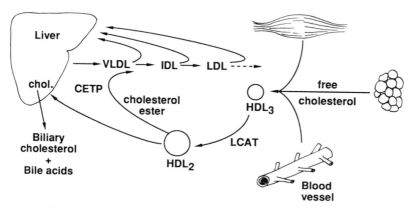

FIG. 3. Possible pathways for reverse cholesterol transport via plasma HDL. CETP, cholesteryl ester transfer protein.

HDL is a complex family of lipoprotein particles that appears to regulate what has been called reverse cholesterol transport in plasma (24). HDL appears to derive its free cholesterol from cell membranes and its cholesteryl ester from the esterification of that cell-derived free cholesterol in plasma. The enzyme lecithin-cholesterol acyl-transferase (LCAT), a 65-kdalton protein, regulates the esterification of HDL free cholesterol (25). HDL phospholipid may be cosecreted with nascent HDL or may associate with circulating HDL after transfer from catabolized chylomicrons and VLDL. Some HDL apolipoproteins such as apo AI, apo AII, and some of the apo E associated with HDL appear to enter the plasma as components of nascent, discoid HDL particles. In contrast, apo CII, apo CIII, and another fraction of apo E associate with HDL only after these apolipoproteins are transferred from catabolized chylomicrons and VLDL. Once formed, it appears that HDL cholesteryl ester is transferred to VLDL, IDL, and LDL via the action of cholesteryl ester transfer protein, a 67,000-kdalton glycoprotein that also regulates lipoprotein triglyceride transfer (26). The fate of this cholesteryl ester is uncertain. HDL cholesterol may also be delivered directly to cells after binding of the HDL particle to poorly defined cell surface receptor sites (27), although the HDL particle may or may not be internalized itself (28). Figure 3 depicts a possible scheme for reverse cholesterol transport via plasma HDL.

PATHOPHYSIOLOGY OF HYPERLIPIDEMIA

Based on the brief outline of lipid and lipoprotein metabolism just described, one can surmise that elevated levels of plasma total triglycerides, total cholesterol, and LDL cholesterol can derive from a variety of disturbances in production and catabolism of each of the major lipoprotein classes or their lipids. Similarly, reduced levels of HDL cholesterol may result from disorders of production and catabolism of lipid and protein components or from derangements in the transfer of cholesteryl ester between lipoproteins.

Hypertriglyceridemia

Elevated levels of fasting plasma triglycerides in the range of 250 to 750 mg/dl are generally associated with increased concentrations of only VLDL triglycerides. When VLDL triglyceride levels are markedly elevated (regardless of etiology) or when LPL is either significantly reduced or totally deficient, chylomicron triglycerides may also be present, even after a 14-hr fast.

Elevations in plasma triglycerides most often are associated with the synthesis and secretion of excessive quantities of VLDL triglyceride by the liver (29). Hepatic triglyceride synthesis is regulated by substrate flow, particularly the availability of free fatty acids; by energy status, particularly the level of glycogen stores in the liver; and by hormonal status, particularly the balance between insulin and glucagon levels. Obesity, excessive consumption of simple sugars and saturated fats, inactivity, alcohol consumption, and glucose intolerance or diabetes mellitus have been commonly associated with hypertriglyceridemia (30). Although no single gene disorder associated with increased hepatic synthesis of triglycerides has been identified, some recent studies have suggested a link between abnormal bile acid metabolism and overproduction of triglycerides in some subjects with hypertriglyceridemia (31). It is believed that in this group of disorders, sometimes referred to as primary hypertriglyceridemia, only triglyceride synthesis is increased and the liver secretes, therefore, a normal number of large, triglyceride-enriched VLDL particles. The secretion of a normal number of VLDL particles limits the rate of production of LDL particles, and these subjects may not necessarily develop coincident elevations of LDL cholesterol. It should be noted, however, that subjects with familial combined hyperlipidemia (see below) can present with isolated hypertriglyceridemia.

The degree of hypertriglyceridemia present in any individual will also depend on the quantity and activity of the two key triglyceride hydrolases, LPL and HTGL. Most data suggest that LPL is normal in the majority of subjects with moderate hypertriglyceridemia (250–500 mg/dl), but that this enzyme activity may be reduced in more severely affected individuals (>750 mg/dl) (11). As noted above, when VLDL triglyceride concentrations are markedly elevated (>1,000 mg/dl), LPL may be either saturated or actually "consumed," so that, in effect, the subject is relatively deficient in

the enzyme during the postprandial period (32). Chylomicron triglycerides may then add to the hypertriglyceridemia in such patients. If LPL is totally deficient, plasma triglyceride concentrations >2,000 mg/dl are commonly seen, with both chylomicrons and VLDL making significant contributions to the hyperlipidemia state (33). HTGL activity is frequently elevated in hypertriglyceridemic subjects, and the meaning of this association is unclear, although it may be relevant to the reduced HDL cholesterol levels found in this condition (21). Deficiencies of HTGL is a rare disorder in humans that results in defective final catabolism and/or abnormal remodeling of small VLDL and IDL (34).

Hypertriglyceridemia with Hypercholesterolemia

Hypertriglyceridemia can also occur in two phenotypes in association with hypercholesterolemia. In the first, called combined hyperlipidemia, both total plasma triglycerides and LDL cholesterol concentrations must, by definition, be greater than the 90th percentiles for age- and sex-matched controls (35). Although it is likely that a variety of combinations of regulatory defects in lipid metabolism account for a significant number of individuals with this phenotype, a familial form of combined hyperlipidemia (FCHL) has been identified in which probands (the initial case discovered) may present with combined hyperlipidemia, with only hypertriglyceridemia, or with only elevated levels of LDL cholesterol (36). In the familial disorder, which appears to be transmitted as an autosomal dominant gene, the diagnosis must rest on the presentation, at some point in time, of combined hyperlipidemia in the proband or, alternatively, the presence of various lipid phenotypes in first-degree family members along with either isolated hypertriglyceridemia or an isolated elevation of LDL cholesterol in the proband.

From available studies, FCHL appears

to be associated with secretion of increased numbers VLDL particles (as determined by the flux of VLDL apo B) (37). Hence, individuals with FCHL would be predisposed to high levels of plasma VLDL triglycerides if, for any other reason (see above) they synthesized triglycerides at an increased rate. Once they had assembled and secreted increased numbers of large, triglyceride-rich VLDL, these individuals would attain varying levels of plasma triglycerides relative to their ability to hydrolyze VLDL triglyceride with LPL and/or HTGL. The ability to hydrolyze VLDL triglycerides would also regulate the generation of LDL in plasma. Thus, subjects with FCHL who had very high VLDL triglyceride concentrations (and were not able to efficiently catabolize VLDL) might have normal or actually reduced numbers of LDL particles in the circulation and a normal LDL cholesterol concentration. If these same individuals were able to efficiently catabolize the increased numbers of VLDL particles that were entering their plasma, they would generate increased numbers of LDL particles and present, therefore, with both hypertriglyceridemia and a high LDL cholesterol level. Finally, subjects with FCHL who were synthesizing only normal quantities of triglycerides and secreting increased numbers of VLDL carrying normal triglyceride loads would generate increased numbers of LDL particles and present with only elevated plasma LDL cholesterol concentrations. FCHL may occur in as many as 1 in 50 to 1 in 100 Americans and is the most common familial lipid disorder found in survivors of myocardial infarction (36).

The second disorder in which elevations of both plasma triglycerides and cholesterol can occur is dysbetalipoproteinemia. In this rare disorder affecting 1 in 10,000 people, mutations in the gene for apo E result in synthesis of defective forms of this apolipoprotein. Because apo E appears to play crucial roles in the catabolism of chylomicron and VLDL remnants (14), subjects with defective apo E accumulate these cholesteryl ester-enriched remnant lipopro-

teins in their plasma. Hence, both VLDL triglyceride and VLDL cholesterol are elevated and chylomicron remnants are present in fasting plasma from dysbetalipoproteinemic subjects (38). LDL cholesterol levels are not elevated in this disorder. Of interest are the data indicating that 1 in 100 people are homozygous for the mutant apo E form (the apo E2 isoform). Of these apo E2/2 subjects, 99% have normal plasma triglyceride and cholesterol levels and actually have reduced LDL cholesterol levels (possibly a consequence of their inability to normally process VLDL). Thus, a second defect in lipid metabolism must be present in the 1 in 10,000 individuals with the clinically relevant entity, dysbetalipoproteinemia.

Isolated Hypercholesterolemia

Elevated levels of fasting plasma total cholesterol are, in general, associated with increased concentrations of plasma LDL cholesterol, because LDL carries approximately 65% to 75% of total plasma cholesterol. If plasma triglyceride levels are markedly increased, VLDL cholesterol, which is usually 5% to 10% of total plasma cholesterol, may be great enough to elevate total plasma cholesterol concentrations. VLDL cholesterol may be a major component of total cholesterol in dysbetalipoproteinemic subjects as well. Finally, the rare patient with significantly elevated HDL cholesterol may appear to have moderately increased total plasma cholesterol.

Elevations of LDL cholesterol can result from single gene defects, polygenic disorders, and environmental effects on lipoprotein metabolism. Familial hypercholesterolemia (FH), which occurs in the heterozygous form in approximately 1 in 500 individuals, is associated with mutations in the gene for the LDL receptor (23). Plasma total and LDL cholesterol concentrations are increased at birth in FH subjects and remain so throughout life. In FH adults, total cholesterol levels range from 300 to 500 in the untreated state, and both tendon xanthomas and premature atherosclerosis with CAD are common. Plasma triglyceride concentrations are typically normal, whereas HDL cholesterol levels may be normal or reduced. Metabolic studies have demonstrated decreased fractional clearance of LDL apo B in subjects with FH, consistent with reduced numbers of LDL receptors, although increased production of LDL has also been observed (39). The latter may be the result of more efficient conversion of VLDL to LDL in the FH patients as a concomitant of reduced LDL receptor function and reduced VLDL remnant removal from plasma. On the other hand, increased assembly and secretion of VLDL (or more dense apo B-containing lipoproteins) may be a concomitant of defective hepatic catabolism of circulating LDL. In any event, markedly elevated levels of LDL cholesterol are the hallmark of FH and are associated with the increased risk for CAD in these patients. The homozygous form of FH occurs in one in one million individuals and is associated with plasma cholesterol levels >500 mg/dl, large tendon and planar xanthomas, and very aggressive, premature CAD.

Recently, a second single gene disorder causing significant elevations of LDL cholesterol has been identified. A mutation in apo B in the region of the protein associated with binding to the LDL receptor has been linked to defective catabolism of LDL *in vivo* and to hypercholesterolemia that is transmitted in an autosomal dominant fashion (40). Finally, as noted above, subjects with FCHL can present with isolated elevations of LDL cholesterol (36).

Polygenic causes of hypercholesterolemia, which are likely to interact with environmental effects on lipoprotein metabolism, are much more common than FH. Most evidence indicates that both overproduction and reduced fractional catabolism of LDL play significant roles in the pathophysiology of this disorder. Both abnormal variables are probably affected by dietary saturated fat and cholesterol consumption,

age, and level of physical activity. Plasma total cholesterol levels usually are in the 250 to 350 mg/dl range. Plasma triglyceride and HDL cholesterol levels are usually normal. Tendon xanthomas are not present in these individuals.

Reduced HDL Cholesterol

Low concentrations of HDL cholesterol are most often seen in subjects with coexistent hypertriglyceridemia (24), although "primary hypoalphalipoproteinemia" has been identified in both individuals and families (41). The pathophysiologic basis of reduced HDL cholesterol concentrations is not well defined and probably quite complex (42). The relationship between hypertriglyceridemia and low HDL levels probably derives from (a) the cholesteryl ester transfer protein mediated transfer of cholesteryl ester from the core of HDL to VLDL, (b) the shift of surface components, particularly phospholipids and apolipoproteins CII and CIII, from HDL to VLDL, and (c) the increased fractional catabolism of the cholesteryl ester-poor, surface-poor HDL that results from the first two processes (25). The complexity of the situation is highlighted by the failure of the HDL levels to normalize when fasting plasma triglycerides are significantly reduced in most subjects with initial hypertriglyceridemia and low HDL cholesterol concentrations.

Primary hypoalphalipoproteinemia refers to the state in which HDL cholesterol concentrations are markedly reduced but plasma triglyceride concentrations are normal. Although this disorder certainly exists, many subjects who present with this phenotype have had hypertriglyceridemia in the past or have an older (or more obese) first-degree relative who has both low HDL and increased triglyceride levels. Hence, carefully conducted family studies and long-term follow-up may be necessary to identify individuals who truly have primary reductions in HDL cholesterol. The basis

TABLE 3. *Characteristics of common hyperlipidemias*

Type signs	Plasma lipid levels	Involved lipoproteins	Clinical
Isolated hypertriglyceridemia			
Mild	TG = 250–750 mg/dl (plasma may be cloudy)	VLDL	Asymptomatic; may be associated with increased risk of vascular disease
Severe	TG >750 mg/dl (plasma may be milky)	VLDL, chylomicrons	Asymptomatic; may be associated with pancreatitis, abdominal pain, hepatosplenomegaly
Hypertriglyceridemia and hypercholesterolemia			
Combined hyperlipidemia TG, LDL	TG = 250–750 mg/dl; total chol = 250–500 mg/dl	VLDL, LDL >95th%	Usually asymptomatic until vascular disease develops; FCHL may present as isolated high TG or as isolated high LDL cholesterol
Dysbetalipoproteinemia	TG = 250–500 mg/dl; total chol = 250–500 mg/dl	VLDL, IDL (LDL normal)	Usually asymptomatic until vascular disease develops; may have palmar or tuboeruptive xanthoma
Isolated hypercholesterolemia			
FH	Heterozygotes: total chol = 300–500 mg/dl Homozygotes: total chol = 400–800 mg/dl	LDL	Usually develop xanthomas in adulthood and vascular disease at 30–50 years Usually develop xanthomas in vascular disease in childhood
Polygenic hypercholesterolemia	Total chol = 225–350 mg/dl	LDL	Usually asymptomatic until vascular disease develops; no xanthomas
Low HDL cholesterol			
Associated with hypertriglyceridemia	HDL = 20–35 mg/dl; total TG >250 mg/dl	HDL	Usually asymptomatic; may increase risk for vascular disease
Primary hypoalphalipoproteinemia	HDL = 5–35 mg/dl; total TG <250 mg/dl	HDL	Depending on etiology; may be asymptomatic; often associated with increased vascular disease

TABLE 4. *NCEP guidelines*

Total cholesterol	Classification	Recommendation
<200 mg/dl	Desirable	Repeat within 5 years or at next regular examination
200–239 mg/dl	Borderline-high	In the absence of CAD or two other risk factors for CAD; receive diet information and repeat exam annually
		In the presence of CAD or two other risk factors for CAD; get a lipoprotein analysis
>240 mg/dl	High	Get a lipoprotein analysis

for such reductions is unknown except for extremely rare situations in which genetic mutations in the area of the apo AI gene have been described (43). Other rare disorders in which HDL cholesterol is severely reduced include Tangier disease and LACAT deficiency.

Table 3 presents a summary of the common types of hyperlipidemia.

THERAPY OF HYPERLIPIDEMIA

General Approach

The Adult Treatment Panel of the National Cholesterol Education Program recently promulgated guidelines for the identification, evaluation, and treatment of individuals with hypercholesterolemia (44). A summary of those guidelines is presented in Table 4. In general, although the cutpoints used to identify individuals who should have a full lipoprotein profile performed are liberal, the guidelines for treat-

ment with pharmacologic agents are conservative. Drug therapy is indicated only for (a) individuals without evidence of CAD or two other risk factors for CAD (Table 5) who, after maximal dietary efforts, have an LDL cholesterol level >190 mg/dl or (b) individuals with CAD or two other risk factors for CAD who, after maximal dietary efforts, have an LDL cholesterol level >160 mg/dl.

Maximal efforts aimed at reaching the initial goals set by the guidelines (Table 4) include use of a lower fat, low cholesterol diet (the Step 1 diet), utilization of registered dietitians when necessary, and progression to a more rigorous diet (the Step 2 diet) if needed. The Step 1 and Step 2 diets are described in Table 6. The length of time that diet therapy is maintained before adding drug treatment will depend on a variety of factors, including the initial lipid values

TABLE 5. *Other risk factors*

Male sex
Family history of premature CAD (definite myocardial infarction or sudden death before age 55 in a parent or sibling)
Cigarette smoking (currently smokes more than 10 cigarettes per day)
Hypertension (either untreated or treated)
Low HDL cholesterol (below 35 mg/dl in several measurements)
Diabetes mellitus
History of definite cerebrovascular or occlusive peripheral vascular disease
Severe obesity (>30% overweight)

TABLE 6. *Recommended diet therapy*

Nutrient	Recommended dietary intake	
	Step 1 diet	Step 2 diet
Total fat	Less than 30% of total calories	
Saturated fatty acids	<10% total calories	<7% total calories
Polyunsaturated fatty acids	Up to 10% of total calories	
Monounsaturated fatty acids	10%–15% of total calories	
Carbohydrates	50%–60% of total calories	
Protein	10%–20% of total calories	
Cholesterol	<300 mg/day	<200 mg/day
Total calories	To achieve and maintain desirable weight	

TABLE 7. *Lipid-lowering drugs*

Generic name	Brand name
Approved drugs (U.S.)	
Cholestyramine	Questran
Colestipol	Colestid
Niacin (nicotinic acid)	
Clofibrate	Atromid
Gemfibrozil	Lopid
Lovastatin	Mevacor
Probucol	Lorelco
Likely to be approved drugs	
Fenofibrate	
Bezafibrate	
Simvastatin	
Pravastatin	
Fluindostatin	

of the subject as well as that individual's overall risk profile for developing CAD. It must be stressed, however, that diet therapy must be attempted prior to drug therapy and that diet treatment must be maintained even after initiation of drug treatment.

The drugs listed in the Adult Treatment Panel Guidelines (Table 7) are ordered according to the Panel's determination of their long-term efficacy, safety, and proven ability (when data were available) to reduce the incidence of CAD events in study populations. The order of priority for use suggested by the Adult Treatment Panel will likely be subject to change over the next few years as more data become available regarding these agents and as newer agents gain approval from the Food and Drug Administration. Those agents not yet approved, but likely to be approved soon, are also listed in Table 7 and will be discussed briefly in the text.

BILE ACID SEQUESTRANT RESINS

Two agents, cholestyramine and colestipol, are currently used in the treatment of hypercholesterolemia. Both have a good record of safety and treatment can be expected to result in dose-related decreases of 15% to 25% in total cholesterol and 20% to 35% decreases in LDL cholesterol. Total plasma triglyceride levels usually remain unchanged in subjects with only hypercholesterolemia. In contrast, plasma triglyceride levels may actually increase in subjects with the combination of hypertriglyceridemia and hypercholesterolemia. HDL cholesterol concentrations may remain the same or increase slightly during therapy with bile acid sequestrants. Both cholestyramine and colestipol have been demonstrated to reduce the risk of having coronary heart disease (CHD) events.

Pharmacology and Metabolism

Cholestyramine is the chloride salt of a basic anion exchange copolymer of styrine and divinylbenzene, which has an average molecular weight $>10^6$ (45). The anion exchange sites are provided by trimethylbenzylammonium groups. Colestipol is a large molecular weight copolymer of diethylpentamine and epichlorohydrin (45). The structures of these two compounds are depicted in Fig. 4. Both drugs are hydrophilic but insoluble in water (>99.7%). Less than 0.05% of radio-labeled colestipol is secreted in the urine. The therapeutic effects of these drugs are due to their actions within the bowel. Neither drug is absorbed from the gastrointestinal tract.

The bile acid binding resins can alter the absorption of concomitantly administered anionic drugs such as digoxin, thyroxine, and warfarin as well as fat-soluble vitamins and folic acid by binding them in the gastrointestinal tract (46). Very few studies of the interaction of the bile acid binding resins and particular drugs have been performed.

Mechanism of Action

These agents are insoluble, nonabsorbable, anion exchange cationic polymer resins that bind bile acids and interfere with their reabsorption by the intestine (47). This interferes with the usually very effi-

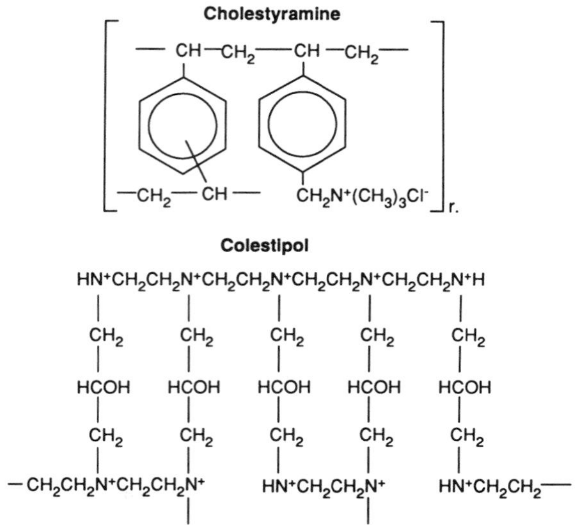

Cholestyramine

Colestipol

FIG. 4. The structures of bile acid binding resins cholestyramine and colestipol.

cient enterohepatic recirculation of bile acids and results in increased conversion of cholesterol to bile acids in hepatocytes. This response may be partially due to the decrease in inhibitory effect of bile acid on the microsomal enzyme, 7α-hydroxylase, the rate-limiting enzyme in the hepatic conversion of cholesterol to bile acids. Reduction of hepatic intracellular free cholesterol ensues, and, in response, the liver increases both the synthesis of cholesterol from mevalonate and the synthesis of LDL receptors. The latter mechanism results in a reduction of the plasma LDL cholesterol level by increasing the fractional removal of LDL from the circulation as demonstrated by *in vivo* kinetic studies of LDL apo B metabolism in humans (48). These drugs are therefore ideally suited to patients with decreased activity of LDL receptors such as patients with heterozygous FH. Conversely, they are ineffective in patients who cannot upregulate their LDL receptors, such as patients with homozygous FH.

Therapy with bile acid sequestrants also results in the generation of smaller, more dense LDL particles that are triglyceride enriched and cholesteryl ester depleted (49). Although there are experimental data

suggesting that such LDL may have reduced ability to interact with LDL receptors, the effects of these changes in LDL composition *in vivo* are not known.

As mentioned above, cholesterol synthesis in the hepatocyte also increases in response to interruption of the enterohepatic circulation (47). This compensatory response probably limits the clinical effectiveness of the resins as LDL-lowering agents. Increased synthesis of triglyceride is another concomitant of increased bile acid synthesis (50) and may lead to increased VLDL triglyceride secretion by the liver and elevations of plasma triglyceride levels. This may be clinically significant in patients with elevated baseline rates of triglyceride synthesis.

Clinical Efficacy

Colestipol and cholestyramine are supplied in packets of 5 and 4 g or in bulk containers of 500 or 372 g, respectively. Therapy is initiated with one packet or one scoop once or twice a day with meals, and the dose is gradually increased as tolerated to a final dose of 30 g/day of colestipol or

24 g/day of cholestyramine. Therapy is associated with 15% to 30% decreases in plasma total cholesterol and LDL cholesterol compared with that achieved with diet alone.

These drugs also tend to cause elevation of plasma triglycerides by increasing the synthesis of VLDL triglyceride, especially in patients with combined hyperlipidemia or familial hypertriglyceridemia who have preexisting elevations of VLDL triglycerides. The resins are actually contraindicated in patients with significantly elevated initial plasma triglycerides (>400 mg/dl). The effects on HDL cholesterol levels have been variable but small increases (3%–5%) may be seen.

Unfortunately, therapy with these two drugs is associated with several side effects that may significantly decrease patient compliance. The gritty texture is unpleasant even when mixed with fruit juice or water. Constipation, nausea, epigastric fullness, flatulence, and abdominal bloating are bothersome to many patients but can be reduced by the addition of bran to the diet or by coadministration of stool softeners such as soluble fiber or glycerine suppositories. Resin therapy may cause exacerbation of rectal hemorrhoids. Recently introduced cholestyramine bars may offer an alternative approach to therapy with this agent.

Toxicity

The resins can theoretically increase the lithogenicity of bile because their use results in reduced availability of bile acids for direct secretion into bile (51). Increased cholelithiasis, however, has not been observed in long-term, controlled trials such as the LRC-CPPT. On the other hand, because these drugs are not absorbed systemically, serious biochemical adverse reactions are rarer than with other hypocholesterolemic drugs although mild elevations of alkaline phosphatase and transaminases may be seen occasionally during treatment with bile acid sequestrants. Overall, the resins have been demonstrated to have excellent long-term safety records in clinical trials.

Effect on Atherosclerosis

These drugs had been the most intensively studied of all cholesterol-lowering drugs with regard to their influence on coronary atherosclerosis. Results from early drug studies that suggested a beneficial effect of resin therapy on coronary atherosclerosis were confirmed in several more recent double-blind, placebo-controlled studies. The effects of cholestyramine therapy on subsequent death from coronary disease and on the incidence of nonfatal myocardial infarction was assessed in the LRC-CPPT (7). This study followed 3,806 males, ages 30 to 59 years, randomized to receive either diet therapy alone or diet therapy plus cholestyramine. After 7.5 years, the cholestyramine group experienced reductions in total cholesterol and LDL cholesterol of 13% and 20%, respectively, compared with the control group, which was treated with diet alone. There was a 19% decrease of nonfatal myocardial infarctions and a 24% decrease in fatal CHD events, as well as a 20% to 25% reduction in new positive stress tests, new angina pectoris, and coronary bypass operations. Although patient compliance with cholestyramine therapy was not ideal, the reductions in CHD events was proportional to the reductions in plasma total cholesterol, which, in turn, correlated to the amount of medication the patients consumed (52).

In another study (The National Heart, Lung, and Blood Institute Type II Coronary Intervention Study), 116 patients with type II hyperlipidemia were randomized to receive either a low-fat, low-cholesterol diet plus placebo or the same diet plus cholestyramine (53). After 5 years, LDL cholesterol decreased by 26%. CAD had progressed in 49% of the placebo group but in only 32% of the cholestyramine group. In both groups progression of coronary disease was inversely correlated with a decrease in LDL cholesterol and an increase in HDL cholesterol (53).

The effect of colestipol in combination with niacin on the progression of coronary atherosclerosis was studied in the Cholesterol-Lowering Atherosclerosis Study (CLAS), which followed 162 nonsmoking men with documented coronary atherosclerosis who had undergone coronary artery bypass surgery (54). After 2 years, therapy was associated with 26% and 43% reductions of total and LDL cholesterol, respectively, and a 37% increase in HDL cholesterol. There was a statistically significant cessation of progression of disease in both native and bypass vessels in the treated subjects. In addition, in 16% of the drug-treated patients coronary atherosclerosis had actually regressed, whereas such regression occurred in only 2% of the control group.

NICOTINIC ACID

The water-soluble vitamin, niacin (Fig. 5), has been used for more than three decades to treat hyperlipidemias. Niacin therapy results in lower plasma levels of total and LDL cholesterol, reductions in total plasma triglyceride concentrations, and significant, often dramatic increases in HDL cholesterol levels. Long-term effects of this treatment have been well described and documented. The use of niacin in middle-aged men with a higher than average plasma cholesterol and increased risk of CHD was

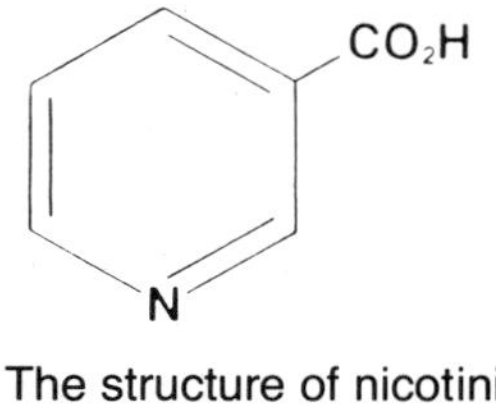

FIG. 5. The structure of nicotinic acid.

associated with a reduction in coronary events (55). A subsequent follow-up study of the men involved in this study showed, furthermore, that the niacin-treated group of men had increased longevity (8).

Pharmacology and Metabolism

Niacin or nicotinic acid is readily absorbed from the gastrointestinal tract, reaching peak blood levels 15 to 40 min after ingestion. Much of the dose is removed via the liver before it reaches the circulation (56). This high first-pass effect on the liver may be responsible for much of the drug's mechanism of action, although (*vide infra*) niacin also has important effects on peripheral tissues. Niacin does not appear to interact with other drugs.

Mechanism of Action

Niacin therapy affects the circulating levels of all major classes of lipoproteins. Marked reductions occur in plasma VLDL concentrations as reflected by decreases in plasma triglyceride levels. LDL cholesterol levels are also reduced, whereas the levels of HDL cholesterol, the putative antiatherogenic lipoprotein, increase.

Niacin decreases circulating levels of free fatty acids due to a decrease in intracellular lipolysis and release of fatty acid from adipose tissue (57). This in turn reduces fatty acid uptake by the liver and may, in part, be responsible for decreased hepatic VLDL production.

Reduced LDL levels appear to be due to decreased synthesis of this particle (58,59), either due to a decrease in hepatic production and secretion of VLDL (58) or to reduced conversion of precursor VLDL to LDL. Decreased production of LDL directly by the liver is another possible basis for niacin's effect on plasma LDL concentrations. Limited data are available on the mechanism responsible for the increase in HDL. Niacin increases plasma HDL levels by decreasing HDL fractional catabolism rather than increasing its production (60). Because hypertriglyceridemia is associated with increased fractional catabolism of HDL, niacin's ability to decrease plasma triglyceride concentrations may result in decreased fractional clearance of HDL from plasma and increased plasma HDL levels (61).

Additional actions of niacin have been described that may relate to its beneficial effects in preventing coronary events. Niacin therapy is associated with release of large amounts of prostaglandins (62), some of which may be associated with the decreased platelet aggregability seen with this drug.

Clinical Efficacy

Unlike other lipid-lowering medications, niacin is available as a nonprescription tablet that can be purchased in most pharmacies or health food stores in 50- to 500-mg tablets. An alternative vitamin form of this compound, niacinamide, is not effective for lipid reduction. Slow-release forms of niacin are available at a significantly increased cost. Although some patients prefer the slow-release forms because they tend to be associated with less flushing, they may cause more gastrointestinal problems. There are limited data relative to the clinical efficacy of the slow-release forms, and what data are available suggest they are less effective than the short-acting agents (63).

Although response to therapy is somewhat variable, reductions of approximately 15% to 25% in total plasma and LDL cholesterol can be expected in most patients. HDL cholesterol increases from 15% to 25% have been reported. In patients with hypertriglyceridemia, niacin therapy may be associated with 30% to 40% decreases in plasma triglyceride concentrations and dramatic reductions in circulating triglycerides to normal levels. Niacin has been used very successfully in combination with bile acid

resins in the treatment of severely affected subjects with FH, in which this combination has reduced LDL cholesterol concentrations by 30% to 50% (54,64).

A most troubling side effect of the medication is a benign vasodilation of peripheral capillary beds associated with niacin administration. To avoid or minimize this flush, it is recommended that small amounts of niacin be taken initially (e.g., 100–250 mg) and that the dose be gradually increased by 250 mg every 3 to 5 days until the level of 1 g two or three times a day is attained. The response to niacin is variable with good cholesterol lowering occurring in some cases at less than 1 g/day, and occasional patients requiring up to 9 g/day. The medication should be taken with meals to decrease flushing and to avoid GI irritation.

Toxicity

Niacin therapy is associated with a number of either inconvenient or potentially harmful side effects, the most common of which is the flush. This sensation, like a mild sunburn, occurs 15 to 30 min after a dose and lasts 30 to 60 min. Occasional patients will complain of light-headedness probably due to postural hypotension. This may be clinically significant if niacin therapy is initiated at full dose. Patients usually develop tachyphylaxis to this effect of niacin and should therefore be told that the worst flushing will occur on initiating the therapy or when increasing the dose. The flushing is thought to be prostaglandin mediated and can be reduced or sometimes totally eliminated by prior ingestion of aspirin or ibuprofen.

Niacin is a gastric irritant and can worsen or precipitate peptic ulcer disease, which we consider to be an absolute contraindication to its use. Increases in liver transaminase levels are common, and up to a threefold increase in the blood levels of these enzymes, in the absence of symptoms, is not considered an indication to stop therapy. An occasional patient will, however, develop a clinical picture compatible with acute hepatitis with fever, fatigue, right upper quadrant pain, and marked elevations of liver function tests. This is dose related and resolves after discontinuation of therapy. For this reason, liver function tests should be obtained several weeks after the patient has been placed on niacin and after increasing the dose. Dry skin and mucous membranes and pruritis occur and may be quite troubling in patients with dermatologic disorders. Blood uric acid levels invariably increase during niacin treatment due to decreased renal clearance, and in predisposed individuals, acute gouty attacks may be precipitated. Additional side effects include decreased glucose tolerance, atrial tachycardia, and toxic amblyopia.

Effect on Atherosclerosis

Niacin alone or in combination with resins has been used in two important secondary prevention studies. Initially shown to reduce the incidence of second myocardial infarctions (55), the Coronary Drug Project Follow-Up study demonstrated 9 years later that niacin treatment was associated with a statistically significant decrease in total and coronary deaths (8). Combined with colestipol, niacin treatment of patients in the CLAS Study was associated with an angiographically proven decrease in CHD progression, and in 16% of cases, a regression of coronary lesions (54).

FIBRATES

The fibric acid derivatives are a widely prescribed group of agents that can significantly reduce plasma total and VLDL triglyceride levels. Their effects on total plasma and LDL cholesterol are more variable, with modest to significant reductions observed in normotriglyceridemic individuals, but unchanged or actually increased LDL cholesterol levels observed in hyper-

triglyceridemic subjects during therapy. HDL cholesterol levels are frequently increased as well, particularly in hypertriglyceridemic subjects.

Pharmacology and Metabolism

The fibrates, or fibric acid derivatives, are a group of hypolipidemic compounds characterized structurally by their phenoxyisobutyrate group. The structures of the approved and likely to be approved fibrates are presented in Fig. 6. Clofibrate, the original compound to be used clinically, gained additional potency with the addition of a Cl at the *para* position of the aromatic ring. Although bezafibrate and fenofibrate both have the *para*Cl functions, gemfibrozil does not. Bezafibrate and gemfibrozil are both in the acid form, and clofibrate and fenofibrate are not. Modification of the benzoyl group in bezafibrate and in fenofibrate appears to have significantly increased hypolipidemic activity, as has chain spacing in the case of gemfibrozil (65).

In general, the fibrates are well absorbed and are bound to plasma albumin, and interestingly, to apo B-containing lipoproteins. The relatively high percentage of binding to circulating proteins has led to significant drug interactions between fibrates and other agents. The most important of these interactions has been with coumarin derivatives and some anti-inflammatory agents. Increased efficacy of coumarin anticoagulants, with the possibility of hemorrhage, must be considered when fibrates are used in patients receiving this class of anticoagulants. Once in the bloodstream, all the fibrates are effectively removed and accumulated by the liver.

Although the modifications of structure of the different fibrates seem modest, their effects on drug metabolism are significant (65). Clofibrate undergoes conversion to free clofibric acid, which is excreted mainly through the kidneys unchanged or after conjugation with glucuronic acid (60%–80%

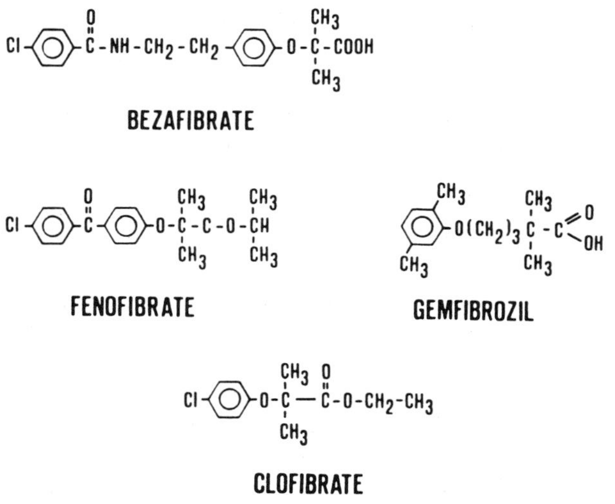

FIG. 6. The structures of the fibrates.

of plasma clofibrate). The half-life of clofibrate is between 13 and 19 hr and may be significantly prolonged in subjects with renal failure. Gemfibrozil is mainly free in plasma, either in the unchanged form or after oxidation to a benzoic form. Plasma half-life is between 1 and 2 hr. Fenofibrate has more extensive metabolic fates, including conversion to both free fenofibric acid and a hydroxylated form of fenofibrate. Fenofibric acid is the major form of the drug in plasma and has a half-life of 20 to 24 hr. Bezafibrate is not significantly metabolized in plasma and has a half-life of only 1.5 hr.

Mechanism of Action

In vitro and *in situ* studies have suggested several effects of the fibrates on both hepatic triglyceride and cholesterol metabolism. The majority of these studies have been conducted in rats, although rabbits have also been used. There are conflicting data regarding differences among the various fibrates as to some of these effects, but because of the reported data for any one drug are from different laboratories using different protocols and methods, no firm conclusions can be drawn.

It appears that fibrates inhibit triglyceride synthesis in the liver. Both reductions in fatty acid synthesis and reduced incorporation of glycerol and oleate into triglycerides have been demonstrated in livers from rats treated with fibrates (66). Fatty acid oxidation also appears to be increased in both mitochondria and in peroxisomes. Decreased incorporation of acetate into cholesterol has also been observed, although it is not clear if reduced mevalonate incorporation into cholesterol also occurs. The activity of hydroxymethyl-glutaryl CoA reductase (HMGCoAR) is reduced in livers from rats treated with fibrates, although direct addition of fibrates to liver cells in culture does not effect HMGCoAR activity (66). Hence, any effect of fibrates on cholesterol synthesis via the rate-limiting enzyme HMGCoAR must be secondary to other direct effects.

In vivo studies of triglyceride and cholesterol metabolism support some of the *in vitro* data cited above. Incorporation of glycerol into VLDL triglyceride, measured in kinetic studies of VLDL triglyceride turnover indicates a modest reduction in the entry of triglycerides into plasma in subjects treated with fibrates (67). Total body sterol balance studies indicate reduced cholesterol synthesis, although there appears to be a concomitant increase in biliary cholesterol excretion (68). Most of the available data from human studies, however, suggest that the major effect of the fibrates on plasma triglyceride and LDL cholesterol levels is via increased activity of LPL and possibly increased LDL receptor activity, respectively (68).

VLDL triglyceride and apo B turnover studies have indicated increased fractional catabolism of VLDL triglycerides during fibrate treatment (67). Direct measurements of postheparin LPL have demonstrated increased activity of this enzyme, consistent with the kinetic data (69). No effects of fibrates on HTGL activity have been noted. Hence, the marked reductions in plasma triglycerides associated with fibric acid therapy results mainly from increased hydrolysis of VLDL triglycerides, with modest, additive reductions in VLDL secretion into plasma.

LDL metabolism during fibrate therapy can be quite complex. In untreated hypertriglyceridemic subjects, LDL cholesterol levels can be normal or even reduced. This steady-state situation seems to arise from the presence of cholesteryl ester-depleted, triglyceride-rich LDL that are removed from the plasma at increased fractional catabolic rates (FCR). During fibrate treatment, the cholesteryl ester content of LDL increases, probably secondary to normalized VLDL metabolism, and the FCR of LDL apo B is reduced to normal (67,68). In hypercholesterolemic subjects who have normal triglycerides in the untreated state, fibrate therapy appears to reduce plasma LDL cholesterol levels by increasing receptor-mediated removal of LDL (67). This finding would be consistent with reduced hepatic cholesterol synthesis during treatment and concomitant increased hepatic LDL receptor activity.

In vitro studies in livers of fibrate treated rats have indicated reduced activity of the enzyme acyl-coenzyme A-cholesterol-acyl-transferase (ACAT) and decreased content of cholesteryl esters (66). Aortae of hyper-cholesterolemic rabbits have been shown to have increased activity of cholesteryl ester hydrolase during therapy as well (66). If both of these mechanisms are active in humans undergoing therapy with fibric acid derivatives, reduced accumulation of cholesteryl ester in vessel walls should result. No studies demonstrating such an effect have been reported.

Increases in HDL cholesterol and apo AI concentrations are commonly seen during fibrate treatment, particularly in subjects presenting initially with hypertriglyceridemia. *In vivo* studies of HDL metabolism have been inconsistent. Gemfibrozil and fenofibrate treatment appear to be associated with increased production of apo AI (67), whereas bezafibrate therapy had no effect on this parameter (67). The FCR of HDL apo AI is frequently increased in hypertriglyceridemic subjects, but there are no data indicating that this abnormality is affected by fibric acid therapy. As in the case of LDL, fibrate therapy does result in reduced HDL triglyceride and increased HDL cholesteryl ester content. Studies of LCAT activity before and during fibrate therapy have been inconsistent (66). It is fair to state at this time that we do not know why HDL cholesterol rises during fibrate treatment.

Clinical Efficacy

In general, there does not seem to be any significant difference between the triglyceride-lowering capabilities of any of these agents. All of these agents can reduce plasma and VLDL triglycerides by 30% to 40%. Their effects on LDL cholesterol do, however, appear to differ in individuals with normal plasma triglyceride levels. Fenofibrate and bezafibrate appear to be significantly more effective in lowering LDL cholesterol in these subjects. When the fibrates are used in hypertriglyceridemic subjects, LDL cholesterol levels, as noted above, either remain unchanged or increase. There do not seem to be any differences among the agents in this regard. Finally, HDL cholesterol levels are increased between 5% and 15% by all the fibric acid derivatives, although the effect of clofibrate appears to be less than that of the other agents.

Toxicity

Animal studies have focused mainly on the proliferation, during fibrate therapy, of peroxisomes and neoplastic nodules in the liver (65). Most of these studies have been conducted in rats, and true carcinomas of the liver have been identified in some studies. The basis of peroxisomal proliferation is unknown but is thought to be secondary to increased beta-oxidation of fatty acids in hepatic mitochondria. These findings have caused concern about potential carcinogenicity of fibrates in humans, but no evidence for hepatic cancer or significant hepatomegaly or liver dysfunction has surfaced in clinical trials.

In the WHO study of clofibrate, however, increased total mortality in the treated group (6) was associated, in part, with an increased incidence of gastrointestinal cancers. In the Helsinki Heart Study, in which gemfibrozil was used, no increase in cancers of any type was seen (9).

Increased lithogenicity of bile appears to be a common concomitant of fibrate therapy, arising from increased delivery of cholesterol to bile simultaneously with reduced conversion of cholesterol to bile acids (70,71). Although there was an increased incidence of gallstones noted in the WHO study treatment group (6), there was no such occurrence in the Helsinki Heart Study (9). In addition, long-term clinical use of fenofibrate and bezafibrate in Europe has failed to uncover significant gallstone disease concomitant with fibrate treatment.

Effect on Atherosclerosis

Two of the fibrates, clofibrate and gemfibrozil, have been used in primary and secondary intervention trials as antiatherogenic agents. Clofibrate was used in several trials with varying results. Overall, there appears to have been reduced numbers of nonfatal myocardial infarctions and/or cardiovascular mortality in these studies, without reduction in total mortality. Some of the variability in results may have derived from varying success in lowering plasma cholesterol levels in different trials. The largest trial was the WHO trial (see above) in which various nonfatal coronary artery ischemic events were reduced in the clofibrate treatment group. Fatal myocardial infarctions were not reduced, however, and total mortality was increased, secondary to increased deaths related to malignant and nonmalignant gastrointestinal disease (6).

By contrast, in the Helsinki Heart Study, in which gemfibrozil was used, treatment was associated with significant reductions in total CAD endpoints, including total cardiovascular mortality (9). In this study, 2,000 males received gemfibrozil and 2,000 males received placebo over a 5-year period. After 3 years, increasingly significant differences in cardiovascular endpoints, including total cardiovascular mortality, became evident (9). At the end of the study, the gemfibrozil-treated group had a 35% reduction in endpoints compared with the placebo group. LDL cholesterol was 11% lower and HDL cholesterol was 12% higher in the treated group versus the placebo group, and multivariate analysis suggested that these changes could account for the differences in endpoint rates. Plasma triglycerides were reduced by 35% in the gemfibrozil group as well.

HMGCoAR INHIBITORS

A new class of powerful agents for reducing plasma cholesterol have recently been introduced in the United States and Western Europe. These competitive inhibitors of HMGCoAR can lower plasma total and LDL cholesterol levels by 25% to 50%. Available data indicate that plasma triglyceride levels fall 15% to 25%, and HDL cholesterol concentrations increase 5% to 10% during therapy with these agents.

Pharmacology

The first of these agents, mevastatin, initially called compactin, is a fungal metabolite that was demonstrated to be a potent inhibitor of cholesterol biosynthesis (72). A series of similar fermentation products and synthetic compounds have since been produced, many of which have been used in humans. The structures of five such compounds are depicted in Fig. 7. Lovastatin and simvastatin differ from mevastatin by the addition of, respectively, 1 or 2 methyl groups. Pravastatin, first identified as a urinary metabolite of mevastatin, differs from the parent compound in that the lactone ring is open, forming the dihydroxycarboxylate form of the compound. This is the active form of the drug. An additional synthesized compound, fluindostatin, is similar to

the acid form of the drug with addition of another benzene ring with an attached fluorine.

As noted above, these agents are administered as either the lactone or the acid salt. Limited available data suggest that at a high dose, the hydroxy acid form of the drug is better absorbed, with only <30% absorption of the lactone form. In the case of the lactone forms, conversion to the active hydroxy acid derivative occurs primarily within the liver. First-pass uptake by the liver of the lactone form is very efficient, and the uptake of this form of the drug by other organs is relatively low (72). Higher levels of the acid salt forms can be measured in the peripheral circulation after oral administration because they are not efficiently removed by the liver. There is evidence, however, that the acid forms are not taken up well by tissues other than the liver. Whether clinically relevant tissue selectivity is a characteristic of any of the available HMGCoAR inhibitors remains to be determined.

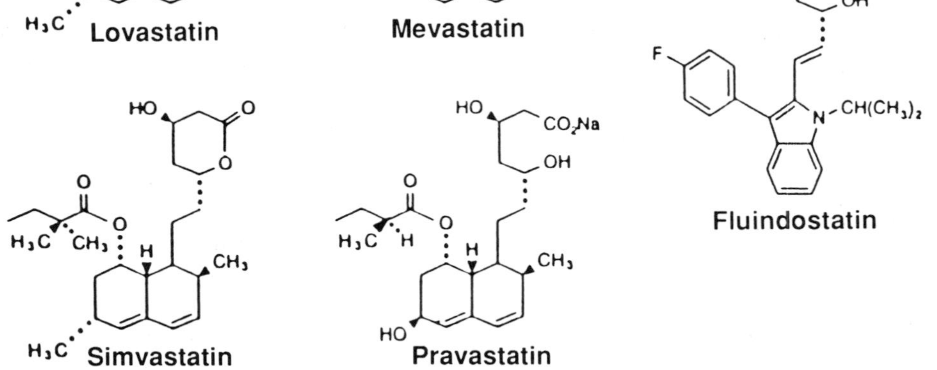

FIG. 7. The structures of the first-generation reductase inhibitors.

These compounds circulate in the bloodstream bound to albumin. The final metabolism of these compounds is primarily in the liver. There is no evidence for enterohepatic recirculation of drug. After oral or intravenous administration, less than 10% of the drug lovastatin was found to be excreted in the urine (72).

Although it was originally reported that these agents did not interfere with other drugs, recent reports indicate that lovastatin may increase the efficacy of coumadin anticoagulants. Further study of this problem is underway.

Mechanism of Action

As their name implies, these compounds are competitive inhibitors of the enzyme HMGCoAR, the rate-limiting enzyme in cholesterol biosynthesis. However, the precise physiologic mechanism whereby these compounds lead to reductions in circulating LDL cholesterol is less straightforward. Studies in animals have suggested that as a response to decreased cholesterol biosynthesis, cells and organs respond by increasing their synthesis of both HMGCoAR (73) and LDL receptors (74). In turn, although a decrease in total body cholesterol biosynthesis may not be apparent (75,76), plasma LDL cholesterol levels are reduced as receptor-mediated fractional removal of LDL by the liver increases (77). This appears to be the major mechanism associated with reduced plasma LDL cholesterol concentrations in subjects with heterozygous FH. In subjects with moderate hypercholesterolemia (polygenic) or with combined hyperlipoproteinemia, however, the benefits of HMGCoAR treatment may derive from decreased hepatic production of apo B-containing lipoproteins without increased fractional catabolism of circulating LDL (78,79). This effect suggests that there may be coordinate regulation of cholesterol synthesis with either apo B synthesis or the assembly and packaging of preformed apo B into VLDL and LDL.

There are no studies focused on the effects of HMGCoAR inhibitors on triglyceride or HDL metabolism. Reduced VLDL assembly and secretion (*vide supra*) may be involved in the decrease in plasma VLDL triglycerides observed, although increased removal of VLDL remnants may also play a role in this effect of these drugs (78,79). HDL concentrations may rise simply as a concomitant of reduced VLDL levels or may indicate some direct effect of HMGCoAR inhibitors on apo AI metabolism.

Clinical Efficacy

The only HMGCoAR inhibitor approved for general use in the United States is lovastatin. The dose-response decrease in total and LDL cholesterol using 5 to 40 mg of this drug twice per day ranged from 21% to 32% and 25% to 39%, respectively (80). The manufacturer supplies the medication in 20- and 40-mg tablets and recommends beginning therapy using 20 mg/day taken in the evening and increasing to 20 mg twice a day and higher doses as needed. Although there was no evidence of tachyphylaxis to the effects of these agents in clinical trials, some physicians have been reporting loss of efficacy after several months of treatment. Although it is likely that reduced patient compliance with drug and diet regimens is the basis for these observations, increased synthesis of HMGCoAR by the liver may be involved.

Aside from the reduction in total and LDL cholesterol, lovastatin therapy is associated with modest reductions of plasma triglyceride (15%–25%), particularly in hypertriglyceridemic subjects, and small increases in HDL (5%–10%).

Toxicity

Lovastatin is associated with increases in liver transaminases, more than three times the upper limit of normal, in approximately 1% of patients. Symptoms compatible with hepatitis are very unusual. The biochemical disorder usually is alleviated after discontinuing the medication. A severe myositis syndrome with fever, myalgias, and creatinine phosphokinase levels of >1,000 I.U. occurs in 0.1% of patients but is more frequent in patients also taking cyclosporin, gemfibrozil, and niacin. Low rates of complaints such as gastrointestinal upset, insomnia, and headache have been reported in clinical trials of lovastatin. There is no evidence of long-term toxicity or oncogenic potential in humans, although long-term data are very limited at this time.

Effect on Atherosclerosis

The limited time since introduction of these agents has not allowed their use in primary or secondary prevention trials. Such studies are, however, currently in progress.

PROBUCOL

Probucol is a lipophilic *bis*-phenol [4,4'-(isopropylidene-dithio)*bis*(2,6-di-ti-t-butyl-phenol)]. Its structure is unrelated to any of the other current hypocholesterolemic agents (Fig. 8). Treatment with probucol results in decreased total plasma cholesterol and LDL cholesterol. However, the reduction in plasma cholesterol is partially due to a decrease in HDL cholesterol. Triglyceride levels usually remain unchanged in patients treated with probucol.

Pharmacology and Metabolism

Probucol is only partially absorbed from the gastrointestinal tract. Following absorption probucol is carried on chylomicrons and VLDL into the circulation and is then distributed between plasma lipoproteins. Probucol is primarily carried on LDL particles and is accumulated by adipose tissue from which it is released slowly over a period of time up to 6 months after discontinuation of therapy. Plasma concentrations plateau after several months. It is mainly excreted through the bile into feces.

Mechanism of Action

The mechanisms by which probucol lowers LDL cholesterol have remained elusive. Probucol has no effect on triglyceride or VLDL metabolism and does not appear to affect the synthesis of LDL apo B (81). *In vivo* studies in animals and *in vitro* studies with cultured cells suggested that probucol causes an increase in LDL apo B clearance via both nonreceptor- and receptor-mediated uptake (82). In rats probucol inhibits cholesterol absorption and in rabbits it causes alterations of the metabolic properties of LDL, but neither effect has been demonstrated consistently in humans (83). Fecal bile acid excretion is transiently increased during probucol therapy, and inhibition of cholesterol synthesis has also been observed in some but not all studies. Notably, probucol may be effective even in LDL receptor-negative patients or animals (84).

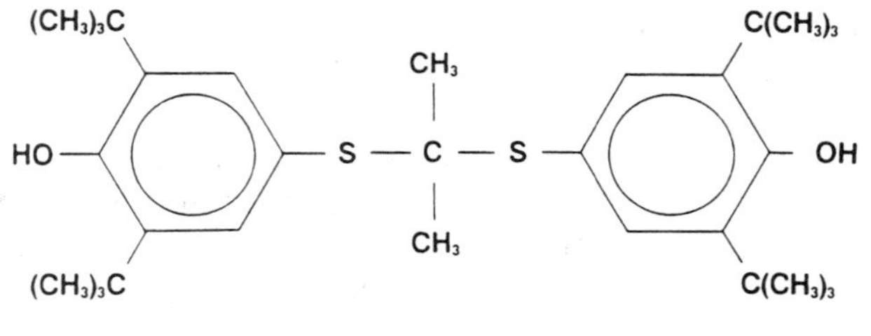

FIG. 8. The structure of probucol.

Another aspect of probucol's activity is prevention of LDL oxidation. Oxidation of LDL has been postulated to be a process that leads to LDL accumulation by macrophages in the arterial wall (85). Studies using very high doses of probucol in animals and cell cultures have demonstrated inhibition of LDL oxidation and foam-cell formation, and recent data suggest that LDL from probucol-treated animals may be taken up and degraded less actively via the scavenger receptor (86–88). The relevance of this mechanism to humans treated with conventional doses is unclear at this time.

It has also been suggested that cholesterol efflux from cells and reverse transport of plasma cholesterol via HDL are more efficient in the presence of probucol, possibly due to increased synthesis of HDL apo E. However, lipoprotein lipase activity is reduced in humans and experimental animals, and this may account for the fall in HDL cholesterol by inhibiting transfer of surface components from triglyceride-rich lipoproteins to HDL (89). In addition, probucol therapy is associated with decreased apo AI synthesis and with smaller, cholesterol- and phospholipid-depleted HDL (81,90).

Efficacy

Probucol is supplied in 250- and 500-mg tablets. The recommended dose is 500 mg twice a day with meals. At this dose one can expect a 10% to 20% reduction in LDL cholesterol and as much as a 25% reduction in HDL cholesterol. Triglyceride levels are usually not altered by probucol therapy (83,91).

Toxicity

Probucol is very well tolerated by patients and side effects are infrequent. Most notable are diarrhea, nausea, and abdominal pain, which caused discontinuation of the drug in 8% of the patients in one study (83,91). A more serious potential adverse effect is the ventricular arrhythmias observed in probucol-treated dogs and monkeys. This effect, however, appears to be species specific and in humans no increase in ventricular arrhythmias has been observed despite statistically significant increases in QT intervals (83,92).

A more relevant concern is the concomitant fall in HDL cholesterol and apo AI seen in most patients. This is disturbing in view of the accumulating evidence of the inverse relationship between HDL concentrations and atherosclerosis. However, in experiments conducted with Watanabe heritable hyperlipidemic rabbits, probucol therapy was associated with reduced atherosclerosis despite reductions in HDL cholesterol (86–88). There appeared to be reduced foam-cell formation in the probucol-treated animals.

Effect on Atherosclerosis

Several studies in humans suggest an antiatherogenic effect for probucol. In a small, controlled primary prevention trial of probucol treatment, either alone or with antihypertensive agents, multivariate analysis suggested decreased incidence of CHD after 5 years of therapy despite reduced HDL cholesterol levels (92). Reduction in the size of xanthalasmas or tendon xanthomas has been reported by several authors during probucol treatment of patients with heterozygous and homozygous forms of FH (84,93). Interestingly, this reversal in cholesterol deposition did not correlate with the degree of cholesterol lowering. A large clinical trial of the effects of probucol treatment on femoral artery atherosclerosis is in progress in Scandinavia (94).

SUMMARY

At the present time, physicians have a varied and effective group of drugs at their disposal for the treatment of severe hyperlipidemia. With either single or combination

TABLE 8. *Hypolipidemic drugs*

Drugs	Mode of action
1. Bile and binding resins colestipol (Colestid); cholestyramine (Questran)	Interruption of the enterohepatic recycling of bile acids; stimulates synthesis of new bile acids from cholesterol. Hepatic LDL receptor increase.
2. Nicotinic acid (niacin)	Decreased synthesis of VLDL and LDL.
3. Fibric acid derivatives clofibrate (Atromid)	Increased activity of lipoprotein lipase; higher rate of triglyceride hydrolysis.
gemfibrozil (Lopid)	Possible decreased synthesis and secretion of VLDL.
fenofibrate (in clinical trials) bezafibrate (in clinical trials)	Fractional catabolism of LDL increases in hypercholesterolemic patients.
4. HMGCoAR inhibitors Lovastatin (Mevacor). Simvastatin, pravastatin, fluindostain, (in clinical trials)	Inhibition of cholesterol synthesis from acetyl CoA at the rate-limiting step HMGCoAR. Reduced cholesterol synthesis by cells results in increased synthesis of LDL receptors. Decreased lipoprotein secretion from liver also possible.
5. Probucol (Lorelco)	Increased clearance of LDL from plasma. Decreased synthesis of apo AI, the major protein in HDL.

Lipoprotein class affected	Dose
1. The fractional removal rate of LDL from plasma increases and plasma LDL can be reduced 20%–30%. HDL cholesterol may increase. VLDL triglycerides may increase particularly in patients with preexisting hypertriglyceridemia.	Cholestyramine 8–12 g b.i.d. (may be taken in three doses as well). Colestipol 10–15 g b.i.d. (may be taken in three doses as well); should be taken 2–3 hr apart from other drugs. Increase dose gradually over 2–4 weeks.
2. Reduced secretion of VLDL triglycerides and proteins into plasma. VLDL levels can be reduced by 25%–35%. LDL can fall by 15%–25%. HDL cholesterol may increase 15%–25%.	1–2.5 g t.i.d. Initial therapy is with small doses: 50–100 mg t.i.d. and increases are small. Full dose reached in 3–4 weeks. A slow-release form is available but may not be as effective.
3. Reduction in triglyceride levels from 20%–30% may occur in Type IV patients and subjects with combined hyperlipidemia. Marked reduction in triglyceride and cholesterol in Type III patients with lower IDL levels. Effects on LDL levels in hypercholesterolemia vary from minimal (clofibrate) to significant (fenofibrate). LDL may increase in hypertriglyceridemic subjects during therapy. Gemfibrozil, fenofibrate, and bezafibrate appear to increase HDL cholesterol levels in many subjects 5%–15%.	Clofibrate 1,000 mg b.i.d.; gemfibrozil 600 mg b.i.d.; fenofibrate (not yet available); bezafibrate (not yet available).
4. Increased clearance of LDL from plasma and reduced cholesterol synthesis results in 30%–40% reduction in plasma LDL cholesterol. Reduced VLDL secretion into plasma may contribute to reduced LDL generation.	20–80 mg/day in one or two equal doses. Single dose (20–40 mg) taken with dinner. Clinical trials have demonstrated significant efficacy. Long-term safety remains to be determined.
5. Increased clearance of LDL from plasma results in 10%–15% reduction in plasma LDL levels. Appears to be effective in subjects with homozygous familial hypercholesterolemia. Reduces plasma HDL cholesterol by 20%–25%. Data suggest reduced apo AI synthesis.	500 mg b.i.d. Probucol is lipid soluble. Full therapeutic effect takes several weeks and lasts several weeks beyond use of drug.

TABLE 8. *Continued*

Side effects	Contraindications
1. Resins not absorbed from gastrointestinal tract. Constipation is main complaint. Gastric pain and nausea; hemorrhoidal bleeding; increased lithogenicity of bile is theoretically possible but increased gallstones have not been seen.	Biliary tract obstruction, gastric outlet obstruction.
2. Flushing of skin: may be relieved by aspirin. Tachycardias, atrial arrhythmias, pruritus, dry skin, nausea, diarrhea, hyperuricemia, peptic ulcer disease, glucose intolerance, hepatic dysfunction.	Peptic ulcer disease, significant cardiac arrhythmias, hepatic disease, gouty arthritis or significant hyperuricemia, glucose intolerance (relative).
3. Increased lithogenicity of bile and increased incidence of gallstones in patients taking clofibrate. Gemfibrozil, fenofibrate, and bezafibrate also increase lithogenicity but have not been shown to increase gallstone formation. Nausea, abnormal liver function tests, myositis occur in less than 1% of patients. Cardiac arrhythmias have been associated with clofibrate use.	Hepatic or biliary disease.
4. Opacities in eye lens may occur: clinical significance unclear. Elevated liver function tests in 1%–2% of patients. Severe myositis in <1% of patients (several cases of rhabdomyolysis).	Risk of myositis may be significantly increased in patients with reduced renal function and in patients receiving cyclosporine, gemfibrozil, or nicotinic acid.
5. Diarrhea, nausea, abdominal pain	None known.

Drug interactions	Combined use
1. Binds fat soluble vitamins (A,D,E,K) although no significant malabsorption has been demonstrated. Decreased absorption of phenylbutazone, phenobarbital, thyroid hormone, digitalis, warfarin, thiazide diuretics, some antibiotics.	Successfully combined with nicotinic acid, lovastatin, fibric acid derivatives, probucol.
2. Synergistic with ganglionic blocking agents used to treat hypertension. Myositis reported (3%) with lovastatin.	Bile acid resins.
3. Increased anticoagulant activity of coumadin. Increased myositis (5%) reported when gemfibrozil combined with lovastatin.	Bile acid sequestrants: fibric acid derivatives may reduce elevated triglycerides that develop in some patients on resins. Resins can reduce LDL that may have risen during treatment of hypertriglyceridemia with fibric acid derivative.
4. 25% incidence of myositis with cyclosporine (in transplant patients). (Possibly coumadin.)	Bile acid resins.
5. None known.	Bile acid resin in combination with probucol resulted in significant reduction in LDL without changes in LDL:HDL ratio.

therapy, plasma lipid levels in almost all individuals can be reduced significantly and often reach the normal range. Problems with compliance and adverse effects remain the major obstacles facing physicians and patients. The availability in the near future of second generation fibrates and reductase inhibitors and the development of third-generation agents of several of the classes of drugs described above should significantly advance the therapy of lipid disorders. As a result, dramatic reductions in CAD in particular and atherosclerotic cardiovascular disease in general can be expected during the next 10 to 20 years.

The indications, efficacy, and adverse effects of each of the agents described above are listed in Table 8.

REFERENCES

1. The Surgeon General's Report on Nutrition and Health. U.S. Department of Health and Human Services. Public Health Service Publication No. 88-50210, Washington, D.C., 1988.
2. Dawber TR. *The Framingham study: the epidemiology of atherosclerotic disease.* Cambridge: Harvard University Press, 1980.
3. Carlson LA, Bottiger LE, Ahfeldt PE. Risk factors for myocardial infarction in the Stockholm prospective study: a 14-year follow-up focusing on the role of plasma triglycerides and cholesterol. *Acta Med Scand* 1979;206:351–360.
4. Zilversmit DB. Atherogenesis: a postprandial phenomenon. *Circulation* 1979;60:473–483.
5. Steinberg D. Current theories of the pathogenesis of atherosclerosis. In: Steinberg D, Olefsky JM, eds. *Contemporary issues in endocrinology and metabolism, vol 3. Hypercholesterolemia and atherosclerosis: pathogenesis and prevention.* New York: Churchill Livingstone, 1987; 5–23.
6. Oliver MF, Heady JA, Morris JN, et al. Report from the committee of principal investigators: a cooperative trial in the primary prevention of ischaemic heart disease using clofibrate. *Br Heart J* 1978;40:1069–1118.
7. Lipid Research Clinics Program. The lipid research clinics coronary primary prevention trial results. I. Reduction in incidence of coronary heart disease. *JAMA* 1984;251:351–364.
8. Canner PL, Berge KG, Wenger NK, et al. Fifteen year mortality in coronary drug project patients: long-term benefit with niacin. *J Am Coll Cardiol* 1968;8:1245–1255.
9. Frick MH, Elo O, Haapa K, et al. Helsinki heart study: primary-prevention trial with gemfibrozil in middle-aged men with dyslipidemia. *N Engl J Med* 1987;317:1237–1245.
10. Green PHR, Glickman RM. Intestinal lipoprotein metabolism. *J Lipid Res* 1980;21:942–952.
11. Olivecrona T, Olivecrona-Bengtsson G. Lipoprotein lipase from milk—the model enzyme in lipoprotein lipase research. In: Borensztajn J, ed. *Lipoprotein lipase.* Chicago: Evener, 1987; 15–58.
12. LaRosa JC, Levy RI, Herbert PN, et al. A specific apoprotein activator for lipoprotein lipase. *Biochem Biophys Res Commun* 1970;21:942–952.
13. Ginsberg HN, Le NA, Goldberg IJ, et al. Apolipoprotein B metabolism in subjects with deficiency of apolipoproteins CII and AI: evidence that apolipoprotein CIII inhibits catabolism of triglyceride-rich lipoproteins by lipoprotein lipase in vivo. *J Clin Invest* 1986;78:1287–1295.
14. Schneider WJ, Kovanen PT, Brown MS, et al. Familial dysbetalipoproteinemia: abnormal binding of mutant apoprotein E to low density lipoprotein receptors of human fibroblasts and membranes from liver and adrenal of rats, rabbits, and cows. *J Clin Invest* 1981;68:1075–1085.
15. Quardfordt SH, Michalopoulos G, Schmirmer B. The effect of human C apolipoproteins in vitro hepatic metabolism of triglyceride emulsions in the rat. *J Biol Chem* 1982;257:14642–14647.
16. Olofsson SO, Bjursell G, Bostrom K, et al. Apolipoprotein B: structure biosynthesis and role in the lipoprotein assembly process. *Atherosclerosis* 1987;68:1–12.
17. Craig WY, Cooper AD. Effects of chylomicron remnants and β-VLDL on the class and composition of newly secreted lipoprotins by HepG2 cells. *J Lipid Res* 1988;29:299–308.
18. Mallory MJ, Kane JP, Hardman DA, Hamilton RL, Dalal KB. Normotriglyceridemic abetalipoproteinemia: absence of the B-100 apolipoprotein. *J Clin Invest* 1981;67:1441–1450.
19. Goldberg IJ, Le NA, Ginsberg HN, Krauss RM, Lindgren FT. Lipoprotein metabolism during acute inhibition of lipoprotein lipase in the cynomolgus monkey. *J Clin Invest* 1988;81:561–568.
20. Chait A, Hazzard WR, Alber JA, et al. Impaired very low density lipoprotein and triglyceride removal and broad beta disease: comparison with endogenous hypertriglyceridemia. *Metabolism* 1978;27:1055–1066.
21. Kinnunen PKJ. Hepatic endothelial lipase: isolation, some characteristics, and physiological role. In: Borgstrom B, Brockman HL, eds. *Lipases.* New York: Elsevier, 1984;308–328.
22. Goldberg IJ, Le NA, Paterniti JR Jr, Ginsberg HN, Lindgren FT, Brown VW. Lipoprotein metabolism during acute inhibition of hepatic triglyceride lipase in the cynomolgus monkey. *J Clin Invest* 1982;70:1184–1192.
23. Brown MS, Goldstein JL. How LDL receptors influence cholesterol and atherosclerosis. *Sci Am* 1984;251:58–66.
24. Eisenberg S. High density lipoprotein metabolism. *J Lipid Res* 1984;25:1017–1058.
25. Kostner GM, Knipping G, Groener JE, Zechner R, Dieplinger H. The role of LCAT and cholesteryl ester transfer proteins for the HDL and LDL structure and metabolism. *Adv Exp Med Biol* 1987;210:79–86.
26. Tall AR. Plasma lipid transfer proteins. *J Lipid Res* 1986;27:361–367.
27. Brinton EA, Oram JF, Chen CH, Albers JJ, Bierman EL. Binding of high density lipoprotein to cultured fibroblasts after chemical alteration of apoprotein amino acid residues. *J Biol Chem* 1986;261:495–503.
28. Pitmann RC, Knecht TP, Rosenbaum MS, Taylor CA Jr. A nonendocytotic mechanism for the selective uptake of high density lipoprotein-associated cholesterol esters. *J Biol Chem* 1987;262:2443–2450.
29. Reaven GM, Hill DB, Gross RC, Farquhar JW. Kinetics of triglyceride turnover of very low density lipoproteins of human plasma. *J Clin Invest* 1965;44:1826–1833.
30. Brown VW, Ginsberg HN. Diabetes and plasma lipoproteins. In: Brodoff BN, Bleicher SJ, eds. *Diabetes mellitus and obesity.* Baltimore: Williams and Wilkins, 1982;192–199.
31. Angelin B, Hershon KS, Brunzell JD. Bile acid

metabolism in hereditary forms of hypertriglyceridemia: evidence for an increased synthesis rate in monogenic familial hypertriglyceridemia. *Proc Natl Acad Sci USA* 1987;84:5434–5438.

32. Goldberg IJ, Kandel JJ, Blum CB, Ginsberg HN. Association of plasma lipoproteins with postheparin lipase activities. *J Clin Invest* 1986; 78:1523–1528.

33. Fredrickson DS, Goldstein JL, Brown MS. The familial hyperlipoproteinemias. In: Stanburg JB, Wyngaarden JB, Fredrickson DS, eds. *The metabolic basis of inherited disease.* New York: McGraw-Hill, 1978;608–617.

34. Breckenridge WC, Little JA, Alaupovic P, et al. Lipoprotein abnormalities associated with a familial deficiency of hepatic lipase. *Atherosclerosis* 1982;45:161–179.

35. The Lipid Research Clinics. *Population Studies Data Book, vol. I: the prevalence study.* Washington, D.C.: U.S. Department of Health and Human Services, Public Health Service National Institutes of Health.

36. Goldstein JL, Schrott HG, Hazzard WR, Bierman EL, Motulsky A. Hyperlipidemia in coronary heart disease: genetic analysis of lipid levels in 176 families and delineation of a new inherited disorder combined hyperlipidemia. *J Clin Invest* 1973; 52:1544–1568.

37. Teng B, Sniderman AD, Soutar AK, Thompson GR. Metabolic basis of hypapobetalipoproteinemia. Turnover of apolipoprotein B in low density lipoprotein and its precursors and subfractions compared with normal and familial hypercholesterolemia. *J Clin Invest* 1986;77:663–672.

38. Morganroth J, Levy RI, Fredrickson DS. The biochemical, clinical and genetic features of type III hyperlipoproteinemia. *Ann Intern Med* 1975;82:158–174.

39. Janus ED, Nicoll A. Wootoon R, Turner PR, Magill PJ, Lewis B. Quantitative studies of very low density lipoprotein: conversion to very low density lipoprotein in normal controls and primary hyperlipidaemic states and the role of direct secretion of low density lipoprotein in heterozygous familial hypercholesterolaemia. *Eur J Clin Invest* 1980;10:149–159.

40. Weiner M. Clinical pharmacology and pharmcokinetics of nicotine acid. *Drug Metab Rev* 1979;9:99.

41. Ordovas JM, Schaefer EJ, Salem D, et al. Apolipoprotein AI gene polymorphism associated with premature coronary artery disease and familial hypoalphalipoproteinemia. *N Engl J Med* 1986;314:671–677.

42. Le NA, Ginsberg HN. Heterogeneity of apolipoprotein A-I turnover in subjects with reduced concentrations of plasma high density lipoprotein cholesterol. *Metabolism* 1988;37:614–617.

43. Schaefer EJ. Clinical biochemical, and genetic features in familial disorders of high density lipoprotein deficiency. *Arteriosclerosis* 1984;4: 303–322.

44. Report of the National Cholesterol Education Program Expert Panel on Detection, Evaluation, and Treatment of High Blood Cholesterol in Adults. The Expert Panel. *Arch Intern Med* 1988;148:36–69.

45. Brown, MS, Goldstein JL. Drug used in the treatment of hyperlipoproteinemias. In: Goodman LS, Gilman AG, eds. *Pharmacological basis of therapeutics,* 7th ed. New York: Macmillan, 1987;827–845.

46. Knodel L, Talbert RL. Adverse effects of hypolipidaemic drugs. *Med Toxicol* 1987;2:10–32.

47. Grundy SM, Aherns EH Jr, Salen G. Interruption of the enterohepatic circulation of bile acids in man: comparative effects of cholestyramine and ileal exclusion on cholesterol metabolism. *J Lab Clin Med* 1971;78:94–121.

48. Shepherd J, Packard CJ, Bicker S, et al. Cholestryamine promotes receptor mediated low density lipoprotein catabolism. *N Engl J Med* 1980;302:1219–1222.

49. Witztum JL, Young SG, Elam RL, Carew TE, Fisher M. Cholestyramine-induced changes in low density lipoprotein composition and metabolism. I. Studies in the guinea pig. *J Lipid Res* 1985;26:92–103.

50. Angelin B, Einarsson K, Hellstrom K, Leijd B. Bile acid kinetics in relation to endogenous triglyceride metabolism in various types of hyperlipoproteinemia. *J Lipid Res* 1978;19:1004–1016.

51. Grundy SM, Mok HYI, Zech L, et al. Colestipol, clofibrate and phytosterols in combined therapy of hyperlipidemia. *J Lab Clin Med* 1977;89:534–566.

52. Lipid Research Clinics Program. The lipid research clinics coronary primary prevention trial results. II. The relationship of reduction in incidence of coronary heart disease to cholesterol lowering. *JAMA* 1984;251:365–374.

53. Brensike JF, Levy RI, Kelsey SF, et al. Effects of therapy with cholestyramine on progression of coronary arteriosclerosis: results of the NHLBI Type II Coronary Intervention Study. *Circulation* 1984;69:313–324.

54. Blankenhorn DH, Nessim SA, Johnson RL, Sanmarco ME, Azen SP, Cashin-Hemphill L. Beneficial effects of combined colestipol-niacin therapy on coronary atherosclerosis and coronary venous bypass grafts. *JAMA* 1987;257: 3233–3240.

55. Coronary Drug Project. Clofibrate and niacin in coronary heart disease. *JAMA* 1975;231:360–381.

56. Marcus R, Coulston AM. Water-soluble vitamins: the vitamin B complex and ascorbic acid. In: Goodman LS, Gilman AG, eds. *Pharmacological basis of therapeutics,* 5th ed. New York: Macmillan, 1551–1572.

57. Carlson LA, Oro L. Effects of treatment with nicotinic acid for one month on serum lipids in patients with different types of hyperlipidemia. *Atherosclerosis* 1973;18:1–9.

58. Grundy SM, Mok HYI, Zech L, et al. Influence of nicotinic acid on metabolism of cholesterol and triglycerides in man. *J Lipid Res* 1981; 22:24–36.

59. Langer T, Levy RI. The effect of nicotinic acid on the turnover of low density lipoproteins in

type II hyperlipoproteinemia. In: Gey KK, Carlson LA, eds. *Metabolic effects of nicotinic acid and its derivatives*. Bern: Hans Huber, 1971;641.

60. Shepherd J, Packard CJ, Patsch JR, Gotto AM Jr, Taunton OD. Effects of nicotinic acid therapy on plasma high density lipoprotein subfraction distribution and composition and on apolipoprotein A metabolism. *J Clin Invest* 1979;63:858–867.

61. Le AN, Gibson JC, Ginsberg HN. Independent regulation of plasma apolipoprotein CII and CIII concentrations in very low density and high density lipoproteins: implications for the regulation of the catabolism of these lipoproteins. *J Lipid Res* 1988;29:669–677.

62. Weisgraber KH, Innerarity TL, Newhouse YM, et al. Familial defective apolipoprotein B-100: enhanced binding of monoclonal antibody MB47 to abnormal low density lipoproteins. *Proc Natl Acad Sci USA* 1988;85:9758–9762.

63. Knopp RH, Ginsberg J, Albers JJ, et al. Contrasting effects of unmodified and time-released forms of niacin on lipoproteins in hyperlipidemic subjects: clues to mechanism of action of niacin. *Metabolism* 1985;34:642–650.

64. Kane JF, Malloy MJ, Tun P, et al. Normalization of low density lipoprotein levels in heterozygous familial hypercholesterolemia with combined drug regimen. *N Engl J Med* 1981;304:251–258.

65. Sirtori CR, Franceschini G. Effects of fibrates on serum lipids and atherosclerosis. *Pharmacol Ther* 1988;37:167–191.

66. Kloer HU. Structure and biochemical effects of fenofibrate. *Am J Med* 1987;83:3–8.

67. Ginsberg HN. Changes in lipoprotein kinetics during therapy with fenofibrate and other fibric acid derivatives. *Am J Med* 1987;83:66–70.

68. Grundy SM, Vega GL. Fibric acids: effects on lipids and lipoprotein metabolism. *Am J Med* 1987;83:9–20.

69. Boberg J, Boberg M, Gross R, Grundy SM, Augustin J, Brown V. The effects of treatment with colfibrate on hepatic triglyceride and lipoprotein lipase activities of postheparin plasma in male patients with hyperlipoproteinemia. *Arteriosclerosis* 1977;267:499–503.

70. Palmer RH. Effects of fibric acid derivatives on bilary lipid composition. *Am J Med* 1987;83:37–43.

71. Pertsemlids D, Penveliwalla D, Aherns EJ Jr. Effects of clofibrate and of an estrogen-progestin combination of fasting biliary lipids and cholic acid kinetics in man. *Gastroenterology* 1974;66:565–573.

72. Alberts AW. HMG-CoA reductase inhibitors—the development. In: Stokes III J, Mancini M, eds. *Atherosclerosis*. New York: Raven Press, 1988.

73. Mehrabian M, Callaway KA, Clarke CF, et al. Regulation of rat liver 3-hydroxy-3-methylglutaryl coenzyme A synthase and the chromosomal localization of the human gene. *J Biol Chem* 1986;261:16249–16255.

74. Kovanen PT, Bilheimer DW, Goldstein JL, Jaramillo JJ, Brown MS. Regulatory role for hepatic low density lipoprotein receptors in vivo in the dog. *Proc Natl Acad Sci USA* 1981;78:1194–1198.

75. Grundy SM, Bilheimer DW. Inhibition of 3-hydroxy-3-methylglutaryl-CoA reductase by mevinolin in familial hypercholesterolemia heterozygotes: effects on cholesterol balance. *Proc Natl Acad Sci USA* 1984;81:2538–2542.

76. Goldberg IJ, Holleran S, Ramakrishnan R, Palmer RH, Dell RB, Goodman DS. Effect of long-term treatment with lovastatin on the parameters of whole body cholesterol metabolism. *Arteriosclerosis* 1988;8:558a.

77. Bilheimer DW, Grundy SM, Brown MS, Goldstein JL. Mevinolin and colestipol stimulate receptor-mediated clearance of low density lipoprotein from plasma in familial hypercholesterolemia heterozygotes. *Trans Assoc Am Physicians* 1983;96:1–9.

78. Grundy SM, Vega GL. Influence of mevinolin on metabolism of low density lipoproteins in primary moderate hypercholesterolemia. *J Lipid Res* 1985;26:1464–1475.

79. Arad Y, Ramakrishnan R, Ginsberg RN. Lovastatin therapy reduces low density lipoprotein apo B levels in subjects with combined hyperlipidemia by reducing the production of apo B-containing lipoproteins. *J Lipid Res* 1990;31:567–582.

80. Therapeutic response to lovastatin (mevinolin) in nonfamilial hypercholesterolemia. A multicenter study. The Lovastatin Study Group II. *JAMA* 1986;256:2829–2934.

81. Nestel PJ, Billington T. Effects of probucol on low density lipoprotein removal and high density lipoprotein synthesis. *Atherosclerosis* 1981;38:203–209.

82. Naruszewicz M, Carew TE, Pittman RC, Witztum JL, Steinberg D. A novel mechanism by which probucol lowers low density lipoprotein levels demonstrated in the LDL receptor-deficient rabbit. *J Lipid Res* 1984;25:1206–1213.

83. Strandberg TE, Vanhanaen H, Miettinen TA. Probucol in long-term treatment of hypercholesterolemia. *Gen Pharmacol* 1988;19:317–320.

84. Baker SG, Joffe BI, Mendelson D, Seftel HC. Treatment of homozygous familial hypercholesterolemia with probucol. *S Afr Med J* 1982;62:7–11.

85. Parasarathy S, Young SG, Witztum JL, Pittman RC, Steinberg D. Probucol inhibits oxidative modification of low density lipoprotein. *J Clin Invest* 1986;77:641–644.

86. Kita T, Nagano Y, Yokode M, et al. Probucol prevents the progression of atherosclerosis in Watanabe heritable hyperlipidemic rabbit, an animal model for familial hypercholesterolemia. *Proc Natl Acad Sci USA* 1987;84:5928–5931.

87. Carew TE, Schwenke DC, Steinberg D. Antiatherogenic effects of probucol unrelated to its hypocholesterolemic effect: evidence that antioxidants in vivo can selectively inhibit low density lipoprotein degradation in macrophages-rich fat

streaks and slow the progression of atherosclerosis in the Watanabe heritable hyperlipidemic rabbit. *Proc Natl Acad Sci USA* 1987;84:7725–7729.

88. Schwartz CJ. Introduction—the probucol experience: a review of the past and a look at the future. *Am J Cardiol* 1988;62;1B–5B.

89. Miettinen TA, Huttunen JK, Kuusi T, et al. Effect of probucol on the activity of postheparin plasma lipoprotein lipase and hepatic lipase. *Clin Chim Acta* 1981;113:59–64.

90. Miettinen TA, Huttunen JK, Ehnholm C, Kumlin T, Mattila S, Naukkarinen V. Effect of long-term antihypertensive and hypolipidemic treatment on high density lipoprotein cholesterol and apolipoproteins AI and AII. *Atherosclerosis* 1980;36:246–259.

91. Illingworth DR. Lipid-lowering drugs. An overview of indications and optimum therapeutic use. *Drugs* 1987;33:259–279.

92. Meittinen TA, Huttunen JK, Naukkarinen V, et al. Multifactorial primary prevention of cardiovascular diseases in middle-aged men. Risk factor changes, incidence and mortality. *JAMA* 1985;254:2097–2102.

93. Yamamoto A, Matsuzawa Y, Yokoyama S, Funahashi T, Yamamura T, Kishino BI. Effects of probucol on xanthomata regression in familial hypercholesterolemia. *Am J Cardiol* 1986;57:29H–35H.

94. Walldius G, Carlson LA, Erikson U, et al. Development of femoral atherosclerosis in hypercholesterolemic patients during treatment with cholestyramine and probucol/placebo: probucol quantitative regression swedish trial (PQRST): a status report. *Am J Cardiol* 1988;62:37B-43B.

Cardiovascular Pharmacology, Third Edition,
edited by Michael Antonaccio.
Raven Press, Ltd., New York © 1990.

Platelets, Thrombosis, and Antithrombotic Therapies

Yves Cadroy and Laurence A. Harker

*Division of Hematology and Oncology, Emory University School of Medicine,
Atlanta, Georgia 30322*

Thrombosis is a leading cause of morbidity and mortality in the western world. Thrombus forms *in vivo* as a pathologic consequence of interactions between blood hemostatic mechanisms and components of the injured vessel wall under variable flow conditions. Arterial thrombotic occlusion complicates atherosclerosis causing acute myocardial or cerebral infarction; venous thromboembolic disease complicates a variety of clinical settings generally characterized by blood stasis, activated blood factors, and vascular dysfunction or damage. Typically, vascular injury with activation of platelet and coagulation mechanisms under high shear flow produces arterial-type thrombus rich in platelets but poor in fibrin and red cells ("white" thrombus). In contrast, the "red" thrombus seen in venous thromboembolic disease is rich in fibrin and red cells and relatively poor in platelets.

The type and intensity of antithrombotic approaches differ for each of these two processes. Antiplatelet agents are effective in the treatment of arterial thrombosis by interfering with platelet recruitment into forming thrombus. Anticoagulants are effective in venous thrombosis by inhibiting the production or the activity of serine proteases comprising the coagulation cascade, particularly thrombin. Fibrinolytic agents remove already formed thrombus by degrading its fibrin network. It may be necessary to administer anticoagulants and/or antiplatelet agents to prevent reformation of thrombus.

PATHOGENESIS OF THROMBUS FORMATION

Intact endothelium maintains the fluidity of blood by multiple mechanisms. For example, the electronegative charge of the endothelial membrane prevents cell deposition on its surface (1). Endothelial cells also rapidly degrade platelet proaggregatory adenosine diphosphate (ADP) (2) and synthesize molecules that potently inhibit platelet reactivity, i.e., prostacyclin (3), nitric oxide (endothelium-derived relaxing factor) (4), and possibly 13-hydroxy octadecadienoic acid (13-HODE) (5). Moreover, endothelium interrupts fibrin deposition by (a) thrombomodulin-dependent production of activated protein C, which down-regulates thrombin generation and (b) heparan sulfate-dependent antithrombin III inhibition of thrombin activity (6–10). Fibrinolytic mechanisms are also up-regulated by thrombin's direct action on endothelium to release tissue plasminogen activator (tPA) (11,12). Furthermore, coagulation is controlled by the action of potent plasma serine-protease inhibitors including antithrombin III, heparin cofactor II, α_2 macroglobulin, and α_1 antitrypsin (13–15). Finally, activated prothrombotic molecules are diluted into flowing blood and then rapidly removed from the circulation by the tissue mononuclear phagocytic system.

Arterial Thrombosis

Arterial thrombosis occurs typically after vascular injury (e.g., mechanical, chemical, immunologic, or thermal). Subendothelial structures are then exposed to circulating blood, and platelets, which normally circulate as single, disc-shaped cells, adhere to and spread over the subendothelium (Fig. 1).

Platelet adhesion, the first step in hemostasis and thrombosis is mediated by the interaction of platelet membrane glycoproteins (GP) with adhesive proteins bound to subendothelial connective tissue structures. The platelet-von Willebrand Factor (vWF) interaction is important for platelet adhesion, particularly at high shear rate (i.e., in small vessels), although it also has detectable effects at lower shear rates (16). This multimeric high molecular weight pro-

tein bridges between platelets and subendothelium (17); vWF in platelets, in plasma, and at the surface of vessels is required for optimal platelet adhesion (18). vWF interacts with connective tissue collagen and/or as yet unidentified microfibrillar noncollagenous substances of the vessel wall to undergo conformational change permitting its interaction with platelet GP Ib/IX (17, 19,20). vWF may also interact with platelet GP IIb/IIIa, the common receptor for several other adhesive proteins, that depends on the tripeptide sequence arg-gly-asp (RGD) (21). Thus, both the interaction vWF-GP Ib/IX and the interaction platelet vWF-GP IIb/IIIa appear to be important in the process of optimal platelet adhesion (22), the former for the initial contact platelet-subendothelium, the latter presumably for the platelet spreading over subendothelial structures (23). Fibronectin, by binding with platelet GP IIb/IIIa or perhaps another platelet receptor (e.g., GP Ic/IIa), is also involved in platelet adhesion, especially at low shear rates (24–26). Vitronectin, nidogen, and laminin may also play roles (27). GP Ia, a putative receptor for collagen, may also have a role for optimal platelet adhesion (28,29). The adhesive protein thrombospondin may not be involved in this process (30,31). The endogenous production of

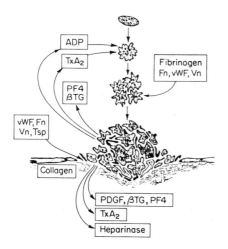

FIG. 1. Platelet adhesion and recruitment. Platelets adhere to subendothelial connective tissue elements at sites of endothelial disruption, primarily through vWF ligand formation between platelet receptor GP Ib and subendothelial collagen. The adhesive proteins, fibronectin, vitronectin, and thrombospondin may also participate in adhesion to subendothelium through platelet receptors GP IIb/IIIa and GP IV. Platelet adhesion initiates a series of complex interactive platelet recruitment reactions comprising (a) release of dense granule ADP, (b) activation of platelet membrane phospholipase complex to form TXA$_2$, and (c) release of alpha granule binding proteins (including fibrinogen, vWF, fibronectin, vitronectin, and thrombospondin). Platelet recruitment requires expression of GP IIb/IIIa as a ligand receptor. Generally, platelet-platelet binding occurs through calcium-dependent bridging with fibrinogen.

platelet 12-hydroxyeicosatetraenoic acid (12-HETE), derived from arachidonic acid via the lipoxygenase pathway, has been reported to be involved in platelet adhesion as an internal regulator of the expression of adhesion moieties on the platelet surface (5).

Adherent platelets change their shape to form irregular spheres that extend pseudopods along the thrombogenic vascular surface. These activated platelets also release their granule contents, contributing to both thrombogenesis (ADP, adenosine triphosphate [ATP], serotonin, Ca^{2+}, adhesive proteins, coagulation factors) and atherogenesis (platelet-derived and other growth factors). Ambient platelets are thus recruited to form an enlarging thrombus (Fig. 2).

Platelet activation depends on an increase in cytoplasmic calcium. Phospholipase C becomes activated probably via stimulation of a regulatory guanine nucleotide binding protein, producing inositol 1,4,5-triphosphate (IP_3) and diacylglycerol. IP_3 mobilizes calcium from the dense tubular system of platelets, and diacylglycerol stimulates protein kinase C (32).

ADP, a potent aggregating agent, is released from the dense granules, binds to its receptor on ambient platelets, decreases cAMP activity, and induces GP IIb/IIIa fibrinogen receptor expression resulting in platelet recruitment (33). An alternative but interactive pathway of platelet recruitment involves arachidonic acid conversion to diacylglycerol and production of cyclic endoperoxides (PGG_2, and PGH_2), the latter serving as substrate for thromboxane A_2 (TXA_2) formation. Both endoperoxides and TXA_2 are potent platelet agonists.

Collagen and thrombin are the most potent inducers of platelet activation. Various receptors appear to participate in platelet-thrombin interactions. Platelet GP V and GP Ib/IX appear to be involved in some as yet undefined way in thrombin activation of platelets (34–36). Serotonin, epinephrine,

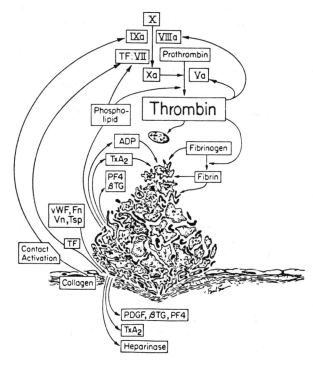

FIG. 2. Central role of thrombin in platelet recruitment. Thrombin is the most important pathophysiologic initiator of platelet recruitment. Whereas thrombin activates platelets independently at concentrations less than that required to convert fibrinogen to fibrin, it also enhances platelet aggregation through ADP- and TXA_2-mediated pathways. Thrombin forms on the platelet surface at a 300,000-fold increased rate through either intrinsic factor VIIIa-dependent or extrinsic factor Va-mediated pathways. Fibrin serves to consolidate the enlarging thrombotic mass.

and platelet-activating-factor are weaker agonists that may facilitate proaggregant activity in combination with other stimulatory agents.

Platelet aggregation proceeds by ligand-mediated, platelet-platelet interactions. The adhesive proteins bind primarily to platelet GP IIb/IIIa. Although this receptor in unstimulated platelets has no ligand-binding activity, receptor expression occurs by some structural, conformational, or microenvironmental changes induced by platelet stimulation. A G-protein-dependent pathway, independent of intracellular Ca^{2+}, has also been implicated (21). Fibrinogen, due to its high plasma concentration, is probably the principal adhesive protein involved in platelet aggregation. However, other adhesive proteins may become involved under some conditions. Thus, vWF may be important in afibrinogenemic patients (37). Similarly, in vascular regions with very high shear stress (e.g., stenosis), vWF may possibly mediate platelet aggregation and thrombus formation (38). In this regard, thrombin has been shown to shift the reactivity of vWF from GP Ib to GP IIb/IIIa (39). Fibronectin, by binding to GP IIb/IIIa or another putative receptor (e.g., GP Ic/IIa) may also play an important role (25). Finally, thrombospondin has been shown to promote platelet aggregation on both unstimulated (via GP IV) and stimulated (via GP IIb/IIIa) platelets (40).

In vivo thrombin plays a central role in thrombus formation (Fig. 2). Thrombin is formed by stimulation of both the intrinsic and extrinsic pathways of coagulation (Fig. 3). Subendothelial tissues and disrupted endothelial cells activate the contact factors of the intrinsic pathway. Injured vascular cells also express tissue factor, which, together with factor VII/VIIa, initiates the activation of extrinsic coagulation. Tissue factor is a glycoprotein that may be expressed by vascular cells, i.e., endothelial cells, smooth muscle cells, and fibroblasts, as well as monocytes/macrophages. Although tissue factor does not circulate, vascular injury induces surface bound tissue factor expression. It complexes with factor VII/VIIa from plasma to convert factor X to Xa and factor IX to IXa. Factor Xa and probably also IXa catalyze factor VII conversion to VIIa, resulting in an increase of some 100-fold in coagulant activity (41). Platelets contribute greatly to the activation of the contact factors (42) by binding XIa via a specific receptor (43) and providing the phospholipid surface for the formation of the "tenase" (IXa-VIIIa-Ca^{2+}-phospholipid) and prothrombinase (Xa-Va-Ca^{2+}-phospholipid) complexes (44). By its membrane content rich in anionic phospholipid, platelets may also augment factor Xa catalyzed factor VII activation (45). Thus, platelets increase the rate at which thrombin is formed by more than 300,000-fold, protect bound coagulation factors from inactivation by plasma inhibitors, and localize the subsequent coagulation reaction to the hemostatic plug.

Because prothrombin is converted to thrombin on platelets by the action of the prothrombinase complex, the prothrombin activation fragment 1.2 remains bound to the platelet surface (44). Meizothrombin, an intermediary compound, is also produced and may mediate platelet activation, despite having only 10% of the clotting activity of thrombin. Indeed, because it is less inhibitable by the complex antithrombin III-heparin, larger amounts of meizothrombin than thrombin may actually be produced (46).

Thrombin greatly amplifies thrombotic processes by positive feedback mechanisms for both platelets and fibrin by activating membrane-bound coagulation factors V and VIII. Finally, the thrombotic mass is consolidated by the thrombin-dependent conversion of fibrinogen into fibrin and the activation of factor XIII, providing a covalent structure to the fibrin clot (47).

Under some circumstances thrombus may form on intact endothelial cells in the absence of morphologically detectable cellular damage or endothelial detachment. For

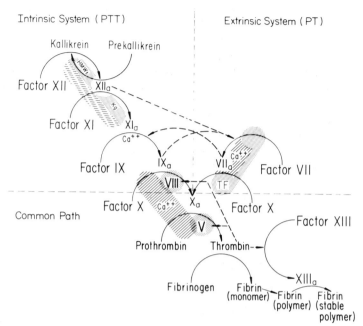

FIG. 3. Mechanisms of clotting factor interactions. Clotting is initiated by either an intrinsic or extrinsic pathway with subsequent factor interactions that converge on a final, common path. The clinical screening tests are indicated as PTT for partial thromboplastin time and PT for prothrombin time. The factors circulate as (a) zymogens that are activated by specific cleavages to highly specific serine proteases, (b) cofactors (*stippled* for protein and *hatched* for phospholipid), or (c) the precursor of the structural protein of the clot (fibrinogen). A separate enzymatic system, generation of factor XIII$_a$, follows for clot stabilization. Protein cofactors include high molecular weight kininogen (HMWt Kg), tissue factor (TF), and factors VIII and V; each of the latter two require modification by thrombin. Other interactions between the intrinsic and extrinsic systems (*arrows* and *dashed lines*) can be demonstrated under some conditions.

example, a low concentration of endotoxin induces tissue factor expression *in vitro* that secondarily results in deposition of fibrin on endothelial cells, especially at low shear rate (48). Interleukin 1 (IL-1) and tissue-necrosis factor (TNF) also induce cultured endothelial cells to generate tissue factor activity (49). Additionally, thrombomodulin-protein C complex activity is decreased (49) and an inhibitor of plasminogen activator is released by endotoxin, IL-1, or TNF in cultured endothelial cells (50,51). The clinical relevance of these cell culture studies is unclear, since *in situ* hybridization studies involving endothelium in human tissue preparations fail to show tissue factor production.

Venous Thrombosis

Stasis is important in the pathogenesis of venous thrombosis. In general thrombi in veins are found at sites of maximum stasis, such as in valve pockets (52) where a captive annular vortex flow results in a prolonged residence time of blood cells and procoagulant material thereby increasing the likelihood that these elements will induce the formation of evolving thrombi (53). Congenital or acquired "hypercoagulability" (deficit in plasma coagulation inhibitors, trauma, surgery) or "hypofibrinolysis" (decrease in tissue-type plasminogen activator or increase in inhibitor of plasminogen activator) (54) predisposed to the development of clinically evident venous thrombosis. Platelets and endothelial cells are less important in venous thrombogenesis. However, thrombosis after hip surgery is unusual in that there is local mechanical damage to the femoral vein produced during the surgical procedure. Presumably this explains why thrombosis occurring after hip surgery is less responsive to standard anticoagulant prophylaxis than other venous thrombotic events associated with surgery (55).

Regulation of Thrombus Formation

A number of mechanisms limit the unwanted extension of thrombosis by modulating activation of platelets and coagulation (Fig. 4). Because thrombin is the pivotal enzyme in the formation of thrombus, it is the principal focus in its regulation. Thrombin initiates antiaggregant (3,4), anticoagulant (6–10), and profibrinolytic properties (11,12) of endothelium. First, thrombin stimulates the release of antiag-

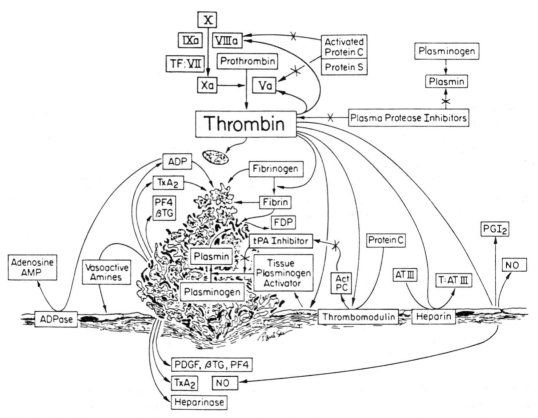

FIG. 4. Regulatory mechanisms limiting the extension of thrombus formation. Intravascular extension of thrombus is limited by multiple protective mechanisms. The most important of these mechanisms is related to the presence of thrombin and/or intact endothelium and include (a) inactivation by complex formation with plasma antithrombin III, (b) facilitation by endothelial heparan sulfate of the inactive thrombin:antithrombin III complex formation, (c) down-regulation of thrombin formation through destruction of surface-bound factor VIII$_a$ and factor V$_a$ by activated protein C formed by thrombomodulin-dependent thrombin cleavage and thrombin-mediated release from endothelium of (d) t-PA, (e) PGI$_2$, and (f) nitric oxide. Additionally, intact endothelium adjacent to forming thrombus inactivates ADP and vasoactive amines released from activated platelets.

gregant molecules, prostacyclin, and nitric oxide (3,4). Second, thrombin complexes with heparin-like glycosaminoglycans at the surface of the endothelium and facilitates complex formation with antithrombin III, inactivating its coagulant and platelet stimulatory capability (6,7). Third, the thrombin-thrombomodulin complex, with protein S as a cofactor, activates protein C. Activated protein C further destroys platelet-bound factors Va and VIIIa activity, thereby down-regulating the production of thrombin (8–10). Fourth, thrombin activity is inhibited by several plasma serine-protease inhibitors, particularly antithrombin (13–15).

Inhibition of the factor VIIa/tissue factor-induced blood coagulation by extrinsic pathway inhibitor or lipoprotein-associated coagulation inhibitor limits thrombus extension associated with tissue injury or inflammation. This inhibitor initially forms a complex with Xa that then inhibits further factor VIIa/tissue factor activation of factor X (56).

Fibrinolysis

The fibrinolytic system enzymatically degrades fibrin, leading to the dissolution of thrombus (Fig. 5). Thus, fibrinolysis rep-

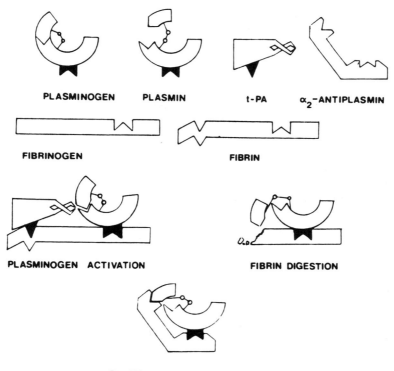

FIG. 5. Schematic visualization of the molecular interactions regulating fibrinolysis. On the fibrin surface, plasminogen is efficiently converted to the proteolytic enzyme plasmin by bound plasminogen activator. The plasmin generated is partially protected from inactivation by α_2-antiplasmin, while free plasmin in the blood is very rapidly inactivated. The lysine-binding sites of plasminogen (represented as ◣) are important for the interaction between plasmin(ogen) and fibrin and between plasmin and α_2-antiplasmin. The active site of plasmin is represented as ▱.

resents a critical regulator of thrombotic mass, as illustrated by the clinical occurrence of thrombosis in patients with constitutive or acquired hypofibrinolysis (54).

Fibrinolysis occurs by the action of plasmin on fibrin, with subsequent release of soluble fibrin degradation products, characteristically D-dimer (57,58). Plasminogen, the circulating zymogen, binds during thrombus formation to the fibrin through lysine-binding sites. Plasminogen is then activated to plasmin by two pathways. The extrinsic pathway occurs via the action of plasminogen activators. First, tissue-type plasminogen activator (t-PA) binds to fibrin, which markedly enhances the activation rate of plasminogen (Fig. 4); t-PA is poorly active in the absence of fibrin (59). Second, urokinase-type plasminogen activator (u-PA), secreted in an inactive form as urinary-type single-chain plasminogen activator (scu-PA), also induces selective activation of fibrin-bound plasminogen by a mechanism yet to be defined (60,61). Intrinsic activation involves formation of contact factors (factor XII, prekallikrein, high molecular weight kininogen). This pathway may be involved in scu-PA activation, but its physiologic role remains unclear (62,63).

Platelets promote fibrinolysis. First, plasminogen binds with platelets, facilitating the conversion of plasminogen activation to plasmin by plasminogen activators; this binding is enhanced by thrombin activation (64,65). Second, scu-PA is also associated with platelet membranes (66). However, plasmin has been reported to inhibit platelet function by blocking the mobilization of arachidonic acid from membrane phospholipid pools (67) and perhaps by destroying platelet membrane GP receptors, especially GP Ib (68). At higher concentrations plasmin has been reported to induce platelet release and platelet aggregation (69).

Normally, plasmin formation is locally confined to the thrombotic mass without escape into the systemic circulation by means of several protective mechanisms

(Fig. 4). First, plasminogen activators are released locally from intact adjacent endothelial cells by the action of thrombin (12). Second, plasminogen activators act within the thrombus because of affinity for fibrin in the case of t-PA and by some less well-defined mechanism for scu-PA. Third, fibrinolysis is regulated by inhibitors. The principal inhibitor of both plasminogen activators (t-PA and scu-PA) present in plasma, PAI-1, potently binds and inactivates the activated molecules reaching the circulation. This inhibitor is also released from platelet α-granules (70,71). Other plasma inhibitors, PAI-2, PAI-3, and protease nexin have also been described (72).

The principal physiologic inhibitor of plasmin is α_2-antiplasmin, which quickly and irreversibly inhibits the enzyme, providing the lysine-binding sites on plasminogen are available (72). Other inhibitors include α_2-macroglobulin, which inactivates, albeit slowly, most of the enzymes of the fibrinolytic pathway, and histidine-rich glycoprotein, a competitive inhibitor of plasminogen (72,73).

ANTITHROMBOTIC THERAPY

The three classes of antithrombotic agents include (a) antiplatelet, (b) anticoagulant, and (c) thrombolytic drugs. Indications for their use differ according to the type of thrombotic process involved. The aim of antithrombotic therapy is to choose agents with an appropriate ratio of antithrombotic efficacy to hemostatic safety. These drugs may be administered separately or combined when broader or more potent antithrombotic effects are required.

Antiplatelet Therapy

This group of therapeutic agents inhibits platelet recruitment into forming thrombus.

Drugs That Inhibit the Arachidonate Pathway

Cyclooxygenase Inhibitors

This group of drugs comprises nonsteroidal anti-inflammatory drugs, e.g., aspirin, indomethacin, phenylbutazone, as well as the uricosuric agent sulfinpyrazone. Although not particularly potent in experimental animal models (74), aspirin is the most efficacious and widely used clinical antiplatelet agent. Aspirin irreversibly acetylates cyclooxygenase (75,76), thereby abolishing both platelet production of TXA_2, the most potent vasoconstrictor and platelet agonist in nature, and endothelial synthesis of prostacyclin (PGI_2), the most potent vasodilator and antiplatelet agent in nature (Fig. 6). Aspirin's inhibitory effect on cyclooxygenase persists throughout the residual life span of exposed platelets. Because endothelial cells resynthesize cyclooxygenase, aspirin's effect on endothelial cells is reversible over approximately 24 to 36 hr.

Clinically, aspirin is an effective antithrombotic agent. Aspirin (300–1,500 mg daily) has been shown to be effective in reducing transient ischemic attacks (TIA), stroke, and death in patients with transient cerebral ischemia (77–80). Similarly, aspirin reduces myocardial infarction and cardiac death in patients with unstable angina and prevents reinfarction and vascular death in patients who have suffered both remote and acute myocardial infarction (81,82). Aspirin also appears to be effective in the primary prevention of myocardial infarction, although the present results are inconclusive (83–85). Aspirin is also effective in the prevention of aortocoronary saphenous vein bypass graft occlusion (86,87) and arteriovenous shunt thrombosis (88).

The choice of aspirin's effective and safe dose is not fully resolved. It has been argued that reducing the doses of aspirin to the least effective dose would maintain endothelial cell synthesis of PGI_2 unaffected while abolishing platelet TXA_2 production. However, even with very low doses (35 mg/day), PGI_2 production, as measured in biopsies of vascular wall tissues is markedly impaired (89). Thus, no differential susceptibility of different tissues has been shown. Nonetheless, it is important to give the lowest effective dose, because aspirin-induced bleeding and other gastrointestinal side effects are dose dependent. Because doses of aspirin between 160 and 1,500 mg daily in adults are probably equally antithrombotic (77,78), and low doses (325 mg or less) have minimal side effects (77,90,91), the current general recommendation is for 325 mg aspirin to be given once daily.

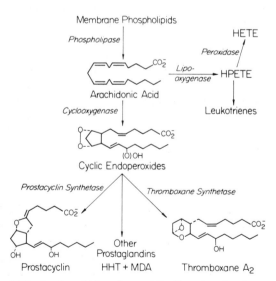

FIG. 6. Arachidonate metabolism in platelets. Note that conversion of PGH_2 to PGI_2 and PGD_2 does not occur within platelets. The eisocanoids listed can be divided into those that stimulate platelet aggregation (TXA_2, PGH_2) and those that inhibit it (PGI_2, PGD_2).

Inhibitors of TXA_2 Production or Action

Blocking TXA_2-mediated activation of platelets by TXA_2 synthetase inhibitor or TXA_2 receptor antagonist (Fig. 6) has the theoretical advantage over cyclooxygenase inhibitors of preserving endothelial prostacyclin production (92). *In vitro,* such agents are weak platelet inhibitors and *in vivo* effects are variable. The weak antithrombotic effects of synthetase inhibitors are ascribed to the continued production of PG endoperoxides that mediate platelet activation (93). Consequently, combining TXA_2 synthetase inhibition with antagonism of the shared TXA_2/PG endoperoxide receptor may produce more potent antithrombotic effects (93). The *in vivo* effects of combined TXA_2 receptor antagonist with 5-HT_2 receptor antagonist is also variable (94–96). Controlled clinical trials will be necessary to establish possible therapeutic benefit.

Drugs That Increase Platelet cAMP Levels

Prostacyclin

Prostacyclin is a potent platelet inhibitor that acts by elevating platelet cAMP through the stimulation of adenylcyclase. However, because of its instability and its potent vasodilator effects at doses that are able to produce useful antiplatelet effects, there is no significant clinical application of prostacyclin at present. A great number of related compounds have been developed with improved stability and claimed reduced vascular effect. However, none of the available agents in this series has been demonstrated to have an improved vasomotor/platelet inhibitor ratio (97).

Although some studies have claimed that prostacyclin or related compounds reduce myocardial injury during acute myocardial infarction (98,99), such results have not been confirmed in controlled trials (100). Although these agents have also been administered in extracorporeal systems to preserve the platelet count (101,102), the hypotensive consequences are prohibitive. Similarly, these agents have been studied in the treatment of atherosclerotic peripheral

vascular disease (97) without benefit evident in controlled trials.

Dipyridamole

Dipyridamole increases cAMP by inhibiting phosphodiesterase activity (103). Experimentally, dipyridamole has been shown to be an effective antithrombotic agent with synergism of action when combined with aspirin (104). However, its clinical indication is limited to the prevention of systemic embolism in patients with prosthetic heart valves, when administered in combination with warfarin (105,106). Dipyridamole is ineffective when given alone and provides no additional benefit when given with aspirin for the treatment of cerebrovascular, coronary thrombotic events or saphenous vein bypass grafts (98).

Ticlopidine

This agent produces a global inhibitory effect on platelet function; however, its mechanism of action remains undefined. It does not affect phosphodiesterase, adenylcyclase, cyclooxygenase, or thromboxane synthetase activities. It modifies platelet receptor signal transduction for ADP, GP IIb/IIIa, etc. (107). Because it is ineffective *in vitro* and requires several days of oral administration to manifest its maximum effect *in vivo,* its activity is due to some as yet unknown metabolites or to some membrane abnormality produced during megakaryocytopoiesis. However, no metabolite has been identified that inhibits platelet function directly. In thrombosis models, ticlopidine is a more potent antithrombotic than aspirin (74). The delay of several days before the drug is fully effective and the persistent effect of ticlopidine for several days after discontinuing treatment complicates its clinical use. Additionally, occasional idiosyncratic neutropenia and gastrointestinal side effects may occur during its use (108).

Clinically, ticlopidine (250 mg twice a day) is effective in the secondary prevention of stroke: recurrence of stroke and cardiovascular death is reduced by 30% compared with placebo (109). At this dosage, ticlopidine is also more potent than aspirin (650 mg twice daily) in preventing the occurrence of nonfatal stroke and death in patients with TIA; these events are reduced by as much as 30% as compared with patients treated with aspirin (110). Other indications of ticlopidine currently under study are in the treatment of peripheral vascular disease, ischemic heart disease, surgical bypass procedures, e.g., postendarterectomy, or extracorporeal procedures (108).

Newer Antiplatelet Strategies

Dietary Omega-3 Fatty Acids

A diet rich in fish oil produces changes in the lipid composition of cell membranes by incorporating accumulating omega-3 polyunsaturated fatty acids instead of arachidonic acid (111). Consequently, stimulated platelets produce TXA_3 rather than TXA_2. TXA_3 is a relatively inactive platelet agonist. Concurrently, endothelial cells release PGI_3, which inhibits platelet function as potently as PGI_2 (112). Thus, inhibitory products are produced by the vessel wall, without stimulator products being generated from platelets. Other antithrombotic effects of fish-oil-rich diets include augmentation of fibrinolytic activity (113) and red blood cell membrane fluidity (114), together with impairment of tissue factor expression by monocytes/macrophages.

Experimentally, dietary omega-3 fatty acids have been shown to reduce *ex vivo* platelet aggregation minimally and prolong bleeding times slightly (111,115). In animal models of arterial thrombosis (116) and ath-

erogenesis, substantial beneficial effects have been reported (117–119). One prospective controlled clinical trial has been reported showing a decreased rate of restenosis after coronary angioplasty, but this effect has not been confirmed in a second study. Studies comparing efficacy and toxicity (hemorrhagic, carcinogenic, or immunosuppressive effects) of such diet supplementation have not been reported.

Drugs That Interfere with Platelet-Adhesive Protein Interactions

A new group of agents has been designed to inhibit platelet recruitment by interrupting platelet binding with adhesive proteins, a process central to the formation of arterial thrombosis. This blockade may be achieved experimentally by peptides or antibodies acting either on the platelet membrane glycoprotein or adhesive proteins. For example, antibodies directed against GP IIb/IIIa produce potent antihemostatic and antithrombotic effects in various animal models (120–123). However, such antibodies have been reported not to be effective in thrombosis models with surgical tissue injury, suggesting that the blockade of adhesive properties of platelets may not be adequate therapy for mechanical vascular interventions (124). Additionally, because of their heterologous source, murine monoclonal antibodies may be immunogenic, precluding further retreatment. Profound thrombocytopenia has also been described in baboons treated with antiplatelet antibodies (121,125). Anti-vWF monoclonal antibody inhibiting the interaction of vWF with GP Ib produces antithrombotic effects in pigs (126,127); this effect is shear rate dependent (125). *In vitro* studies suggest that the interaction of vWF and GP Ib is increased when combined with antibodies against the GP IIb/IIIa receptor and with the collagen receptor (22).

An alternative and interesting approach

may be the utilization of peptides containing the cytoadhesion recognition peptide sequence, RGD, common to most of the adhesive proteins. Such peptides have been shown to inhibit platelet aggregation *in vitro* and have potent antithrombotic effects in baboons (128). This area of research is under active development (129–131).

Anticoagulants

Anticoagulants act by inhibiting thrombin formation, thrombin activity, or coagulation serine proteases participating in the events giving rise to thrombin generation. They are mainly used in the prevention and treatment of fibrin-dependent thrombotic events, including venous thrombosis, pulmonary embolism, and other situations involving venous thromboembolic risk or complications. However, because thrombin has a pivotal role in platelet-dependent thrombosis, some of these agents have been proposed for the treatment of arterial thrombosis.

Drugs Accelerating Antithrombin III Action

Heparin

Standard unfractionated heparin is the most widely used antithrombotic agent in clinical practice. Heparin is a heterodisperse mixture of polysaccharides of a molecular weight ranging between 3,000 and 40,000 daltons and averaging approximately 15,000 daltons. Heparin catalyzes bimolecular complex formation between plasma antithrombin III (AT III) and serine proteases of the coagulation pathway; thrombin inhibition by heparin is primarily responsible for its anticoagulant action. At higher concentrations, heparin induces thrombin inhibition through heparin cofactor II (HC II), another specific plasma antithrombin. A minor anticoagulant effect independent of both AT III and HC II has been also described (132). Heparin has been reported to

inhibit, stimulate, or have no effect on platelets (133).

Clinical studies have shown that both antithrombotic efficacy and bleeding complications are dose dependent. Heparin monitoring by coagulation tests is critical because there is great variability in the anticoagulant response to heparin among individuals and within the same individual at different times during the course of thromboembolic diseases (134,135). Because the activated partial thromboplastin time (APTT), a global coagulation test, correlates relatively well with *ex vivo* plasma heparin levels (136), it is generally used to monitor therapy (Fig. 7). Laboratory monitoring of the platelet count is also important because heparin-induced thrombocytopenia has been reported in approximately 1% to 5% of patients receiving therapeutic heparin (137).

Heparin may be administered by continuous intravenous injection or by intra-

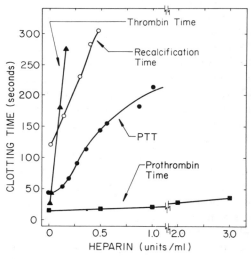

FIG. 7. Effect of heparin on coagulation screening tests. When dilutions of heparin are added to normal plasma, the relative susceptibility of the screening tests is apparent. Note the extreme sensitivity of the thrombin time compared with the relative insensitivity of the prothrombin time. Intrinsic system tests average around twice prolonged at therapeutic levels (0.2–0.5 units/ml).

venous or subcutaneous bolus injection. Subcutaneous administration is usually reserved for prophylaxis of venous thrombosis during surgery or medical patients at bed rest. A recent review of more than 70 randomized trials in 16,000 patients reported that the perioperative use of low-dose heparin (5,000 U twice daily) prevents approximately half of all pulmonary emboli and approximately two-thirds of all deep-vein thromboses appearing after urologic, orthopedic, or general surgery (138). Although this result may be achieved using a fixed low dose of heparin, the prevention of deep-vein thrombosis in patients undergoing elective hip surgery requires subcutaneous heparin in doses producing APTT values in the high normal range rather than fixed doses (139).

The route of administration is not critical in the initial treatment of deep venous thrombosis provided the *ex vivo* APTT is prolonged 1.5 to two times the control value within the first few hours. The total daily dose of heparin to achieve this result is generally greater with intermittent intravenous injection than with continuous infusion. Thus, a greater risk of bleeding has been described in patients treated with intermittent injection (140–142). Also, the amount of heparin required to obtain an adequate anticoagulant response is larger when heparin is given subcutaneously than by continuous infusion (143). When initial doses are adequate to achieve immediate therapeutic levels, adjusted subcutaneous heparin is as potent as continuous intravenous heparin in patients with acute deep-vein thrombosis (144). For example, full therapeutic doses of subcutaneous heparin prevent left ventricular mural thrombosis in patients with acute transmural anterior myocardial infarction (145).

Experimentally, heparin is also effective in the treatment of platelet-dependent thrombotic events, albeit at doses markedly higher than those required to block fibrin-dependent venous thrombosis (146). Also, heparin reduces the development of acute platelet-thrombus deposition during angioplasty in pigs. In this model, a number of antiplatelet agents tested are less or not effective (147). Clinically, heparin has been reported to be more potent than aspirin in reducing the frequency of myocardial infarction in patients with unstable angina (148). Finally, heparin may be capable of inhibiting the proliferation of vascular smooth muscle cells, a process fundamental to atherosclerosis (149).

Low Molecular Weight Heparins

Low molecular weight heparins (LMWHs) are prepared by fractionation or depolymerization of unfractionated heparin; these agents are quite heterogeneous. However, compared with unfractionated heparin, LMWHs are all characterized by a decreased capacity to prolong the APTT and a reduced ratio of antithrombin activity to antiactivated factor X (anti-Xa) activity. Indeed, this ratio is inversely related to molecular weight. Consequently, anti-Xa activity is generally used for laboratory monitoring. Experimentally, LMWHs (mean molecular weight of approximately 5,000) have antithrombotic effects that are comparable with unfractionated heparin but with reduced antihemostatic activities. These findings suggest that LMWHs have a more favorable therapeutic ratio (150).

Although most clinical studies have failed to confirm improved hemostatic safety for LMWHs, preliminary results indicate that LMWHs injected subcutaneously may also be effective in the treatment of established deep-vein thrombosis (150,151). Additionally, LMWHs have a longer half-life than standard heparin, with better bioavailability over the usual therapeutic range (152). Thus, a single subcutaneous injection per day of LMWHs has been reported to be at least as effective as two or three injections per day of subcutaneous standard heparin in prophylaxis for patients undergoing general or orthopedic surgery.

Vitamin K Antagonists

Vitamin K is necessary for the gamma-carboxylation during postribosomal synthesis of clotting factors II, VII, IX, and X and also of the anticoagulant proteins C and S. The gamma-carboxylated glutamyl residues are necessary for the binding of calcium ions, an essential step in the generation of the procoagulant and anticoagulant activities of these proteins. Vitamin K antagonists prevent gamma-carboxylation and therefore produce biologically inactive proteins (132). There are various types of vitamin K antagonists, and all are absorbed orally. Warfarin is the most widely used in United States because of its intermediate rate of metabolism (half-life approximately 35 hr) and good bioavailability (153,154). The anticoagulant effect of vitamin K antagonists is fully manifest 36 to 72 hr after drug administration and is optimal when factors are reduced to approximately 10% of normal. There is, however, a great individual variability of the response to vitamin K antagonists (155).

To monitor warfarin therapy the prothrombin time (PT) is generally used (Fig. 7). In the past, laboratory monitoring has been complicated by variable sensitivities of the thromboplastins used in the procedure. Therefore, to standardize the PT, an international reference preparation of thromboplastin has been designated and the observed PT ratio is now converted into an International Normalized Ratio (INR) using an International Sensitivity Index (ISI), different for each thromboplastin (156).

The optimal therapeutic range has thus been established. Less intense oral anticoagulant regimens (INR = 2.0–3.0) have been documented to be as effective with less hemorrhagic effects than the standard regimen (INR = 2.5–5.0) in the prevention of venous thrombosis, the treatment of venous thrombosis after an initial course of heparin, and the prevention of systemic embolism in patients with acute myocardial infarction or atrial fibrillation. A more intense therapeutic regimen (INR = 3.0–4.5) is still recommended for patients with mechanical prosthetic valves or recurrent systemic embolism (157).

Newer Anticoagulants

A number of agents that directly or indirectly inhibit thrombin formation or activity are currently under study. Natural hirudin, a peptide found in medicinal leeches, is the most potent inhibitor of thrombin found in nature. It acts by forming a tight, stoichiometric complex with thrombin (158). Although newly available recombinant forms of hirudin are less potent by an order of magnitude, they have been shown to be very effective in animal venous thrombosis models (159). Importantly, recombinant hirudin is also potent in interrupting thrombus formation in arterial thrombosis models resistant to standard heparin (160,161). A synthetic antithrombin, D-phenylalanyl-L-prolyl-L-arginyl-chloromethylketone (D-FPRCH$_2$C1), is equally potent (162). Interestingly, a hirudin peptide, encompassing the minimal hirudin sequence exhibiting antithrombin activity, is inactive with respect to platelets but effective in preventing fibrin-dependent thrombus formation (163).

Activated protein C produces potent antithrombotic effects in the prevention of platelet-dependent thrombosis without significantly increasing the risk of bleeding, as determined by template bleeding time measurements (164). Newly available recombinant activated protein C is also effective (165). These results are of particular interest because of the favorable ratio of antithrombotic efficacy to hemostatic safety.

Dermatan sulfate is a natural glycosaminoglycan recently proposed as an antithrombotic drug. In contrast to heparin, dermatan sulfate catalyzes specifically the HC II-thrombin interaction but has no affect on AT III-serine proteases interactions (166). Experimentally, dermatan sulfate is an attractive antithrombotic agent as therapy for venous thrombotic events because it is antithrombotic without exhibiting antihemostatic effects (167). Also, the association of standard heparin and dermatan sulfate has been experimentally shown to be effective at doses that are not antithrombotic when the agents are used singly (168). Clinical trials currently underway will determine potential efficacy/safety.

Fibrinolytic Therapy

Although fibrinolytic mechanisms are initiated during thrombus formation, natural fibrinolysis is both delayed and variable. Fibrinolytic therapy consists of the administration of exogenous fibrinolytic molecules capable of rapidly dissolving already formed thrombus. Fibrin-rich, recently formed thrombi are more responsive than platelet-rich, older thrombi (169). A great number of fibrinolytic agents have been developed. Newer molecules are more fibrin specific, thereby reducing systemic fibrinogenolysis. However, because the fibrinolytic agents currently available do not discriminate between fibrin in thrombi from fibrin in hemostatic plugs, fibrin selectivity does not appear to improve hemostatic safety. In general, bleeding complications associated with thrombolytic therapy occur mainly at sites of vascular injury (170,171). In a preliminary study the template bleeding time has been reported to predict spontaneous bleeding (172).

Agents Directly Cleaving Plasminogen

Streptokinase

Streptokinase, a bacterial product, was the first fibrinolytic agent widely available for clinical purposes. Streptokinase acts by combining in a stoichiometric fashion with plasminogen to convert circulating plasminogen to plasmin (173). In humans, streptokinase has a circulating half-life of approximately 25 min and, depending on clinical indication, is generally given in a loading dose (250,000 units) followed by a maintenance dose (100,000 units hourly for 12 to 48 hr). For acute myocardial infarction, 1.5 million units of streptokinase are infused over 1 hr (170). Streptokinase has poor thrombus specificity and in therapeutic doses produces fibrinolysis and fibrinogenolysis in concert.

Because of its bacterial origin, streptokinase is both antigenic and immunogenic. To reduce its immunogenicity, streptokinase has been experimentally coupled to low molecular weight polyethylene glycols to block its capacity to bind with immunoglobulins while retaining its fibrinolytic activity. Interestingly, the *in vivo* half-life of the complex is prolonged (174).

An acylated plasminogen-streptokinase activator complex (APSAC) has been designed that binds to fibrin through lysine-binding sites of plasminogen in order to improve fibrin selectivity (175,176). The *in vivo* deacylation of the catalytic center of plasminogen molecules sustains the fibrinolytic effect. Compared with streptokinase, the circulating half-life of APSAC is prolonged (90 min) (170). Although APSAC is significantly more antithrombotic than streptokinase experimentally (176), the systemic activation of the fibrinolytic system at therapeutically effective doses in humans (30 units) is similar to that described for streptokinase (170).

Urokinase

At present, urokinase is produced from human urine or fetal kidney cells in tissue culture or by recombinant technology. Unlike streptokinase, urokinase cleaves plasminogen directly and is not antigenic. In therapeutic doses, it is not more fibrin selective than streptokinase. The *in vivo* half-life of urokinase is approximately 15 min. Urokinase is classically given in a loading dose (4,400 units/kg) followed by a maintenance dose (4,400 units/kg/hr for 12 to 48 hr) (170). It appears to be therapeutically equivalent to streptokinase without the immunologic complications.

Biologic Plasminogen Activators

t-PA

Previously obtained from conditioned cell culture media, t-PA is now produced by recombinant procedures. Single-chain and double-chain t-PA are distinguished: double-chain t-PA has a slightly longer half-life (170) and seems clinically more effective (177). Commercial t-PA is a mixture of these two chains. Because of its binding specificity for fibrin, t-PA activates fibrin-bound rather than circulating plasminogen. Consequently, infused t-PA produces less plasma fibrinogenolysis. However, t-PA has a short circulating half-life of 5 to 10 min. Currently, for treatment of acute myocardial infarction, a total of 100 mg over 3 hr is infused (10 mg bolus, 60 mg over the first hour, and 10 mg for each of the next 2 hr) (170). Although t-PA is sparing of fibrinogenolysis, it is not clear whether it is either more effective or safer than streptokinase (see below).

scu-PA

scu-PA is produced by cell culture or recombinant DNA methods. Its circulating half-life is also short, approximately 5 to 10 min. Although experience is limited, intravenous administration of 40 to 70 mg has been used. In contrast to urokinase, scu-PA is relatively fibrin specific (61,62) and therefore produces less systemic fibrinogenolysis (178). However, the specific thrombolytic activity of t-PA has been found experimentally to be higher than that of scu-PA (179,180). Interestingly, in vivo, t-PA and scu-PA, administered simultaneously (181) or sequentially (182) in certain combinations and by mechanisms not yet entirely determined (183), have been reported to act synergistically. However, this combination does not appear to be synergistic for systemic destruction of fibrinogen (181,182). This experimental finding has been reproduced in a limited number of patients with myocardial infarction (184,185).

Newer Fibrinolytic Strategies

New molecules are being designed that have both a longer half-life and greater fibrin specificity. This approach has used the strategy of forming molecular hybrids (186–188) or mutants of t-PA (189) and scu-PA (190) and the development of fibrin-targeted, antibody-directed fibrinolytic agents (191). Fibrinolytic agents administrable by intramuscular (192,193) or oral routes are also under study. No modification has yet emerged with clearly superior characteristics suitable for clinical development. Finally, synergistic combinations of fibrinolytic agents are also under investigation.

Clinical Thrombolytic Therapy

At present, fibrinolytic therapy is largely limited to patients with acute myocardial infarction. Coronary angiography in patients with acute myocardial infarction has shown that occlusive coronary thrombus is present in at least 85% of cases (194), with an early spontaneous reperfusion rate of 10% (195–197). Fibrinolytic therapy administered in the first few hours after the onset of symptoms achieves coronary reperfusion in 50% to 80% of treated patients (198). This result is associated with improvement in both ventricular function and in short- and long-term mortality. Thus, mortality is reduced by 20% to 60% (198). The best results occur in patients that receive thrombolytic therapy early (<1 hr after the onset of symptoms) (199), in combination with aspirin (200), and in association with successful reperfusion (201). Systemic therapy with t-PA appears to be comparable with intracoronary streptokinase with respect to reperfusion and substantially more sparing of plasma fibrinogen levels. Although systemic t-PA has been reported to be more effective than systemic streptokinase or systemic APSAC (198), this question remains to be definitively resolved. When the results of the four currently available studies are combined in which t-PA and streptokinase are directly compared, early mortality (21–30 days) is less in patients treated with t-PA than in those treated with streptokinase (198). However, left ventricular function appears to be equally improved by streptokinase (202). Early reocclusion after t-PA therapy appears to take place in approximately 10% to 20% of reperfused arteries (170) consequent to severe residual stenosis (203). Unfortunately, percutaneous transluminal coronary angioplasty does not appear to reduce the rate of reocclusion (204–206), despite the inclusion of routine aspirin and heparin therapy after acute thrombolysis (170). Studies in experimental animals suggest that potent antiplatelet therapy (including prostaglandins [207], antiplatelet monoclonal antibodies [122,123], combination of TXA_2 synthetase inhibitor with antagonists of the TXA_2 receptor [93] or the $5-HT_2$ receptor [94,95]) may reduce reocclusion following thrombolytic reperfusion. Although heparin does not prevent the formation of platelet-rich thrombus, other agents that inhibit thrombin action or its production, e.g., synthetic antithrombins, recombinant hirudin, or activated protein C, may be substantially more effective. Low-dose heparin is recommended in these patients to prevent the complication of deep venous thrombosis and pulmonary and systemic embolism. Recurrent reinfarction is reduced by early β-blockade therapy (206) and chronic aspirin administration (170).

Major bleeding complications in patients treated with thrombolytic therapy occur in 5% to 15%, primarily at sites of invasive procedures. The incidence of bleeding complications unrelated to vascular injury (particularly intracranial bleeding) is low but dose dependent. For equipotent regimens, t-PA and streptokinase have similar frequencies of intracranial bleeding (170).

Thrombolytic agents have been less extensively studied in patients with unstable angina. Whereas 70% of patients with unstable angina are claimed to show coronary thrombus (210), the usefulness of fibrinolytic therapy regimen has not been conclusively determined (211–213). Thrombolytic therapy in acute thrombotic and thromboembolic stroke (214–216) and other acute peripheral vascular occlusion (171) is being actively investigated.

Deep venous thrombosis may be successfully treated with fibrinolytic agents. Compared with heparin, fibrinolytic therapy has been reported to have the advantage of preventing the postphlebitic syndrome (171); however, this result has not been confirmed by controlled clinical trials. Unfortunately, because treatment periods are long (12–72 hr), bleeding risk is increased threefold by thrombolytic agents over heparin alone (217). For pulmonary embolism, thrombolytic agents followed by heparin therapy are also effective; this form of therapy is currently recommended for treatment of massive life-threatening pulmonary embolism (171).

In the future, combination of agents may optimize efficacy and safety for the agents currently available. Thus, effective treatment of acute myocardial infarction involves the combination of aspirin, streptokinase, and low-dose heparin. Also, combinations of warfarin and dipyridamole, heparin and aspirin, and heparin and prostacyclin have been successfully used in patients with prosthetic heart valves (105), unstable angina (148), and hemodialysis (102), respectively.

Thrombosis is a complex process with many sites for potential intervention. With the development of new understanding of the complex systems for activation and inactivation of various pathways and the capability of molecular biology to produce many new specific and potent, genetically engineered therapeutic molecules, antithrombotic therapy is likely to undergo substantial innovation in the immediate future.

ACKNOWLEDGMENT

This work was supported in part by grants HL 41619, HL 41346, and HL 31950 from the National Institutes of Health.

REFERENCES

1. Sawyer S, Srinivasan S. The role of electrochemical surface properties in thrombosis at vascular interfaces: cumulative experience of studies in animals and man. *Bull NY Acad Med* 1972;48:235–256.

2. Pearson JD, Carlton JS, Gordon JL. Metabolism of adenine nucleotides by ectoenzymes of vascular endothelial and smooth-muscle cells in culture. *Biochem J* 1980;190:421–429.

3. Moncada S, Vane JR. Arachidonic acid metabolites and their interactions between platelets and blood vessel wall. *N Engl J Med* 1979; 300:1142–1147.

4. Moncada S, Palmer RMJ, Higgs EA. Prostacyclin and endothelium-derived relaxing factor: biological interactions and significance. In: Verstraete M, Vermylen J, Lijnen R, Arnout J, eds. *Thrombosis and haemostasis 1987.* Leuven: Leuven University Press, 1987;505–523.

5. Buchanan MR, Bastida E. The role of 13-HODE and HETE's in vessel wall circulating blood interactions. *Agents Actions* 1987;22:1/2.

6. Marcum JA, McKenny JB, Rosenberg RD. Acceleration of thrombin antithrombin complex formation in rat hindquarters via heparin like molecules bound to the endothelium. *J Clin Invest* 1984;74:341–350.

7. Lollar P, Owen WG. Clearance of thrombin from the circulation in rabbits by high-affinity binding sites on the endothelium: possible role in the inactivation of thrombin by antithrombin III. *J Clin Invest* 1980;66:1222–1230.

8. Esmon CT, Owen WG. Identification of an endothelial cell cofactor for thrombin-catalyzed activation of protein C. *Proc Natl Acad Sci USA* 1981;78:2249–2252.

9. Owen WG, Esmon CT. Functional properties of an endothelial cell cofactor for thrombin-catalyzed activation of protein C. *J Biol Chem* 1981;256:5532–5535.

10. Esmon NL, Owen WG, Esmon CT. Isolation of a membrane-bound cofactor for thrombin-catalyzed activation of protein C. *J Biol Chem* 1982;257:859–864.

11. Levin EG, Loskutoff DJ. Cultured bovine endothelial cells produce urokinase and tissue-type plasminogen activators. *J Cell Biol* 1982; 94:631–636.

12. Levin EG, Marzec UM, Anderson J, Harker LA. Thrombin stimulate tissue plasminogen activator release from cultured human endothelial cells. *J Clin Invest* 1984;74:1988–1995.

13. Harpel P. Blood proteolytic enzyme inhibitors: their role in modulating blood coagulation and fibrinolytic pathways. In: Colman RW, Hirsh J, Marder VJ, Salzman EW, eds. *Hemostasis and thrombosis: basic principles and clinical practice,* 2nd ed. Philadelphia: Lippincott, 1987;219–234.

14. Rosenberg RD, Lam LH. Correlation between structure and function of heparin. *Proc Natl Acad Sci USA* 1979;76:1218–1222.

15. Tollefsen DM, Blank MK. Detection of a new heparin-dependent inhibitor of thrombin in human plasma. *J Clin Invest* 1981;68:589–596.

16. Badimon L, Badimon JJ, Turitto VT, Fuster V. Role of von Willebrand factor in mediating platelet-vessel wall interaction at low shear rate: the importance of perfusion condition. *Blood* 1989;73:961–967.

17. de Groot PG, Sixma JJ. Role of von Willebrand factor in the vessel wall. *Semin Thromb Hemost* 1987;13:416–424.

18. Fressinaud E, Baruch D, Rothschild C, Baumgartner HR, Meyer D. Platelet von Willebrand factor: evidence for its involvement in platelet adhesion to collagen. *Blood* 1987;70:1214–1217.

19. Sakariassen KS, Bolhuis PA, Sixma JJ. Human blood platelet adhesion to artery subendothelium is mediated by factor VIII-Von Willebrand factor bound to the subendothelium. *Nature* 1979;279:636–638.

20. Kao KJ, Pizzo SV, McKee PA. Demonstration and characterization of specific binding sites for factor VIII/von Willebrand factor of human platelets. *J Clin Invest* 1979;63:656–664.

21. Phillips DR, Charo IF, Parise LV, Fitzgerald LA. The platelet membrane glycoprotein IIb-IIIa complex. *Blood* 1988;71:831–843.

22. Fressinaud E, Baruch D, Girma JP, Sakariassen KS, Baumgartner HR, Meyer D. von Willebrand factor-mediated platelet adhesion to collagen involves platelet membrane glycoprotein IIb-IIIa as well as glycoprotein Ib. *J Lab Clin Med* 1988;112:58–67.

23. Lawrence JB, Gralnick HR. Monoclonal antibodies to the glycoprotein IIb-IIIa epitopes involved in adhesive protein binding: effects on platelet spreading and ultrastructure on human arterial subendothelium. *J Lab Clin Med* 1987;109:495–503.

24. Houdijk WPM, Sixma JJ. Fibronectin in artery subendothelium is important for platelet adhesion. *Blood* 1985;65:598–604.

25. Bastida E, Escolar G, Ordinas A, Sixma JJ. Fibronectin is required for platelet adhesion and thrombus formation on subendothelium and collagen surfaces. *Blood* 1987;70:1437–1442.

26. Nievelstein PFEM, Sixma JJ. Glycoprotein IIb-IIIa and RGD(S) are not important for fibronectin-dependent platelet adhesion under flow conditions. *Blood* 1988;72:82–88.

27. Ill CR, Engvall E, Ruohslahti. Adhesion of

platelets to laminin in the absence of activation. *J Cell Biol* 1984;99:2140–2145.

28. Nieuwenhuis HK, Akkerman JWN, Houdijk WPM, Sixma JJ. Human blood platelets showing no response to collagen fail to express surface glycoprotein Ia. *Nature* 1985;318:470–472.

29. Nieuwenhuis HK, Sakariassen KS, Houdijk WPM, Nievelstein PFEM, Sixma JJ. Deficiency of platelet membrane glycoprotein Ia associated with a decreased platelet adhesion to subendothelium: a defect in platelet spreading. *Blood* 1986;68:692–695.

30. Houdijk WPM, de Groot PG, Nievelstein PFEM, Sakariassen KS, Sixma JJ. von Willebrand factor and fibronectin but not thrombospondin are involved in platelet adhesion to the extracellular matrix of human vascular endothelial cells. *Arteriosclerosis* 1986;6:24–33.

31. Lahav J. Thrombospondin inhibits adhesion of platelets to glass and protein-covered substrata. *Blood* 1988;71:1096–1099.

32. Holmsen H. Platelet secretion. In: Colman RW, Hirsh J, Marder VJ, Salzman EW, eds. *Hemostasis and thrombosis: basic principles and clinical practice*, 2nd ed. Philadelphia: Lippincott, 1987;606–617.

33. Colman RW, Walsh PN. Mechanisms of platelet aggregation. In: Colman RW, Hirsh J, Marder VJ, Salzman EW, eds. *Hemostasis and thrombosis: basic principles and clinical practice*, 2nd ed. Philadelphia: Lippincott, 1987;594–605.

34. Phillips DR, Agin PP. Platelet plasma membrane glycoproteins: evidence for the presence of nonequivalent disulfide bonds using nonreduced-reduced two-dimensional gel electrophoresis. *J Biol Chem* 1977;252:2121–2126.

35. Tollefsen DM, Majerus PW. Evidence for a single class of thrombin-binding sites on human platelets. *Biochemistry* 1976;15:2144–2149.

36. Okumura J, Hasitz M, Jamieson GA. Platelet glycocalicin: interaction with thrombin and role as thrombin receptor of the platelet surface. *J Biol Chem* 1978;253:3435–3443.

37. De Marco L, Girolami A, Zimmerman TS, Ruggeri ZM. von Willebrand factor interaction with glycoprotein IIb/IIIa complex. Its role in platelet function as demonstrated in patients with congenital afibrinogenemia. *J Clin Invest* 1986;77:1272–1277.

38. Weiss HJ, Hawiger J, Ruggeri ZM, Turitto VT, Thiagarajan P, Hoffman T. Fibrinogen-independent platelet adhesion and thrombus formation on subendothelium mediated by glycoprotein IIb-IIIa complex at high shear rate. *J Clin Invest* 1989;83:288–297.

39. George JN, Torres MM. Thrombin decreases von Willebrand factor binding to platelet glycoprotein Ib. *Blood* 1988;71:1253–1259.

40. Tuszynski GP, Rothman VL, Murphy A, Siegler K, Knudsen KA. Thrombospondin promotes platelet aggregation. *Blood* 1988;72:109–115.

41. Nemerson Y. Tissue factor and hemostasis. *Blood* 1988;71:1–8.

42. Walsh RN, Griffin JH. Contributions of human platelets to the proteolytic activation of blood coagulation factors XII and XI. *Blood* 1981;57:106–118.

43. Sinha D, Seaman FS, Koshy A, Knight LC, Walsh PN. Blood coagulation factors XIa binds specifically to a site on activated human platelets distinct from that for factor XI. *J Clin Invest* 1984;73:1550–1556.

44. Mann KG, Tracy PB, Krishnaswamy S, Jenny RJ, Odegaard BH, Nesheim ME. Platelets and coagulation. In: Verstraete M, Vermylen J, Lijnen R, Arnout J, eds. *Thrombosis and haemostasis 1987*. Leuven: Leuven University Press, 1987;505–523.

45. Rao LVM, Rapaport SI. The effect of platelets upon factor Xa-catalyzed activation of factor VII in vitro. *Blood* 1988;72:396–401.

46. Rosing J, Tans G. Meizothrombin, a major product of factor Xa-catalyzed prothrombin activation. *Thromb Haemost* 1988;60:355–360.

47. Lorand L, Konishi K. Activation of the fibrin-stabilizing factor of plasma by thrombin. *Arch Biochem Biophys* 1964;105:58–67.

48. Clozel M, Kuhn H, Baumgartner HR. Procoagulant activity of endotoxin-treated human endothelial cells exposed to native human flowing blood. *Blood* 1989;73:729–733.

49. Moore KL, Andreoli SP, Esmon NL, Esmon CT, Bang NU. Endotoxin enhances tissue factor and suppresses thrombomodulin expression of human vascular endothelium in vitro. *J Clin Invest* 1987;79:124–130.

50. Colucci M, Paramo JA, Collen D. Generation in plasma of a fast-acting inhibitor of plasminogen activator in response to endotoxin stimulation. *J Clin Invest* 1985;75:818–824.

51. Emeis JJ, Kooistra T. Interleukin-1 and lipopolysaccharide induce an inhibitor of tissue-type plasminogen activator in vivo and in cultured endothelial cells. *J Exp Med* 1986;163:1260–1266.

52. Sevitt S. The structure and growth of valve-pocket thrombi in femoral veins. *J Clin Pathol* 1974;27:517–528.

53. Kareno T, Motoniya M. Flow through a venous valve and its implication for thrombus formation. *Thromb Res* 1984;36:245–257.

54. Nilsson IM, Ljunger H, Tengborn L. Two different mechanisms in patients with venous thrombosis and defective fibrinolysis: low concentration of plasminogen activator or increased concentration of plasminogen activator inhibitor. *Br Med J* 1985;290:1453–1456.

55. Thomas DP. Overview of venous thrombogenesis. *Semin Thromb Hemost* 1988;14:1–8.

56. Rapaport SI. Inhibition of factor VIIa/tissue factor-induced blood coagulation: with particular emphasis upon a factor Xa-dependent inhibitory mechanism. *Blood* 1989;73:359–365.

57. Francis CW, Marder VJ, Martin SE. Plasmic degradation of crosslinked fibrin. I. Structural analysis of the particulate clot and identification of new macromolecular soluble complexes. *Blood* 1980;56:456–464.

58. Francis CW, Marder VJ, Barlow GH. Plasmic

degradation of crosslinked fibrin. Characterization of new macromolecular soluble complexes and a model of their structure. *J Clin Invest* 1980;66:1033–1043.

59. Bachmann F, Kruithof EKO. Tissue plasminogen activator: chemical and physiological aspects. *Semin Thromb Hemost* 1984;10:6–17.

60. Pannell R, Gurewich V. Pro-urokinase—a study of its stability in plasma and of a mechanism for its selective fibrinolytic effect. *Blood* 1986; 67:1215–1223.

61. Lijnen HR, Zammarron C, Blaber M, Winkler ME, Collen D. Activation of plasminogen by pro-urokinase. I. Mechanism. *J Biol Chem* 1986;261:1253–1258.

62. Ichinose A, Fujikawa K, Sumaya T. The activation of pro-urokinase by plasma kallikrein and its inactivation by thrombin. *J Biol Chem* 1986;261:3486–3489.

63. Kluft C, Dooijewaard G, Emeis JJ. Role of the contact system in fibrinolysis. *Semin Thromb Hemost* 1987;13:50–68.

64. Miles LA, Plow EF. Binding and activation of plasminogen on the platelet surface. *J Biol Chem* 1985;260:4303–4311.

65. Miles LA, Ginsberg MH, White JG, Plow EF. Plasminogen interacts with human platelets through two distinct mechanisms. *J Biol Chem* 1986;77:2001–2009.

66. Park S, Harker LA, Marzec UM, Levin EG. Demonstration of single chain urokinase-type plasminogen activator of human platelet membrane. *Blood* 1989;73:1421–1425.

67. Schafer AI, Adelman B. Plasmin inhibition of platelet function and arachidonic acid metabolism. *J Clin Invest* 1985;75:456–461.

68. Adelman B, Michelson AD, Loscalzo J, Greenberg J, Handin RI. Plasmin effect of platelet glycoprotein Ib-von Willebrand factor interactions. *Blood* 1985;65:32–40.

69. Niewiarowski S, Senyi AF, Gillies P. Plasmin-induced platelet aggregation and platelet release reaction. *J Clin Invest* 1973;52:1647–1659.

70. Sprengers ED, Kluft C. Plasminogen activator inhibitors. *Blood* 1987;69:381–387.

71. Erickson LA, Ginsberg MH, Loskutoff DJ. Detection and partial characterization of an inhibitor of plasminogen activator in human platelets. *J Clin Invest* 1984;74:1465–1472.

72. Aoki N, Harpel PC. Inhibitors of the fibrinolytic enzyme system. *Semin Thromb Hemost* 1984;10:24–41.

73. Lijnen HR, Hoylaerts M, Collen D. Isolation and characterization of a human plasma protein with affinity for the lysine binding sites in plasminogen. *J Biol Chem* 1980;255:10214–10222.

74. Hanson SR, Harker LA. Baboon models of acute arterial thrombosis. *Thromb Haemost* 1987;58:801–805.

75. Burch JW, Stanford PW. Inhibition of platelet prostaglandin synthetase by oral aspirin. *J Clin Invest* 1979;61:314–319.

76. Majerus PW. Arachidonate metabolism in vascular disorders. *J Clin Invest* 1983;72:1521–1525.

77. UK-TIA Study Group. The UK-TIA Aspirin Trial: interim results. *Br Med J* 1987;296: 316–320.

78. Bousser MG, Eschwege E, Haguenau M, et al. "AICLA" controlled trial of aspirin and dipyridamole in the secondary prevention of atherothrombotic cerebral ischemia. *Stroke* 1983; 14:5–14.

79. The Canadian Cooperative Study Group. A randomized trial of aspirin and sulfinpyrazone in threatened stroke. *N Engl J Med* 1978; 299:53–59.

80. Fields WS, Lemak NA, Frankowski RF, Hardy RJ. Controlled trial of aspirin in cerebral ischemia. *Stroke* 1977;8:301–314.

81. Antiplatelet Trialists' Collaboration. Secondary prevention of vascular disease by prolonged antiplatelet treatment. *Br Med J* 1988; 296:320–331.

82. ISIS-2 Collaborative Group. Randomised trial of intravenous streptokinase, oral aspirin, both or neither among 17,187 cases of suspected acute myocardial infarction; ISIS-2. *Lancet* 1988;2:349–352.

83. The Steering Committee of The Physicians Health Study Research Group. Special report: preliminary report: findings from the aspirin components of the ongoing physicians' health study. *N Engl J Med* 1988;318:262–264.

84. Peto R, Gray R, Collins R, et al. Randomised trial of prophylactic daily aspirin in British male doctors. *Br J Med* 1988;296:313–316.

85. Hennekens CH, Peto R, Hutchinson GB, Doll R. An overview of the British and American Aspirin Studies. *N Engl J Med* 1988;318:923–924.

86. Lorenz RL, Schacky CV, Weber M, et al. Improved aortocoronary bypass patency by low-dose aspirin (100 mg daily). *Lancet* 1984;1:1261–1264.

87. Goldman S, Copeland J, Moritz T, et al. Improvement in the early saphenous vein graft patency after coronary artery bypass surgery with antiplatelet therapy: results of a Veterans Administration cooperative study. *Circulation* 1988;77:1324–1332.

88. Harter HR, Burch JW, Majerus PW, et al. Prevention of thrombosis in patients on hemodialysis by low-dose aspirin. *N Engl J Med* 1979;301:577–579.

89. Kyrle PA, Eichler HG, Jager U, Lechner K. Inhibition of prostaglandin and thromboxane A_2 generation by low-dose aspirin at the site of plug formation in man in vivo. *Circulation* 1987;75:1025–1029.

90. Levy M. Aspirin use in patients with major upper gastrointestinal bleeding and peptic ulcer disease. *N Engl J Med* 1974;290:1158–1162.

91. Lewis HD, Davis JW, Archibald DG, et al. Protective effects of aspirin against acute myocardial infarction and death in men with unstable angina. *N Engl J Med* 1983;309:396.

92. FitzGerald GA, Reilly IAG, Pedersen AK. The biochemical pharmacology of thromboxane synthase inhibition in man. *Circulation* 1985;72:1194–1201.

93. Fitzgerald DJ, Fragetta J, FitzGerald GA. Prostaglandin endoperoxydes modulate the response to thromboxane synthase inhibition during coronary thrombosis. *J Clin Invest* 1988;82: 1708–1713.

94. Golino P, Ashton JH, Glas-Greenwalt P, Mc-Natt J, Buja LM, Willerson JT. Mediation of reocclusion by thromboxane A$_2$ and serotonin after thrombolysis with tissue-type plasminogen activator in a canine preparation of coronary thrombosis. *Circulation* 1988;77:678–684.

95. Golino P, Ashton JH, McNatt J, et al. Simultaneous administration of thromboxane A$_2$- and serotonin S$_2$-receptor antagonists markedly enhances thrombolysis and prevents or delays reocclusion after tissue-type plasminogen activator in a canine model of coronary thrombosis. *Circulation* 1989;79:911–919.

96. Lam JYT, Chesebro JH, Badimon L, Fuster V. Serotonin and thromboxane A$_2$ receptor blockade decrease vasoconstriction but not platelet deposition after deep arterial injury. *Circulation* 1986;74(suppl):II-97(abstr).

97. Moncada S, Higgs EA. Prostaglandins in the pathogenesis and prevention of vascular disease. *Blood Rev* 1987;1:141–145.

98. Henriksson P, Edajg O, Wennmaln A. Prostacyclin infusion in patients with acute myocardial infarction. *Br Heart J* 1985;53:173–179.

99. Chiariello M, Golino P, Cappelli-Bigazzi M, Ambrosio G, Tritto I, Salvatore M. Reduction in infarct size by the prostacyclin analogue iloprost (ZK 36374) after experimental coronary artery occlusion-reperfusion. *Am Heart J* 1988;115:499–504.

100. Armstrong PW, Langevin LM, Watts DG. Randomized trial of prostacyclin infusion in acute myocardial infarction. *Am J Cardiol* 1988;61:455–457.

101. Malpass TW, Hanson SR, Savage B, Hessel II EA, Harker LA. Prevention of acquired transient defect in platelet plug formation by infused prostacyclin. *Blood* 1981;57:736–740.

102. Turney JH, Williams LC, Fewell MR, Parsons V, Weston MJ. Platelet protection and heparin sparing with prostacyclin during regular dialysis therapy. *Lancet* 1980;2:219–222.

103. FitzGerald GA. Dipyridamole. *N Engl J Med* 1987;316:1247–1257.

104. Hanson SR, Harker LA, Bjornsson TD. Effect of platelet-modifying drugs on arterial thromboembolism in baboons: aspirin potentiates the antithrombotic actions of dipyridamole and sulfinpyrazone by mechanism(s) independent of platelets cyclo-oxygenase inhibition. *J Clin Invest* 1985;75:1591–1599.

105. Sullivan JM, Harken DE, Gorlin R. Pharmacologic control of thromboembolic complications of cardiac-valve replacement. *N Engl J Med* 1971;284:1391–1394.

106. Chesebro JH, Fuster V, Elveback LR, et al. Trial of combined warfarin plus dipyridamole or aspirin therapy in prosthetic heart valve replacement: danger of aspirin compared with dipyridamole. *Am J Cardiol* 1983;51:1537–1541.

107. Maffrand JP, Defreyn G, Bernat A, Delebassee D, Tissinier AM. Reviewed pharmacology of ticlopidine. *Angiologie* 1988;77(suppl):6–13.

108. Saltiel E, Ward A. Ticlopidine. A review of its pharmacodynamic and pharmacokinetic properties, and therapeutic efficacy in platelet-dependent disease states. *Drugs* 1987;34:222–262.

109. Gent M, Blakely JA, Easton JD, et al. The Canadian American ticlopidine study (cats) in thromboembolic stroke. *Lancet* 1989;1:1215–1220.

110. Hass WK, Easton JD, Adams HP, et al. A randomized trial comparing ticlopidine hydrochloride with aspirin for the prevention of stroke in high-risk patients. *N Engl J Med* 1989;321: 501–507.

111. Goodnight SH Jr, Harris WS, Connor WE. The effects of dietary omega-3 fatty acids on platelet composition and function in man: a prospective, controlled study. *Blood* 1981;58:880–885.

112. Dyerberg J, Bang HO, Stoffersen E, Moncada S, Vane JR. Eicosapentanoic acid and prevention of thrombosis and atherosclerosis? *Lancet* 1978;2:117–119.

113. Barcelli U, Glas-Greenwalt P, Pollack VE. Enhancing effect of dietary supplementation with omega-3 fatty acids on plasma fibrinolysis in normal subjects. *Thromb Res* 1985;39:307–312.

114. Popp-Snijders C, Schouten JA, van der Meer J, van der Veen EA. Fatty fish-induced changes in membrane lipid composition and viscosity of human erythrocyte suspensions. *Scand J Clin Lab Invest* 1986;46:253–258.

115. Goodnight SH Jr, Harris WS, Connor WE, Illingworth DR. Polyunsaturated fatty acids, hyperlipidemia, and thrombosis. *Arteriosclerosis* 1982;2:87–113.

116. Lam JYT, Chesebro JH, Badimon L, Badimon JJ, Bowie EJW, Fuster V. Cod liver oil alters the platelet arterial wall response to injury by angioplasty. *Circulation* 1987;76(suppl):IV-601.

117. Weiner BH, Ockene IS, Levine PH, et al. Inhibition of atherosclerosis by cod-liver oil in a hyperlipidemic swine model. *N Engl J Med* 1986;315:841–846.

118. Davis HR, Bridenstine RT, Vesselinovitch D, Wissler RW. Fish oil inhibits development of atherosclerosis in rhesus monkeys. *Arteriosclerosis* 1987;7:441–447.

119. Hollander W, Hong S, Kirkpatrick BJ, Lee A, Colombo M, Prusty S. Differential effects of fish oil supplements on atherosclerosis. *Circulation* 1987;76(suppl):IV-1245.

120. Coller BS, Folts JD, Scudder LE, Smith SR. Antithrombotic effect of a monoclonal antibody to the platelet glycoprotein IIb-IIIa receptor in an experimental animal model. *Blood* 1986;68:783–786.

121. Hanson SR, Pareti FI, Ruggeri ZM, et al. Effects on monoclonal antibodies against the platelet glycoprotein IIb/IIIa complex on thrombosis and hemostasis in the baboon. *J Clin Invest* 1988; 81:149–158.

122. Gold HK, Coller BS, Yasuda T, et al. Rapid and sustained coronary artery recanalization with combined bolus injection of recombinant tissue-type plasminogen activator and monoclonal antiplatelet Gp IIb-IIIa antibody in a canine preparation. *Circulation* 1988;77:670–677.

123. Yasuda T, Gold HK, Fallon JT, et al. Monoclonal antibody against the platelet glycoprotein (Gp) IIb-IIIa receptor prevents coronary artery reocclusion after reperfusion with recombinant tissue-type plasminogen activator in dogs. *J Clin Invest* 1988;81:1284–1291.

124. Torem S, Schneider PA, Hanson SR. Monoclonal antibody-induced inhibition of platelet function: effects on hemostasis and vascular graft thrombosis in baboons. *J Vasc Surg* 1988; 7:172–180.

125. Cadroy Y, Kelly AB, Marzec UM, et al. Effects on hemostasis and thrombosis of monoclonal antibodies against platelet glycoprotein receptors Ib, IIb-IIIa, and against von Willebrand factor in the primate. *Circulation* 1989;80 (suppl):II-24 (abstr.).

126. Bellinger DA, Nichols TC, Read MS, et al. Prevention of occlusive coronary artery thrombosis by a murine monoclonal antibody to porcine von Willebrand Factor. *Proc Natl Acad Sci USA* 1987;84:8100–8104.

127. Badimon L, Badimon JJ, Chesebro JH, Fuster V. Inhibition of thrombus formation: blockage of adhesive glycoprotein mechanisms versus blockage of the cyclooxygenase pathway. *J Am Coll Cardiol* 1988;11:30A (abstr).

128. Cadroy Y, Houghten RA, Hanson SR. RGDV peptide selectively inhibits platelet-dependent thrombus formation in vivo. Studies using a baboon model. *J Clin Invest* 1989;84:939–944.

129. Huang TF, Holt JC, Lukasiewicz H, Niewiarowski S. Trigramin. A low molecular weight peptide inhibiting fibrinogen interaction with platelet receptors expressed on glycoprotein IIb-IIIa complex. *J Biol Chem* 1987;262:16157–16163.

130. Gan ZR, Gould RJ, Jacobs JW, Friedman PA, Polokoff MA. Echistatin. A potent platelet aggregation inhibitor from the venom of the viper, Echis Carinatus. *J Biol Chem* 1988;263: 19827–19832.

131. Cook JJ, Huang TF, Rucinski B, Tuma RF, Williams JA, Niewiarowski S. Inhibition of platelet hemostatic plug formation by Trigramin, a novel RGD containing peptide. *Circulation* 1988;78(suppl):II-313 (abstr).

132. Hirsh J. Mechanism of action and monitoring of anticoagulants. *Semin Thromb Hemost* 1986;12:1–11.

133. Moelker HCT. Heparins and platelet function. *Prog Pharmacol* 1982;44:99–133.

134. Simon TL, Hyers TM, Gaston JP, Harker LA. Heparin pharmacokinetics: increased require-

ments in pulmonary embolism. *Br J Haematol* 1978;39:111–120.

135. Hirsch J, van Aken WG, Gallus AS, Dollery CT, Cade JF, Yung WL. Heparin kinetics in venous thrombosis and pulmonary embolism. *Circulation* 1976;53:691–695.

136. Basu D, Gallus A, Hirsh J, Cade J. A prospective study of the value of monitoring heparin treatment with the activated partial thromboplastin time. *N Engl J Med* 1972;287:324–327.

137. King DJ, Kelton JG. Heparin-associated thrombocytopenia. *Ann Intern Med* 1984;100:536–540.

138. Collins R, Scrimgeour A, Yusuf S, Peto R. Reduction in fetal pulmonary embolism and venous thrombosis by perioperative administration of subcutaneous heparin. *N Engl J Med* 1988;318:1162–1173.

139. Leyvraz PF, Richard J, Bachman F, et al. Adjusted versus fixed-dose subcutaneous heparin in the prevention of deep-vein thrombosis after total hip replacement. *N Engl J Med* 1983; 309:954–958.

140. Salzman EW, Deykin D, Shapiro RM, Rosenberg R. Management of heparin therapy: controlled prospective trial. *N Engl J Med* 1975; 292:1046–1050.

141. Glazier RL, Crowell EB. Randomized prospective trial of continuous versus intermittent heparin therapy. *JAMA* 1976;236:1365–1367.

142. Wilson JR, Lampman J. Heparin therapy: a randomized prospective study. *Am Heart J* 1979;97:155–158.

143. Hull R, Raskob G, Hirsh J, et al. Continuous intravenous heparin compared with intermittent subcutaneous heparin in the initial treatment of proximal-vein thrombosis. *N Engl J Med* 1986;315:1109–1114.

144. Doyle DJ, Turpie AGG, Hirsh J, et al. Adjusted subcutaneous heparin or continuous intravenous heparin in patients with acute deep vein thrombosis. *Ann Intern Med* 1987;107:441–445.

145. Turpie AGG, Robinson JG, Doyle DJ, et al. Comparison of high-dose with low-dose subcutaneous heparin to prevent left ventricular mural thrombosis in patients with acute transmural anterior myocardial infarction. *N Engl J Med* 1989;320:352–357.

146. Cadroy Y, Harker LA, Hanson SR. Inhibition of platelet-dependent thrombosis by low molecular weight heparin (CY222): comparison with standard heparin *J Lab Clin Med* 1989; 114:349–357.

147. Heras M, Chesebro JH, Penny WJ, et al. The importance of adequate heparin dosage in arterial angioplasty in a porcine model. *Circulation* 1988;78:654–660.

148. Theroux P, Ouimet H, McCans J, et al. Aspirin, heparin, or both to treat acute unstable angina. *N Engl J Med* 1988;319:1105–1111.

149. Castellot JJ Jr, Cochran DL, Karnovsky MJ. Effect of heparin on vascular smooth muscle cells. 1: Cell metabolism. *J Physiol* 1984;124: 21–29.

150. Hirsh J, Ofosu FA, Levine M. The develop-

ment of low molecular weight heparins for clinical use. In: Verstraete M, Vermylen J, Lijnen R, Arnout J, eds. *Thrombosis and haemostasis 1987*. Leuven: Leuven University Press, 1987; 325–348.

151. Samama M, Boissel JP, Combe-Tamzali S, Leizorovicz A. Clinical studies with low molecular weight heparins in the prevention and treatment of venous thromboembolism. *Ann NY Acad Sci (in press)*.

152. Boneu B, Caranobe C, Cadroy Y. Pharmacokinetic studies of standard unfractionated heparin, low molecular weight heparins in the rabbit. *Semin Thromb Hemost* 1988;14:18–27.

153. Deykin D. Warfarin therapy. *N Engl J Med* 1970;283:691–694.

154. Deykin D. Warfarin therapy. *N Engl J Med* 1970;283:801–803.

155. Kelly JG, O'Malley K. Clinical pharmacokinetics of oral anticoagulants. *Clin Pharmacokinet* 1979;4:1–15.

156. Poller L. Laboratory control of anticoagulant therapy. *Semin Thromb Hemost* 1986;12:13–19.

157. Hirsh J, Poller L, Deykin D, Levine M, Dalen JE. Optimal therapeutic range for oral anticoagulants. *Chest* 1989;95(suppl):5S–11S.

158. Bagdy D, Barbas E, Graf L, Petersen TE, Magnusson S. Hirudin. *Methods Enzymol* 1976; 45:669–678.

159. Markwardt F, Fink E, Kaiser B, et al. Pharmacological survey of recombinant hirudin. *Pharmazie* 1988;43:202–207.

160. Kelly AB, Hanson SR, Marzec U, Harker LA. Recombinant hirudin (r-H) interruption of platelet-dependent thrombus formation. *Circulation* 1988;78(suppl)II:1242 (abstr).

161. Heras M, Chesebro JH, Penny WJ, Bailey KR, Badimon L, Fuster V. Effects of thrombin inhibition on the development of acute platelet-thrombus deposition during angioplasty in pigs. Heparin versus recombinant hirudin, a specific thrombin inhibitor. *Circulation* 1989;79: 657–665.

162. Hanson SR, Harker LA. Interruption of acute platelet-dependent thrombosis by the synthetic antithrombin D-phenylalanyl-L-prolyl-L-arginyl chloromethylketone. *Proc Natl Acad Sci USA* 1988;85:3184–3188.

163. Cadroy Y, Maraganore JM, Hanson SR, Harker LA. Antithrombotic effects of a synthetic hirudin peptide in baboons (*submitted*).

164. Gruber A, Griffin JH, Harker LA, Hanson SR. Inhibition of platelet-dependent thrombus formation by human activated protein C in a primate model. *Blood* 1989;73:639–642.

165. Gruber A, Hanson SR, Kelly AB, et al. Recombinant activated protein C (r-apC) inhibition of platelet-dependent thrombosis. *Circulation* 1988;78(suppl)II:1250.

166. Tollefsen DM, Pestka CA, Monafo WJ. Activation of heparin cofactor II by dermatan sulfate. *J Biol Chem* 1983;258:6713–6716.

167. Fernandez F, van Ryn J, Ofosu F, Hirsh J, Buchanan MR. The haemorrhagic and antithrombotic effects of dermatan sulphate. *Br J Haematol* 1986;64:309–317.

168. Cadroy Y, Dol F, Caranobe C, et al. Standard heparin enhances the antithrombotic activity of dermatan sulfate in the rabbit but CY216 does not. *Thromb Haemost* 1988;59:295–298.

169. Jang I, Gold HK, Ziskind AA, et al. Differential sensitivity of erythrocyte-rich and platelet-rich arterial thrombi to lysis with recombinant tissue-type plasminogen activator. A possible explanation for resistance to coronary thrombolysis. *Circulation* 1989;79:920–928.

170. Marder VJ, Sherry S. Thrombolytic therapy: current status (first of two parts). *N Engl J Med* 1988;318:1512–1520.

171. Marder VJ, Sherry S. Thrombolytic therapy: current status (second of two parts). *N Engl J Med* 1988;318:1585–1595.

172. Gimple LW, Gold HK, Leinbach RC, Yasuda T, Johns JA, Ziskind AA, Collen D. Bleeding time measurement predicts spontaneous bleeding during thrombolysis with recombinant tissue-type plasminogen activator (rt-PA). *J Am Coll Cardiol* 1988;11:231A (abstr).

173. McClintock DK, Bell PH. The mechanism of activation of human plasminogen by streptokinase. *Biochem Biophys Res Commun* 1971;43: 694–702.

174. Rajagopalan S, Gonias SL, Pizzo SV. A nonantigenic covalent streptokinase-polyethylene glycol complex with plasminogen activator function. *J Clin Invest* 1985;75:413–419.

175. Smith RAG, Dupe RJ, English PD, Green J. Fibrinolysis with acyl-enzymes: a new approach to thrombolytic therapy. *Nature* 1981;290:505–508.

176. Smith RAG, Dupe RJ, English PD, Green J. Acyl-enzymes as thrombolytic agents in rabbit model of venous thrombosis. *Thromb Haemost* 1982;47:269–274.

177. Mueller HS, Rao AK, Forman SA, and the TIMI investigators. Thrombolysis in myocardial infarction (TIMI): comparative studies of coronary reperfusion and systemic fibrinogenolysis with two forms of recombinant tissue-type plasminogen activator. *J Am Coll Cardiol* 1987;10:479–490.

178. Loscalzo J, Wharton TP, Kirshenbaum JM, et al., and the Pro-urokinase for Myocardial Infarction Study Group. Clot-selective coronary thrombolysis with pro-urokinase. *Circulation* 1989;70:776–782.

179. Gurewich V, Pannell R, Louie S, Kelley P, Suddith RL, Greenlee R. Effective and fibrin-specific clot lysis by a zymogen precursor form of urokinase (pro-urokinase). A study in vitro and in two animal species. *J Clin Invest* 1984;73:1731–1739.

180. Collen D, Stassen JM, Blaber M, Winkler M, Verstraete M. Biological and thrombolytic properties of proenzyme and active forms of human urokinase-III. Thrombolytic properties of natural and recombinant urokinase in rabbits with experimental jugular vein thrombosis. *Thromb Haemost* 1984;52:27–30.

181. Ziskind AA, Gold HK, Yasuda T, et al. Synergistic combinations of recombinant human tissue-type plasminogen activator and human single-chain urokinase-type plasminogen activator. Effect on thrombolysis and reocclusion in a canine coronary artery thrombosis model with high-grade stenosis. *Circulation* 1989; 79:393–399.

182. Collen D, Stassen JM, De Cock F. Synergistic effect on thrombolysis of sequential infusion of tissue-type plasminogen activator (t-PA) single-chain urokinase-type plasminogen activator (scu-PA) and urokinase in the rabbit jugular vein thrombosis model. *Thromb Haemost* 1987; 58:943–946.

183. Pannell R, Black J, Gurewich V. Complementary modes of action of tissue-type plasminogen activator and pro-urokinase by which their synergistic effect on clot lysis may be explained. *J Clin Invest* 1988;81:853–859.

184. Collen D, Stump DC, van de Werf F. Coronary thrombolysis in patients with acute myocardial infarction by intravenous infusion of synergic thrombolytic agents. *Am Heart J* 1986;112: 1083–1084.

185. Collen D. Synergism of thrombolytic agents: investigational procedures and clinical potential. *Circulation* 1988;77:731–735.

186. Nelles L, Lijnen HR, Collen D, Holmes WE. Characterization of a fusion protein consisting of amino acids 1 to 263 of tissue-type plasminogen activator and amino acids 144 to 411 of urokinase-type plasminogen activator. *J Biol Chem* 1987;262:10855–10862.

187. Robbins KC, Tanaka Y. Covalent molecular weight—92,000 hybrid plasminogen activator derived from human plasmin amino-terminal and urokinase carboxyl-terminal domains. *Biochemistry* 1986;25:3603–3611.

188. Robbins KC, Boreisha IG. A covalent molecular weight—92,000 hybrid plasminogen activator derived from human plasmin fibrin-binding and tissue plasminogen activator catalytic domains. *Biochemistry* 1987;26:4661–4667.

189. Collen D, Stassen JM, Larsen G. Pharmacokinetics and thrombolytic properties of deletion mutants of human tissue-type plasminogen activator in rabbits. *Blood* 1988;71:216–219.

190. Nelles L, Lijnen HR, Collen D, Holmes WE. Characterization of recombinant human single chain urokinase-type plasminogen activator mutants produced by site specific mutagenesis of lysine 158. *J Biol Chem* 1987;262:5682–5689.

191. Runge MS, Quertermous T, Matsueda GR, Haber E. Increasing selectivity of plasminogen activators with antibodies. *Clin Res* 1988;36:501–506.

192. Sobel BE, Fields LE, Robison AK, Fox KAA, Sarnoff SJ. Coronary thrombolysis with facilitated absorption of intramuscularly injected tissue-type plasminogen activator. *Proc Natl Acad Sci USA* 1985;82:4258–4262.

193. Sobel BE, Saffitz JE, Fields LE, et al. Intramuscular administration to tissue-type plasminogen activator in rabbits and dogs and its implication for coronary thrombolysis. *Circulation* 1987;75:1261–1272.

194. DeWood MA, Spores J, Notske R, et al. Prevalence of total coronary occlusion during the early hours of transmural myocardial infarction. *N Engl J Med* 1980;303:897–902.

195. Khaja F, Walton JA, Brymer JF, et al. Intracoronary fibrinolytic therapy in acute myocardial infarction. Report of a prospective randomized trial. *N Engl J Med* 1983;308:1305–1311.

196. Leiboff RH, Katz RJ, Wasserman AG. A randomized angiographically controlled trial of intracoronary streptokinase in acute myocardial infarction. *Am J Cardiol* 1984;53:404–407.

197. Rentrop KP, Feit F, Blanke H, et al. Effects of intracoronary streptokinase and intracoronary nitroglycerin infusion on coronary angiographic patterns and mortality in patients with acute myocardial infarction. *N Engl J Med* 1984;311:1457–1463.

198. Tiefenbrunn AJ, Sobel BE. The impact of coronary thrombolysis on myocardial infarction. *Fibrinolysis* 1989;3:1–15.

199. Gruppo Italiano per lo Studio Della Streptochi-Nasi Nell'Infarto Miocardico (GISSI). Long-term effects of intravenous thrombolysis in acute myocardial infarction: final report of the GISSI study. *Lancet* 1987;2:871–874.

200. ISIS-2 (Second International Study of Infarct Survival). Collaborative Group 1988. Randomised trial of intravenous streptokinase, oral aspirin, both, or neither among 17,187 cases of suspected acute myocardial infarction: ISIS-2. *Lancet* 1988;2:349–360.

201. Kennedy JW, Ritchie JL, Davis KB, Stadius ML, Maynard C, Fritz JK. The Western Washington randomized trial of intracoronary streptokinase in acute myocardial infarction. A 12 month follow-up report. *N Engl J Med* 1985; 312:1073–1078.

202. White HD, Rivers JT, Maslowski AH, et al. Effective of intravenous streptokinase as compared with that of tissue plasminogen activator on left ventricular function after first myocardial infarction. *N Engl J Med* 1989;320:817–821.

203. Harrison DG, Ferguson DW, Collins SM, et al. Rethrombosis after reperfusion with streptokinase: importance of geometry of residual lesions. *Circulation* 1984;69:991–999.

204. Topol EJ, Califf RM, Georges BS, et al. and the Thrombolysis and Angioplasty in Myocardial Infarction (TAMI) Study Group. A multicenter randomized trial of intravenous recombinant tissue plasminogen activator and immediate angioplasty in acute myocardial infarction. *N Engl J Med* 1987;317:581–588.

205. Simoons ML, Arnold AER, Betriu A, et al. for the European Cooperative Study Group for Recombinant Tissue-Type Plasminogen Activator (rt-PA). Thrombolysis with tissue plasminogen activator in acute myocardial infarction: no additional benefit from immediate percutaneous coronary angioplasty. *Lancet* 1988;1:197–202.

206. The TIMI Study Group. Comparison of inva-

sive and conservative strategies after treatment with intravenous tissue plasminogen activator in acute myocardial infarction. Results of the Thrombolysis in Myocardial Infarction (TIMI) Phase II Trial. *N Engl J Med* 1989;320:618–627.

207. Vaughan DE, Plavin SR, Schafer AI, Loscalzo J. Prostaglandin E₁ markedly accelerates thrombolysis by tissue plasminogen activator. *Blood* (*in press*).

208. Williams DO, Borer J, Braunwald E, et al. Intravenous recombinant tissue type plasminogen activator in patients with acute myocardial infarction: a report from the NHLBI thrombolysis in myocardial infarction trial. *Circulation* 1986;73:338–346.

209. Topol EJ, George BS, Kereiakes DJ, et al. and the TAMI Study Group. A randomized controlled trial of intravenous tissue plasminogen activator and early intravenous heparin in acute myocardial infarction. *Circulation* 1989; 79:281–286.

210. Sherman CT, Litvack F, Grundfest W, et al. Coronary angioscopy in patients with unstable angina pectoris. *N Engl J Med* 1986;315: 913–919.

211. Gold HK, Johns JA, Leinbach RC, et al. A randomized, blinded, placebo-controlled trial of recombinant human tissue-type plasminogen

activator in patients with unstable angina pectoris. *Circulation* 1987;75:1192–1199.

212. Nicklas JM, Topol EJ, Kander N, Walton JA, Gorman L, Pitt B. Randomized double-blind placebo-controlled trial of rt-PA in unstable angina. *Circulation* 1987;76(suppl)IV;1212 (abstr).

213. Ambrose JA, Hjemdahl-Monsen C, Burrico S, et al. Quantitative and qualitative effects of intracoronary streptokinase in unstable angina and non-O wave infarction. *J Am Coll Cardiol* 1987;9:1156–1165.

214. Del Zoppo GJ, Zeumer H, Harker LA. Thrombolytic therapy in acute stroke: possibilities and hazards. *Stroke* 1986;17:595–607.

215. Del Zoppo GJ, Ferbert A, Otis S, et al. Local intraarterial fibrinolytic therapy in acute carotid territory stroke: a pilot study. *Stroke* 1988;19:307–313.

216. Hacke W, Zeumer H, Ferbert A, Bruckmann H, Del Zoppo CJ. Intraarterial fibrinolytic therapy improves outcome in patients with acute vertebrobasilar occlusive disease. *Stroke* 1988;19:1216–1222.

217. Goldhaber SZ, Burning JE, Lipnick RJ, Hennekers CM. Pooled analyses of randomized trials of streptokinase and heparin in phlebographically documented acute deep vein thrombosis. *Am J Med* 1984;76:393–397.

Subject Index

A

A23187, 92
A64662, 217–218
Acebutolol, 446
    action mechanisms, 321
    pharmacokinetics, 452
    as selective β_1-blocker, 63
Acetylcholine
    adenosine triphosphate interaction, 3
    autonomic regulatory function, 190
    as cotransmitter, 232,251,257
    enkephalin interaction, 3
    endothelium-dependent relaxing factor
        interaction, 90–92,93,271
    as excitatory transmitter, 6
    location, 234
    morphine interaction, 3,268
    muscarinic autoreceptor effects, 251
    norepinephrine interaction, 4,254–255,256
    as nucleus tractus solitarius neurotransmitter,
        181
    parasympathetic nervous system release, 2–3
    prostaglandin interaction, 3
    sympathetic nervous system release, 2–3,
        230–231
    sympathetic stimulation effects, 4–5
    vasoactive intestinal peptide interaction, 239
Acetylcholine esterase, 2
AcetylCoA, 297
N-Acetylcysteine, 316
N-Acetylprocainamide, 402–403,404
N-Acetyltransferase, 402
Actin, 11,78,323
Action potentials
    normal cardiac, 369–371
    of vascular muscular smooth muscle, 11
Acylcarnitine, 114
AcylCoA, 114
AcylCoA-carnitine transferase system, 297
AcylCoA-cholesterol-acyl-transferase, 502
AcylCoA-fatty acid, 297
Adenosine
    coronary blood flow effects, 309–310
    as endothelium-dependent vasodilator, 93
    norepinephrine interaction, 4
    transjunctional modulatory action, 260–262
Adenosine diphosphate (ADP)
    as endothelium-dependent vasodilator, 93
    in myocardial metabolism, 297,298,299
    platelet effects, 515,517
Adenosine monophosphate (AMP), in myocardial
        metabolism, 297,298,299
Adenosine monophosphate, cyclic (cAMP)
    β-adrenergic agonist interaction, 324
    as endothelium-dependent vasodilator, 93

    formation, 9
    G-protein interaction, 345
    platelet, 524
    as second messenger, 84–86,87–88,116
Adenosine triphosphatase (ATPase), 323,345
Adenosine triphosphate (ATP)
    as cotransmitter, 231–232,236–237
        automodulation, 245–246
        cholinergic, 239
    endothelium-dependent relaxing factor
        interaction, 258
    as endothelium-dependent vasodilator, 93
    excitatory junction potential effects, 237,257
    intracellular calcium and, 112,114
    in ischemia, 330
    in myocardial metabolism, 297,298,299
    noradrenergic-regulated release, 245
    as purinergic inhibitor, 10
    in systolic heart failure, 345
    vasoconstriction action, 258
    vasodilation action, 93,258
        indirect, 236–237
Adenyl compounds, neuroeffector transmission
        effects, 261–262,269–270
Adrenal medulla, 6,30
Adrenergic nerves, 3–6
    autonomic control and, 15–16
    transmission mechanisms, 5–6
Adrenergic receptor, 8,9
Adrenergic receptor antagonists, 54
α-Adrenergic receptor
    classification, 39–44,319
    prejunctional, 242–244
α-Adrenergic receptor agonists, sympathetic
        nervous system effects, 185–189
α-Adrenergic receptor antagonists
    antihypertensive effects, 55–60
    sympathetic nervous system effects, 185–189
α_1-Adrenergic receptor
    activation, 9
    automodulatory function, 243
    calcium channel antagonist interaction, 130
    distribution, 43–44
    postsynaptic, 42,43
    presynaptic, 41
α_1-Adrenergic receptor agonists, 40–41
α_1-Adrenergic receptor antagonists, 40–41
    sympathetic nervous system effects, 173,
        185–186
α_2-Adrenergic receptor
    clonidine interaction, 185,186
    distribution, 43–44,242,243
    postjunctional, 43,244–245
α_2-Adrenergic receptor agonists, 40–41
    as antihypertensive agents, 44–53

α_2-Adrenergic receptor antagonists, 40–41
β-Adrenergic receptor
  angiotensin II synthesis effects, 266
  cholinergic neuroeffector transmission and,
    255–256
  classification, 39–44,319
  class II antiarrhythmic drug blockage, 378–379
  in congestive heart failure, 348–349
  prejunctional, 249–251
  renin interaction, 204
β-Adrenergic receptor agonists
  antihypertensive actions, 60–68
    action mechanisms, 60–63
    adverse effects, 64–66
    ancillary properties, 63–64
    therapeutic use, 66–67
    withdrawal syndrome, 66
  cyclic nucleotide interaction, 84
β-Adrenergic receptor antagonists, 326,446
  action mechanisms, 319–323
  adverse effects, 322–323
  antiarrhythmic actions, 385,391
  as calmodulin inhibitor, 83
  as congestive heart failure therapy, 349,357–358
  as ischemic heart disease therapy, 319–323
  as left ventricular diastolic dysfunction therapy,
    344
  myocardial contractility and, 299–301
β_1-Adrenergic receptor, distribution, 43–44
β_1-Adrenergic receptor agonists, 41,42
β_1-Adrenergic receptor antagonists, 41
β_2-Adrenergic receptor
  distribution, 43–44
  postsynaptic, 42–43
  presynaptic, 40,41
β_2-Adrenoreceptor agonists, 41,42
β_2-Adrenoreceptor antagonists, 41
Ajmaline, 390,391
Alacepril, 219
Aldosterone
  atrial natriuretic factor interaction, 352
  plasma volume effects, 26
  renin release and, 204
  sodium-retaining properties, 206–207
Aldosteronism, secondary, 356
Alkaloids
  rauwolfian, 54–55
  veratrum, 29
Alkyxanthines, 310
Amine cotransmitters, 234–236
γ-Aminobutyric acid
  autonomic regulatory function, 190,191
  medullary depressor response effects, 174–175
  as nucleus tractus solitarius neurotransmitter
    inhibitor, 181–182
  sympathetic neuron effects, 178,183–184
  transneuronal modulatory activity, 257
Aminoglycosides, 118
Amiodarone
  adverse effects, 464–465,466
  antiarrhythmic action, 385–386,390–391,
    461–466
  drug interaction, 325
  electrophysiologic actions, 379,380

Amlodipine
  action sites/mechanisms, 123,129,145,146
  structure, 123,144
Amphetamines, 5
Amrinone, 354,355
Anaphylaxis, slow-reacting substances of, 18
Angina
  exertional, 314–315,320,324
  myocardial oxygenation and, 293
  therapy, 316–328
    β-adrenergic blocking agents, 319–323
    antithrombotic therapy, 326–328
    calcium channel antagonists,
      134–135,142,323–325
    nitrates, 316–319
Angiotensin
  antagonists, 222–223
  autonomic regulatory function, 184–185, 190
  definition, 201
Angiotensin-converting enzyme, 201,208,209
  blood pressure effects, 218–219,221–222
  localization, 201
  synthesis, 265
Angiotensin-converting enzyme inhibitors,
    201,203,218,219–222,264
  angiotensin-II interaction, 68–69
  as congestive heart failure therapy, 361–362
  hemodynamic effects, 221–222
  as left ventricular diastolic dysfunction therapy,
    344
  substrates, 218
  sympathetic nervous system effects, 37
Angiotensin I
  congestive heart failure and, 349,350
  formation, 17,201,349,350
  inhibition, 218,266
Angiotensin II, 207,208
  cardiovascular effects, 10,263–267,351
  congestive heart failure and, 349,350
  formation, 17,201,202,349,350
  hypertensinogenic effect, 206–207
  noradrenergic neuroeffector transmission
    effects, 263–267
  norepinephrine interaction, 4,264,266–267
  prostaglandin interaction, 264
  renin antibody interaction, 210
  renin release and, 204–205
  sympathetic nervous system effects, 263
Angiotensinogen, 201,207,210
Angiotonin, 201
Anipamil, 144,145,147
Antianginal agents
  action mechanisms, 316–328
    antithrombotic therapy, 326–328
    β-adrenergic blocking agents, 319–323
    calcium channel blocking agents,
      134–135,323–325
    nitrates, 316–319
    thrombolytic therapy, 326–328
Antiarrhythmic drugs. *See also* specific
    antiarrhythmic drugs
  as calmodulin inhibitors, 83
  class I, 369,377
    action mechanisms, 377–378

class II, 369,377
   action mechanisms, 378–379
class III, 369,377
   action mechanisms, 379–380
class IV, 369,377
   action mechanisms, 380–381
electropharmacology, 377–391
Anticoagulants, 515,526–529
Antidepressants
   as calmodulin inhibitors, 83
   tricyclic, 46–47,53
Antidiarrheal opiates, 125
Antidiuretic hormone. *See* Vasopressin
Antihypertensive agents, 369–483. *See also*
      Vasodilators; specific antihypertensive
      agents
   centrally acting, 185–189
   α-adrenoreceptor interaction, 45–46
   classification, 369
   sympathetic nervous system effects, 37–73
   as α_2-adrenoceptor agonists, 44–53
   neuronal pathways, 38–39
   vascular contractile protein effects, 81–84
α_2-Antiplasmin, 522
Antiplatelet therapy, 515,522–526
Antithrombin III, 526
Antithrombin III-heparin, 515,518
Antithrombotic therapy, 326–328,522–532
   anticoagulants, 526–529
   antiplatelet therapy, 522–526
   fibrinolytic therapy, 529–532
α_1-Antitrypsin, 516
Apolipoproteins
   AI, 486,487
      fibrate effects, 502
      high-density lipoprotein metabolism and, 489
      primary hypoalphalipoproteinemia and, 494
   AII, 486,487,489
   AIV, 486,487
   B, 486,487
      fibrate effects, 500,502
      hydroxymethyl-glutaryl CoA reductase
         inhibitor effects, 505
      hypercholesterolemia and, 492
      probucol effects, 506
   characteristics, 487
   CII, 486,487,488,489
   CIII, 486,487,488,489
   E, 486–487,488,489,491
Arachidonic acid, 17–18,114
Arginine vasopressin
   atrial natriuretic factor interaction, 352
   autonomic regulatory function, 190
   congestive heart failure and, 346–347,349,
      350–351
   as nucleus tractus solitarius neurotransmitter,
      182
   sympathetic preganglionic neuron effects,
      178–179
   sympathoinhibitory effects, 185
Arginine vasotocin, 350
Arrhythmia. *See also* Antiarrhythmic drugs;
      Bradycardia, Tachycardia
   calcium channel antagonist therapy, 135

in congestive heart failure, 349,361
electrophysiologic mechanisms, 371–377
   abnormal conductance, 374–377
   ectopic impulse formation, 371–374
Arteriography, coronary, 294
Aspartyl protease, 202
Aspirin
   as angina therapy, 328
   antiplatelet effects, 326
   an antithrombotic agent, 523,531
   as myocardial infarction therapy, 328
   for rethrombosis prevention, 328
Atenolol, 446
   action mechanisms, 321
   as angina therapy, 326
   as lipophilic drug, 61
   pharmacokinetics, 452
   as selective β-blocker, 63
Atherosclerosis, 310–315
   bile acid sequestrant resin therapy, 497–498
   calcium channel antagonist therapy, 137–138
   chylomicron metabolism and, 487
   hydroxymethyl-glutaryl CoA reductase
      inhibitor therapy, 506
   hyperlipidemia and, 485
   niacin therapy, 500
   platelets and, 517
   premature, 492
Atrial flutter, 382,397–398,405
Atrial muscle fiber, as fast-response fiber,
      369–370
Atrial natriuretic factor
   calcium interaction, 77
   in congestive heart failure, 347,351–352
   guanylate cyclase interaction, 85
   vasodilator actions, 92–93
Atriopeptins, 85
Atrioventricular node
   drug effects
      amiodarone, 462
      bretylium, 456
      encainide, 431
      flecainide, 436,438,439
      lidocaine, 411
      mexiletine, 426
      phenytoin, 417–418
      procainamide, 400
      propafenone, 441,443
      propranolol, 444,447,450,453
      quinidine, 393–394
      tocainide, 422,423,424
      verapamil, 468,469,470,471,472–473
   slow-response fibers, 371
   in supraventricular arrhythmia, 381,382–391
Atropine, 7,8
Autonomic nervous system
   activation, 6
   anatomy, 1–2
   cardiac innervation, 24–25
   cardiovascular function effects, 1–10
   neuroeffector transmission modulation. *See*
      Neuroeffector transmission
   peripheral blood flow control, 15–17
Azacyclotridecan-2-imine, 125

B

Bainbridge reflex, 28
Barbiturates, 125
Baroreceptors, 27–28
    afferent nerves, 26
        neurotransmitters, 179–181
    in congestive heart failure, 348
    intrarenal, 204
    location, 163–164
    of nucleus tractus solitarius, 181–184
Bay K 8644, 92
Benzodiazepines, 83,125
Bepridil, 83
Bezafibrate, 500,501,502
Bezold-Jarisch reflex, 29
Bile acid, abnormal metabolism, 490
Bile acid sequestrant resins, 495–498
Bisoprolol, 63
Blood-brain barrier, 15
Blood flow
    in atherosclerosis, 311,313
    coronary, 25
        endothelium and, 301–303
        endothelium-dependent relaxing factor and,
            302,303–305
        neural control, 26–29
    peripheral, 10–19
        autonomic control, 15–17
        autoregulation, 14–15
        vascular beds, 12–15
Blood pressure
    angiotensin-converting enzyme and, 218–219,
        221–222
    central neurotransmitters and, 161–199
    renin-angiotensin system and, 201,202,205–207
Blood vessels, characteristics, 12–13
Blood volume, 25–26
Botulism toxin, 3
Bradycardia
    clonidine and, 48
    neuropeptide Y and, 256
Bradykinin, 92,269
Brain, blood flow, 14,15
Bretylium, 54
    adverse effects, 458,460
    antiarrhythmic actions, 455–461
    electrophysiologic actions, 379–380
    norepinephrine interaction, 5
BRL 36878, 220
Bryostatin, 89
Bumetanide, 353
Butyrophenone, 83
BW A575C, 222

C

Calciosome, 111
Calcitonin, 110
Calcitonin gene-related peptide, 92,232,260
Calcitriol. *See* Vitamin D
Calcium
    cardiovascular effects, 323–324
        cellular excitability, 108–109
        contractility, 11–12
    depolarization, 19
    endothelium-dependent relaxing factor and,
        92
    heart failure, 345
    neurotransmitter release, 241
    platelet activation, 517
    renin release, 205
    sympathetic vesicle effects, 4
    vascular smooth muscle cell membrane
        regulation, 75–78
    cytoplasmic concentration, 323–324
    regulation, 108–115
        absorption, 108–109
        deposition, 108–109
        excretion, 108–109
        at intracellular surfaces, 111–112,113,114
        metabolism, 112–113
        at plasmalemma level, 110–111,112
Calcium antagonists, 107–160
    action mechanisms, 127–130
        at noncalcium channel systems, 130–131
        selectivity, 131–134
    action sites, 122–127
    α-adrenoceptor interaction, 68
    classification, 120–122
    inactivity, 83
    neuropeptide Y interaction 238
    sales of, 107
    second-generation, 107
    therapeutic applications, 107,108,134–138
        angina, 134–135,142
        atherosclerosis, 137–138
        cardiac arrhythmia, 135
        cardiomyopathy, 137
        cerebral vascular disorders, 136–137
        congestive heart failure, 137,361
        contraindications, 140–141
        drug interactions, 141–142
        hypertension, 135–136
        ischemic heart disease, 323–325
        left ventricular diastolic dysfunction, 344
        peripheral disorders, 137
        pharmacologic considerations, 138–140
        side effects, 140–141
    third-generation, 107
    vasodilator properties, 96
    withdrawal, 143
Calcium-ATPase, calmodulin-dependent, 111,112
Calcium binding proteins, 108–109
Calcium blockers, *See* Calcium antagonists
Calcium channel antagonists. *See* Calcium
        antagonists
Calcium channels, 115–120
    classification, 116–118
    G proteins and, 116,118,119,120,129–130
    intracellular, 115–116
    plasmalemmal, 115–116
    regulation, 142–144
    in disease, 143–144
Calcium paradox, 113–115
Caldesmon, 78,81
Calmidazolium, 83
Calmodulin, 78,86,109
Calmodulin antagonists, 82–84

Captopril
  angiotensin II interaction, 68–69
  as chronic heart failure therapy, 355
  as congestive heart failure therapy, 359–360,361
  structure, 219
Cardiac cells, normal action potentials, 369–371
Cardiac output, 23–24
Cardiomyopathy, calcium channel regulation and, 137,143–144
Catalase, 329
Catecholamines
  adrenal release, 6
  as arrhythmia cause, 378
  blood pressure effects, 186
  clonidine interaction, 185–186
  in congestive heart failure, 349
  myocardial contractility and, 299
  renin release and, 204
  sympathetic vesicle uptake, 3–4
Catechol-*o*-methyl transferase, 6
Cathepsin D, 266
Cell death, calcium-related, 113–114
Cerebral vascular disorders, therapy, 136–137
CGS 13928, 220
CGS 14824-A, 220
CGS 16617, 220
Chemoreceptors, 28–29
Chlorisondamine, 53
Cholesterol, 486,489. *See also* Lipoproteins
Cholesteryl ester, 485,502
Cholesteryl ester transfer protein, 489
Cholestyramine, 495–498
Choline acetyltransferase, 2,92
Cholinergic neurons, 16–17
  neuroeffector transmission
    automodulation, 251
    cotransmitters, 239–240
    false transmitters, 231
    noradrenergic modulation, 255–256
    purinergic transmission effects, 257
Cholinergic receptor, 7–9
  muscarinic, 7,9,253–255,257
  nicotinic, 7
Chromakalim, 95
Chromogranin, 5,6
Chylomicron
  atherosclerosis and, 487
  function, 486,487
  hypertriglyceridemia and, 489,490
  triglyceride content, 485
CI-925, 220
Cilazapril, 220
Cimetidine, 442
Cinchonism, 396
Cinnarizine, 83
Cirazoline, 41
CL 242,817, 219
Clofibrate, 500–501,503
Clonidine
  antihypertensive action, 45,46,48–50,51,52,53
  central nervous system effects, 38,185
  norepinephrine inhibitory effects, 243–244
  sympathetic preganglionic neuron effects, 173
  withdrawal syndrome, 52–53

Clopimozide, 125
Cocaine, 5,46–47
Colestipol, 495–497,498
Collagen, platelet activation and, 517
Compactin. *See* Nevastatin
Congestive heart failure, 341–367
  acute heart failure, 353–355
  β-adrenergic receptors, 345
  chronic heart failure, 355,357
  couterregulatory adaptive mechanisms, 351–353
  diastolic dysfunction, 341–344
  excitation-contraction coupling, 345
  exercise response, 348
  incidence, 341
  loading conditions, 345–346
  myocardial contractility and, 345
  myocardial oxygen demand and, 314
  neuroendocrine abnormalities, 346–347
  precursors, 341
  renin-angiotensin-aldosterone system and, 202,346–347,349–351
  sodium retention in, 346–347,348,349
  sympathetic nervous system and, 347–349
  systolic dysfunction, 344–345
  treatment
    β-adrenergic blockers, 357–358
    angiotensin-converting enzyme inhibitors, 361–362
    calcium channel antagonists, 137
    digitalis, 356
    diuretics, 355–356
    inotropic agents, 357
    nitrates, 360
    nitric oxide inducers, 360
    nitroglycerin, 318
    partial β-agonists, 357–358
    procainamide, 403–404
    vasodilators, 358–361
Conotoxin, 117–118
Contractile proteins, vascular smooth muscle effects, 78–84
Coronary artery(ies)
  anatomy, 294–295
  blood flow, 25,300,301
    adenosine and, 309–310
    β-adrenergic blocker effects, 320
    in atherosclerosis, 311,313
    endothelium and, 301–309
    endothelium-dependent relaxing factor and, 302,303–305
  bypass surgery, 294
  innervation, 15
  occlusion, 28
  stenosis, 310
Coronary artery disease
  atherosclerosis, 310–315
  as congestive heart failure precursor, 341
  familial hypercholesterolemia and, 492
  hyperlipidemia and, 485–486
    therapy, 494–495,497–498,503
  as mortality cause, 293
  preventive diet therapy, 494–495
Coumarin, 500
Creatine phosphate, 297,345

Cyclazenine, 54
Cyclohexyladenosine, 309–310
Cyclooxygenase, 17–18
Cyclooxygenase inhibitors, 523
Cyclopentyladenosine, 309–310
Cyclopropane, 378
5'-N-Cyclopropylcarboxamido-adenosine, 310
Cyclosporin, 506

D

D600, action sites/mechanisms, 107,127,128,
    129–131
Debrisoquine, 54
Delapril, 220
Dermatan sulfate, 528–529
Diabetes mellitus, 341
Diacylglycerol
    binding antagonists, 89
    as calcium channel second messenger, 116,120
    platelet activator and, 517
    smooth muscle formation, 81
Diazoxide, 94
Diet therapy, for hypocholesterolemia, 494–495
Digitalis, 299,356,421
Digitalis glycosides, antiarrhythmic actions,
    384–385,388,391
Digitoxin, 142
Digoxin
    as congestive heart failure therapy, 356
    drug interactions, 142,325,442,495
1,4-Dihydropyridine
    activation enantiomers, 129
    calcium channel sensitivity, 120
    structure-activity relationship, 121,123–126
3,4-Dihydroxyphenylalanine, 3,4
Diltiazem
    action selectivity, 132,133
    action sites/mechanisms,
        121,124,125,127,128,129–130,131,326
    adverse effects, 139,324–325
    cardiodepressant effects, 107
    as myocardial infarction prophylaxis, 325
    pharmacokinetics, 139
    therapeutic applications
        angina, 134–135
        cardiac arrhythmia, 135
        cardiomyopathy, 137
        congestive heart failure, 137
        hypertension, 135–136
Diphenylbutylpiperidine, 83,125
Dipyridamole
    adenosine interaction, 310
    antiplatelet effects, 524,531
Disopyramide
    adverse effects, 407–408,409–410
    antiarrhythmic actions, 386,390,405–410
    calcium antagonist interaction, 142
    pharmacokinetics, 408–409
Diuretics
    calcium antagonist interaction, 142
    as congestive heart failure therapy, 355–356
Dobutamine, 41,353–355

Dopamine
    as acute heart failure therapy, 353,354
    agonists, 8
    antagonists, 8
    in congestive heart failure, 347,351,352–353
    as cotransmitter, 234,248–249
    functions, 10
    norepinephrine interaction, 4
    receptors, 10,234
        prejunctional, 248–249
    renin interaction, 17
Dopamine β-hydroxylase, 3,234
Dopexamine, 357
Doxazosin, 41,56,58,59
Dynorphin, 232
Dysbetalipoproteinemia, 491

E

Echocardiography, 343
Edema, pulmonary, 343,345,353–354
Electrocardiographic changes, drug-related,
    463–464
    disopyramide, 407,408
    encainide, 432,434
    flecainide, 437
    lidocaine, 412
    procainamide, 401
    propafenol, 441
    propranolol, 448
    quinidine, 395
Embolism, pulmonary, 531
Enalapril
    angiotensin II interaction, 69
    as chronic heart failure therapy, 355,361
    as coronary heart failure therapy, 359–360
    structure, 220
Encainide
    adverse effects, 432–433,434–435,439–440
    antiarrhythmic actions, 429–435,439–440
Endoperoxides, 517
Endothelin, 271–272
Endothelin-1, 307–309
Endothelium
    coronary blood flow and, 301–309
    neuroeffector transmission and, 270–272
    smooth muscle cell interface, 89–94
    thrombin effects, 520
    in thrombosis, 515
    vasoconstrictive activity, 307–309
Endothelium-dependent relaxing factor, 302,
    303–305
    acetylcholine interaction, 90–92,93,251,255,
        271
    ATP interaction, 236,258
    calcium interaction, 92
    as guanylate cyclase activator, 84–85
    norepinephrine interaction, 94
    serotonin interaction, 94
    vasoconstrictor agent interaction, 94
Endothelium-derived hyperpolarizing factor, 91
Endotoxin, 519
Endoxin, 19

Enkephalins
  acetylcholine interaction, 3
  as cotransmitters, 237,240,268
    prejunctional receptors, 249
  sympathetic preganglionic neuron effects,
    177–178
Enoximone, 357
Epinephrine
  autonomic regulatory function, 189,190
  as cotransmitter, 234–235
    α₂-adrenergic receptor effects, 245
    β-adrenergic receptor effects, 249–251
  as nonselective adrenergic receptor blocker,
    41
  as nucleus tractus solitarius neurotransmitter,
    181
  platelet activation and, 517–518
  rostral ventrolateral medulla content, 166–168
Esmolol, 64
Estrogen, 143
Ethacrinic acid, 356
5'-N-Ethylcarboxamidoadenosine, 310
Ethynybenzalkanamines, 125
EU-5476, 219
Excitatory junction potentials
  ATP effects, 237,257
  postsynaptic, 6
Exercise stress testing, 315–316
Exocytosis, 234
EXP6155, 223
EXP6803, 223

F

Factor II, 528
Factor IX, 528
Factor IXa, 518
Factor Va, 520,521
Factor VII, 518,528
Factor VIIa, 518
Factor VIIIa, 520,521
Factor X, 521,528
Factor Xa, 518
Felodipine, 83,120,145,146
Fenofibrate, 500,501,502
Fenoldopam, 352
Fentiapril, 219
Fibrates, 500–503
Fibrillation, atrial, 382,398
Fibrinogen, 518
Fibrinolysis, 521–522
Fibrinolytic therapy, 529–532
Fibronectin, 516,518
Flecainide
  adverse effects, 438,439–440
  antiarrhythmic actions, 435–440
Fleckenstein, Albrecht, 107
Flesinoxan, 187
Flordipine, 144
Flosequinan, 360–361
Fluindostatin, 504
Flunarizine, 83,136–137
Fluspirilene, 125

Folic acid, 495
Forskolin, 84
Fosfopril, 221
Free fatty acids, 490
Free radicals
  calcium paradox and, 114
  in reperfusion injury, 328,329,331–332
Furosemide, 353,354,356

G

Gallopamil, 144,147
Ganglion-blocking agents, 39,53–54
Gemfibrozil 500,501,502,503,506
Glossopharyngeal nerve, 164
Glucose, 490
Glutamate, 169,189,190
Glyceryl trinitrate, 305,306
Glycine xylidide, 414
Glycogen, 490
Glycoprotein(s), platelet membrane, 516
Glycoprotein Ia, 516
Glycoprotein Ib, 522
Glycoprotein Ib/IX, 517
  antibodies, 517
Glycoprotein IIb/IIIa, 328,516
  antibodies, 525
  fibrinogen receptor, 517
Glycoprotein V, 517
Glycoprotein Mo 1, 331
Glycosaminoglycans, heparin-like, 521
Glycosides
  antiarrhythmic actions, 387–388
  digitalis, 384–385,388,391
G proteins
  β-adrenergic receptor coupling, 345
  calcium channel regulation and,
    116,118,119,120,129–130
  phospholipase C interaction, 517
G-substrate proteins, 88
Guanabenz, 51
Guanethidine, 5,54,256
Guanfacine, 45,51,53
Guanine nucleotide regulatory proteins. *See* G
  proteins
Guanosine diphosphate (GDP), 9
Guanosine monophosphate, cyclic (cGMP)
  nitrate interaction, 360
  as vascular smooth muscle second messenger,
    84,85,86–88
  vasodilator interaction, 301–302,305
Guanosine triphosphate (GTP), 9
Guanylate cyclase, vasodilator interaction,
  84–85,303,305,307

H

Halothane, 378
Heart, 19–25
  atrial function, 23
  autonomic innervation, 24–25
  cardiac muscle fiber properties, 19–20
  cardiac output, 23–24

Heart (*contd.*)
  inotropic factors, 22–23
  mechanical properties, 20–23
  oxygen consumption, 25
Heart rate, myocardial oxygen consumption and, 300
Hemicholinium, 3
Heparan sulfate, 515
Heparin, 526–527,529,531
  action mechanism, 326
  low-molecular weight, 527
  for rethrombosis prevention, 328
Heparin cofactor II, 516,526
Hepatic triglyceride lipase, 488,490,491,502
Hering-Breuer reflex, 28
Hexamethonium, 7,53
Hip surgery, thrombosis following, 520
Hirudin, 528
His-Purkinje system
  drug effects
    amiodarone, 463
    bretylium, 546–547
    disopyramide, 406–407
    encainide, 431
    flecainide, 436–437
    lidocaine, 411–412
    mexiletine, 426–427
    phenytoin, 418
    procainamide, 400–401
    propafenone, 441
    propranolol, 447
    quinidine, 394–395
    tocainimide, 422–423
  in supraventricular arrhythmia,
    381,382,383,384,385,387,389
Histamine, 10
  neuroeffector transmission effects, 232,268–269
  vasodilator system, 17
Hormones. *See also* specific hormones
  neurotransmitter modulatory action, 263–272
Humeral mechanisms, sympathetic nervous
    system, 164–165
Hydralazine
  action mechanisms, 96
  as chronic heart failure therapy, 355
  as congestive heart failure therapy, 358–359,360
6-Hydroxydopamine, 5
12-Hydroxyeicosatetraenoic acid, 517
Hydroxylase-7α, 496
Hydroxyl radical, 329
Hydroxymethyl-glutaryl CoA reductase
    inhibitors, 501,503–506
13-Hydroxy octadecadienoic acid, 515
Hydroxperoxy eicosatetraenoic acid, 18
5-Hydroxytryptamine, 125
Hypercholesterolemia. *See also* specific
    lipoproteins
  familial, 491–492,493
  hypertriglycidemia with, 490–491
  isolated, 491–492,493
  therapy, 495–498
Hypercoagulability, 519–520
Hyperlipidemia, 485–513
  β-adrenergic blocker-related, 322

  combined, 490,493
    familial, 490–491,492,496
  pathophysiology, 489–494
    hypercholesterolemia, 490–491
    hypertriglyceridemia, 489–491
    isolated hypercholesterolemia, 491–492,493
    reduced high-density cholesterol, 492,494
  therapy, 494–509
    bile acid sequestrant resins, 495–498
    diet therapy, 494–495
    fibrates, 500–503,508–509
    hydroxymethyl-glutaryl CoA reductase
      inhibitors, 503–506,508–509
    nicotinic acid, 498–500,508–509
    probucol, 506–507,508–509
Hypertension, 201
  angiotensin-converting enzyme inhibitor
    effects, 221–222
  baroreceptors and, 27–28
  calcium channel antagonist therapy, 135–136
  calcium channel regulation in, 113,144
  as congestive heart failure precursor, 341
  myocardial oxygen demand effects, 314
  renin-angiotensin system and, 201,202
  renin inhibitor therapy, 210–218
  vascular smooth muscle in, 75
Hypertriglyceridemia, 489–491
  hypercholesterolemia with, 490–491
  primary, 490
Hypoalphalipoproteinemia, primary, 492,493,494
Hypofibrinolysis, 519–520,522
Hypotension, angiotensin-converting enzyme
    inhibitor-related, 361–362
Hypoxanthine, 297,309,330
Hypoxia, medullary, 28,29

I

Ibopamine, 357
Idazoxan, 41,186
Imipramine, 5
Indalapril, 220
Indolapril, 220
Indomethacin, 523
Inhibitory postsynaptic potentials, 6
Inosine, 297,309
Inositol phosphate, 120
Inositol triphosphate, antagonists, 88–89
Inositol-1,4,5-triphosphate, 111,116,517
Inotropic agents, as congestive heart failure
    therapy, 357
Integral membrane calcium binding protein, 113
Interleukin-1, 519
Ischemia. *See also* Ischemic heart disease
  acute myocardial, 343
  calcium channel regulation in, 144
  myocardial contractility and, 298–299
  oxidative phosphorylation and, 297–298,299
  silent, 293
  β-adrenergic blocker effects, 320–321
Ischemic heart disease, 293–340
  clinical detection, 315–316
  coronary atherosclerosis and, 310–315
  coronary blood flow and, 301–310

myocardial/coronary anatomy and, 293–297
myocardial metabolism and, 297–299
myocardial oxygen consumption and, 299–301
therapy, 316–328
  adjunctive, 328–332
Isoamyl nitrite, 305
Isoproterenol, 266–267
Isoquinolinesulfonamides, 82,87
Isosorbide dinitrate
  action mechanisms, 317
  as chronic heart failure therapy, 355
  as congestive heart failure therapy, 358–359,360
    resistance, 360
Isradipine, 145,146

J

Juxtaglomerular apparatus, renin release,
  17,204,205

K

K252A, 89
Ketanserin
  action mechanisms, 59–60
  catecholamine interaction, 187
  structure, 56
Kidney
  blood pressure regulatory function, 29
  renin gene transcription, 203
  renin release, 204–206
Kinin(s), 18,201,310
Kininase II, 201
Krebs cycle, 297
KR1-1314, 217
KRI-1230, 216–217
KT362, 89
Kynurenic acid, 169

L

Labetalol, 59,67,321
Laminin, 516
Lecithin-cholesterol acyltransferase, 489
Left ventricular chamber stiffness, 341–343
Left ventricular dysfunction
  diastolic, 341–344
  systolic, 344–345
  measurement, 343
  treatment, 343–344
Leiotonin, 81
Leu-enkephalin, precursor, 245
Leukotrienes, 17
Levodopa, 357
Lidocaine
  adverse effects, 413,416
  antiarrhythmic actions, 388–389,410–413,
    415–416,419
  pharmacokinetics, 413–415
Lipoproteins
  high-density
    bile acid sequestrant resin effects, 498
    as coronary artery disease risk factor, 485
    fibrate effects, 500,502,503

hydroxymethyl-glutaryl CoA reductase
      inhibitor effects, 504,505
    metabolism, 489
    niacin therapy effects, 498–499
    primary hypoalphalipoproteinemia and,
      492,493,494
    probucol effects, 506,507
  intermediate-density, 486,487,488
  low-density
    bile acid sequestrant resin effects, 496,
      497–498
    as coronary artery disease risk factor, 485
    fibrate effects, 500,502–503
    hydroxymethyl-glutaryl CoA reductase
      inhibitor effects, 503–504,505
    hypertriglyceridemia and, 490,491
    isolated hypercholesterolemia and,
      491–492,493
    metabolism, 486,487,488
    niacin therapy effects, 498–499,500
    probucol effects, 506,507
  normal metabolism, 486–489
  very-low density
    beta, 485
    bile acid sequestrant resin effects, 496,497
    as coronary artery disease risk factor, 485
    fibrate effects, 500,501,502
    hydroxymethyl-glutaryl CoA reductase
      inhibitor effects, 505
    hypertriglyceridemia and, 489–490,491
    isolated hypercholesterolemia and, 492
    metabolism, 487–488
    niacin therapy effects, 498,500
    probucol effects, 506
Lipoxygenase pathway, 18
Lisinipril, 220
Lofexidine, 51
Lovastatin, 504,505–506
Lymphoid tissue, sympathetic innervation, 163
Lysophospholipids, calcium paradox and, 114

M

α_2-Macroglobulin, 516,522
Macrophage, monocyte-derived, 485
Magnesium, renin release effects, 205
MC 838, 219
Mecamylamine, 53
Medulla
  raphe nucleus
    depressor response, 174–175
    pressor response, 175–178
  tonic sympathetic activity, 162
  ventrolateral, caudal
    arginine vasopressin release, 171–172
    baroreceptor reflexes, 182–183
    cardiovascular regulatory function, 170
  ventrolateral, innervation, 182
  ventrolateral, rostral
    cardiovascular regulatory function, 165
    clonidine action site, 186
    neurotransmitters, 166–179
    organization, 162,163

Medulla (*contd.*)
    sympathetic preganglionic neuron regulation
        by, 189
Meizothrombin, 518
Mesudipine, 144
Met-enkephalin analog, 268
Methoxamine, 41
α-Methyldopamine
    antihypertensive action, 45,46,47,
        50–51,52,53,185
    as false transmitter, 506
α-Methylnorepinephrine, 6,243–244
Metolazone, 356
Metoprolol
    action mechanisms, 321,322
    drug interactions, 442
    pharmacokinetics, 452
    as selective β_1-blocker, 63
    structure, 445
Mexiletine
    adverse effects, 427,429
    antiarrhythmic actions, 425–429
Milrinone, 357
Minoxidil, 94–95
Mitochondria, calcium-regulating, 111–112,
    114
Mitral valve leaflet, slow-response fibers, 371
Molsidomine, 360
Monoamine oxidase, 6
Monoamine oxidase inhibitors, 46–47
Monoclonal antibody
    antithrombotic effects, 328
    renin, 210–211
Monoethylglycine xylidide, 414
Morphine
    acetylcholine interaction, 3
    histamine interaction, 10
    neuroeffector transmission effects, 267,268
Myocardial infarction
    reperfusion injury prevention, 328–332
    therapy, 326–328
        adjunctive, 328–332
        β-adrenergic blocking agents, 319–320
Myocardium
    anatomy, 293–297
    blood flow, in atherosclerosis, 311,313
    in congestive heart failure, 341–346
    contractility
        G proteins and, 345
        during ischemia, 298–299
    metabolism, 297–299
    oxygen demand
        β-adrenergic blocking agents and, 319,320
        in atherosclerosis, 313–315
        determinants, 299–301
        nitrates and, 316
    in systolic heart failure, 344–345
Myocyte, β-adrenergic receptors, 345
Myosin, 11,79,323
Myosin kinase, 324
Myosin light-chain kinase, 11,79–84
    inhibition, 81–84
Myosin light-chain kinase phosphatase, 11

N
Nadolol, 321,446,452
Naphthalene sulfonamide, 83
Naphthazoline, 255
α-Neoendorphin, 245
Neuroeffector transmission, 229–291
    automodulation, 240–251
        cholinergic transmission modulation, 251
        noradrenergic transmission modulation,
            241–251
        physiological role, 241
    cotransmission, 230–240
        cholinergic cotransmitters, 239–240
        cotransmitter system properties, 232–234
        noradrenergic cotransmitters, 234–239
    hormonal modulation, 263–272
    transjunctional modulation, 260–263
    transneuronal modulation, 251–260
        cholinergic modulation, 252–256
        nonadrenergic, noncholinergic mediator
            modulation, 256–257
        noradrenergic modulation, 253–256
        sensory neuron transmitters, 257–260
Neurohypophyseal hormone, 350
Neurokinins, 258–260
Neuropeptide(s)
    axonal transport, 233
    as calmodulin inhibitors, 83
    perivascular, 232
Neuropeptide Y
    as cotransmitter, 237,238–239
        α_2-adrenergic receptor effects, 245
        cholinergic transmission effects, 256
        prejunctional receptors, 246–247
    perivascular, 232
    rostral ventrolateral medulla content, 167
Neurotransmitters. *See also* specific
        neurotransmitters
    biosynthesis, 233
    intraneuronal location, 234
    release, 234
    sympathetic nervous system-regulatory,
        161–199
        antihypertensive agents and, 185–189
        of caudal ventrolateral medulla, 170–172
        of dorsal raphe nuclei, 178
        of medullary raphe nuclei, 174–178
        neurohumeral control, 184–185
        of nucleus tractus solitarius, 179–184
        of paraventricular nucleus, 178–179
        of rostral ventrolateral medulla, 166–169
    types, 232–233
Nevastatin, 504
Niacin, as hyperlipidemia therapy, 498–500,
    506
Nicardipine
    action selectivity, 133
    endothelin-1 interaction, 309
    pharmacokinetics, 139–140
    as receptor inhibitor, 131
Nicorandil, 96
Nicotinic acid, 498–500
Nidogen, 516

Nifedipine
  action selectivity, 132,133
  action sites/mechanisms, 121,124,125,
    129–130,131,324
  adverse effects, 140–141
  cardiodepressant effects, 107
  contraindications, 134,135
  drug interactions, 141–142
  pharmacokinetics, 138
  structure, 123
  therapeutic applications
    cardiac arrhythmia, 135
    cerebral vascular disorders, 136–137
    congestive heart disease, 137
    hypertension, 135–136
    left ventricular diastolic dysfunction, 343
  withdrawal, 143
Niludipine, 144
Nimodipine, 131,145,146
  pharmacokinetics, 139–140
Nisoldipine, 145,146
  pharmacokinetics, 139–140
Nitrates
  action mechanisms, 316–319
  calcium interaction, 77
  combination therapy, 326
  as congestive heart failure therapy, 360
  as left ventricular diastolic dysfunction therapy,
    344
Nitrendipine, 131,145,146
  pharmacokinetics, 139–140
Nitric oxide
  endothelial-cell derived, 307–308
  as endothelium-dependent relaxing factor,
    90–91,303–304,305–306,360
Nitric oxide inducers, 360
Nitroglycerin
  action mechanisms, 316–317,318
  as acute heart failure therapy, 353
  as left ventricular diastolic dysfunction therapy,
    343
Nitroprusside
  action mechanisms, 96,305,306
  as acute heart failure therapy, 353,354,355
  calcium blockage by, 77
  as left ventricular diastolic dysfunction therapy,
    343
Nitrovasodilators. *See also* specific
    nitrovasodilators
  action mechanisms, 305–307
  endothelium-dependent, 307–309
Nonadrenergic, noncholinergic autonomic
    transmission, 231–232,236
  transneuronal modulation, 252,256–257
Noradrenergic neurons
  A1, 170–171
  A5, 162,163,172–174
  cotransmitters, 234–239
    automodulation, 240–251
    cholinergic modulation, 230,252–255
Norepinephrine
  acetylcholine interaction, 4,254–255,256
  adrenal methylation, 6

  adrenergic mechanisms, 3–6
  α-adrenergic receptor interaction, 9,39–40,
    243–244
  β-adrenergic receptor interaction, 41,249
  adrenocorticotrophic hormone interaction,
    267
  angiotensin II interaction, 264,266–267
  arginine vasopressin neuron effects, 172
  ATP interaction, 236,237
  autoinhibition, 242
  autonomic regulatory function, 189,190
  blood pressure effects, 26–27
  calcium antagonist interaction, 77
  calcium channel effects, 119–120
  cholinergic transmission effects, 255,256
  cholinomimetic drug-related modulation,
    252–255
  in congestive heart failure, 346–347,348
  depolarization effects, 11,372
  endothelium-dependent relaxing factor
    interaction, 94
  negative feedback, 4
  neuropeptide Y interaction, 245,247
  as nucleus tractus solitarius neurotransmitter,
    181
  peripheral resistance effects, 16
  sympathetic nervous system release, 231
  sympathetic preganglionic neuron effects,
    173–174
  synthesis, 3–6
Nucleotides, cyclic. *See also* specific cyclic
    nucleotides
  as vascular smooth muscle second messengers,
    84–88
Nucleus reticularis lateralis, as clonidine action
    site, 186
Nucleus tractus solitarius anatomy, 38,39,48
  as hypertensive agent action site, 38
  baroreceptor afferent pathway, 164
  circumventricular organs and, 165
  neurotransmitters, 179–184
    baroreceptor interactions, 179–182

O

Octopamine, 6,232
Omega-3 fatty acids, 525
Opioid peptides
  as cotransmitters, 237,240
    α₂-adrenergic receptors, 245
    neuroeffector transmission, 267–268
    prejunctional receptors, 249
  norepinephrine interaction, 4
Organum vasculosum, of the lamina terminalis,
    164,185
Ouabain, 5
Oxidative metabolism, calcium-mediated, 112
Oxodipine, 144
Oxprenolol, 321
Oxygen demand, myocardial, 297–301
  β-adrenergic blocking agents and, 319,320
  in atherosclerosis, 313–315
  determinants, 299–301

Oxygen demand (*contd.*)
  nitrates and, 316
Oxymetazoline, 255
Oxytocin, 178–179

P

Pacemaker cells, 372–373,374
Parasympathetic nervous system, 2–3
Parathyroid hormone
  calcium regulatory function, 109–110,113
  endothelium-related vasodilatory effects, 92
Paraventricular nucleus
  arginine vasopressin release, 171
  neurotransmitters, 178–179
  organization, 163,164,178
  pressor response, 179
Penfluridol, 125
Pentolinium, 53
Pentopril, 220
Pepstatin, 211
  analog, 213
Peptide(s)
  analogs
    as angiotensin antagonists, 222–223
    as renin inhibitors, 214–216
  as cotransmitters, 237–239
  cytoadhesion recognition sequence, 526
  as renin inhibitors, 210–212,214–216
  vasodilator response, 92–93
Peptide histidine isoleucine amide, 232
Perhexiline, 83
Perindopril, 220
Peripheral vascular disorders, therapy, 137
Perivascular nerve fibers, neuropeptides,
    232,258,259
Phenethylamines, 5
Phenothiazine, 83
Phenoxybenzamine, 58–59,245
Phentolamine
  as nonselective adrenergic receptor antagonist,
    41,245
  therapeutic use, 58–59
  vasodilatory action, 56
D-Phenylalanyl-L-prolyl-L-arginyl-
    chloromethylketone, 528
Phenylbutazone, 523
Phenylephrine, 9,41
Phenylethanolamine-*N*-methyltransferase, 6
(R)-Phenylisopropyladenosine, 309–310
Phenytoin
  adverse effects, 419–420,421
  antiarrhythmic actions, 416–420
  drug interactions, 142
  pharmacokinetics, 420–421
Phorbol esters, 120
Phosphatidylinositol cycle, 84,85,88–89
Phosphodiesterase, 9
Phosphodiesterase inhibitor, 355,357
Phosphorylation, oxidative, 297–298,299
Physostigmine, 171
Pimozide, 125
Pinacidil, 95

Pindolol, 446
  action mechanisms, 321,322
  as congestive heart failure therapy, 357
  pharmacokinetics, 452
Pirenzepine, 254
Pivalopril, 219
Plasmin, 522
Plasminogen
  cleaving agents, 529–530
  in fibrinolysis, 522
Plasminogen activator
  as myocardial infarction therapy, 327
  single-chain, 522,530
  tissue-type, 515,530-531
  urokinase-type, 522,530
Platelet
  arachidonate metabolism, 523
  endothelium-dependent relaxing factor and, 305
  fibrinolysis effects, 522
  in neurovascular transmission, 269–270
  in thrombosis, 516–518
Platelet-activating factor, 517–518
Platelet-adhesive protein inhibitors, 525–526
Platelet aggregation
  in acute ischemic syndromes, 326
  propranolol effects, 321–322
Platelet-derived growth factor, 89
Polymorphonuclear leukocyte, in reperfusion
    injury, 328–329,331–332
Pons, tonic sympathetic activity, 162
Potassium
  renin release effects, 205
  repolarization effects, 19
  vascular smooth muscle effects, 76,77,310
Potassium channel openers, 94–97
Practolol, 321
Pravastatin, 504
Prazosin
  adverse effects, 58
  antihypertensive activity, 56–58
  catecholamine interaction, 187
  therapeutic use, 59
Prenylamine, 4,107
Pre-prorenin, 204,218
Prioximone, 357
Probucol, 506–507,508
Procainamide, 142
  adverse effects, 402,404–405
  antiarrhythmic actions, 386,389–390,391,
    398–402,404–405
  calcium antagonist interaction, 142
  pharmacokinetics, 402–404
Propafenone, antiarrhythmic actions, 440–444
Propanetriol trinitrate, 317
Propranolol
  action mechanisms, 321,322
  adverse effects, 449–450,453–454
  antiarrhythmic actions, 385,388,389,444–455
  electrophysiologic actions, 378–379,445–448
  heart rate effects, 24–25
  hemodynamic profile, 62
  pharmacokinetics, 451–453
Prorenin, 204

Prostacyclin
  angiotensin II-related synthesis, 205,209
  antiplatelet effects, 524
  cyclic nucleotide interaction, 84
Prostaglandins
  acetylcholine interaction, 3
  angiotensin II interaction, 205,208–209,264
  aspirin-related inhibition, 523
  in congestive heart failure, 347,351,352
  coronary vascular muscle effects, 310
  cyclic nucleotide interaction, 85–87,88
  endothelium-dependent relaxing factor
      interaction, 305
  formation, 17–18
  functions, 10,18
  neuroeffector transmission effects, 271
  neutrophil-inhibiting, 331
  norepinephrine interaction, 4
  renin interaction, 17,204,205
  transjunctional modulatory action,
      260–261,262–263
Protease, 329
Protein C
  activated, 520,521,528
  antithrombotic effects, 328
  thrombomodulin-dependent, 515
Protein kinase
  activation, 9
  cAMP-dependent, 87,88,324
  cGMP-dependent, 87,88
  modulators, 89
  vascular smooth muscle contraction effects, 80
Protein kinase C
  calcium channel effects, 120
  inhibitors, 82
  vascular smooth muscle contraction effects,
      80,81
Prothrombin, 518
Prothrombinase, 518
Purinergic nerves, 10
Purinergic receptor
  prejunctional, 245–246
  subtypes, 236,237
Purinergic transmission, 257
Purkinje fibers. *See also* His-Purkinje system
  action potentials, 371,375
  automaticity, 373

Q

Quinapril, 220
Quinidine, 142
  adverse effects, 395–396,398
  antiarrhythmic actions, 385,386,389–390,
      391–398
  pharmacokinetics, 396–397
Quinidine-like activity, 63–64

R

Ramipril, 220
Raubasine, 54
Rauwolfia alkaloids, 54–55

Rauwolscine, 41
Receptors, 6–7. *See also* Adrenergic receptors;
      Cholinergic receptors
  agonists, 7,8
  antagonists, 7,8
Renin, 207–208,209
  antibodies, 209–210
  definition, 201
  function, 202
  gene, 203
  inhibitors, 210–218
    novel moiety-containing, 216–218
    peptide analogs, 214–216
    peptides, 210–212
    prosegment analog, 218
    statine-containing, 211–214
    substrate cyclic analogs, 218
  molecular forms, 204
  plasma activity, 17
  purification, 202
  release, 17,201,202,204
    β-adrenergic receptor-stimulated, 319
    drug effects, 205,206
    physiological control, 204–205
  species differences, 202–203
  substrate, 211
  synthesis, 203,204
  vasoconstrictive action, 201
Renin-angiotensin-aldosterone system, 17,201–228
  blood pressure effects, 29,201,202,205–207
  congestive heart failure and, 202
  hemorrhage and, 30
  hypertension effects, 201,202,205–208,210
    renin inhibitors and, 209–218
  sodium depletion and, 30
  vascular wall in, 207–209
Rescinnamine, 54
Reserpine
  action mechanisms, 54–55
  adverse effects, 55
  antihypertensive action, 45,46–47
  norepinephrine interaction, 3–4,6
Revascularization, coronary, 343
mRibonucleic acid (mRNA), renin, 203,204
Rilmenidine, 51,52
Ryodipine, 144

S

Salbutamol, 41
Sarcoplasmic reticulum, calcium-regulatory
      mechanisms, 11–12,76–77,111,112,131
Sensory neurons, neuroeffector transmission
      effects, 257–260
Serine-protease inhibitors, 516
Serotonin
  autonomic regulatory function, 190
  as cotransmitter, 232,235–236
    prejunctional receptors, 248
  endothelium-dependent relaxing factor
      interaction, 94
  functions, 10
  medullary pressor response effects, 175–178

Serotonin (*contd.*)
   neuroeffector transmission effects, 269
   norepinephrine interaction, 4
   perivascular, 232
   platelet activation and, 517–518
   subtypes, 235–236
   sympathetic preganglionic neuron effects,
      176,177–178
   vasoactive function, 18
Serotonin agonists, sympathetic preganglionic
   neuron effects, 186
Shock, cardiogenic, 327
Simvastatin, 504
Sinoatrial node
   automaticity, 372
   drug effects
      amiodarone, 462
      bretylium, 455–456
      disopyramide, 406
      encainide, 431
      flecainide, 436
      lidocaine, 410–411
      mexiletine, 426
      phenytoin, 416–417
      procainamide, 399
      propafenone, 441
      propranolol, 446
      quinidine, 392–393
      verapamil, 467
   slow-response fibers, 371
Sodium-calcium exchanger, 111,112,114
Sodium channels, 1,4-dihydropyridine effects, 131
Sodium nitroprusside. *See also* Nitroprusside
   platelet function effects, 305
Sodium transport, cardiac transmembrane, 370
Somatostatin, 237,240,257
Sotalol, 61,379,380
SQ 29,852, 221
Starling's law of the leart, 19,21–22
Statine, 211–214
Statone, 213
"Steal syndromes," 313
Stenosis, coronary, 310
Straurosporine, 89
Streptokinase, 327,328,529,531
Stroke, hemorrhagic, 328
Subfornical organ, 164,165,185
Substance P
   autonomic regulatory function, 189,190
   as baroreceptor neurotransmitter, 179–181
   enkephalin interaction, 240
   neuroeffector transmission effects, 258–259
   perivascular, 232,258,259
   rostral ventrolateral medulla content, 167,
      168–169
   sympathetic preganglionic neuron effects, 177
   vascular smooth muscle effects, 271
   vasodilator actions, 92
Sudden death, 293
Superoxide anion, 329
Superoxide dismutase, 303,329–331
Sympathetic nervous system. *See also* Adrenergic
   nerves; Adrenergic receptor; Autonomic
   nervous system; Parasympathetic nervous
   system

   adrenergic mechanisms, 3–6
   anatomy, 3,161–165
   as antihypertensive agent action site, 39
   congestive heart failure and, 347–349
   as ganglionic blocking agent action site, 39
   vasodilator fibers, 16
Sympathetic preganglionic neurons
   blood flow regulatory effects, 161–162
   clonidine effects, 173,186
   8-OH DPAT effects, 188–189
   epinephrine effects, 166–167
   excitatory amino acid effects, 169
   norepinephrine effects, 173–174
   rostral ventrolateral medulla interaction,
      166–168
   serotonin effects, 176,177–178
Sympatholytic drugs, cardiovascular effects, 30
Sympathomimetic drugs, myocardial oxygen
   demand effects, 314
Syrosingopine, 54

T
Tachycardia
   atrioventricular nodal reentry and, 384–386
   paroxysmal atrial, 405
   paroxysmal supraventricular
      pharmacological management, 381–391
      Wolff-Parkinson-White syndrome and,
      383,386–391
Tangier disease, 494
Terazosin, 41,56,58,59
Terbutaline, 41
Tetrabenazine, 4
Tetraethylammonium, 53
Thiazides, 355–356
Thrombin
   inhibition, 521
   platelet activation and, 517
   thrombosis regulatory function, 520–521
   vasodilator actions, 92–93
Thromboembolic disease, venous, 515
Thrombolytic therapy, 326–328
Thrombosis
   acute ischemic syndromes and, 326
   coronary, 312–313
   endothelium-dependent relaxing factor and, 305
   pathogenesis, 515–522
      arterial, 516–519
      fibrinolysis and, 521–522
      regulatory mechanisms, 520–521
      venous, 519–520
Thrombospondin, 516,517,518
Thromboxane, inhibition, 326
Thromboxane A_2
   analog, 270
   endoperoxide substrate, 517
   platelet aggregation effects, 18
   receptor antagonist, 523–524
Thromboxane, A_3, 525
Thromboxane antagonist, 331
Thromboxane synthetase inhibitor, 331
Thyrotropin-releasing hormone, 167,177
Thyroxine, 464,495
Tiamenidine, 51

Tiapamil, 144,145,147
Ticlopidine, 524–525
Timolol, 321,446,452
Tissue factor, 518,519
Tissue factor antagonists, 328
Tissue-necrosis factor, 519
Tocainide, 422–425
Tolazoline, 56
Tonin, 266
Tricuspid valve leaflet, slow-response fibers,
   371
Tricyclic antidepressants, hypotensive activity,
   46–47,53
Triglycerides
   hepatic synthesis, 490
   lipoprotein-related regulation, 486
Triiodothyronine, 464
Trimazosin, 41,56,58,59
Trimetaphan, 53
Tropomyosin, 11
Troponin, 11,78,323
Troponin C, 19,109
d-Tubocurarine, 7
Tyramine, 5,46–47
Tyrosine hydroxylase, 5,234

U
U46619, 270
Uptake-1, 5
Urapidil, 56,59
Urokinase, 327,529–530,531

V
Vagal fibers, myelinated, 28
Vagus nerve, 164,296
Vascular beds, 12–15
   blood flow control, 13–15
Vascular smooth muscle
   adenosine effects, 309–310
   1,4-dihydropyridine activity, 126,128,131
   calcium antagonist effects, 132–134
   calcium channels, 119–120
   characteristics, 11–12
   endothelium, 301–309
   platelet modulatory effects, 269,270
   vasodilator effects, 75–105
      calcium regulatory mechanisms, 75–84
      contractile proteins, 78–84,97
      endothelium-smooth muscle cell interface,
         89–94
      potassium regulatory mechanisms, 76,77
      second messenger systems, 84–89
      vascular smooth muscle cell membrane and,
         75–78
Vascular wall, renin-angiotensin system,
   207–209
Vasoactive intestinal peptide
   as cotransmitter, 251
      cholinergic, 239–240
      sympathetic modulation, 256–257
   location, 234
   perivascular, 232
   vasodilator actions, 92

Vasoconstriction, 11–12
   in acute ischemic syndromes, 326
   adenosine and, 261,262
   α-adrenergic receptors and, 9
   angiotensin and, 201,265–266
   arginine vasopressin and, 350
   ATP and, 258
   endothelin and, 271–272
   neuropeptide Y and, 238–239
   prostaglandin and, 263
Vasodilation, 12
   ATP and, 258
   cholinergic, 251,255
   metabolic, 14
   vasoactive intestinal peptide and, 239–240
Vasodilators. *See also* specific vasodilators
   as congestive heart failure therapy, 358–361
   direct-acting, 360–361
   endothelium-dependent, 91–94,97
   potassium channel openers, 94–97
   vascular smooth muscle effects, 75–105
      calcium regulatory mechanisms, 75–84
      contractile proteins and, 78–84,97
      endothelium-smooth muscle cell interface,
         89–94
      potassium regulatory mechanisms, 76,77
      second messenger systems, 84–89
      vascular smooth muscle cell membrane and,
         75–78
Vasopressin
   plasma volume effects, 26
   renin interaction, 17,204,205
   vasoactive function, 18
Venom, 83
Ventricular muscle fiber, as fast-response fiber,
   370
Ventriculography, radionuclide left, 343
Verapamil
   action selectivity, 132,133
   action sites/mechanisms,
      121,124,125,127,128,130–131,324
   adverse effects, 140–141,324–325,470,472
   analogs, 126–127
   antiarrhythmic actions, 385,390,466–473
   calcium blockage by, 77
   cardiodepressant effects, 107,110
   dosage, 471–472
   drug interactions, 141,142
   electrophysiologic actions, 380–381,467–468
   hemodynamic actions, 468–469
   pharmacokinetics, 138–139,470–471
   structure, 109
   therapeutic applications
      angina, 134–135
      cardiac arrhythmia, 135
      cardiomyopathy, 137
      cerebral vascular disorders, 136–137
      hypertension, 135–136
   withdrawal, 143
Vitamin(s), fat-soluble, 495
Vitamin D, 110,113
Vitamin K antagonist, 528
Vitronectin, 516
von Willebrand factor, 516,518
   monoclonal antibodies, 525

W
Warfarin, 442,528,531
Wolff-Parkinson-White syndrome, 383,
 386–391,473
WY-44,221, 219

X
Xamoterol, 358
Xanthine oxidase, 329,330
Xanthoma, tendon, 491–492,507

Y
Yohimbine, 41,52,244,245
YS 980, 219

Z
Zaprinast, 86–87
Zofenopril, 219